NEUROLOGIC REHABILITATION

CONTEMPORARY NEUROLOGY SERIES AVAILABLE:

NEUROLOGIC REHABILITATION

BRUCE H. DOBKIN, M.D.
Professor of Neurology
Director, Neurologic Rehabilitation and Research Unit
University of California Los Angeles School of Medicine
and Medical Center
Los Angeles, California

 F. A. DAVIS COMPANY • Philadelphia

F. A. Davis Company
1915 Arch Street
Philadelphia, PA 19103

Printed in the United States of America

Last digit indicates print number: 10 9 8 7 6 5 4 3 2 1

Medical Editor: Robert W. Reinhardt
Medical Developmental Editor: Bernice M. Wissler
Production Editor: Roberta Massey
Cover Designer: Steven Ross Morrone

Library of Congress Cataloging-in-Publication Data

Dobkin, Bruce H.
    Neurologic rehabilitation / Bruce H. Dobkin.
      p. cm.—(Contemporary neurology series ; 47)
    Includes bibliographical references and index.
    ISBN 0-8036-0169-7 (alk. paper)
    1. Nervous system—Diseases—Patients—Rehabilitation. I. Title.
  II. Series.
    [DNLM: 1. Nervous System Diseases—rehabilitation.   2. Brain
  Injuries—rehabilitation.   3. Spinal Cord Injuries—rehabilitation.
  4. Movement Disorders—rehabilitation.   W1 C0769N v.47 1996 / WL
  100 D633n 1996]
  RC350.4.D63 1996
  616.8'043—dc20
  DNLM/DLC
  for Library of Congress   95-46567
                                                                                CIP

We shall not cease from exploration
And the end of all our exploring
Will be to arrive where we started
And know the place for the first time.
    T. S. Eliot
    "Little Gidding"
    in *Four Quartets*

And for allowing me that indulgence, to Barbara, Jessica, and Rebecca.
And for his new adventure, to Craig.

PREFACE

Unquestioned answers and unanswered questions fill every nook of the sprawling turf that is home to the diverse professionals who practice neurologic rehabilitation. The time has come to balance our therapeutic enthusiasm for the unquestioned answers with a dose of skepticism. We need to prove that what we do works best. The good experiences of physical, occupational, and speech therapists; of neuropsychologists, nurses, and social workers; and of physicians, especially neurologists, physiatrists, and orthopedists, require continued formalizing and testing.

We should also pursue the unanswered questions. Here, the borders that might define the theories and practices of neurologic rehabilitation keep expanding.

I have marked some arbitrary borders in this survey of the concerns, practices, and scientific grounding of the rehabilitation specialists who care for people with diseases and injuries of the nervous system. They are Imaginot Lines, not meant to serve as unscalable intellectual boundaries. This monograph encompasses sites from clinical research and basic science that underpin present and future efforts in neurorestoration. It emphasizes a few of the ideas about how we learn, one of the essences of rehabilitation. For our purposes, learning is "a set of processes associated with practice or experience leading to relatively permanent changes in the capability of responding."[14] As researchers explore these processes, they are finding functionally and regionally dissociable groups of neurons that participate in modules and in parallel pathways. These subdivisions of the cerebral landscape present opportunities to understand brain activities and to develop theory-based and pharmacologic treatments. The growing body of neuroscientific knowledge about motor control, motor learning, and cognitive processing challenges us to consider how we might provide patients with the best of all possible interventions.

In a more traditional way, my surveyor's chain reaches into the issues of impairments, disabilities, and handicaps (Table 1). Operationally, clinical efforts take into account *impairments*, such as a hemiparesis. However, the clinical members of the rehabilitation team primarily try to limit any associated *disabilities*, such as not being able to walk across a room without assistance because of the hemiparesis. In

Table 1. 1980 WORLD HEALTH ORGANIZATION'S INTERNATIONAL CLASSIFICATION OF IMPAIRMENTS, DISABILITIES AND HANDICAPS

Impairment: Any loss or abnormality of psychological, physiological or anatomical structure or function.

Disability: Any restriction or lack (resulting from an impairment) of ability to perform an activity in the manner or within the range considered normal for a human being.

Handicap: A disadvantage for a given individual, resulting from an impairment or disability, that limits or prevents the fulfillment of a role that is normal for that individual.

Source: World Health Organization. WHO International Classification of Impairments, Disabilities and Handicaps: A Manual of Classification Relating to the Consequences of Disease. Geneva: World Health Organization, 1980.

addition, rehabilitationists are concerned about resulting *handicaps*, such as no longer being able to make social visits because the hemiparesis impedes the person's ability to climb the steps to a friend's home. Disabilities are usually explained by premorbid and new neurologic impairments. Handicaps are much less directly related to impairments. The most traditional aim of medical rehabilitation has been to try to decrease the handicaps of patients by improving function at the level of disability. We can aim, however, to draw upon new notions about neuroplasticity and to consider ways to lessen impairments.

THE PREVALENCE OF DISABILITY

A physical impairment limits the activities of many Americans. Using the World Health Organization's definition of disability, the National Health Interview Surveys, 1983–1985, found that 22 million Americans were restricted or unable to perform the major activity for their age.[12] From ages 18 to 69, this restriction applies to work or keeping house. The 1990 census revealed that 13 million Americans over the age of 16 have difficulty in mobility or self-care.[10] About 60 percent of these disabled people are under the age of 65. From a broader perspective, it is estimated by the United Nations that 500 million persons worldwide endure physical disabilities. More than 80 percent live in Third World countries.[1]

Nervous system diseases are among the leading causes of disability in noninstitutionalized people in the United States. In 1992, the National Foundation for Brain Research estimated that the annual direct and indirect costs of neurologic disorders, excluding alcohol and other substance abuse and psychiatric illness, are $252 billion.[13]

Neurologic diseases account for 80 percent of first-time and repeat rehabilitation inpatient admissions at most facilities that do not specialize in orthopedic rehabilitation. Insight into the distribution of first-time admissions after onset of

Table 2. **UNIFORM DATA SYSTEM DIAGNOSES FOR FIRST ADMISSIONS FOR REHABILITATION IN 1992**

Diagnosis	% of Total
Stroke	34
Orthopedic conditions	31
Brain dysfunction	
Nontraumatic	2
Traumatic	5
Spinal cord dysfunction	
Nontraumatic	3
Traumatic	3
Other neurologic	
conditions	5

Source: Adapted from Granger C, Hamilton B.[8]

impairments comes from the Unified Data System for Medical Rehabilitation (UDS).[8] For 1992, this database reported descriptor information and serial scores on a measure of disability called the Functional Independence Measure (FIM) from 256 medical rehabilitation hospitals and units in 44 states. Table 2 shows the five most common impairment groups among these 83,000 patients. Repeat admissions and other diagnoses accounted for 16 percent of admissions.

THE BUSINESS OF REHABILITATION

The push by insurers and Medicare to get patients discharged from an acute hospitalization as soon as possible means that clinicians must make quick decisions about whether a rehabilitation effort is needed and what intensity of services is most appropriate. In the United States, the high cost of inpatient programs has led to a trend to try to offer supportive and rehabilitative therapy services in the home, in a skilled nursing facility, or in an outpatient program. European rehabilitation services, particularly those in Great Britain, have emphasized home management. However, the specialized free-standing or in-hospital rehabilitation unit is still the most common acute hospital discharge in the United States for functionally dependent patients who are likely to become independent enough in the short run to return home.

Acute neurologic rehabilitation is a big business, although it accounts for only 1 percent of the US health care budget. The 1982 Tax Equity and Fiscal Responsibility Act (TEFRA) created financial incentives for the growth of rehabilitation facilities. They have been, so far, excluded from the Prospective Payment System. These facilities receive from 45 to 75 percent of their income from Medicare. Between 1984 and 1994, the number of free-standing rehabilitation hospitals rose from 49 to more than 187, while rehabilitation units in acute hospitals increased from 308 to 804.[16] Approximately 25,000 beds are available for neurologic rehabilitation. More than 11,000 skilled nursing facilities also provide rehabilitation services. So far, the hospitals are exempted from payment under the Diagnostic Related Group scheme, because, for example, the diagnosis of stroke itself is a poor predictor of the total charges for rehabilitation services.[11] Studies are under way to create a payment system based upon Functional Related Groups.[15] Where beds are in overabundance, marketing claims by rehabilitation facilities and national chains tend to drown out real efforts at developing better outcome measures and specific interventions that have been proven to be efficacious by rigorous testing.

The work of rehabilitationists does not end with discharge from an acute hospital or inpatient therapy service. The American Hospital Association estimated that at least 2.6 million outpatient visits are made to rehabilitation hospitals.[16] Some care takes place in the more than 235 specially designated Comprehensive Outpatient Rehabilitation Facilities (CORFs) that meet certain federal guidelines for care and reimbursement. Other patients receive services at home, at private clinics, in nursing homes, and in coma stimulation programs, transitional living centers, and community reintegration programs. The value of these organized services is generally unproven. All, however, can provide the psychosocial milieu that assists patients and families through difficult transitions. Medical and emotional problems often arise during chronic care. These can increase disability and the long-term cost of care if not anticipated and corrected.

THE REHABILITATIONIST'S ROLE

When does rehabilitation begin? It is most responsible to start by promoting preventive measures. Ethical issues and politicized health care policies repeatedly touch the considerations of rehabilitation specialists. The troubling morbidity of stroke demands that the rehabilitation team educate people about risk factors, vigorously treat them, and participate in clinical trials of primary and secondary prevention. The poor cognitive outcomes in so many of the survivors of serious traumatic brain injury drive rehabilitationists to push for helmet laws for bikers, programs to curb alcohol and drug abuse, and technologies to improve highway safety. The growing numbers of spinal cord–injured youths call out for stricter gun possession laws and smarter social programs that may circumvent acts of violence.

For diseases with an acute onset, rehabilitation may begin at the moment of injury to neurons and their pathways. After an hypoxic-ischemic neuronal injury, we might be able to do more than manage neuromedical complications. Physicians may soon also have pharmacologic interventions that limit cell death.[4] In the longer view of recovery of function, we will have to understand more about how these new therapies might affect the potential agonists and antagonists of neural plasticity.

What is done by rehabilitationists? The borders of their activities are rather fluid. Rehabilitation has been defined as "the development of a person to the fullest physical, psychological, social, vocational, avocational, and educational potential consistent with his or her physiological or anatomical impairment and environmental limitations."[6] In general, rehabilitation efforts have been bounded by the functional consequences of nervous system injury and disease. The strategy of care has been an interdisciplinary or multidisciplinary effort led by physiatrists and orthopedists, and, increasingly, by neurologists. The past 50 years of physiatry have emphasized the role of the physician as one who helps relieve disability and handicap and maximizes functional independence. This differs from the doctor's role in the acute medical model. Instead, rehabilitation physicians evaluate and prognosticate; interact with the team of therapists over compensatory physical and cognitive strategies and assistive devices; try drug interventions mostly for spasticity, pain, and mood disorders; and serve as networking administrative brokers to gather the resources and services the patient and family need.

Physician and team practices since World War II gradually migrated from an early emphasis on caring for joints and muscles to empirical approaches that drew upon selected studies in neurophysiology. Recently, therapists have begun to move onto the turf researched by neuroscientists and psychologists who study the activity-dependent neuroplasticity that accompanies motor and cognitive learning. In the next 10 years, rehabilitationists must develop and test scientific theories about neurorestoration and merge fruitful approaches with clinical practices.

Research and scientific training are said to have lagged in American physiatry.[2,5] The National Institute of Disability and Rehabilitation Research had been the main federal supporter of rehabilitation medicine's clinical, especially psychosocial, research. Attempts to encourage basic and clinical studies and correct the lag have led to the legislated National Center for Medical Rehabilitation Research within the National Institute of Child Health and Human Development (NICHHD). At the same time, the National Institutes of Health has encouraged better research efforts through the 1990 report[3] from its "Task Force on Medical Rehabilitation Research," its 1992 strategic plan, and by growing support from its agencies. The National Institute of Neurological Diseases and Stroke (NINDS), National Institute on Aging (NIA), NICHHD, and National Institute of Arthritis and Musculoskeletal Disorders (NIAMS) have fostered collaborative research among basic and clinical scientists in neurorehabilitation-related studies.

Because most inpatient rehabilitation diagnoses are for neurologic diseases, neurologists have had a growing interest in the subacute and chronic care of their patients. Their background in neuroscience, imaging, neurophysiology, and neuropharmacology gives neurologists special insights into how rehabilitation could proceed in the future. Rehabilitation has become an increasing part of their clinical work, teaching, and research over the past 20 years.[7] For example, the American Society of Neurologic Rehabilitation has over 500 members and the American Academy of Neurology has a large neurorehabilitation section. Both offer annual symposia. Some controversy over who should undertake neurologic rehabilitation has arisen in both the United States and the United Kingdom.[9] Similar political and training issues intermittently envelop therapists among the other rehabilitation professions. This is a healthy debate that will stimulate productivity. The value added by physicians and other rehabilitation specialists to the neurorestoration of patients will depend in coming years on the ability of all kinds of clinicians to direct, interpret, and apply basic and clinical research.

THE BOUNDARIES OF THIS BOOK

This monograph emphasizes approaches to the clinical disorders that commonly arise during the rehabilitation of diseases of the central and peripheral nervous systems. When the actual and potential changes associated with the adaptability of assemblies of neurons and interlinked pathways could affect how we might facilitate motor, cognitive and behavioral recovery, I describe some of the most relevant findings. The book appropriates some of the property of disciplines such as neuroanatomy and neurophysiology, developmental neurobiology, neuropharmacology, kinesiology and biomechanics, muscle physiology, and cognitive psychology. I place special emphasis on studies that use the neuroimaging techniques listed in Table 3. Functional imaging appears to offer an especially robust approach to assess the potential for gains after brain injury and for understanding how physical, pharmacologic, and biologic interventions might affect the physiologic architecture of the brain.

While reviewing the assessments and practices of the rehabilitation team, I will suggest how these efforts might be improved by input from basic and applied neuromedical and psychosocial science researchers, as well as by experimental designs for scientifically sound interventions. The dearth of outcome studies that have been designed well enough to show whether a particular intervention is better than another makes it difficult to evaluate much of an individual therapist's and the interdisciplinary team's accomplishments. Sometimes, rehabilitationists must wonder whether any physical or cognitive training procedure carried out in a particular fashion accomplishes its goal in a cost-effective way and generalizes to other important activities. We are still a long way from knowing which of our interventions are acceptably safe, can work, or will work for the patient at hand.

Much clinical neurorehabilitation research has been invested in the study of predictors of outcome after an acute injury. Although these need to be reviewed,

Table 3. NEUROIMAGING TECHNIQUES

Structural
    Arteriography
    Computed tomography (CT)
    Magnetic resonance imaging (MRI)

Functional
    Positron emission tomography (PET)
    Functional magnetic resonance imaging (fMRI)
    Single-photon emission computed tomography (SPECT)
    Magnetic resonance spectroscopy
    Transcranial electrical and magnetic stimulation
    Quantitative electroencephalography (EEG)
    Magnetoencephalography (MEG)
    Transcranial Doppler
    Optical imaging

Integrated
    PET, SPECT, or fMRI superimposed upon MRI
    EEG or MEG superimposed upon MRI

mostly to help us understand the natural history of recovery, I pay special attention to the positive and negative outcomes for specific interventions. These outcomes especially contribute to a rational approach to the practice of neurorehabilitation. To monitor progress and regression during acute and chronic care, rehabilitation specialists need measures of impairments, disabilities, and quality of life. Tools for these measures should be valid, reliable, and sensitive to clinically important changes. I describe some practical tools and outline, in a broad fashion, research strategies suitable for studies of neurorehabilitation efficacy.

After examining the theories and practices of the members of the neurorehabilitation team without regard to any specific disease, the book moves to a framework for the management of the medical rehabilitation problems that tend to cut across diseases. Then, it offers details about the rehabilitation problems posed by individual diseases with an emphasis on epidemiology, predictors of overall functional outcome, and approaches and expected outcomes for the specific impairments and disabilities that are managed during inpatient and outpatient care. These chapters also review the effectiveness of what is done and offer speculations about what might be done.

Much of what is practiced could be distilled into a set of fixed coordinates for the trainee, practitioner, or researcher. Instead, this monograph will try to step a bit beyond the state of the art, drawing upon practical insights and techniques from a range of rehabilitation-related fields. These mutable boundaries of knowledge are expanding at a dizzying rate, especially in the neurosciences relevant to recovery. Perhaps this approach will encourage physicians and therapists to set off on their own to push the boundaries toward sound interventions that merge basic and clinical research with the practical arts of therapy.

Only one surveyor writes over this landscape. I have been influenced and intrigued over the last 15 years of my own research and practice in neurologic rehabilitation at UCLA, by those referenced in these chapters, and by many others who cannot be acknowledged in a short monograph. So personal biases and space restrictions will set the final Imaginot Line for this book. That should not limit the reader's imagination about the rich future for those who contribute to the practices of neurologic rehabilitation.

Bruce H. Dobkin

REFERENCES

1. Bowe F. Disabled and elderly people in the First, Second and Third Worlds. Int J Rehabil Res 1990; 13:1–14.
2. Braddom R. Why is physiatric research important? Am J Phys Med Rehabil 1991;70(suppl):S2–S3.
3. Cole T, Edgerton V. Report of the Task Force on Medical Rehabilitation Research. National Institutes of Health, 1990.
4. Collins R, Dobkin B, Choi D. Selective vulnerability of brain: New insights into the pathophysiology of stroke. Ann Intern Med 1989;110:992–1001.
5. DeLisa J, Jain S, Yablon S. Resident interest in physical medicine and rehabilitation fellowships. Am J Phys Med Rehabil 1991;70:290–292.
6. DeLisa J, Martin G, Currie D. Rehabilitation medicine: Past, present and future. In: DeLisa J, ed. Rehabilitation Medicine. Philadelphia: JB Lippincott, 1988, p 3.
7. Editorial. Why the Journal of Neurologic Rehabilitation? Journal of Neurologic Rehabilitation 1987; 1:1–2.
8. Granger C, Hamilton B. The Uniform Data System for Medical Rehabilitation report of first admissions for 1992. Am J Phys Med Rehabil 1994;73:51–55.
9. Greenwood R. Neurology and rehabilitation in the United Kingdom: A view. J Neurol Neurosurg Psychiatry 1992;55(Suppl):48–53.
10. LaPlante M. Disability Statistics Report: State estimates of disability in America. In US Department of Education, NIDRR, 1993.
11. McGinnis G, Osberg J, DeJong G, et al. Predicting charges for inpatient medical rehabilitation using severity, DRG, age and function. Am J Public Health 1987;77:826–829.
12. NIDRR. Data on Disability From the National Health Interview Surveys, 1983–1985. Washington, DC, 1988.
13. Rubin R, Gold W, Kelley D, et al. The Cost of Disorders of the Brain. National Foundation for Brain Research, 1992.
14. Schmidt R. Motor Control and Learning. Champaign, IL: Human Kinetics, 1988.
15. Stineman M, Escarce J, Granger C, et al. A case mix classification system for medical rehabilitation. Med Care 1994;32:60–67.
16. Wolk S, Blair T. Trends in Medical Rehabilitation. American Rehabilitation Association, 1994.

CONTENTS

PART 1

Neuroscientific Foundations for Rehabilitation

PLASTICITY IN MOTOR AND COGNITIVE NETWORKS

After an ischemic, hypoxic, or traumatic injury to the central nervous system, physical and cognitive impairments and accompanying disabilities usually lessen over a few months. A few clinically recognizable influences account for some of these gains (Table 1–1). Reversibly injured, edematous, and metabolically depressed nervous system tissue regains its normal properties: neuronal excitability recovers and activity in partially spared pathways resumes. Functional brain imaging by positron emission tomography (PET) has revealed patterns of cerebral perfusion and oxygen metabolism that help to predict, within less than 24 hours of an infarction, whether tissue recovery and clinical recovery are likely.[129] Gains also arise from compensatory behavioral strategies that are learned through formal and informal rehabilitative efforts.

For example, after a left thalamic parenchymatous and intraventricular hemorrhage, seen on the computed tomographic (CT) scan in Figure 1–1A, the patient had right hemiplegia, hemianopia, hemianesthesia, and aphasia after recovering from obtundation. Six months later, the magnetic resonance imaging (MRI) scan in Figure 1–1B showed a much smaller area of encephalomalacia in the thalamus and internal capsule. The visual-field and language impairments had resolved. With rehabilitation efforts over much of that time, the patient's self-care was possible with supervision, but he walked only 30 feet, and walking required moderate assistance from another person. Over the next 3 months, a rehabilitation program that used a task-oriented approach with body weight–supported treadmill training led to his ability to walk independently in the community with an ankle-foot orthosis and cane, despite little selective movement and no sensation on the right. The patient's gains, then, were associated with resolution of the toxic and compressive effects of the blood on neighboring tissue and adaptations learned during his rehabilitation. Was his progress owed to luck that critical tissue was spared and to success in skirting residual impairments? Can some credit be given to

3

Table 1–1. **POTENTIAL MECHANISMS FOR SUBSTITUTION OR RESTITUTION OF FUNCTION**

Network Plasticity
- Recovery of neuronal excitability
  - Resolution of cellular toxic or metabolic dysfunction
  - Resolution of edema; resorption of blood products
  - Resolution of diaschisis
- Activity in partially spared pathways
- Alternate behavioral strategies
- Representational mutability of neuronal assemblies
  - Expansion of representational maps
  - Recruitment of cells not ordinarily involved in an activity
- Recruitment of parallel and subcomponent pathways
  - Altered activity of the distributed functions of cortical and subcortical neural networks
  - Activation of pattern generators, such as for stepping
  - Inhibition and disinhibition of functional groups of neurons
  - Recruitment of networks not ordinarily involved in an activity
- Dependence on task-related stimulation

Neuronal Plasticity
- Altered efficacy of synaptic activity
  - Activity-dependent unmasking of previously ineffective synapses
  - Learning and memory tied to activity-dependent changes in synaptic strength
  - Increased neuronal responsiveness from denervation hypersensitivity
  - Change in number of receptors
  - Change in neurotransmitter release and uptake
- Synaptic sprouting
- Axonal and dendritic regeneration
  - Signaling gene expression for cell viability, growth, and remodeling proteins
  - Modulation by neurotrophic factors
  - Actions of chemoattractants and inhibitors in the milieu
- Remyelination
- Transsynaptic degeneration
- Ion channel changes on fibers for impulse conduction
- Actions of neurotransmitters and neuromodulators
- Tissue grafts

rehabilitation methods that modulated nervous system pathways?

This patient's partial recovery might also have been mediated by some of the growing number of mechanisms that allow for structural and functional reorganization within gray and white matter (see Table 1–1). These mechanisms are the subject of the first two chapters of this book, but mechanisms of neuroplasticity interact with many other variables that carry uncertain weights. Recovery from an acquired brain injury also depends on the strength of connections in neural networks, which seem to have a protective effect against the loss of what was learned and affect how readily a subject might relearn. For example, better outcomes after stroke and traumatic brain injury are predicted by a higher premorbid level of education. Other variables, such as age, number of lesions, timing of sequential lesions, and genetic factors, contribute to a patient's final outcome.[74,100]

The potential to enhance neurologic recovery by manipulating the biologic adaptability of the brain and spinal cord has become relevant to clinical practice. Medical rehabilitation routines have begun to apply techniques that can build on this neuroplasticity to optimize the recovery process. In relation to studies of neurologic rehabilitation, *neuroplasticity* generally refers to use-dependent neuronal network modifications. Changes include short-term modulations of function and long-term structural changes. Knowledge about neuroplasticity is drawn from growing information that ranges from the molecular aspects of developmental neurobiology to functional cerebral imaging in normal persons and in patients with brain injury.

When considering how patients change over time after injury, we may find it difficult to distinguish among strict definitions of *recovery, sparing,* and *compensation*[5] (Table 1–2). Other terminology considers two processes that interact to affect the degree of recovery during rehabilitation.[43] The first process, *restitution,* is relatively independent of external variables such as physical and cognitive stimulation. It includes the biochemical events that tend to recover in neural tissue. The second process, *substitution,* depends on external stimuli such as rehabil-

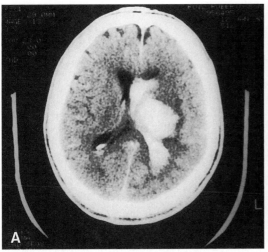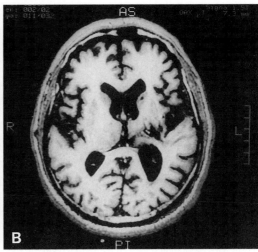

Figure 1–1. (*A*) This computed tomography (CT) scan shows an acute left thalamic intracerebral hemorrhage with mass effect and intraventricular blood. (*B*) The magnetic resonance imaging (MRI) scan performed 6 months later shows encephalomalacia of the thalamus and subcortical tissue, including the internal capsule.

itative interventions. It includes the functional adaptations of defective, but partially restored neural networks that compensate for components lost or disrupted by the injury. Functional neuroimaging has helped to reveal these adaptations. However, these processes can be difficult to distinguish when we observe our patients. Motor functions can appear to have recovered when, in

Table 1–2. **TERMINOLOGY FOR POSTINJURY GAINS**

Term	Definition
Recovery	Complete return of identical functions that were lost or impaired
Restitution	Tendency of a neural network to recover after an interruption as a consequence of internal, biologic events
Substitution	Functional adaptation of a defective but partially restored neural network that depends on external stimulation
Sparing	Adequate function through residual neural pathways
Compensation	Functional adaptation for an impairment or disability

fact, residual neural activity is actually supporting behavioral plasticity. For example, in rodents and monkeys with an experimentally induced unilateral pyramidal lesion, the ability to reach for a pellet of food gradually improves and, at first glance, may appear to have fully recovered. A closer analysis by slow-motion videotaping of the movement reveals better control of the proximal than the distal limb. The animal reaches with a grasp, brings the pellet to its mouth without the normal supination of the hand and forearm, turns its head to chase after the food, and cannot easily release its grip.[213] The hand-to-mouth pattern of the patient with hemiparesis is similar to the injured animal's alternate strategy.

One of the most challenging goals in neurologic rehabilitation is to enhance the recovery of motor control for walking and for the reaching and fine coordinated movements of the upper extremity. This chapter emphasizes mechanisms of sensorimotor plasticity for movement over adaptations associated with the recovery of cognitive processes, mostly because experimental studies of motor functions have been more complete. Principles of special interest for rehabilitation are common to both sensorimotor and cognitive functions. This selective review of the relevant neuroscience of today aims to provide leads for a science of neurorehabilitation for tomorrow.

MOTOR CONTROL

Movement is more than simply an efferent activity. Posture, coordination, orientation to the environment, perceptual information, drives, and goals help to formulate a particular action by means of various movement strategies. The mechanisms that allow humans to acquire complex motor skills are critical to understanding how purposeful movements may be reacquired in patients with neurologic diseases.

Mountcastle wrote: "The brain is a complex of widely and reciprocally interconnected systems" and "The dynamic interplay of neural activity within and between these systems is the very essence of brain function." He proposed: "The remarkable capacity for improvement of function after partial brain lesions is viewed as evidence for the adaptive capacity of such distributed systems to achieve a goal, albeit slowly and with error, with the remaining neural apparatus."[149] What are some of the "essences" of brain function and adaptive capacity?

Many neuronal clusters, pathways, and neurophysiologic and molecular mechanisms contribute to the expression of postures and movements. No one theory has yet explained the details of the controls for normal motor behavior, let alone the abnormal patterns and synergies that emerge secondary to a lesion at any level of the neuraxis. Many models successfully predict various aspects of motor performance, although few have been biologically plausible and behaviorally relevant. Neural network modeling and mathematic concepts for dynamic pattern generation in complex biologic systems have been offered both as theoretic organizing principles and as a way to foster experimentation.[182] Motor programs can also be conceptualized as cortical cell assemblies that are stored in the form of strengthened synaptic connections between pyramidal neurons and their outputs, especially to the basal ganglia, for the preparation and ordered sequence of movements.[214] Great progress has been made in understanding what small groups of cells code and how ever larger groups might interact to carry out a learned or novel action.[56,73] Electrophysiologic and functional brain imaging studies, discussed later in this chapter, show that movements are represented in the brain before they are executed. Subjects select and activate a stored neural program that coordinates a task. The motor representation includes the mental content that relates to the goal or consequences of an action, as well as the neural operations that take place before the action starts.

Various neural architectures with distinct and overlapping circuitry characteristics presumably underlie adaptive behaviors.[148] Although we do not know the details of these molecular and physiologic processes, most studies support the observations of Mountcastle and others that the motor system learns and performs, with the overriding object being to achieve movement goals. Goal-oriented learning should be the essence of rehabilitation strategies.

Most motor functions are controlled in a distributed fashion at multiple interconnected sites of the cortex, subcortical and brainstem nuclei, and spinal motor pools.[18] Regions that contribute to a motor or a cognitive activity are not so much functionally localized as they are functionally specialized. Higher levels seem to integrate subcomponents such as reflexes and oscillating neural networks or pattern generators without directly designating the details of parameters such as the timing, intensity, and duration of the sequences of muscle activity among synergist, antagonist, and stabilizing muscle groups. For certain motor acts, the motor cortex needs only to set a goal; preset neural routines in the brainstem and spinal cord are then capable of carrying out the details of movements. This process helps to explain how an equivalent motor act can be accomplished by variations in movements that depend on the demands of the environment, prior learning, and rewarded experience. Having achieved a behavioral goal, the reinforced sensory and movement experience is learned by the motor network. This learning results from increased synaptic activity that assembles neurons into functional groups with preferred lines of communication.[53] At a cellular level, activity-dependent changes in synaptic strength have been related to motor learning and memory. For example, in the cerebellum, repetitive and simultaneous excitatory inputs at the parallel-fiber/Purkinje-cell synapse cause a so-called long-term depression of synaptic strength. Cerebellar long-term depression (LTD) appears to be a fundamental mediator of aspects of motor learning.[128] These forms of adaptability or neural plasticity, superimposed on intact circuits for task subroutines, could permit improvements and new motor learning after a neurologic injury.

Many different adaptations within the nervous system and in outward behaviors can occur after a central or peripheral injury. Many of these adaptations have their roots in normal mechanisms of learning and in developmental neurobiology.[219] Increasing evidence from neurophysiologic and functional imaging studies points especially to intercoordinated, functional assemblies of cells distributed throughout the neuraxis that initiate and carry out complex movements. These neuronal sensorimotor assemblies show considerable plasticity in the maps of the dermatomes, muscles, and movements that they represent. In addition, these assemblies form multiple parallel systems that cooperate to manage the diverse information necessary for the rapid, precise, and yet highly flexible control of multijoint movements. This organization subsumes many of the neural adaptations that contribute to normal learning of skills and, perhaps, to at least partial recovery after a neural injury.

Theories underlying neurorehabilitative motor training must account for the interdependency and reciprocity of neuronal networks and the distributed control of movement throughout these systems. Until recently, most of what physical therapists have practiced was based on two rather limited models of motor control.[96] In one model, chains of reflexes are the units of movement. Sensory inputs are used to direct motor outputs. In another, the hierarchic model, motor control is derived in steps from cortical voluntary, brainstem intermediate, and spinal reflex levels. These notions depict an elegantly wired machine that performs stereotyped computations on sensory inputs. These models have led to the so-called neurodevelopmental therapy strategies that progress from attempts to elicit reflexively driven and then internally commanded patterns of muscle activation (see Chapter 3, Team Practices). The movements are often not related to a task that is meaningful to the patient. Both concepts are being overtaken by programs that consider how subjects learn goal-oriented tasks. This shift in focus will lead to alternative, testable therapeutic approaches for neurologic rehabilitation.

Despite the uncertainty at times about whether we are observing mechanisms of recovery, restitution, substitution, sparing, or compensation, one can discuss some of the potential means for restorative reorganization in cortical, subcortical, and spinal circuits. These reverberating circuits calibrate motor control. To consider their role in plasticity, I selectively review some of the anatomy and physiology of their switches and rheostats. This discussion takes a top-down anatomic approach, because diseases and injuries tend to involve particular levels of the neuraxis. Within each level, but with an eye on the potential for interactive reorganization throughout the neuraxis, I consider some aspects of the biologic adaptability of the substrates for sensorimotor functions within the neuronal assemblies and distributed pathways for improvements in walking and in the use of a paretic arm.

Cortical Networks

PRIMARY MOTOR CORTEX

The primate primary motor cortex (M_1) in Brodmann's area 4 (Fig. 1–2) has an overall somatotopic organization; however, separable islands of cortical motoneurons with similar representations intermingle to create a more complex map for movement than those portrayed by the traditional drawings of the homunculus.[183] For example, M_1 has separate clusters of output neurons that can facilitate the activity of a single spinal motoneuron. For the upper extremity, at least two spatially separate regions of area 4 project corticospinal outputs, primarily to the lower cervical segments.[93] At least seven in-

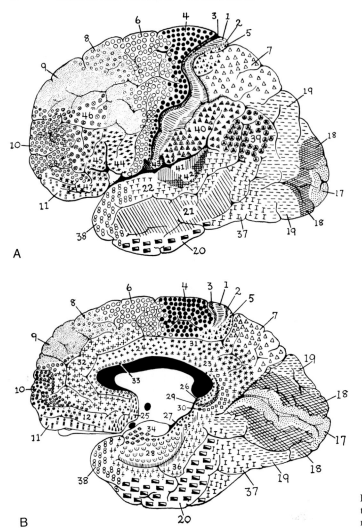

Figure 1–2. Brodmann's cytoarchitectural map of the (A) lateral and (B) medial surfaces of the brain.

dependent arm fields have somatotopic representation in areas 4 and 6.[24] In addition, a single corticospinal neuron can project to the spinal motoneurons for different muscles and precisely adjust the amount of muscle coactivation.[94a] The individual and integrated actions of these representations reflect important aspects of motor control. For example, the mosaic of cortical neuronal patches that activate muscles of the fingers are separated by patches of neurons that activate muscles of the shoulder and the elbow. Some individual neurons in the zones in which these patches overlap control muscles of the wrist, elbow, and shoulder.[179a]

Also, representations for movements of each finger overlap with each other and with patches of neurons for wrist action.[181]

Thus, a cortical motoneuron or an assembly of interacting motoneurons can represent the selective activation of one muscle or can activate a set of muscles that carry out a complex movement. This overlapping organization contributes to the control of the complex muscle synergies needed for fine coordination and forceful contractions.[123] When M_1 is lesioned in the monkey, the upper extremity is initially quite impaired. The hand can be retrained to perform simple movements that activate single muscles. Although this rehabilitation leads to flexion and extension of the wrist, the monkey cannot learn to make a smooth diagonal wrist movement using muscles for flexion and radial deviation.[94a] It accomplishes this motion only in a step-wise sequence, which suggests that M_1 is critical for activating and inactivating muscles in a precise spatial and temporal pattern that also includes making fractionated finger movements.

Some investigators have suggested that M_1 might be a computational map for sensorimotor transformations rather than a map of muscles or particular movement patterns.[111] The details of these computations, the neural correlates for features of upper extremity function, and the relationships among neurons during movement are under study in primates and other animals. For example, single-cell activity in the motor cortex is most intense for reaching with a particular magnitude and direction of force.[72] The direction of an upper extremity movement may be coded by the sum of the vectors of the single-cell activities in motor and related cortex in the direction of the movement.[184] Neurons in parietal area 7 have been shown to become preferentially activated for the preshaping of a hand movement and seem to match the pattern of a movement to the shape of the object that is to be manipulated.[196] The degree to which the motor cortex discharge represents the extrinsic attributes of movements versus joint- and muscle-centered intrinsic variables is unclear, however. Cortical cells involved in a particular movement may make a smaller contribution to an unrelated movement. Potentially, these cells can functionally shift to take over some aspects of an impaired movement in the event a cortical or subcortical injury removes the primary cortical activators from their input to spinal motoneurons. As described later in this chapter, these motor and neighboring cortical sensory neurons can adapt in remarkable ways during training. In addition, functional imaging with PET in normal subjects has revealed the somatotopic distribution of activation during upper extremity tasks in M_1 as well as in supplementary and cingulate motor cortices.[83] Functional imaging techniques can be used to try to assess whether this somato-topic distribution within the limb changes after a brain injury that affects arm movement, particularly in relation to improved function during a specific rehabilitation strategy.

Pyramidal Projections. M_1 contributes about 40 to 60 percent of the 1 million corticospinal fibers that enter each medullary pyramid.[40] From 70 to 90 percent of pyramidal fibers decussate into the lateral corticospinal tract, and 10 to 30 percent remain uncrossed and form the ventral corticospinal tract.[151] The asymmetry in the corticospinal tracts, in which the ventral and lateral tracts are larger on the right side in about 75 percent of spinal cords, might offer a clue about sparing after an injury and about plasticity.[152]

The fibers of the ventral corticospinal tract synapse especially with motoneurons for axial and girdle muscles. These fibers reach the lumbar spinal cord minimally, if at all, and some fibers cross in the anterior commissure to connect with motoneurons of the opposite ventral horn.[40] Ipsilateral corticospinal pathways may be involved in the control of distal and proximal upper limb movements.[2] Corticospinal neurons from area 4, as well as from the caudal portion of area 6, project to the spinal intermediate zone and onto spinal motoneurons. In the macaque and probably in humans, these projections are distributed to the dorsal horn and to the dorsal and lateral parts of the intermediate zone, mainly contralaterally, and to the contralateral motoneurons for the muscles of the distal extremity. In addition, the corticospinal tracts synapse bilaterally in the ventromedial parts of the intermediate zone.[121] Thus, the primary motor cortex has connections that could modulate some proximal and distal ipsilateral as well as contralateral movements. PET studies show that the ipsilateral inputs can play a role in recovery after an injury to one hemisphere.

M_1 outputs are also integrated into brainstem controls for motor activities. For example, the cortical projections from the hand and foot areas to the spinal intermediate zone coincide with projections from the rubrospinal tract. The red nuclei seem to help control the extremities and digits for skillful steering and fractionated movements. These functions overlap those of the motor cortex.[180] M_1 and other motor cortices project directly and by collateral fibers to the ipsilateral red nucleus, so these midbrain neurons, which also receive cerebellar projections, may independently subserve some aspects of the motor control of the distal limbs despite a hemispheric injury.[115]

Other precentral motor projections, particularly those that project bilaterally to the ventromedial parts of the intermediate zone, seem to contribute to steering movements of the body axis, such as postural and orienting movements of the head and body and synergistic movements of the body and limbs. Kuypers has suggested that the interneurons of the ventromedial intermediate zone represent a diffuse system of widespread connections among a variety of motoneurons, whereas the dorsal and lateral areas are a focused system with a limited number of connections.[121] Other corticomotoneurons project directly and by collateral fibers to the upper medullary medial reticular formation. These motoneurons overlap the descending reticulospinal pathway to the same gray matter of the spinal cord in the intermediate zone. Within these pathways, then, some potential redundancy could, after an injury, allow partial sparing or reorganization of motor functions, especially for axial and proximal movements.

M_1 neurons receive different types of sensory input before converging on their target motoneurons.[98] The dorsal horn inputs from the pyramidal tract found in the macaque and presumably in humans modulate sensory inputs from the periphery. In turn, sensory receptors, especially for proprioception from the distal limb muscles, have topographically organized inputs to the primary motor cortex. For example, primary and secondary somatosensory and thalamocortical inputs, among their other duties, help to adjust the gain of M_1 neurons according to output requirements. The modulation of motor output by sensory inputs appears to be important at every level of the neuraxis, starting from segmental spinal cord inputs. Rehabilitation strategies should include testing ways to find which sensory inputs optimize movements during training for a task.

Sparing of the Corticospinal Pathway. Bucy and colleagues report an instructive clinicopathologic correlation between corticospinal tract sparing and recovery.[20] To relieve a patient's hemiballismus, these investigators incised the central 10 mm of the right cerebral peduncle to a depth of 7 mm just above the pons. Within 24 hours, the patient's flaccid hemiplegia began to improve. He regained a hand grasp and toe movements. By the 10th day, he bore weight on the leg. By the 29th day, he ambulated with a walker and executed fine movements of the fingers "fairly well." He plateaued by 7 months, with a "very mild" hemiparesis, independent gait, and the ability to hop on the left leg almost as well as on the right. At autopsy 2½ years later, the only intact corticospinal fibers were in the medial and lateral peduncle, descending from the frontal and parietal areas, respectively. Corticopontine fibers persisted in the upper lateral pons, which includes fibers of parietal origin. Only 17 percent of the axis cylinders in the right medullary pyramid persisted, and an estimated 90 percent of precentral giant cells of Betz suffered retrograde degeneration.

Another study relates the severity of chronic hemiparesis in patients who had suffered a stroke to the magnitude of shrinkage of the cerebral peduncle measured by CT. Sparing of more than 60 percent of the peduncle, including the medial portion, predicted the recovery of a precision grip and, to a lesser degree, the force of the grip.[205] The typical hemiplegic posture of elbow, wrist, and finger flexion followed 60 percent shrinkage, which roughly corresponded to a loss of 88 percent of the descending fibers. For example, Figure 1–3 reveals wallerian degeneration from a cortical infarction (Fig. 1–3A) through the internal capsule (Fig. 1–3B) and pons (Fig. 1–3D), with about 30 to 40 percent shrinkage of the cerebral peduncle (Fig. 1–3C) on the left. The patient in Figure 1–3 could slowly grasp and release a cone and oppose his thumb to his fifth digit. Of course, studies of the pyramidal tract at the level of the peduncle may produce different results than studies of lesions of the internal capsule, in which corticostriate, corticothalamic, corticopontine, and other corticofugal fibers may be damaged.

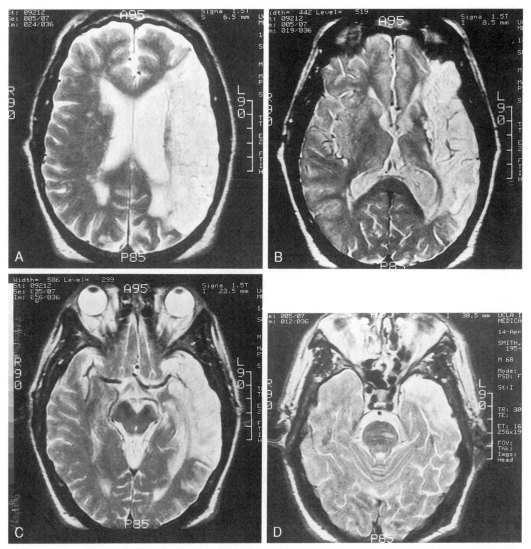

Figure 1–3. T_2-weighted magnetic resonance imaging (MRI) scans of a large, chronic left cerebral cortical infarction reveals partial involvement of the corticospinal tract by wallerian degeneration and relative sparing of subcortical tissue. (*A*) The MRI scan at the uppermost axial level shows a left middle cerebral artery distribution of ischemia. (*B*) A linear area of demyelination is seen within the posterior limb of the left internal capsule. (*C*) The left cerebral peduncle is atrophic from loss of descending tracts. (*D*) A horizontal, linear region of degeneration appears within the belly of the left pons.

OTHER MOTOR AREAS

The premotor cortex and supplementary motor area (SMA), along with M_1, exert what Hughlings Jackson called "the least automatic" control over voluntary motor commands, which are issued according to the task required. The premotor area 6 has been divided into a dorsal area, in and adjacent to the precentral sulcus, and a ventral area, which is in and adjacent to the caudal bank of the arcuate sulcus at its inferior limb. In the dorsal premotor area, separate arm and leg representations are found, along with both distal and proximal upper extremity representations.[93] In the monkey, after an M_1 lesion these premotor areas may contribute to upper extremity movements, short of coordinated co-contractions and fractionated wrist and finger actions.[94a] In this model, improved limb function could be related to sparing of or substitution by the premotor cortex.

At least three nonprimary motor areas also contribute from their locations in areas 23 and 24 of the ventral bank of the cingulate cortex and from immediately rostral to the SMA.[120] The posterior portion of area 24 in cingulate cortex sends dense projections to the spinal cord, M_1, and the caudal part of the SMA.[157] This posterior portion also interacts with area 6. The rostral portion targets mostly the SMA. Indeed, each of the six distinct cortical motor areas has a separate and independent set of inputs from adjacent and remote regions, as well as parallel, separate outputs to the brainstem and spinal cord.[192]

The roles of these multiple generators for movement are just beginning to be understood. For example, area 24 is activated in PET studies mainly when a subject is forced to choose from a set of competing oculomotor, manual, or speech responses.[157] This area presumably participates in motor control by facilitating an appropriate response or by suppressing the execution of an inappropriate response when behavior has to be modified in a novel or challenging, nonautomatic situation.

The SMA plays a particularly intriguing role within the mosaic of anatomically connected cortical areas involved in the execution of movements. When electrically stimulated, complex and sequential multijoint, synergistic movements of the distal and proximal limbs are produced, so the area has important spinal connections. Surface electrode stimulation over the mesial surface of the cerebral cortex in patients before the surgical excision of an epileptic focus has revealed the somatotopy within the SMA and suggests its involvement not only in the control of muscle contractions but also in the intention to perform a motor act. Moreover, stimulation of the right SMA has produced both contralateral and ipsilateral movements, whereas left-sided stimulation has led mostly to contralateral activity.[65] In humans, the SMA is involved in initiating movements triggered by sensory cues. Bilateral activation occurs during tasks that are more difficult, such as novel, isolated finger movements, consistent with the role of this area in motor planning.[81]

The contributions of the other motor areas account for some of the nuances of impairments in motor control after a cortical injury. For example, lesions of the arcuate and superior precentral motor areas over the lateral convexity cause proximal weakness and apraxia. The region is important to the preparation of a movement, especially if previously learned, when cued by visual, auditory, and tactile sensory information.[91] Lesions of the SMA can cause akinesia and impaired control of bimanual and sequential movements, especially of the digits.

Knowledge is accruing regarding motor area interaction with cortex that does not have direct spinal motoneuron connections. A sensory-triggered response, for example, may be guided by sensory association areas, a conditional sensory response by premotor neurons, and a representational or memory-based response by motor regions.[77] Although prefrontal areas do not directly control a muscle contraction, they play a role in the initiation, selection, inhibition, and guidance of behavior by representational knowledge. These areas have this effect by means of somatotopically arranged prefrontal to premotor, corticostriatal, corticotectal, and thalamocortical connections.[76]

Rehabilitation specialists can begin to consider the contribution of these other motor systems to motor control, to anticipate how their activation may vary in relation to different tasks, to test for their dysfunction, and to adapt appropriate interventions. For example, patients with lesions that interrupt the corticocortical projections from somatosensory cortex to the primary motor cortex may have difficulty in learning new motor skills, but they may be able to execute existing motor skills.[158] In the presence of a lesion that destroys or disconnects some motor areas, a part of the distributed functional network for relearning a movement or learning a new, compensatory skill may be activated best by a particular strategy. Therapists may work around the disconnection with a strategy that is visually directed, auditorily cued, self-paced, proximal limb–directed, mentally planned, or sequenced or unsequenced movement–based.

ACTIVATION STUDIES OF DISTRIBUTED MOTOR NETWORKS

Activation and subtraction studies with PET and functional MRI (fMRI) have broadened our understanding of some of the specific operations within the distributed neural systems for movement, language, attention, memory, perception, and other aspects of cognition.[133,165,166] The fMRI signal arises when neuronal activity increases local blood flow and volume with little or no change in oxygen consumption. This situation increases the oxygen content of local venous blood, which increases the intensity of the magnetic resonance signal.[199] The two techniques have begun to reveal the functional anatomy of processes often impaired by stroke.[38,64,160] Of great interest for rehabilitation, PET and fMRI can help to reveal the areas involved in learning a variety of motor tasks.[102,114] These studies show how the nature of a task, such as its difficulty, whether it is internally or externally cued, and how it is learned, alters which cerebral regions come into play.[169,172] For example, functional neuroimaging studies show that the recovery of prelearned finger movements requires the activation of the same primary sensorimotor and SMA cortices as the learning of a novel, difficult task.[172] These studies reveal that a high level of synaptic activity accompanies the early stages of motor skill learning.[82] Functional imaging of the motor areas during the rehabilitative training of an important task may potentially be used to show whether critical tissue for learning is activated by the training strategy. Despite some potential limitations,[64] PET and fMRI allow the generation and testing of hypotheses about motor and cognitive processes and about adaptive functional changes after a cerebral injury.

Regional cerebral blood flow (rCBF) studies of normal subjects by PET reveal the cortical areas that are most highly activated during simple upper extremity motor tasks. Activity increases in the contralateral M_1 and the premotor, SMA, arcuate, and parietal cortical areas that are linked to it during proximal and distal arm, fine finger, and whole hand movements.[45] In one experiment that helps to define this distributed motor system, subjects were studied under four conditions. These persons moved a joystick (1) after a tonal cue according to a previously trained sequence, (2) in random directions, (3) when the correct movement was specified by one of the four tones they heard, and (4) when the correct movement was the opposite of that specified by the tones on the previous task.[45] The rCBF during these tasks was compared with that during simple movement of the joystick forward at the same rate as the other tasks after a sound. The SMA had greater metabolic activity in the first two conditions, presumably because it is important in planning. These tasks required internal generation of a movement, whereas the second two were directed by external cues. Activity within the left superior parietal cortex increased in all four conditions, suggesting that the process by which movement is selected is coded here. The bilateral premotor cortices were also activated in all cases. In the random condition, several frontal areas and the cingulate sulcus were activated; this finding points to the contribution of these areas to self-initiated acts.

Another experiment points to the contribution of parallel, cortical networks in a distributed motor system. Skeletal muscle strength was shown to increase by having individuals imagine that they were contracting a particular muscle.[221] Indeed, when the abductor digiti quinti was exercised to increase its strength and when subjects only imagined that they practiced abduction against resistance, the abductor of the contralateral, untrained hand also increased in strength. This neural, as opposed to muscular, origin of muscle strengthening also seems to occur during physical exercise before any muscle hypertrophy is evident. PET and other techniques suggest that the strengthening is derived from the activation of central motor planning areas outside of M_1. These areas increase the coordination of outputs to spinal motoneurons.[176] The transfer of the motor program to the nonexercised digit may have been through the corpus callosum or by bilateral activation of the SMA.[106]

Studies of mental imagery of a movement reveal the basis for a potential rehabilitative strategy. When a three-dimensional object was presented visually, PET showed that motor representations arise during the conditions of observing a grasping movement as well as while imagining the same movement.[44] During the PET study, rCBF increased in extrastriate visual and cingulate cortices and in the cerebellum and basal ganglia during observational learning, which is a powerful learning strategy for acquiring motor skills. Imagining the same movement increased rCBF in the premotor, prefrontal, and cingulate cortices and in the caudate nucleus. Premotor neurons are activated in other visually guided tasks, whereas, as described earlier, the SMA is more active during internally generated, remembered, and self-determined movements. The differences in the network activations between observing and imagining raise the possibility that training a behavior by mental imagery may contribute to a functionally adaptive substitution after a central or peripheral neural injury. This strategy could be tested in a combined functional neuroimaging and clinical trial to, for example, improve disuse muscle weakness or affect the recovery of a motor skill such as reaching or stepping.

Metabolic imaging studies provide a sense of which cortical networks are special contributors to movement under various conditions. How variations in the force, speed, or kinematics of a new or well-learned movement affect the amount of activation is not yet clear. By understanding the task-related conditions that mediate these shifts, rehabilitation specialists may be able to design and to study physical, cognitive, and pharmacologic interventions that enhance, inhibit, and modulate pathways to lessen disability.

CORTICAL SENSORIMOTOR REPRESENTATIONAL PLASTICITY

Cortical motor and sensory neurons are not permanently fixed in the way they subserve their limb functions. On the contrary, they quickly adapt to changing demands. In the adult and developing animal and in humans, the topographic maps of sensory and motor neuronal representations are capable of physiologic and structural reorganization.[7] Electrophysiologic and metabolic imaging experiments also reveal changes in the cortical maps for visual, auditory, and olfactory representations induced by central and peripheral lesions and by experience. This apparently ubiquitous property of adult cortical output and receptive fields offers insight into the training and other input conditions that might optimize remodeling and, in turn, the recovery of motor control and higher cognitive activities. How these modifications of functional pathways are modulated and how they may be manipulated to enhance, as well as to avoid inhibiting, recovery are among the most important applications of basic neuroscience to human neurorestoration.

Sensory Maps. In a series of primate studies (Experimental Case Study 1–1), Merzenich and colleagues have found that cortical representational changes are especially likely to arise during training paradigms that involve learning and the acquisition of specific skills. The more a set of neurons was activated by a sensory stimulus, as when a primate learned to perform a task with repeated use of the same skin surface, the more widespread the cortical sensory representation became for the most stimulated area of skin. The investigators could not always correlate an enlargement of the map with an increase in the primate's skill at the task. The improvements these investigators observed as a result of the primates' training could also have been derived from enhancement in the neural representation of the stimulus at another cortical or a subcortical area that was not mapped. It is also possible that a physiologic variable more closely associated with the greater skill was coded by a property of the neurons other than the spatial and temporal responses that were measured.[170]

In humans, cortical sensory reorganization has been postulated from clinical observations. For example, when the same side of the face was touched within 4 weeks of amputation of an arm, the amputee experienced the sensation in the missing hand. This finding suggests that the sensory input from the face had invaded the cortical hand area, perhaps by the unmasking of previ-

---

EXPERIMENTAL CASE STUDY 1–1
Cortical Somatosensory Representational Changes

Using a mapping technique with an array of microelectrodes over the cortical surface of monkeys, Merzenich and colleagues conducted a series of experiments demonstrating the mutability of somatosensory representations.[104] Following the amputation of a digit in adult monkeys, the sensory representation of adjacent digits in cortical areas 3b and 1 enlarged topographically by about 1 mm to occupy the territory that had been filled by the sensory neurons associated with the lost digit.[103] The change evolved over several weeks. Moreover, the details of the animals' touch maps improved in neighboring fingers.

In another experiment, monkeys were rewarded for touching with the tip of a digit for about ½ hr a day a rotating disk that had an uneven surface.[104] Compared with control subjects and with touching a static disk, reorganization of the parietal receptive field in areas 3a and 3b rapidly evolved in the monkeys that touched the rotating disk. The cortical representation of the stimulated phalanx enlarged immediately after stimulation in a complex distribution. The phalanx representation returned to the prestimulation size within 30 days. In other paradigms, stimulation of a small skin surface during a behavioral task also led to the emergence of a greatly expanded zone of a coherent response that correlated with the improvement in the animal's ability to make relevant discriminations about the applied stimuli.[171]

Their focal brain lesion model in the monkey is of special interest to specialists in rehabilitation. A cortical lesion in area 3b was induced where stimulation of one of the fingers had produced neuronal activation. These investigators induced the primate to use the same skin area of the hand in a reinforcing behavioral task by having the animal manipulate food pellets that it could then eat. By the time the primate was able to do so efficiently, the cortical region that represented the lesioned finger had shrunk, the map of surrounding finger areas had enlarged, and a separate representation of the lesioned finger's skin had arisen in area 3a.[105] These investigators suggested that behaviorally important stimulation at a constant skin location led to an increase in the synaptic effectiveness for the related thalamocortical inputs, which produced a larger thalamic receptive field. In addition, changes in synaptic effectiveness within the local intracortical somatosensory neural network seemed to account for some of the observed variations in representations. Horizontal connections that link cortical neurons over 6 to 8 mm have been found in the visual system. Axons of primary sensorimotor cortex pyramidal cells have as many as five intracortical collateral axons that form synapses over distances of 6 mm.[101] This increase in synaptic efficacy is equivalent to the neuroplasticity mechanism of unmasking of synaptic connections after an injury.

---

ously silent synapses from thalamocortical and intracortical circuits.[168]

Manipulations that lead to alterations in cortical somatosensory maps also change the organization of representational maps in the thalamus, brainstem, and spinal cord (Experimental Case Study 1–2).[204] The possibility of both subcortical and spinal changes raises the issue of the relative contribution of each to cortical plasticity. A particular rehabilitative intervention might modify these contributions differentially.

Another phenomenon related to the plasticity of representational sensory maps was revealed in a study of denervation by amputation or anesthesia of one digit in monkeys. A rapid expansion of the parietal sensory field occurred in both the contralateral cortex and the ipsilateral homotopic cortex.[23] The neurons that showed this dynamic change did not respond to stimulation of the ipsilateral digit. The mechanism and pathway mediating this transfer are uncertain, but they presumably maintain integration between the bilateral fields. A possibly related phenomenon of bilateral homotopic change is found in the observation of ipsilateral sensory impairment in light touch

---

EXPERIMENTAL CASE STUDY 1–2
Subcortical Somatosensory Representational Changes

Subcortical representational maps are also mutable. Local anesthetic injected into dorsal column nuclei resulted in the emergence of a new receptive field for each affected neuron within minutes, a finding suggesting that new fields arise from unmasking previously ineffective inputs.[163] This model looks at the effect of abolishing afferent activity. In another model of tactile learning, neurons of different cortical layers responded rapidly to changes in sensory experience of the rat whisker receptive fields.[46] Additional cortical layer and thalamic changes followed. Unmasking appeared less important than specific synaptic strengthening.

Staging these somatosensory changes at each level of the neuraxis remains a researcher's challenge. Somatotopic reorganization can occur at the earliest stages of somatosensory processing. Stimulation of peripheral afferents extends a cell's receptive field beyond the boundaries usually found in electrophysiologic studies. For example, after a peripheral nerve lesion, the reorganization in the somatotopic map shown in the ventroposterior lateral nucleus of the thalamus in adult monkeys was as complete as that found in the parietal cortex.[70]

Many other lines of research suggest that compensation after a central or peripheral injury can be due to a functional shift to neighboring neurons. Pons and colleagues found an extensive amount of cortical reorganization 12 years after 4-year-old monkeys underwent peripheral deafferentation of the dorsal roots from C-2 to T-4.[164] The normal border of the face and hand representations in the somatosensory areas had been stretched along a line 10 to 14 mm long, the length of the deafferented zone. The expanded face area included the chin and lower jaw and met the adjacent normal trunk map. These distances are far greater than one would expect if the mechanism were the unmasking of the synaptic arbors of thalamocortical axons. The mechanism is still open to debate.[126] The investigators suggest that the extensive reorganization arose from subcortical changes, because maps of body parts are represented in a much smaller neural region in the brainstem, even less than in the thalamus, and far less than in the cortex itself. Axonal sprouting, perhaps in the brainstem, or multiple somatosensory cortical representations that overlapped may also have led to the recorded changes.

---

threshold, point localization, or two-point discrimination in up to 40 percent of patients after a hemispheric injury. In a study of patients with a single lesion from a stroke, 30 percent had a significantly impaired light touch threshold compared with age-matched control subjects over the web space between the first and second digits in the "unaffected" ipsilateral hand.[59]

Motor Maps. Representational plasticity has been induced in a variety of animal models. Studies of enlarging neuronal assemblies have been combined with a search for the neurotransmitters and morphologic changes that may accompany reorganization (Experimental Case Study 1–3; see also Chapter 2).

In patients, evidence of cortical reorganization, such as enlarging representational motor maps and participation of distributed neural networks during normal motor learning and after a nervous system injury, comes from studies by magnetic scalp stimulation, PET, fMRI, and, to a more modest extent, transcranial Doppler ultrasonography of the intracranial arteries.[187] Magnetic and electrical scalp stimulation, like the other techniques, have revealed changes in the size of representations in cognitive[161] and sensorimotor[30] investigations. In magnetic stimulation, a transient clockwise current in a magnetic stimulating coil placed on the scalp in an optimal position induces a counterclockwise current in the brain. This current painlessly activates cortical neurons and, in turn, excites single bulbar and spinal motoneurons. The technique evoked larger motor responses from a greater number of scalp positions in the abdominal muscles rostral to a thoracic spinal cord lesion than were evoked

EXPERIMENTAL CASE STUDY 1–3
Cortical Motor Representational Changes

Motor maps also show functional reorganization. Merzenich and colleagues mapped the motor cortical zones that represented the digital, hand, wrist, elbow, and shoulder movements of monkeys before and after 11 hours of behavioral training.[139] The primates retrieved food pellets from small food wells without using their thumbs. The area 4 territories evoked by the digit movements required for the task increased significantly (Fig. 1–4). New movement relationships emerged in the map between digit and wrist extensor activity that were inherent to success in the task. The cortical surface over which this increased coupling of neurons evolved corresponded to a network as great as or greater than the spread of the axonal arbors of intracortical pyramidal cells.

Other experiments by this research group support long-held notions about the plasticity of the movement maps of the primary motor cortex.[122] They also extend the work of others who found that the cortex of primates is composed of multiple representations of distal forelimb movements. For example, these investigators recorded from the hand area of M_1 as squirrel monkeys performed a task that required skilled use of the arm and digits. In the hemisphere contralateral to the preferred hand, the researchers found representations, especially for digit flexion, wrist extension, and forearm supination, to be greater in number, to cover a larger area, and to show greater spatial complexity compared with the nondominant hand's cortical representations for the same task.[153] The investigators concluded that the number of re-representations and the types of movements that overlap are variable among individuals and between the hemispheres of an individual. These differences derive in part from ontogenetic development and from experiences such as coactivating muscles or by using them in a particular sequence to reach a goal.

Several neurotransmitters may participate in the changes in representational maps with experience and activity. A reduction in intracortical inhibitory pathways mediated by GABA permits the expression of new receptive fields.[110] Cholinergic and N-methyl-D-aspartate (NMDA) receptor modulation is also required.[112] These messengers apparently unmask pre-existing synapses that had been functionally ineffective. For example, following deafferentation, tonic inhibition decreased in rat and cat somatosensory cortex, and the responsiveness of neurons to acetylcholine increased. This finding uncovered new receptive fields and strengthened existing ones.[52] Drugs used in clinical practice may alter these transmitters and receptors and affect plasticity.

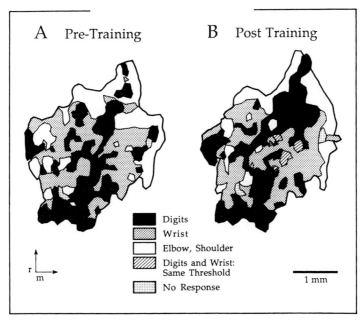

Figure 1–4. Movement maps derived by recording from a grid placed over area 4 of the macaque before and after the animal was trained in a food-retrieval task. The upper cortex shows territorial gains for the neuronal assemblies of the digits (black) and new evocations by combined digit and wrist movements (parallel lines) that were needed to learn the motor task. (From Marzenich, M, Recanzone, G, Jenkins, W, et al,[140] with permission.)

in the abdominal muscle groups of normal subjects.[198] This finding suggested to the investigators that the cortical motor map had expanded after the injury. These investigators could not exclude a change at the level of the affected spinal motoneurons, such as an increase in their excitatory response to a descending volley or sprouting of corticospinal axons.

In normal subjects, magnetic stimulation has shown representational plasticity during skill acquisition. Persons who practiced a five-finger piano exercise for 2 hours a day for 5 days showed an enlarging motor cortical area targeting the long finger flexor and extensor muscles and a decreased threshold for activation as they learned the skill.[155] In another experiment, cortical output maps to the muscles involved in a serial-reaction time task, in which subjects had to learn from ongoing experience which buttons to push, enlarged as subjects learned the task.[156] Up to that point, these persons had had implicit or unconscious knowledge of the task. When they achieved explicit knowledge or knowledge they could put into words of how to do the task, the map of cortical output returned to baseline. These examples of rapid motor learning with enlarging maps suggest that synaptic connections are unmasked and the motoneurons form new movement associations. Once the procedure is overlearned and automatic, the cortical excitation for learning is no longer needed, and the knowledge is at least partly stored elsewhere. Similar observations have been made with PET.[82]

FUNCTIONAL REORGANIZATION AFTER CEREBRAL INJURY

Studies by Magnetic Cortical Stimulation. Investigators have met with variable success in their attempts to demonstrate the actions of the undecussated corticospinal pathway by cortical transcranial magnetic or electrical stimulation in healthy persons and in those who have had a stroke.[154,206] In patients with mirror movements in the unaffected hand when the paretic fingers move, onset of a brain injury early in life is more likely to be associated with corticospinal tract adaptations than is adult-onset injury.

Magnetic stimulation of the motor cortex ipsilateral to the affected side of subjects with hemiplegic cerebral palsy produced hand movements in some of the subjects.[26] This finding correlated with a prenatal injury occurring before about 32 weeks' gestation and with intense mirror movements. Corticospinal axons apparently branched from the normal hemisphere to bilateral homologous spinal motoneuron pools during the time of normal developmental axonal elongation. Other studies that included PET suggested to the investigators that such persons had an aberrant cortical motor organization, as well as corticospinal pathways with prominent ipsilateral and contralateral actions.[31] The short-latency muscle compound action potentials typical of fast fiber conduction in corticospinal pathways have been elicited bilaterally in children with infantile hemiplegia; this finding suggests a spared function of the ipsilateral ventral tract. These action potentials have generally not been observed after adult-onset hemiparesis.[10,154]

Five patients in one study had residual hemiparesis, independent finger motion, and mirror movements after an internal capsule lacunar stroke. MRI showed antegrade wallerian degeneration of the affected pyramidal tract. Suprathreshold magnetic stimulation of the hemisphere ipsilateral to the infarct elicited bilateral responses in the patients' fingers.[66] Stimulation of the undamaged hemisphere caused only a contralateral response. Stimulation of the affected side could have produced bilateral movement through surviving axons in the degenerated pyramidal tract or through a nonpyramidal pathway that was facilitated as a consequence of the injury. The investigators suggest that the bilaterally organized corticoreticulospinal tract, mentioned previously, may be responsible for this effect. Loss of transcallosal inhibition could be another mechanism.[27] The findings parallel the PET studies described earlier of bilateral activation for recovered finger movements after a striatocapsular infarct.

Subcortical lesions that only partially damage the corticospinal and other motor tracts are especially likely to allow some degree of recovery. This sparing may not be appreciated by clinical examination. Magnetic stimulation studies in patients with pyramidal lesions reveal three mechanisms for weakness[144]:

1. When the number of corticospinal fibers that synapse with a motoneuron falls too short to generate adequate-sized excitatory postsynaptic potentials (EPSPs), a descending volley does not excite the spinal neuron.
2. The conduction velocity of a demyelinated corticospinal fiber may be slowed, and this change may delay and disperse the fiber's excitatory stimuli to the point at which the spinal neuron is not excited.
3. A dysfunctional descending pathway may allow one impulse to pass, but the next volley may find the fiber to be refractory. A subsequent volley may pass, but the relative blocking of the required train of volleys would impede spinal neuron excitation. This mechanism may also cause fatigability with repetitive attempts to use a paretic muscle group.

Recovery of an adequate EPSP may depend on the recovery of ion channels, remyelination, increased strength of output from undamaged cortical and brainstem neurons that also descend onto spinal neurons to the same muscle, and other inputs to the spinal neuron that increase the threshold for excitation. These cumulative changes alter the cell properties of spinal motoneurons in complex and unpredictable ways, however.[136] This complexity makes future manipulation for rehabilitative purposes difficult, but possible.

Studies by Functional Imaging. Studies of human rCBF and metabolism also reveal anatomic and functional reorganization after injury. The capacity for functional reorganization has been especially apparent in infants and children after hemispherectomy for epilepsy and after stroke.[29] Ipsilateral cortical efferent pathways can come to subserve hand activity, for example.[179] This action correlates with the maturational changes of human sensorimotor cortex through age 15 years, before the natural, perhaps activity-dependent regression of neurons and synapses in the developing brain.[28]

Hemiparetic adults who were able to squeeze a ball repeatedly about 4 weeks after a cortical stroke were found, compared with normal subjects, to activate their bilateral inferior parietal regions (areas 3, 1, and 2) during a xenon 133 study of rCBF.[15] The investigators speculated that these areas would participate in motor recovery because up to 40 percent of corticospinal fibers arise from there and a small proportion do not decussate.

Regional CBF studies by PET in a group of patients who recovered from a motor stroke showed considerable functional adaptation. At least 3 months after a striatocapsular infarction, patients were tested under the conditions of rest, repeated thumb-to-finger opposition of the recovered right hand, and the same movement for the left hand.[209] During the motor task with either hand, the contralateral motor cortices and ipsilateral cerebellum were activated to the same degree as in unaffected persons. For the patients with recovered hand function, however, rCBF was greater than in normal subjects in the bilateral ventral premotor (area 6), SMA, anterior insula, and parietal (area 40) cortices, as well as in the ipsilateral premotor cortex and basal ganglia and in the contralateral cerebellum. These nonprimary cortical motor areas seem to have served a compensatory function. The bilateral recruitment may also explain the associated or mirror movements in the left hand that often accompanied a right-handed task.

Indeed, in a related study of patients with lesions within the striatocapsular complex, the ipsilateral primary sensorimotor cortex was significantly activated only in subjects who exhibited associated movements of the unaffected hand during the finger opposition task by the recovered hand.[210] Moreover, activation sites differed in relation to the precise localization of the subcortical lesion. For example, one subgroup of patients with lesions limited to the posterior limb of the internal capsule showed a 1-cm extension of activation within the contralateral primary sensorimotor cortex. This change corresponded to a spread from the hand area into the cortex for the face. This metabolically visualized enlargement of the contiguous cortical sensorimotor field is consistent with the multiple representations of muscles and movements within the motor cortex and with the mutability of neuronal representational maps. Lesions confined to the anterior limb did not show this pattern, perhaps because the disrupted frontopontine or corticostriatal fibers that initially caused the hand paresis recovered or were compensated for by a parallel motor pathway.

These PET studies of recovery offer other insights. Opposition of the fingers of the normal left hand activated the right insula, the anterior cingulate, the striatum, and the lateral prefrontal, premotor, and inferior parietal (area 40) cortices more than normally. This activation may reflect the need for a greater effort by these patients. Mild impairment of movements of the ipsilateral upper extremity has been reported in patients with cerebral infarcts and is perhaps related to bilateral changes in pathway function induced by a unilateral lesion.[16,33,107] The experiments also showed that the lateral prefrontal and cingulate cortices and the angular gyrus were activated by a simple task after the stroke, a finding that suggests that these interconnected areas related to selective attention and intention must come into play when an automatic movement reorganizes. Thus, this study with PET revealed at least three mechanisms for recovery: (1) sparing of pathways in the case of anterior limb capsular lesions, (2) representational expansion, and (3) activation of distributed pathways that would not ordinarily have been as metabolically active.

Metabolic imaging studies are yielding many instances of compensatory shifts in neuronal systems, especially in primary sensory and association cortex. These shifts are most evident as the paretic patient carries out and monitors difficult motor activities.[11] Activation patterns may also have predictive meaning. For example, a poor performance in discriminating the size of an object with the recovering hand after a striatocapsular infarct correlated with low rCBF in the contralateral sensorimotor cortex at rest and bilateral activation during the task.[208]

As metabolic maps of cognitive and sensorimotor functions are defined for tasks carried out by unaffected persons and by those who have suffered a focal injury, specialists in rehabilitation will better understand the pathways that subserve recovery and the effects of physical and pharmaco-

logic interventions on plasticity. Some of the potential uses of functional imaging in rehabilitation are listed in Table 1–3. PET, fMRI, and other neuroimaging techniques can become the tools of rehabilitation specialists for the study of these and other hypotheses about training and recovery. Carefully designed experiments and clinical trials that incorporate these tools may provide insights for a scientific approach to neurorehabilitation.

Representational Plasticity in Neurorestoration. Work in sensorimotor cortical neuronal plasticity suggests designs for rehabilitative strategies. Cortical representational changes follow paradigms of learning and the acquisition of specific skills. The greater the number of sources of inputs that can be correlated by their timing and the greater the convergence of their distribution within the cortex, the more likely their representations are to show plasticity. This adaptivity is time based rather than strictly anatomically based in the sense that, for example, adjacent skin surfaces are represented in adjacent cortical regions especially because of the high probability that they are excited coincidentally.[138] Parts that work together enlarge their representations. Indeed, one may reasonably conclude that coupled assemblies of cortical neurons continually compete to dominate the neurons along their borders. The demand placed on a sensorimotor network expands its territory. Better function for the task at hand tends to accompany this more cohesive synaptic activity.

The improved hand functions and map changes in the primate studies of Merzenich and colleagues (see Experimental Case Study 1–1) depend on use of the limb during a learning paradigm. More and different neighboring neurons then adapt to the task. After an injury, neuronal groups have the potential to learn discrimination if at least some nearby cells that were involved in representing the function regain their signal-processing abilities. This phenomenon is an example of what some investigators have called *vicariation;* neurons not usually involved in a lost behavior take over part of it.

Can rehabilitation specialists incorporate the modulation of cortical assemblies into treatment strategies? Studies of dynamic neuronal cell assemblies suggest that specific training paradigms and drugs that increase

Table 1–3. POTENTIAL USES OF FUNCTIONAL NEUROIMAGING IN RECOVERY OF FUNCTION

- Characterize the natural history of resting metabolic activity and degree of recovery.
- Relate metabolic patterns, at rest or by an activation study for a specific task, to readiness for rehabilitation. Determine whether functional prerequisites within a neural network must be fulfilled before effective adaptive change can occur and before rehabilitative therapy can affect outcomes.
- Characterize predictors of recovery from resting and from activation studies for specific movements and cognitive functions. Determine the presence of spared tissue.
- Characterize neural mechanisms of recovery of specific functions. Determine whether normal task-dependent functional imaging networks change after an injury and reorganize with recovery.
- Understand how a lesion in one region alters transneuronal activity and the patient's behavior.
- Compare the response of a patient with brain injury to normal responses in an activation paradigm during a task. This could help therapists to develop new interventional strategies that circumvent defunct processes.
- Map the initial response to a particular training intervention for a new patient. Compare with studies correlating early patterns of activation with long-term functional gains. Use the patient's response to predict whether that intervention is likely to be of benefit. If the training technique does not elicit the predicted activations, then perhaps it may be modified to do so. This strategy may reduce the number of subjects needed to study the efficacy of a new intervention.
- Determine whether an intervention engages areas that usually need activation for success in carrying out a task. Develop treatments based on knowledge of areas in which the desired behavior is represented.
- Correlate activation patterns with variations in the type, duration, and intensity of physical and cognitive therapies.
- Study the effects of medications on levels of activation and changes in patterns of engaged regions.
- Assess strategies for hemi-inattention and aphasia that engage or suppress the activity of the uninjured hemisphere.
- Monitor the effects of implants that replace neurons and glia, produce neurotransmitters, and provide trophic factors or other substances that protect cells from degeneration or that enhance axonal and dendritic growth.

local synaptic activity may optimize remodeling and, in turn, improve sensorimotor and higher cognitive activities. If the movement or sensory stimulation is part of an act that is important to the subject, such as supinating the arm to feed oneself, then the relearned action is more likely to lead to widespread neuronal activation, to enlarge its representation, and to play a role in restitution of function. Goal-oriented training also appears to be a means to induce the activation of the distributed pathways that may participate in partial recovery of function.

The experiments suggest that training for a behavioral compensatory technique that promotes nonuse of an arm may inhibit recovery. Improved function has followed the forced use and functional training of the experimentally deafferented arm of monkeys and the paretic arm of patients after stroke.[197] In experiments with adult cats that have undergone hemispherectomy, it took about eight 2-hour training sessions with restraint of the normal limb and food deprivation before the animals successfully learned to use their paretic forepaws to retrieve food from a narrow feeding device. This "intensive remedial therapy" strategy produced a stereotyped pattern of motor activities that differed from an intact cat's motor strategy for food retrieval.[201] If such plasticity exists after human nervous system injuries, the challenge is to define the optimal sensorimotor stimulation and learning paradigm to enhance the recovery of a specific activity. Rehabilitative strategies for sensory re-education that apply the concept of behaviorally relevant, repetitive sensory inputs to promote the emergence of larger-than-normal receptive fields have been proposed to lessen impairments after a cerebral[39] or peripheral nerve injury.[127] Single-case studies in patients with stroke show task-specific improvements in the appreciation of textures and wrist proprioception with one such strategy.[25]

Functional imaging may show which cortical areas must be activated to accomplish a motor task in patients with particular impairments and structural lesions. Based on prior imaging and outcome trials, PET and fMRI activation studies performed during the early stages of retraining for a task can be used to show whether synaptic activity is as high as expected in relevant cortical areas. If a training strategy does not elicit the predicted activations, then it can be modified to do so.

Subcortical Systems

STRIATUM

Distributed, parallel loops characterize the subcortical volitional movement circuits that involve the basal ganglia and the cerebellum. Basal ganglia outputs project mostly to the motor and prefrontal areas and to brainstem motor sites. Many anatomic and physiologic studies have shown the basic parallel and segregated arrangement, rather than a convergent integration, of the motor pathways in the cortico-striato-nigro-thalamo-cortical circuits. Whereas dysfunction in the striatum causes Parkinson's and Huntington's diseases, these circuits are also of interest to rehabilitation specialists because of their importance during sensorimotor learning and the possibility that uninjured cortical circuits may reorganize to help substitute for injured circuits.

The frontal lobe–basal ganglia–thalamocortical circuits include a motor circuit from the precentral motor fields, the oculomotor circuit from the frontal and supplementary eye fields, the prefrontal circuit from the dorsolateral prefrontal and lateral orbitofrontal cortex, and the limbic circuit from the anterior cingulate and medial orbitofrontal cortex.[3] Within the skeletomotor pallidothalamocortical system, localized regions of the globus pallidus are organized into discrete channels. At least in the primate arm, these channels project to particular positions in M_1, SMA, and the ventral premotor area through the ventrolateral thalamus.[95] These channels presumably process different variables for movement. The path to M_1 seems to affect parameters such as the direction and force of movement, whereas paths to premotor areas tend to higher-order programming tasks, such as the internal guidance and sequence of a movement.

The input and output architecture of the sensorimotor striatum has a modular design that remaps cortical inputs onto distributed local modules of striatal projection neurons.[84] One type of striatal interneuron, a *tonically active neuron*, appears to bind these modular networks temporally during behavioral learning. Dopamine and possibly cholinergic influences mediate the response properties of these neurons. This organization allows the basal ganglia to participate in concurrent skeletomotor, oculomotor, cognitive, and limbic drive activities. Together, the circuits internally generate a movement, automatically execute a motor plan, and acquire and retain a motor skill. Instead of synchrony of all networks, they are coordinated within the striatum by distributed sets of the tonically active neurons that are sensitive to *motivation-related signals*.[84] These frontal-subcortical circuits also participate in a range of human behaviors. In considering rehabilitation strategies, task-oriented therapies that carry significance to the patient and are rewarding are most likely to activate these circuits. Pharmacologic agents that affect the neurotransmitters of the striatum, including dopamine, glutamate, and γ-aminobutyric acid (GABA), could alter the net excitatory and inhibitory activities of these systems after a central injury.

OTHER PARALLEL CIRCUITS

Parallel arrangements hold as well for the cerebellar projections that connect to separate target zones of the ventrolateral thalamus. Indeed, anatomic studies reveal almost no convergence of lemniscal, cerebellar, pallidal, or substantia nigral afferents in the thalamus. Separate channels are maintained within the somatic sensory and motor thalamus for cutaneous sensation, for deep, slowly adapting and rapidly adapting inputs, for each of the cerebellar nuclei, and for the vestibular and spinothalamic systems.[106] Each thalamocortical projection is independent. Thus, individual channels can control separate functional units of motor cortex, and, in turn, each is independent in its control of subcortical motor nuclei. Although these systems are not likely to be highly redundant, they may provide a partially reiterative capacity for sparing or substitution after a sensorimotor network injury.

FUNCTIONAL IMAGING OF CIRCUITS

Some of the functional relationships of these circuits have been visualized by autoradiography in studies of lesions in animal models (Experimental Case Study 1–4). The recovery of metabolic activity has been associated with behavioral recovery. In patients studied at least 3 months after a left-sided striatocapsular infarction who had recovered contralateral hand function, resting rCBF was significantly lower in the left basal ganglia; the thalamus; the primary sensorimotor, insular, and dorsolateral prefrontal cortices; the left cerebral peduncle; and the ipsilateral right cerebellum, compared with unaffected subjects.[209] This pattern cor-

responds to the parallel circuits among the basal ganglia, the thalamus, and the cortical projections (Fig. 1–5). The remote effects of the striatocapsular lesion were postulated to be related either to a transsynaptic functional deactivation or to structural changes from transsynaptic or retrograde degeneration. Moreover, rCBF was increased in the left posterior cingulate and premotor cortices and ipsilateral caudate nucleus. The investigators speculated that a loss of the functional inhibition of these areas by homotopic regions of the opposite hemisphere had developed.

Brainstem Pathways

In the patient with hemiplegia, the uncrossed pyramidal pathways and the bilateral extrapyramidal pathways probably participate in the recovery of enough use of truncal and antigravity muscles on the paralyzed side to aid walking and proximal arm func-

---

EXPERIMENTAL CASE STUDY 1–4
Network Associated with Motor Changes

Functional imaging in animals with induced lesions has provided insight into the distributed networks associated with changes in motor function. Autoradiography was performed on the macaque monkey after unilateral ablation of cortical areas 4 and 6 on the left. Partial recovery of the local cerebral metabolic rate for ^{14}C-2-deoxyglucose in certain subcortical structures accompanied partial motor recovery.[185] At 1 week, when the animal was hemiplegic, hypometabolism was found in the ipsilateral thalamus and the basal ganglia, structures that receive direct and indirect input from the motor cortex. Activity was also diminished in the contralateral cerebellar cortex and, less so, in the thalamus and the bilateral brainstem and deep cerebellar nuclei. This finding was consistent with the unilateral and bilateral projections of the ablated cortex and with a decrease in transsynaptic activity. This deafferentation remote from the lesion is a functional depression called *diaschisis*. At 8 weeks, before maximal recovery, the animals used the affected hindlimb for ambulation and made incomplete extension movements for reaching with the right forelimb. The investigators found partial recovery of metabolic activity in some of the ipsilateral thalamic nuclei, complete recovery in the contralateral thalamus, and up to moderate restoration in the other regions. The vestibular nuclei increased their activity at 1 and 8 weeks, perhaps as a compensatory mechanism that increased extensor postural reflexes. The investigators suggest that connections from other cortical areas that project to the caudate nucleus and putamen may have accounted for the increase in glucose utilization and improved function. Other mechanisms that may have contributed to these effects include enhanced activity of interneurons within the affected striatal neuronal groups, increased activity from subcortical projections, and sprouting of fibers from undamaged axons within the caudate nucleus and putamen or from projections from other sites.[75]

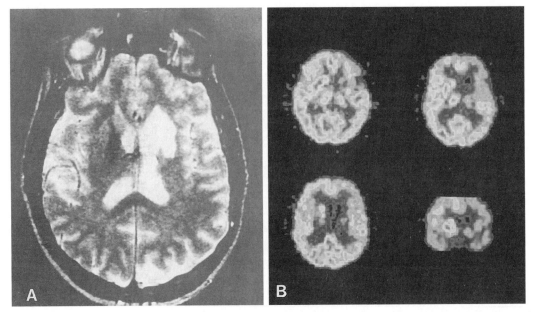

Figure 1–5. (*A*) A T$_2$-weighted-magnetic resonance imaging (MRI) scan shows an infarction of the left caudate and anterior limb of the internal capsule in a patient who suffered an occlusion of the recurrent artery of Heubner. (*B*) A positron emission tomography (PET) scan shows the regional metabolic activity for 2-deoxyglucose. The brighter areas are at higher levels of activity. The top two axial cuts show hypometabolism within the left striatum, thalamus, and dorsolateral frontal lobe. The bottom right coronal cut also shows the marked asymmetry, with hypometabolism of the left subcortical gray matter and frontal cortex.

tion.[71] As noted earlier, the ipsilateral motor cortex, by way of the uncrossed ventral corticospinal tract, has often been invoked as a pathway that may compensate for a contralateral cerebral injury.

The vestibulospinal and reticulospinal tracts, which connect to bilateral spinal motoneurons associated mostly with axial and girdle muscles, may also contribute to this recovery. These two brainstem pathways receive corticofugal inputs that are both crossed and uncrossed within the pontine and medullary reticular formations. Rudimentary synergistic movements such as opening and closing the hand persist after pyramidectomy, probably through the activity of the descending rubrospinal, vestibulospinal, and reticulospinal systems.[180] The rubrospinal tract provides a potential path for independent, flexion-biased movements, especially for the elbow and hand.[115] The more individuated a movement, the greater the amount of corticomotoneuronal activity needed to superimpose control on subcortical centers and directly on spinal motoneu-

rons to multiple muscles. Substitution of one pathway for another may allow some compensatory motor recovery. In the cat, for example, selective destruction of the corticospinal and rubrospinal tracts initially abolishes the animal's ability to grab food and bring it to its mouth.[6] Three weeks later, food-taking behavior with the affected forepaw has recovered by activation of the interneuronal and propriospinal pools of the forelimb by the descending bulbospinal pathway.

LOCOMOTOR REGIONS

One of the most common goals of rehabilitation is to recover the ability to walk. Anatomic and physiologic studies reveal some of the hierarchic controls and distributed pathways that seem to play important roles after an injury to cortical and subcortical senosorimotor structures.

Functional imaging provides an overview of the most metabolically active cortical and subcortical regions during normal casual locomotion at approximately 2 mph on a treadmill. Subtraction images that compared supine rest and treadmill walking after injection with a glucose tracer (fluorodeoxyglucose [FDG]) showed increased activity in the cerebellar vermis and the bilateral occipital and paramedian motor cortices.[100a] Increases in activation were also observed in Brodmann's areas 4, 18, 22, 40, and 43 and within the superior vermis. This activity presumably reflects the integration of visual, auditory, and somatosensory information with motor activity in the leg region for motor control during rather rhythmic stepping. The UCLA PET imaging group has done FDG studies (unpublished) and others have used SPECT[84a] to compare treadmill walking with standing. Bilateral primary sensorimotor and SMA cortices were especially active during walking, as fits with their motor functions. The cingulate and prefrontal cortices were active, perhaps especially in relation to the rhythmic movement and attention needed for treadmill locomotion, along with the occipital, inferior parietal, and superior temporal cortices needed for multimodality sensory integration. In addition, the amygdala; caudate nuclei; ventral striatum; dorsolateral thalami; dorsal midbrain; and cerebellum, particularly the vermis, were significantly more active with walking. In a study in which normal subjects imagined performing locomotive leg movements while supine during a PET with [15]Oxygen-labeled water, significant increases in activation were found compared with rest in the sensorimotor cortex, SMA, cingulate gyrus, and cerebellar vermis, similar to activations during flexing and extending the feet while supine.[94b] Rehabilitation specialists will be able to apply PET, fMRI, and other functional imaging techniques that lend themselves to either supine or upright activation studies to detect and promote the reorganization of cortical networks for walking after a cerebral injury and to better understand the contributions of subcortical locomotor regions.

Locomotion often improves despite damage to the corticofugal pathways. The brainstem, particularly the reticular formation, is one of the most important structures for automatic and volitional control of features of posture and movement. Interacting with the cortex, deep cerebellar nuclei, substantia nigra, and globus pallidus, the brainstem has a convergent region for locomotion (Fig. 1–6). The descending message for the initiation of locomotion seems to be carried by reticulospinal pathways from specific areas of the midbrain and pons that synapse with lumbar spinal neurons.[109] Indeed, ventral root potentials are induced by reticular formation stimulation. Many animal studies have provided a map for the location of this activity. Chemical and electrical stimulation of the mesencephalic locomotor region (MLR) of the decerebrate cat and other species, especially in and around the pedunculopontine nucleus, causes the animal to step when placed on a treadmill. The step rate can be modulated by the intensity of stimulation.[69] Neurons in the cuneiform nucleus, ventrolateral central gray matter, and locus coeruleus are functional parts of this locomotor pathway. Reticulospinal cells in the medial pontomedullary reticular formation (MPRF) receive this bilateral information along with hypothalamic and other converging inputs and send it to motoneurons through the ventrolateral funiculus in the spinal cord. This input modulates spinal pattern generators for stepping in many animal models and, presumably, in humans. A hemisection of the low thoracic spinal cord is followed by considerable recovery of locomotion in monkeys and cats, a recovery mediated at least in part by descending reticulospinal fibers on the intact side that cross at a segmental level below the transection.[57]

Cholinergic agonists, excitatory amino acids, and substance P elicit or facilitate locomotion when they are injected into the MPRF. Cholinergic antagonists and GABA abolish MLR-evoked locomotion. Dopamine and amphetamine also initiate locomotion by modulating amygdala and hippocampal inputs to the nucleus accumbens, which projects to the MLR through the ventral pallidal area.[147] The clinical use of systemic drugs that increase or block the neurotransmitters of this network may enhance or inhibit the automatic patterns of stepping.

These locomotor regions can become impaired by a variety of neurologic diseases. Patients with Parkinson's disease and progressive supranuclear palsy lose neurons in the pedunculopontine nucleus. Their gait devi-

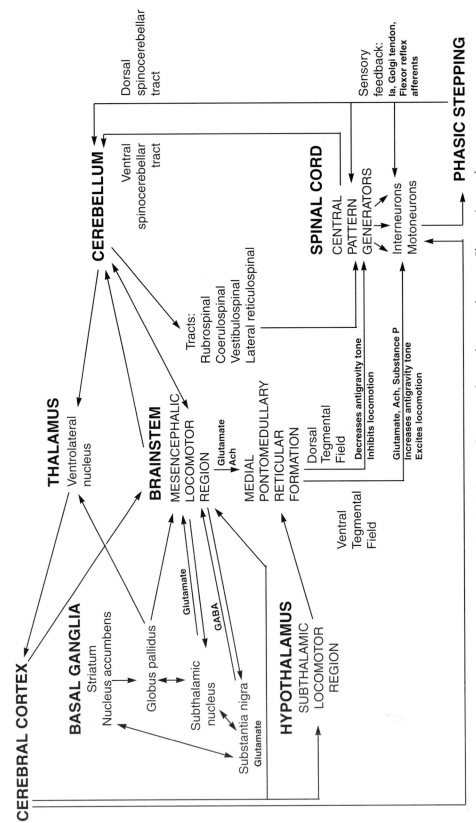

Figure 1–6. Cortical, subcortical, and spinal neuronal groups and tracts that control aspects of locomotion are shown in their relationship to central pattern generators for stepping.

ations include difficulty in the initiation and rhythmicity of walking. In a case report, a patient who suffered a small hemorrhagic stroke in this dorsal region on the right side abruptly lost the ability to stand and to generate anything but irregular, shuffling steps while supported, despite the absence of paresis and ataxia.[130]

Of course, locomotor activity also requires constant processing of information from the environment. Brainstem circuits help to mediate this information. For example, cells of the superior colliculus that project to the motor and premotor cortex manage the task of coordinating the sensory cues for orientation behaviors during ambulation and other activities. Physiologic studies of the superior colliculus reveal a sensory convergence system in which motor responses are not irrevocably linked to a particular stimulus but vary with visual, auditory, somatosensory, and other stimuli.[137] The output message from what are mostly multimodal cells is a synthesis of the spatial and temporal characteristics of the stimuli. This synthesis allows a remarkably simple neural mechanism for a flexible range of motor responses in a changing environment. In clinical practice, visual input can help to compensate for proprioceptive impairments during gait retraining, but it may impede stepping and postural adjustments when associated with perceptual deficits. Visual, auditory, vestibular, and cognitive cues can be given to help to initiate and continue stepping in the patient with hypokinetic manifestations of Parkinson's disease.

Spinal Motor Activity

CENTRAL PATTERN GENERATORS

The spinal cord, like the brainstem, has intrinsic systems for locomotion. Although cortical and peripheral sensory input is essential for normal locomotion under disparate environmental conditions, the initiation and timing of synergist and antagonist muscle activity for stepping appear to be primarily the task of a self-oscillating lumbar interneuronal network. Even an isolated section of lumbar spinal cord can produce cyclic outputs that rhythmically flex and extend a joint.[85,97] This primitive locomotor circuit is called a "central pattern generator (CPG)" (see Fig. 1–6).

Elementary burst-generating networks probably control different muscles around a joint. For example, when one group of interacting neurons fires, a withdrawal reflex may result. A different pattern that allows stepping emerges when another partially overlapping combination of neurons becomes activated. Many neural circuits that produce rhythmically recurring motor patterns have been described.[86,188,211] The recurrent burst patterns arise by combining into a network such common cellular mechanisms as reciprocal inhibition, mutual excitation, spike frequency adaptation, and pacemaker-like or plateau properties.[86] Amine and peptide neuromodulators modify the properties of these neuronal circuits. These neuromodulators can tonically facilitate or depress ongoing motor acts, can initiate and prime the circuits to respond more effectively to inputs, and can alter the cellular and synaptic properties of neurons within a network, allowing the same CPG or group of CPGs to generate different motor patterns for different behaviors.[159]

Computer simulations of locomotion that model neural oscillators for each leg joint, along with inputs from proprioceptors and the senses and rhythmic movements of the musculoskeletal system, show the relative simplicity of a locomotor system designed around centrally generated patterns.[195] This organization allows flexibility and stability in an unpredictable environment and permits a change in a single parameter, such as a cortical or brainstem signal, to make a change from walking to running.

DESCENDING INPUTS

The vertebrate brainstem and spinal cord contain the neural circuitry needed to generate the flexor and extensor motor output necessary for locomotion in the absence of other descending and afferent sensory information. The CPGs must alter their output in response to even simple changes in conditions, however, such as variations in the characteristics of the surface walked. For effective stepping, as for upper limb movements, the motor output has to be timed precisely to changing positions, forces, and movements of the limbs. Descending and afferent sensory input timed to the gait cycle can transform a group of oscillatory networks into coordinated activity. The lumbar stepping motoneurons are especially influenced by descending serotonergic and noradrenergic brainstem pathways. These pathways may set the gain for sensory and motor output and may modulate the oscillatory behavior of spinal neurons and specific aspects of the locomotor pattern.[190] In electrophysiologic studies of the cat, cortical motoneurons discharged modestly during locomotion over a flat surface under constant sensory conditions. They increased their discharges when a task required more accurate foot placement for walking along a horizontally positioned ladder, compared with overground or treadmill locomotion. Changing the trajectory of the limbs to step over obstacles also increased cortical output.[51] These studies suggest that the flexor input of the

corticospinal tract and its widespread branching within the spinal cord can facilitate the collection of potentially interacting unit pattern generators, each regulating the muscle activity around a single joint. In addition, afferent inputs appear to make a large contribution to stepping. This finding has a potential impact on techniques of gait retraining.

SEGMENTAL AFFERENT INFLUENCES

The lumbar spinal cord of the adult cat, in the absence of supraspinal input, but with peripheral sensory input, retains the ability to generate hindlimb stepping (Experimental Case Study 1–5). In this model, static physical therapies can impede recovery, whereas rhythmic alternating movements of the limbs during treadmill training with joint loading seem critical to the recovery of locomotor output.[94] Thus, sensory input to

---

EXPERIMENTAL CASE STUDY 1–5
Spinal Locomotor Circuit Plasticity

The cat's deafferented spinal cord below a low thoracic transection can generate alternating flexor and extensor muscle activity a few hours after surgery when dihydroxyphenylalanine (DOPA) or clonidine is administered intravenously or when the dorsal columns or dorsal roots are continuously stimulated. This phenomenon is called *fictive locomotion*. Several weeks after a complete lower thoracic spinal cord transection without deafferentation, adult cats and other mammals were trained on a treadmill so that their paralyzed hindlimbs fully supported their weight, rhythmically stepped, and adjusted their walking speed to that of the treadmill belt in a manner similar to normal locomotion.[125,177] Postural support alone was detrimental to subsequent locomotion, whereas rhythmic alternating movements of the limbs with joint loading seemed critical to the recovery of locomotor output.[54] Serotonergic and noradrenergic drugs enhanced the stepping pattern, and strychnine, through a glycinergic path, quickly induced it.[55] The step phase transitions from stance to swing are triggered by afferent feedback related to extension at the hip and the unloading of leg extensor muscles.[159] One possible basis for these critical-phase transitions is that group Ib Golgi tendon input during early stance inhibits the generation of flexor activity. As this input wanes near the end of stance, it releases the flexor burst-generating system and permits the initiation of the swing phase.

Fictive locomotion has been demonstrated in marmoset monkeys.[97] Methods that elicited spinal stepping in cats, dogs, and rabbits, including supported treadmill training, skin stimulation, DOPA, 4-aminopyridine, and clonidine, however, did not result in stepping in macaque monkeys tested immediately and 4 months after thoracic spinal cord transection.[58] When some reticulospinal and vestibulospinal descending pathways were spared in these experiments, locomotion did recover to varying degrees.[200]

the spinal cord has a critical role in modulating motor output for locomotion. Studies of pattern generation and step training in animals after spinal cord transection have led to a search in patients with a spinal cord injury (SCI) for pharmacologic and physical therapy tools to trigger and modulate the expression of rhythmic locomotor patterns. Although some uncertainty remains about whether humans have CPGs for locomotion, studies of spontaneous cyclic leg movements and of the effects of sensory inputs related to stepping in patients with SCI suggest that such CPGs may exist.

In a remarkably detailed clinical study of patients with operative verification of complete versus incomplete transection after traumatic SCI, Riddoch could not elicit rhythmic flexion-extension movements below the complete thoracic lesions. He found almost exclusively a flexor response to cutaneous stimulation.[174] Reflexive extension followed by flexion was found in patients with partial preservation of anatomic continuity. Some subjects with operative verification of complete transection after traumatic SCI, however, have reported spontaneous slow, irregular alternating steppinglike or bicycling-like movements when supine that lasted up to 10 minutes.[119] Involuntary lower extremity steppinglike movements were recorded from a patient with an incomplete cervical SCI of long standing.[22] These movements were evoked when the patient was supine with the hips and knees in extension and when suspended over a treadmill belt. Noxious afferent input from one hip appeared to initiate the rhythmic locomotor activity. I have recorded similar spontaneous locomotor-like movements and electromyographic (EMG) activity in a patient with an incomplete thoracic SCI.[50a] The movements also developed by placing the hip in extension. This source of afferent input is consistent with the sensory stimulation that enables some cats that have undergone spinal transection to learn to perform hindlimb stepping on a treadmill.

Other evidence for a CPG in humans comes from the finding of rhythmic myoclonic activity generated by a patient's transected spinal cord that was sensitive to peripheral stimulation of flexor reflex afferents.[21] The electrical stimuli could induce, slow, or interrupt the subject's symmetric 0.3 to 0.6-Hz rhythmic activity in extensor muscles. In addition, a long-latency flexion reflex that seems to be related to the interneuronal network responsible for spinal stepping has been found in 13 patients with a clinically diagnosed complete SCI.[175]

Using a protocol similar to that which elicited stepping in the cats that underwent thoracic spinal transection, several groups of investigators have studied patients with paraplegia who had minimal sensorimotor function in the legs but who clearly had some residual supraspinal influence. EMG activity similar to that seen during normal stepping was found when these patients' feet were placed in contact with a moving treadmill over which they were suspended as the investigators moved the legs to simulate locomotion.[49,202,212] With this body weight–supported treadmill training (BWSTT), some patients achieved independent treadmill walking and became able to step overground. During training, the level of loading during stance and the angular velocity and degree of extension at the hip altered the EMG output.[50a,73] Serotonergic and noradrenergic drugs were shown to influence this motor output, mostly by altering some signs of spasticity.[68]

Patients with complete thoracic SCIs often show rhythmic flexor and extensor EMG activity in their leg muscles during assisted stepping with BWSTT (see Fig. 7–4).[48,50a] One report suggested that some patients with complete SCI can be trained to step independently during BWSTT.[47] Greater sensory input, such as increased loading of the joints, the degree of hip extension, and cutaneous electrical stimulation timed to the gait cycle, can enhance EMG output and can evoke hip flexion.[50,173] These reports suggest that spinal neuronal circuits can be trained to produce stereotyped stepping outputs in the absence of voluntary movement at single joints. Extensor and flexor afferent inputs appear to be critical to training when central connections are severely reduced or absent.

Most physical therapies emphasize standing and static balance early after the onset of hemiplegia and paraparesis before the patient is trained in walking. Subsequent chapters look at techniques such as BWSTT and task-oriented training in relation to mechanisms of recovery of stepping.

SPINAL REFLEX ACTIVITY

Many theories of physical therapy focus on the use of brainstem and spinal reflexes as a way to retrain voluntary movement and to affect hypotonicity and hypertonicity (see Chapter 3). Tonic and phasic stimuli are used to modify the excitability of spinal motor pools, postural reflexes, and co-contractions. Physical therapists may try to activate or suppress a stretch reflex, the asymmetric and symmetric tonic neck reflexes, the tonic labyrinthine reflex, and the withdrawal and extensor reflexes. They use stimuli that include muscle or tendon vibration, joint compression, skin stroking, and other sensory inputs that elicit reflexive movement and positive and negative supporting reactions.

These reflexes seem like static control devices for individual muscles and joints. A moving, multisegmented limb has more dynamic mechanical properties that require more complex circuits for motor control; however, considerable potential for plasticity exists within the determinants of muscle tone and stretch reflexes. The response to muscle stretch during passive movement, postural adjustment, and voluntary movement is not inflexible. The dynamic properties of reflexes were demonstrated during locomotion in cats after thoracic spinal cord transection.[63] During the swing phase of stepping, an electrical stimulus over the dorsum of a paw elicited a flexion response and extension in the other hindlimb, but during stance, it caused further extension of the stimulated limb.

Moment-to-moment adjustments in reflexes have been partly accounted for by a variety of mechanisms.[41,136] Most of these mechanisms also play a role in the development of spasticity. They include the following:

1. The mechanical, viscoelastic properties of muscle that vary in part with changes in actinomycin crossbridges and alterations in connective tissues.
2. Peripheral sensory receptors that respond to a perturbation from primary and secondary muscle spindles and Golgi tendon organs but are regulated over a wide range of responsiveness by central commands.
3. The convergence of segmental and descending inputs on Renshaw cells and other motor and interneurons that can summate in many ways, so that excitation of one peripheral receptor does not always produce the same stereotyped reflex response.
4. Joint and cutaneous flexor reflex afferents that are activated during limb movements and vary in the degree to which they set the excitability of interneurons.
5. Presynaptic inhibition of afferent proprioceptive inputs to the spinal cord that are constantly affected by the types of afferents stimulated, as well as by descending influences.
6. Long-latency responses to muscle contraction that supplement the short-latency, segmental monosynaptic component of the stretch reflex to compensate especially for a large change in mechanical load.
7. The variety of sources of synaptic contracts on alpha motoneurons, along with the intrinsic membrane properties that affect their excitability and their pattern of recruitment of muscle fibers.

Wolpaw and Carp demonstrated activity-driven plasticity within the spinal stretch reflex in experiments in which the H-reflex was operantly conditioned in monkeys to increase or decrease in amplitude.[218] An 8 percent change began within 6 hours of conditioning and then gradually changed by 1 to 2 percent per day. This change required at least 3000 trials daily. The alteration persisted for several days after spinal transection, a finding suggesting that the circuitry involved had learned and had held a memory trace. A long-term change in presynaptic inhibition mediated by the Ia terminal presumably mediated this learning. With EMG biofeedback, the stretch reflex in the human biceps has been successfully conditioned to increase or decrease, using about 400 trials per session.[60] Task-specific modulation of the gain of reflexes is found in persons whose strength of the stretch reflex in leg extensors is high during standing, low during walking, and lower during running.[191] A higher gain with standing presumably provides greater postural stability. The gain also changes with the phase of the step cycle.

Thus, coupled spinal input and output activity can be trained, although it takes considerable practice within a highly specific paradigm. This adaptive plasticity could be of value in developing therapies for spasticity and abnormal spinal reflex activity and to modulate movements such as stepping.[217] Whether the facilitation, inhibition, and disinhibition techniques used by therapists optimize the use of this neurophysiologic plasticity is not clear.

Neurotransmitter Effects

Animal studies and one small clinical trial have provided preliminary evidence that a variety of pharmacologic agents may facilitate or inhibit the rate or degree of recovery of sensorimotor function and walking after a cerebral injury (Experimental Case Study 1–6). Although studies of neurotransmitter manipulations in animal lesion models are intriguing, the results are not readily applicable to clinical trials in patients undergoing rehabilitation.

Amphetamine improved motor function

EXPERIMENTAL CASE STUDY 1–6
Modulation of Neurotransmitters

After d-amphetamine administration, both rats and cats that underwent a unilateral or bilateral ablation of the sensorimotor or frontal cortex exhibited an accelerated rate of recovery of the ability to walk across a beam. This recovery endured well past the single or intermittent dosing schedule of the drug.[194] In a rat primary somatosensory cortex infarction model, d-amphetamine augmented the rate and completeness of recovery in a T-maze sensorimotor integrative task.[99] In these instances, the drug worked only when combined with physical activity and practice, the equivalent of training and motor experience. A dopamine blocker, haloperidol, prevented this recovery in the animal studies. Yohimbine, an alpha-2–noradrenergic antagonist, accelerated recovery. Both the alpha-1–noradrenergic antagonist prazosin and the alpha-2–noradrenergic agonist clonidine reinstated deficits in recovered rats.[193] Clonidine inhibits locus coeruleus neuronal activity, reducing norepinephrine synthesis and release. It did not delay early recovery, as had been expected. The drug has at least one other potential effect, however; it can activate the lumbar neural circuitry for stepping. In this model, then, norepinephrine played a role in both promotion and maintenance of recovery, although not always in a predictable fashion. The investigators suspected that the noradrenergic drug alleviated a functional depression, or diaschisis, in remote, transsynaptically connected regions of the brain.

Other neurotransmitters, including acetylcholine, dopamine, GABA, and serotonin have enhanced motor recovery. Phenytoin, scopolamine, clonidine, neuroleptic agents, and benzodiazepines have retarded gains in specific experimental designs in animals. In the rat sensorimotor cortex lesion model described in Experimental Study 2–1, treatment with a benzodiazepine led to ipsilateral loss of neurons in the corpus striatum and substantia nigra and interfered with behavioral recovery of the affected limb.[108] As noted earlier, acetylcholine may play a key role in modulating the reorganization of the somatosensory representational map, and serotonergic and noradrenergic agents enhance the lumbar neural circuits for stepping. Some drugs may enhance one function but reinstate or cause another type of motor or cognitive dysfunction.[8]

Other experiments reveal how surviving connections can inhibit recovery after a brain injury. By abolishing the inhibiting influence, function can improve.[100] One classic example is the Sprague experiment. The temporo-occipital visual cortex of the cat was destroyed unilaterally. The induced hemianopia decreased when either the contralateral superior colliculus was destroyed or the bridge between the two colliculi was split.[189] This finding suggests that depression of the ipsilateral colliculus by inhibition from its homologous structure was partly responsible for the visual field loss. Although surgical "corrections" are unlikely to have clinical applications, pharmacologic attempts at disinhibition may have such applications.

in a small group of selected patients shortly after their stroke, although these results have not yet been duplicated.[35] The drug worked only when combined with physical activity and practice, the equivalent of training and motor experience. Other drugs have been associated with poorer and slower 30-day recovery of sensorimotor function in patients with stroke.[79]

Just how a drug may affect recovery is speculative. The reduction of diaschisis associated with collateral sprouting and denervation supersensitivity to neurotransmitters,[14] the unmasking of latent connections, and the facilitation of the cellular bases for new learning have been suggested.[61,78] Other possible mechanisms include replacement of a normally present transmitter, provision of a mediator for cortical representational plasticity, stimulation of a pattern generator, and modulation of other substances such as growth factors. Some drugs have more clear-cut mechanisms of action. For example, the conduction of action potentials along demyelinated axons may be partially restored by pharmacologic agents such as 4-aminopyridine (4-AP) and tetraethylammonium, which block potassium channels, prolong the action potential, and improve impulse conduction.[42,207] In patients with multiple sclerosis, 4-AP has found use and may work at the level of an incomplete SCI or subcortical ischemic lacunae.

MUSCLE PLASTICITY

Skeletal muscle has dynamic functional and molecular properties. The molecular diversity of the fiber population is reflected in the many phenotypes that have been characterized.[162] Although the functional significance of this diversity is uncertain for the subtler fiber type differences, the factors that create diversity are becoming clear. They include genetic programs, hormones, and usage patterns.

Atrophy

NEURAL INFLUENCES

Results of biopsies of muscle after hemiplegia in human patients have shown atrophy of type II fibers,[17] which have larger axons, fatigue rapidly and recover slowly, and use glycogen for anaerobic metabolism. Type I fibers have high levels of oxidative metabolic enzymes that allow fatigue resistance. These fibers tend to dominate in antigravity muscles. Many myosin isoforms exist between these two broad categories.

Muscle fiber type grouping and end-plate changes seen on occasion have raised the possibility of collateral sprouting and reinnervation after an upper motoneuron injury. Neurogenic changes in paralyzed muscles have been suggested by the finding of fibrillation potentials and positive sharp waves by EMG. These changes peak at 4 to 10 weeks after a stroke or cervical SCI and are evident even a year later.[1,19] Nerve conduction studies have not identified any peripheral nerve injury as the cause of these findings. Transsynaptic degeneration of anterior horn cells has been invoked as the cause, but this idea was based on the study of only a few cervical and thoracic spinal injuries associated with a loss of lumbar spinal neurons believed not due to a peripheral nerve injury.[1]

Another pathology study revealed no loss of anterior horn motoneurons after stroke; however, the cross-sectional area of the lower motoneurons on the affected side was significantly less in patients with hemiparesis than that of the opposite side and in control subjects.[167] Indeed, the degree of degeneration of the medullary pyramid and of muscular weakness paralleled the decrease in the size of the motoneurons. The decrease in cell area may follow the loss of a transsynaptic trophic influence from the upper motoneuron, from the muscle target organ that atrophies, or from both.

Skeletal muscles change their properties not only after alterations in their connectivity but also with functional demands. The neural control of the phenotypic expression of muscle is most striking. Fast, phasic type II muscle can convert to slow, continuously active type I muscle by a change in its activity level, which induces the expression of genes that code for the shift in contractile proteins. A change from fast to slow activity pattern leads, during 1 to 3 weeks, to changes in capillary density, sarcoplasmic reticulum adenosine triphosphatase (ATPase), hexokinase, oxidative and anaerobic metabolism, and alteration of the myosin molecule.[203]

The regulation of acetylcholine receptors in developing muscle and in adult muscle also depends on activity, innervation, and probably other trophic influences. For example, some signal causes agrin to be synthesized by motoneurons, transported down the axon, and released into the synaptic cleft. It binds to the basal lamina and triggers the muscle fiber to aggregate acetylcholine, acetylcholinesterase, and other postsynaptic components.

HORMONAL INFLUENCES

Receptors for hormones are present on the muscle membrane and contribute to plasticity. Fiber features are altered by thyroid and growth hormones and by testosterone and beta-2 agonists,[88] which may stimulate muscle growth or may prevent disuse atrophy. For example, experimental animal models show that high and low levels of thyroid hormone contribute to the adaptive changes of myosin heavy-chain isoforms when skeletal muscle experiences altered contractile activity, such as non–weight bearing.[13] Growth hormone combined with exercise can have a synergistic effect on limiting muscle atrophy and increasing muscle mass and strength in elderly patients.[220] The beta-2–adrenergic agonist metaproterenol significantly increased muscle mass and strength in patients with atrophy from chronic SCI.[186] The drug probably exerts an anabolic effect on protein structures in the muscle.[117] Larger clinical trials that include dose-response paradigms are needed to determine the place of these potential medical manipulations for rehabilitation. Finally, as the genetic defects for muscle diseases come to be recognized, specific interventions such as myoblast implants, dystrophin gene insertions, and alterations in ion channels will offer ways to modulate neuromuscular plasticity.

DISUSE

Muscle atrophy from disuse is a common problem in neurorehabilitation. Paresis, limitations in mobility, and poor fitness open the door to this potentially preventable contributor to additional weakness, fatigue, and disability. Muscle wasting can be attributed more to changes in muscle length and loading than to a fall in neuromuscular activity. Disuse atrophy tends to be most pronounced in paralyzed slow fatigue-resistant muscle fibers that normally bear weight and cross single joints.[80] The most severe atrophy is found in unloaded muscles that are immobilized at a shortened length. Muscle in persons at complete rest is said to atrophy initially at the rate of 1 to 6 percent daily for the first week, and strength in an immobilized limb can fall 30 to 40 percent in 6 weeks.[90] A simple, linear relation is unlikely to exist between inactivity and consequent changes in mass, force, and endurance. More recent data offer clues about possible interventions for disabled patients.

Many of the properties of skeletal muscle can be modulated by the pattern and level of both active and passive mechanical activity. Passive stretch alone can produce muscle enlargement. The mechanical transduction of stretch into a cellular signal is accomplished by several mechanisms.[12] When neuromuscular activation was reduced in animal experiments by suspension of the hindlimbs, by thoracic transection of the spinal cord, by isolation of the spinal cord by transection and deafferentation of lumbar roots, or by space flight, certain observations were made that are relevant to rehabilitation of the suddenly bedridden patient.[178] Atrophy was greatest in the slow extensor muscles and in the deeper portions of muscles that contained the greatest proportion of slow twitch and high oxidative fibers. Limb unloading, as in the hindlimb suspension model, led to a rapid phase of atrophy in the first 1 to 2 weeks, so countermeasures are perhaps most important in this phase after the onset of paresis and bedrest. For a muscle fiber to maintain or to increase its usual size, it had to produce some minimum level of force for some minimum time each day. This goal was accomplished better by mechanical loading than by electrical stimulation, perhaps because protocols for the latter did not allow the development of enough tension. The expression of myosin forms adapted partly in response to the mechanical stress imposed on fibers. Mitochondrial and glycolytic enzymes were also affected.

In patients with chronic complete and incomplete SCI who were undergoing BWSTT for gait, preliminary data suggest that manually assisted stepping can increase the mass of some leg muscles, presumably through the influence of mechanical loading and intrinsic spinal neural influences.[92] A combination of early weight bearing, even modest isometric strength training, and electrical stimulation of muscle using optimal stimulation parameters[118] may limit atrophy until greater volitional activity recovers. Noninvasive techniques that include CT and MRI of muscle can help to monitor the effects of interventions on muscle volume.[62,67]

Fatigability

Muscle fatigability, defined as the inability to sustain a constant or repetitive force at the desired level, often accompanies weakness with central and peripheral diseases of the motor pathways. In normal subjects, some aspects of fatigue have been elucidated. During high-intensity exercise, metabolic alterations, especially in H^+ and $H_2PO_4^-$, determine fatigue, and restoration of muscular force generation depends especially on $H_2PO_4^-$.[143] Low-intensity, intermittent exercise that causes fatigue at low levels of voluntary activity for hours afterward is related to impaired excitation-contraction coupling. Fatigue that accompanies rapid, repetitive, low-intensity activity, such as playing the piano, has a central and metabolic cause. The central component involves impairment that evolves in the firing rate of motor units.

In peripheral neurogenic diseases, muscle weakness tends to correlate with fatigability. The mechanism involves an accelerated reduction in muscle membrane excitation and propagation during a sustained contraction.[145] In amyotrophic lateral sclerosis (ALS), functional and structural abnormalities of the neuromuscular junction may explain clinical fatigability and impaired neuromuscular transmission, which includes low-amplitude miniature end-plate potentials.[132] The plasticity of muscle, a change from fatigue-resistant fibers to fibers fatigable from disuse in patients with multiple sclerosis and SCI, has been suggested as a cause of exertional fatigue.[124]

Miller and colleagues have related biochemical changes in the muscles of patients with spastic paraparesis to their greater-than-normal fatigability.[142] With repetitive electrical stimulation of the peroneal nerve, the tetanic decline in tension of the tibialis anterior muscle and the decline in phosphocreatine and intracellular pH were greater than in healthy control subjects. In addition, the half-relaxation time was prolonged; this parameter is the number of milliseconds from the time of the last stimulus to the time at which the peak tension has decayed by half. The investigators believe that this time reflects a reduced rate of ATP production and slowed calcium ATPase activity in the membrane of the sarcoplasmic reticulum. This finding suggests that at least some aspects of fatigability seen with central lesions arise from secondary changes in muscle fibers associated with altered metabolism. Secondary changes in muscle may also contribute to stretch-related hypertonicity in patients with spastic paresis.

Early and specific drug and physical rehabilitative interventions may prevent or reverse atrophy, fiber type change, and fatigability. For example, the pattern of weight bearing and stepping early after injury may affect muscle plasticity. Electrical stimulation of paretic muscle by parameters that enhance muscle twitch properties can decrease fatigability. Optical imaging and spectroscopy can be used to measure important muscle adaptations and responses to interventions.[135]

COGNITIVE PROCESSES

Between the sensory inputs and the motor outputs that control the execution of motor acts dwell the even more challenging black boxes of attention, perception, memory, thought, recognition, language, and executive and other cognitive activities. Rehabilitative approaches to impairments of these functions are proposed in later chapters.

Overview of a Network Model

Cognitive functions are represented by neural networks that show great adaptability.

This plasticity is derived from the anatomically distributed, parallel processing of these networks, as well as from the projections of neurotransmitters from subcortical nuclei that modulate arousal, motivation, and emotional impact.[134,141] In addition, patterns of connectivity within a network reveal circuitry that possesses great flexibility.[146] A further potential for compensation after disruption of a network derives from the finding that multiple associational, sensory, and motor areas of the brain contain some of the learned features of, for example, what we later recognize, though a particular modality may carry the highest weight and be especially important.[37] These areas, then, are regions of functional specialization rather than of functional localization. Many cognitive rehabilitation strategies have been developed based on the notion that impairments might be ameliorated by tapping into one or more of the distributed grids that remain connected.

Because cognitive domains appear to be mapped at multiple sites that are highly connected with feedbacks, the coordination among networks can be interrupted by lesions at multiple sites, as in traumatic brain injury (TBI) or multi-infarct dementia, or by a generalized toxic or metabolic insult. Poor sleep patterns, which are common in patients undergoing rehabilitation, can interfere with cognitive processing at many levels. Inadequate sleep can diminish attention and concentration. Some reports suggest that disruption of slow wave and rapid eye movement (REM) sleep interferes with the consolidation of memory, including the storage of declarative and procedural or skills-related long-term recall.[113,216]

In the context of cognitive therapy, Chapter 9 describes the modules involved in the serial and parallel processing of memory. This chapter looks briefly at a few other networks that are frequently altered by a cerebral injury, namely, spatial, language, and behavioral functions.

REPRESENTATIONS OF SPACE: VISUOSPATIAL IMPAIRMENTS

Various spatial impairments result from stroke and TBI. These impairments range from right posterior parietal lesions that cause a hemineglect to left parietal lesions that produce Gerstmann's syndrome, which includes left-right confusion and finger agnosia, with inability to report on which finger is touched. Poor spatial localization by vision or touch may occur on the patient's body, within peripersonal space, or beyond the patient's reach. Short-term or long-term spatial memory may be affected. The neural network for these distributed functions includes the posterior parietal cortex, especially Brodmann's area 7, which receives visual, touch, and proprioceptive stimuli. Spatial information in this area is represented by the patterns of firing of neuronal groups, which are sensitive, for example, to where a visual image falls on the retina, the angle of the head, and the location of the eyes in their orbits.[87] The parietal regions project to the premotor cortex and putamen to an arm-centered and head-centered spatial coordinate system. They also project to the frontal eye fields, superior colliculi, and other areas to control saccadic eye movements to locate objects in space. In addition, these regions send information to the entorhinal cortex and into the hippocampus and to the dorsolateral prefrontal cortex to hold memories about the location of items in space.

The sum of these functions allows the perception and recall of space and permits the visual and body-centered guidance of reaching and other visual guidance behaviors. These multiple coordinate systems, divided among at least a few bilateral brain regions, offer the potential for therapists to design interventions that work around a focal disruption of one part of the spatial architecture. Strategies for treating hemi-inattention and related phenomena are discussed in Chapter 7.

LANGUAGE NETWORK: APHASIA

Aphasia studies reveal examples of how rehabilitationists must readdress the way they conceptualize complex functions. The traditional aphasia syndromes correlate in a general way with damage to specific sites, but the loss of function is not from a single region of injury. Indeed, many aphasiologists have questioned the extent to which the traditional aphasia subtype classification relates to localization[215] (see Table 3–5). In the terms of a neurocognitive network for language, Mesulam has described Wernicke's area as a nodal bottleneck for accessing a distributed grid of connections that holds information about sound-word-meaning relationships, whereas Broca's area is the bottleneck for transforming neural word representations from Wernicke's and other areas into their corresponding articulatory sequences.[141] Wernicke's region in Brodmann's areas 37, 39, and 40 and Broca's region in areas 44 and 45 and their surrounds are tissues of relative specialization. They cannot be simply dichotomized as receptive and expressive language zones.

Damasio and Tranel have proposed that the systems that support concepts, language, and the two-way access between them are anatomically separate.[38] A mediational set of neural structures uses convergence zones and feedforward-feedback connections to link separate regions. To support this proposal, these investigators found patients who had impaired verb retrieval and normal noun retrieval associated with a left frontal cortical injury. In contrast, these researchers described other patients who had impaired retrieval of proper nouns and certain classes of common nouns with normal verb retrieval from a lesion in the left anterior and middle temporal lobe.[38] They also found a segregation of systems for different categories of nouns. Backed up by neuroimaging studies, these investigators suggest that systems that mediate access to concrete nouns are close to systems that support concepts for concrete entities. Systems that access verbs are elsewhere, close to the neural entities that support concepts of movement and relationships in time and space. Within these systems, parallel and interlocking streams of corticocortical projections build the levels of complexity of our knowledge of words.

From the point of view of plasticity and aphasia treatment, these findings support the approach that word forms can be reactivated from their highly distributed and fragmentary base representations in auditory, kinesthetic, and motor cortices.[38] Thus, small differences in the amount and location of damage to the inputs and outputs of the distributed network for language produce demonstrable differences in neurolinguistic

impairments, or aphasia subtypes. These differences affect the degree of eventual recovery.[4,150] Detailed knowledge about these systems should lead to more theory-based aphasia therapy.

Other notions about plasticity and recovery of language are similar to those of motor recovery. Some of the gains in language functions after acute onset of aphasia have been related to right hemisphere participation[9] and to sparing of left hemisphere structures. Other data suggest that left-sided cortical and subcortical networks are important for the recovery of motor output and phonemic assembly in Broca's aphasia, whereas the right hemisphere may partially compensate for auditory comprehension and semantic processing in fluent aphasia.[116] The evaluation and therapy of the aphasias must continue to seek pathways through the architecture of information flow when stroke and head trauma close some routes.

BEHAVIOR AND MOOD

Behavioral and mood dysfunction often accompany stroke, TBI, multiple sclerosis, the cortical and subcortical dementias, and other cerebral disorders. As noted earlier, at least five parallel, segregated circuits link the frontal lobe and subcortical structures that include the corpus striatum and the thalamus. Behavioral and mood syndromes due to frontal lobe injury are recapitulated by lesions of the subcortical member structures of these circuits. Three distinct neurobehavioral syndromes have been described.[36]

1. The *dorsolateral prefrontal syndrome* includes deficits in motor programming, evident in alternating, reciprocal, and sequential motor tasks. Executive function impairments include the inability to generate hypotheses and to show flexibility in maintaining or shifting sets required by changes in the demands of a task. Patients also exhibit poor organizational strategies for learning tasks and for copying complex designs, as well as diminished verbal and drawing fluency. Lesions span the dorsolateral caudate nucleus, the globus pallidus, and the ventral anterior and dorsomedian thalamus (see Fig. 1–5).

2. The *orbitofrontal syndrome* especially affects personality. The range of characteristics includes altered interests, initiative and conscientiousness, disinhibition, tactless words, irritability, lability, and euphoria. Patients tend to be enslaved by environmental cues. They may automatically imitate the gestures and actions of others. Lesions span the same structures as in the dorsolateral syndrome but in different sectors.

3. The *anterior cingulate syndrome* includes profound apathy, even akinetic mutism. Lesions range from the cortex to the nucleus accumbens, globus pallidus, and dorsomedian thalamus.

Both dorsolateral prefrontal and orbitofrontal subcortical circuits appear to have a role in depression. Mixed behavioral features suggest the involvement of more than one circuit. Rehabilitation approaches to disconnections within these behavior and mood circuits are discussed in Chapters 7 and 9.

Imaging Studies

Although many problems have yet to be solved, functional imaging techniques offer the possibility of map making at every level of function, from the behavioral to the neural network, to the cellular, and to the level of protein synthesis and electrochemical reactions. So far, PET studies of blood flow and metabolism have advanced our understanding of some of the specific operations within the distributed neural systems for language, attention, memory, perception, and other aspects of cognition.[133,166]

PET activation studies can reveal the location of important parallel, component computations orchestrated to complete a cognitive task. To observe these components, subtraction studies have come into common use. The subject is given at least two cognitive tasks that are related but differ by a presumed psychologic or behavioral process. Each process differentially activates cerebral regions. By subtracting the activation produced by one from the other, the anatomic basis for one process is isolated.

These studies can be misleading for many reasons.[64] Unrecognized subprocesses may be at work. Automatic, subconscious processing may activate regions. For example, anterior language areas can be activated by preparation for speech, in the absence of articulation. Instructions, practice, habituation, level of difficulty, attentional demands, emotional state, rate and order of stimulation, and other features of experimental design all affect metabolic localization. Other limitations on rapid cognitive processes include the relative slowness of scanning, measured in seconds rather than in milliseconds; the relative insensitivity of detecting changes in regional perfusion of, at best, a few percentage points; the adequacy of statistical methods used to compare two or more activation states; and errors in mapping a PET image onto an MRI scan to combine exact anatomic structures with physiologic activity. Of course, regional brain activity measures cannot reflect the fine details of local neural activity and connectivity. Despite these potential limitations, functional imaging allows the generation and testing of hypotheses about cognitive processes and about adaptive functional changes after a cerebral injury.

Other techniques, such as single-photon emission computed tomography (SPECT),[131] high-resolution optical imaging,[89] fMRI, magnetoencephalography (MEG), computed electroencephalography, and noninvasive scalp electric and magnetic stimulation are also revealing physiologic and anatomic maps of activated higher brain functions. These technologies vary considerably in their time resolution and spatial localization.[34] The signals of fMRI peak within several seconds and have a resolution that approaches 1 to 2 mm during visual, motor, sensory, and cognitive activation studies.[32] Thus, this imaging technique, which is far less expensive than PET, may become a key method for evaluating the topographic organization and reorganization of the brain. Indeed, it offers the potential of becoming the best noninvasive tool for three-dimensional localization of distributed processing networks.

MEG reveals changes in magnetoelectrical fields associated with neuronal activity over milliseconds. Although the time resolution of PET and fMRI is longer, for example, than that of MEG and cortical depth electrode recordings, PET and fMRI have the spatial attributes that are especially likely to transform our understanding of what the brain does normally and after injury.[165] Research efforts will try to combine techniques such as fMRI and MEG to gain the best qualities and resolution of each.

These indices of synaptic and neuronal activity could play an important role in the rehabilitation of higher cognitive functions (see Table 1–3). For example, in patients with stroke and TBI, PET and fMRI can detect the evolution of functional reorganization throughout the involved network. They manifest a whole circuit reverberating with a learning task or show the increase in synchrony along the parts of a distributed pathway as a subject performs. Imaging may reveal how specific pharmacologic agents and cognitive rehabilitative tasks affect motor and mental processes. Mapping the initial response to a particular training intervention for a new patient after having performed studies that correlate early patterns of activation with long-term gains may predict whether that intervention is likely to be of benefit. Moreover, imaging protein synthesis or another marker of metabolism may help to determine the optimal timing for training, if studies show, for example, that a specific pattern of hypometabolism correlates with a lesser likelihood of learning within the affected network. Comparing the response of a patient with brain injury with the responses of normal subjects in an activation paradigm for a cognitive activity may also help therapists to develop new interventional strategies that put less demand on processes that appear defunct in their patients. PET and fMRI can become the tools of rehabilitation specialists for the study of these and other hypotheses about training and recovery.

Neurotransmitter Effects

Neurotransmitters modulate the distributed, parallel networks for the cognitive processes that sit between sensory inputs and motor outputs. At least five neurotransmitter pathways are differentially distributed to cortical and thalamic sensorimotor sites. Among their activities, the cholinergic pro-

jections from the nucleus basalis may serve as a gate for behaviorally relevant sensory information. Noradrenergic projections may increase the signal-to-noise ratio and may modulate resistance to distraction. Dopaminergic projections from the ventral tegmental tract may relate a reward to the cognitive effort. Histaminergic projections from the hypothalamus and serotonergic projections from the raphe nuclei, along with the others, play roles in attention, mood, motivation, learning, and vigilance.[141]

Clinical trials of drugs that aim to improve cognition in patients undergoing rehabilitation will have to consider potentially confounding problems. The following must be determined:

1. The type, location, extent, and age of the lesion.
2. The specific drug, its dosage, time of initiation, duration of use, and adverse effects.
3. The accompanying physical or cognitive therapy that may add to a drug's effectiveness in inducing activity-dependent plasticity.

Subsequent chapters look at agents that, in specific settings, can help to ameliorate disorders of cognition, behavior, and mood. Clinicians should select medications with special care in the months following a cerebral injury so they do not iatrogenically impede the course toward improvement.

SUMMARY

Patients who suffer acute injuries and diseases of the brain and spinal cord often have a progressive lessening of their impairments and disabilities. Recovery of neuronal function, activity within partially spared tissue, and compensation by new behavioral strategies account for much of this improvement. Studies of animal models during learning and after a lesion made at any level of the neuraxis point to gains associated with at least two other mechanisms. Multiple loci of neurons that represent aspects of a sensorimotor or cognitive behavior can expand their representations to neighboring cells that then participate in the behavior. These neuronal assemblies, with their local circuitry, receptive fields, and stimulus-response characteristics, are connected to other assemblies by relative hierarchic controls. Many of the details of motor activities, such as stepping, can be carried out by components of the hierarchy and can be evoked with little cortical input. In addition, assemblies that provide features for the performance of a task are often highly distributed and run in parallel pathways, which can potentially assume some aspects of the behavior of injured pathways.

Goal-oriented behaviors, along with paradigms that optimize learning, induce representational plasticity and may increase the beneficial output from the anatomic networks that participate in a behavior. Rehabilitation strategies can be tested for their ability to make use of this plasticity. Physical and drug therapies, perhaps monitored by functional neuroimaging, must be tested for their ability to drive activity-dependent plasticity and to enhance the function of patients.

REFERENCES

1. Aisen M, Brown W, Rubin M. Electrophysiologic changes in lumbar spinal cord after cervical cord injury. Neurology 1992;42:623–626.
2. Aizawa H, Mushiake H, Inase M, et al. An output zone of the monkey primary motor cortex specialized for bilateral hand movement. Exp Brain Res 1990;82:219–221.
3. Alexander G, Crutcher M. Functional architecture of basal ganglia circuits: Neural substrates of parallel processing. Trends Neurosci 1990; 13:266–271.
4. Alexander M, Naeser M, Palumbo C. Broca's area aphasias. Neurology 1990;40:353–362.
5. Almli C, Finger S. Toward a definition of recovery of function. In: Finger S, LeVere T, Almli C, et al, eds: Brain Injury and Recovery. New York: Plenum Press, 1988:1–13.
6. Alstermark B, Lundberg A, Pettersson L. Integration in descending motor pathways controlling the forelimb in the cat. Exp Brain Res 1981; 42:299–318.
7. Asanuma C. Mapping movements within a moving motor map. Trends Neurosci 1991;14:217–218.
8. Barth T, Grant M, Schallert T. Effects of MK801 on recovery from sensorimotor cortex lesions. Stroke 1990;21(Suppl III):153–157.
9. Baynes K. Language and reading in the right hemisphere: Highways or byways of the brain? Journal of Cognitive Neuroscience 1991;2:159–178.
10. Benecke R, Meyer B, Freund H. Reorganisation of the descending motor pathways in patients af-ter hemispherectomy and severe hemispheric lesions demonstrated by magnetic brain stimulation. Exp Brain Res 1991;83:419–426.
11. Blood K, Perlman S, Bailliet R, et al. Visual cortex hyperactivity during arm movements in brain injured individuals: Evidence of compensatory shifts in functional neural systems. Journal of Neurologic Rehabilitation 1991;5:211–217.
12. Booth F, Thomason D. Molecular and cellular adaptation of muscle in response to exercise: Perspectives of various models. Physiol Rev 1991; 71:541–585.
13. Booth F, Tseng B. Molecular and cellular approaches to understanding muscle adaptation. News in the Physiological Society 1993;8:165–169.
14. Boyeson M, Jones J, Harmon R. Sparing of motor function after cortical injury. Arch Neurol 1994; 51:405–414.
15. Brion J-P, Demeurisse G, Capon A. Evidence of cortical reorganization in hemiparetic patients. Stroke 1989;20:1079–1084.
16. Brodal A. Self-observations and neuroanatomical considerations after a stroke. Brain 1973;96:675–694.
17. Brooke M, Engel W. The histographic analysis of human muscle biopsies with regard to fibre types: Diseases of the upper and lower motor neurons. Neurology 1969;19:378–393.
18. Brooks V. The Neural Basis of Motor Control. New York: Oxford University Press, 1986:24–34.
19. Brown W, Snow R. Denervation in hemiplegic muscles. Stroke 1990;21:1700–1704.
20. Bucy P, Keplinger J, Siqueira E. Destruction of the "pyramidal tract" in man. J Neurosurg 1964; 21:385–398.
21. Bussel B, Roby-Brami A, Biraben A, et al. Myoclonus in a patient with spinal cord transection. Brain 1988;111:1235–1245.
22. Calancie B, Needham-Shropshire B, Green B, et al. Involuntary stepping after chronic spinal cord injury. Brain 1994;117:1143–1159.
23. Calford M, Tweedale R. Interhemispheric transfer of plasticity in the cerebral cortex. Science 1990;249:805–807.
24. Camarda R, Matelli M, Luppino G, et al. Multiple representation of body parts in the agranular frontal cortex of the macaque monkey. Neurology 1993;43(Suppl):A158.
25. Carey L, Matyas T, Oke L. Sensory loss in stroke patients: Effective training of tactile and proprioceptive discrimination. Arch Phys Med Rehabil 1993;74:602–611.
26. Carr L, Harrison L, Evans A, et al. Patterns of central motor reorganization in hemiplegic cerebral palsy. Brain 1993;116:1223–1247.
27. Chiappa K, Cros D, Kiers L, et al. Crossed inhibition in the human motor system. J Clin Neurophysiol 1995;12:82–96.
28. Chugani H, Phelps M, Mazziotta J. Positron emission tomography study of human brain functional development. Ann Neurol 1987;22:487–497.
29. Chugani H, Shewmon D, Peacock W, et al. Surgical treatment of intractable neonatal-onset seizures: The role of PET. Neurology 1988;38:1178–1188.

30. Cohen L, Brasil-Neto J, Pascual-Leone A, et al. Plasticity of cortical motor output organization following deafferentation, cerebral lesions, and skill acquisition. In: Devinsky O, Beric A, Dogali M, eds: Electrical and Magnetic Stimulation of the Brain and Spinal Cord. New York: Raven Press, 1993:187–200.

31. Cohen L, Meer J, Tarkka I, et al. Congenital mirror movements. Brain 1991;114:381–403.

32. Cohen M, Bookheimer S. Localization of brain function using magnetic resonance imaging. Trends Neurosci 1994;17:268–277.

33. Colebatch J, Gandevia S. The distribution of muscular weakness in upper motor neuron lesions affecting the arm. Brain 1989;112:749–763.

34. Crease R. Biomedicine in the age of imaging. Science 1993;261:554–561.

35. Crisostomo E, Duncan P, Propst M, et al. Evidence that amphetamine with physical therapy promotes recovery of motor function in stroke patients. Ann Neurol 1988;23:94–97.

36. Cummings J. Frontal-subcortical circuits and human behavior. Arch Neurol 1993;50:873–880.

37. Damasio A. Category-related recognition defects as a clue to the neural substrates of knowledge. Trends Neurosci 1990;13:95–98.

38. Damasio A, Tranel D. Nouns and verbs are retrieved with differently distributed neural systems. Neurobiology 1993;90:4957–4960.

39. Dannenbaum R, Dykes R. Sensory loss in the hand after sensory stroke: therapeutic rationale. Arch Phys Med Rehabil 1988;69:833–839.

40. Davidoff R. The pyramidal tract. Neurology 1990;40:332–339.

41. Davidoff R. Skeletal muscle tone and the misunderstood stretch reflex. Neurology 1992;42:951–963.

42. Davis F, Stefoski D, Rush J. Orally administered 4-AP improves clinical signs in multiple sclerosis. Ann Neurol 1990;27:186–192.

43. Decety J. Can motor imagery be used as a form of therapy? Journal of NIH Research 1995;7:47–48.

44. Decety J, Perani D, Mazziotta J, et al. Mapping motor representations with positron emission tomography. Nature 1994;371:600–604.

45. Deiber M, Passingham R, Colebatch J, et al. Cortical areas and the selection of movement: A study with positron emission tomography. Exp Brain Res 1991;84:393–402.

46. Diamond M, Huang W, Ebner F. Laminar comparison of somatosensory cortical plasticity. Science 1994;265:1885–1888.

47. Dietz V, Colombo G, Jensen L. Locomotor activity in spinal man. Lancet 1994;344:1260–1263.

48. Dobkin B, Edgerton V, Fowler E. Sensory input during treadmill training alters rhythmic locomotor EMG output in subjects with complete spinal cord injury. In: Proceedings of the Annual Meeting of the Society for Neuroscience. Anaheim, CA, 1992:1403.

49. Dobkin B, Edgerton V, Fowler E, et al. Training induces rhythmic locomotor EMG patterns in subjects with complete SCI. Neurology 1992; 42(Suppl 3):207–208.

50. Dobkin B, Fowler E, Edgerton V, et al. Step-like electromyographic activity in the legs in subjects with complete and severe incomplete thoracic spinal cord injury. Ann Neurol 1994;36:298.

50a. Dobkin B, Harkema S, Requejo P, et al. Modulation of locomotor-like electromyographic activity in subjects with complete and incomplete chronic spinal cord injuries. Journal of Neurologic Rehabilitation 1995;9:183–190.

51. Drew T. The role of the motor cortex in the control of gait modification in the cat. In: Shimamura M, Grillner S, Edgerton V, ed. Neurobiological Basis of Human Locomotion. Tokyo: Japan Scientific Societies Press, 1991:201–212.

52. Dykes R, Metherate R. Sensory cortical reorganization following peripheral nerve injury. In: Finger S, Levere T, Almli C, et al, eds. Brain Injury and Recovery. New York: Plenum Press, 1988: 215–234.

53. Edelman G, Finkel L. Neuronal group selection in the cerebral cortex. In: Edelman G, Gall W, Cowan W, ed. Dynamic Aspects of Neocortical Function. New York: John Wiley, 1984:653–696.

54. Edgerton V, Roy R, Hodgson J, et al. Recovery of full weight-supporting locomotion of the hindlimbs after complete thoracic spinalization of adult and neonatal cats. In: Wernig A, ed. Plasticity of Motoneuronal Connections, vol 5. Amsterdam: Elsevier, 1991:405–418.

55. Edgerton V, Roy R, Hodgson J, et al. Potential of the adult mammalian lumbosacral spinal cord to execute and acquire improved locomotion in the absence of supraspinal input. J Neurotrauma 1991;9(Suppl 1):S119–S128.

56. Eichenbaum H. Thinking about brain cell assemblies. Science 1993;261:993–994.

57. Eidelberg E, Nguyen L, Deza L. Recovery of locomotor function after hemisection of the spinal cord in cats. Brain Res Bull 1986;16:507–515.

58. Eidelberg E, Walden J, Nguyen L. Locomotor control in macaque monkeys. Brain 1981; 104:647–663.

59. Essing J, Gersten J, Yarnell P. Light touch thresholds in normal persons and cerebral vascular disease patients. Stroke 1980;11:528–533.

60. Evatt M, Wolf S, Segal R. Modification of human spinal stretch reflexes. Neurosci Lett 1989; 105:350–355.

61. Feeney D. Pharmacologic modulation of recovery after brain injury: A reconsideration of diaschisis. J Neuro Rehabil 1991;5:113–128.

62. Fleckenstein J, Weatherall P, Bertocci L, et al. Locomotor system assessment by muscle magnetic resonance imaging. Magn Reson Q 1991;7:79–103.

63. Forssberg H, Grillner S, Rossignol S. Phasic gain control of reflexes from the dorsum of the paw during spinal locomotion. Brain Res 1977; 132:121–139.

64. Frackowiak R. Functional mapping of verbal memory and language. Trends Neurosci 1994; 17:109–115.

65. Fried I, Katz A, McCarthy G, et al. Functional organization of human supplementary motor cortex studied by electrical stimulation. J Neurosci 1991;11:3856–3866.

66. Fries W, Danek A, Witt T. Motor responses after transcranial electrical stimulation of cerebral hemispheres with a degenerated pyramidal tract. Ann Neurol 1991;29:646–650.

67. Fukunaga T, Roy R, Edgerton V, et al. Physiological cross-sectional area of human leg muscles based on magnetic resonance imaging. J Orthop Res 1992;10:926–934.

68. Fung J, Stewart J, Barbeau H. The combined effects of clonidine and cyproheptadine with interactive training on the modulation of locomotion in spinal cord injured subjects. J Neurol Sci 1990; 100:85–93.

69. Garcia-Rill E, Skinner R. Modulation of rhythmic function the posterior midbrain. Neuroscience 1988;27:639–654.

70. Garraghty P, Kaas J. Functional reorganization in adult monkey thalamus after peripheral nerve injury. Neuroreport 1991;2:747–750.

71. Gazzaniga M, Bogen J, Sperry R. Dyspraxia following division of the cerebral commissures. Arch Neurol 1967;16:606–612.

72. Georgopoulos A, Ashe J, Smyrnis N, et al. The motor cortex and the coding of force. Science 1992;256:1692–1695.

73. Georgopoulos A, Taira M, Lukashin A. Cognitive neurophysiology of the motor cortex. Science 1993;260:47–52.

74. Geschwind N. Mechanisms of change after brain lesions. In: Nottebohm F, ed: Hope for a new neurology. Ann N Y Acad Sci 1985;457:1–11.

75. Gilman S, Dauth G, Frey K, et al. Experimental hemiplegia in the monkey: Basal ganglia glucose activity during recovery. Ann Neurol 1987; 22:370–376.

76. Goldman-Rakic P. Motor control function of prefrontal cortex. In: Porter R, ed: Motor areas of the cerebral cortex. Ciba Found Symp 1987;132; 187–197.

77. Goldman-Rakic P, Selemon L. New frontiers in basal ganglia research. Trends Neurosci 1990; 13:241–244.

78. Goldstein L. Pharmacology of recovery after stroke. Stroke 1990;21(Suppl III):139–142.

79. Goldstein L, Matchar D, Morgenlander J, et al. Influence of drugs on the recovery of sensori-motor function after stroke. Journal of Neurologic Rehabilitation 1990;4:137–144.

80. Gordon T, Mao J. Muscle atrophy and procedures for training after spinal cord injury. PT 1994; 74:50–60.

81. Grafton S. Cortical control of movement. Ann Neurol 1994;36:3–4.

82. Grafton S, Mazziotta J, Presty S, et al. Functional anatomy of human procedural learning determined with regional cerebral blood flow and PET. J Neurosci 1992;12:2542–2548.

83. Grafton S, Woods R, Mazziotta J. Within-arm somatotopy in human motor areas determined by PET imaging of cerebral blood flow. Exp Brain Res 1993;95:172–176.

84. Graybiel A, Aosaki T, Flaherty A, et al. The basal ganglia and adaptive motor control. Science 1994;265:1826–1831.

84a. Greenstein JJ, Gastineau B, Siegel B, et al. Cerebral hemisphere activation during human bi-pedal locomotion. Human Brain Mapping 1995; 2(suppl 1):320.

85. Grillner S. Neurobiological bases for rhythmic motor acts in vertebrates. Science 1985;228:143–149.

86. Grillner S, Matsushima T. The neuronal network underlying locomotion in lamprey: Synaptic and cellular mechanisms. Neuron 1991;7:1–15.

87. Gross C, Graziano M. Multiple representations of space in the brain. The Neuroscientist 1995;1:43–50.

88. Gupta K, Shetty K, Agre J, et al. Human growth hormone effect on serum IGF-I and muscle function in poliomyelitis survivors. Arch Phys Med Rehabil 1994;75:889–894.

89. Haglund M, Ojemann G, Hochman D. Optical imaging of epileptiform and functional activity in human cerebral cortex. Nature 1992;358:668–671.

90. Hakkinen K. Neuromuscular adaptation during strength training, aging, detraining, and immobilization. Critical Reviews in Physical and Rehabilitation Medicine 1994;6:161–198.

91. Halsband U, Freund H. Premotor cortex and conditional learning in man. Brain 1990; 113:207–222.

92. Harkema S, Dobkin B, Requejo P, et al. Effect of assisted treadmill step training on EMG patterns and muscle volumes in spinal cord injured subjects. In: Twelfth Annual Neurotrauma Symposium. Miami, 1994.

93. He S-Q, Dum R, Strick P. Topographic organization of corticospinal projections from the frontal lobe: Motor areas on the lateral surface of the hemisphere. J Neurosci 1993;13:952–980.

94. Hodgson J, Roy R, Dobkin B, et al. Can the mammalian spinal cord learn a motor task? Med Sci Sports Exerc 1994;26:1491–1497.

94a. Hoffman DS, Strick P. Effects of a primary motor cortex lesion on step-tracking movements of the wrist. J Neurophysiol 1995;73:891–895.

94b. Honda M, Freund H-J, Shibasaki H, et al. Cerebral activation by locomotive movement with the imagination of natural walking. Human Brain Mapping 1995;2(suppl 1):318.

95. Hoover J, Strick P. Multiple output channels in the basal ganglia. Science 1993;259:819–821.

96. Horak F. Assumptions underlying motor control for neurologic rehabilitation. In: Lister M, ed: Contemporary Management of Motor Control Problems: Proceedings of the II Step Conference. Alexandria, VA: Foundation for Physical Therapy, 1991:11–27.

97. Hultborn H, Petersen N, Brownstone R, et al. Evidence of fictive spinal locomotion in the marmoset. In: Proceedings of the Annual Meeting of the Society for Neuroscience. Washington, DC, 1993:530.

98. Humphrey D. Representation of movements and muscles within the primate precentral motor cortex. Fed Proc 1986;45:2687–2699.

99. Hurwitz B, Dietrich W, McCabe P, et al. Amphetamine promotes recovery from sensory-motor integration deficit after thrombotic infarction of the primary somatosensory rat cortex. Stroke 1991;22:648–654.

100. Irle E. Lesion size and recovery of function: Some new perspectives. Brain Res Brain Res Rev 1987; 12:307–320.

100a. Ishii K, Senda M, Toyama H. Brain function in bipedal gait: A PET study. Human Brain Mapping 1995;2(suppl 1):321.

101. Jacobs K, Donoghue J. Reshaping the motor cortical maps by unmasking latent intracortical connections. Science 1991;251:944–947.

102. Jenkins I, Brooks J, Frackowiak R, et al. Motor sequence learning: A study with positron emission tomography. J Neurosci 1994;14:3775–3790.

103. Jenkins W, Merzenich M. Reorganization of neocortical representations after brain injury. In: Seil F, Herbert E, Carlson B, eds: Progress in Brain Research. Amsterdam: Elsevier, 1987:249–266.

104. Jenkins W, Merzenich M, Ochs M, et al. Functional reorganization of primary somatosensory cortex in adult owl monkeys after behaviorally controlled tactile stimulation. J Neurophysiol 1990;63:82–104.

105. Jenkins W, Merzenich M, Recanzone G. Neocortical representational dynamics in adult primates: Implications for neuropsychology. Neuropsychologia 1990;28:573–584.

106. Jones E. Ascending inputs to, and internal organization of, cortical motor areas. In: Porter R, ed: Motor Areas of the Motor Cortex. Chichester: John Wiley & Sons, 1987:21–39.

107. Jones R, Donaldson I, Parkin P. Impairment and recovery of ipsilateral sensory-motor function following unilateral cerebral infarction. Brain 1989; 112:113–132.

108. Jones T, Schallert T. Subcortical deterioration after cortical damage: Effects of diazepam and relation to recovery of function. Behav Brain Res 1992;51:1–13.

109. Jordan L. Brainstem and spinal cord mechanisms for the initiation of locomotion. In: Shimamura M, Grillner S, Edgerton V, eds: Neurobiological Basis of Human Locomotion. Tokyo: Japan Scientific Societies Press, 1991:3–20.

110. Juliano S, Ma W, Eslin D. Cholinergic depletion prevents expansion of topographic maps in somatosensory cortex. Proc Natl Acad Sci USA 1991;88:780–784.

111. Kalaska J, Crammond D. Cerebral cortical mechanisms of reaching movements. Science 1992; 255:1517–1523.

112. Kano M, Ino K, Kano M. Functional reorganization of adult cat somatosensory cortex is dependent on NMDA receptors. Neuroreport 1991; 2:77–80.

113. Karni A, Tanne D, Rubenstein B, et al. Dependence on REM sleep of overnight improvement of a perceptual skill. Science 1994;265:679–682.

114. Kawashima R, Roland P, O'Sullivan B. Fields in human motor areas involved in preparation for reaching, actual reaching, and visuomotor learning: A PET study. J Neurosci 1994;14:3462–3474.

115. Kennedy P. Corticospinal, rubrospinal and rubroolivary projections: A unifying hypothesis. Trends Neurosci 1990;13:474–479.

116. Kertesz A. What do we learn from recovery from aphasia. In: Waxman S, ed: Functional Recovery in Neurological Disease. New York: Raven Press, 1988:277–292.

117. Kjaer M, Mohr T. Substrate mobilization, delivery, and utilization in physical exercise: Regulation by hormones in healthy and diseased humans. Critical Reviews in Physical and Rehabilitation Medicine 1994;6:317–336.

118. Kramer J. Muscle strengthening via electrical stimulation. Critical Reviews in Physical Rehabilitation Medicine 1989;1:97–133.

119. Kuhn R. Functional capacity of the isolated human spinal cord. Brain 1950;73:1–51.

120. Kurata K. Somatotopy in the supplementary motor area. Trends Neurosci 1992;15:159–160.

121. Kuypers H. Some aspects of the organization of the output of the motor cortex. In: Porter R, ed: Motor Areas of the Cerebral Cortex. Chichester: John Wiley & Sons, 1987:63–82.

122. Lashley K. Temporal variation in the function of the gyrus precentralis in primates. Am J Physiol 1923;65:585–602.

123. Lemon R. The output map of the primate cortex. Trends Neurosci 1988;11:501–506.

124. Lenman A, Tulley F, Vrbova G, et al. Muscle fatigue in some neurological disorders. Muscle Nerve 1989;12:938–942.

125. Lovely R, Gregor R, Roy R, et al. Weight-bearing hindlimb stepping in treadmill-exercised adult spinal cats. Brain Res 1990;514:206–218.

126. Lund J, Sun G-D, Lamarre Y, et al. Cortical reorganization and deafferentation in adult macaques. Science 1994;265:546–548.

127. Mackinnon S, Dellon A. Surgery of the Peripheral Nerve. New York: Thieme, 1988:521–533.

128. Malenka R. Mucking up movements. Nature 1994;372:218–219.

129. Marchal G, Serrati C, Baron J, et al. PET imaging of cerebral perfusion and oxygen consumption in acute ischaemic stroke: Relation to outcome. Lancet 1993;341:925–927.

130. Masdeu J, Alampur U, Cavaliere R, et al. Astasia and gait failure with damage of the pontomesencephalic locomotor region. Ann Neurol 1994; 35:619–621.

131. Masdeu J, Brass L, Holman L, et al. Brain singlephoton emission computed tomography. Neurology 1994;44:1970–1977.

132. Maselli R, Wollman R, Leung C, et al. Neuromuscular transmission in amyotrophic lateral sclerosis. Muscle Nerve 1993;16:1193–1203.

133. Mazziotta J, Gilman S. Clinical Brain Imaging: Principles and Applications. Philadelphia: FA Davis, 1992.

134. McCormick D. Cholinergic and noradrenergic modulation of thalamocortical processing. Trends Neurosci 1989;12:215–220.

135. McCully K, Kakihira H, Vandenborne K, et al. Noninvasive measurements of activity-induced changes in muscle metabolism. J Biomech 1991; 24:153–161.

136. Mendell L. Modifiability of spinal synapses. Physiol Rev 1984;64:260–324.

137. Meredith M, Stein B. Descending efferents from the superior colliculus relay integrated multisensory information. Science 1985;227:657–659.

138. Merzenich M, Recanzone G, Jenkins W, et al. Cortical representational plasticity. In: Rakic P, Singer W, eds: Neurobiology of Neocortex. New York: John Wiley & Sons, 1988:41–67.

139. Merzenich M, Recanzone G, Jenkins W, et al. Adaptive mechanisms in cortical networks underlying cortical contributions to learning and nondeclarative memory. In: Cold Spring Harbor Symposia on Quantitative Biology. Cold Spring Harbor, NY: Cold Spring Harbor Laboratory Press, 1990:873–887.

140. Merzenich M, Recanzone G, Jenkins W, et al. How the brain functionally rewires itself. In: Arbib M, Robinson J, eds: Natural and Artificial Parallel Computations. Cambridge, MA: MIT Press, 1990:190.

141. Mesulam M-M. Large-scale neurocognitive networks and distributed processing for attention, language, and memory. Ann Neurol 1990; 28:597–613.

142. Miller R, Green A, Moussavi R, et al. Excessive muscular fatigue in patients with spastic paraparesis. Neurology 1990;40:1271–1274.

143. Miller R, Moussavi R, Green A, et al. The fatigue of rapid repetitive movements. Neurology 1994; 43:755–761.

144. Mills K. Magnetic brain stimulation: A tool to explore the action of the motor cortex on single human spinal motoneurones. Trends Neurosci 1991;14:401–405.

145. Milner-Brown H, Miller R. Increased muscular fatigue in patients with neurogenic muscle weakness: Quantification and pathophysiology. Arch Phys Med Rehabil 1989;70:361–366.

146. Morecraft R, Geula C, Mesulam M-M. Architecture of connectivity within a cingulo-fronto-parietal neurocognitive network for directed attention. Arch Neurol 1993;50:279–284.

147. Morgenson G. Limbic-motor integration. Progress in Psychobiology and Physiological Psychology 1987;12:117–170.

148. Morton D, Chiel H. Neural architectures for adaptive behavior. Trends Neurosci 1994;17:413–420.

149. Mountcastle V. An organizing principle for cerebral function: The unit module and the distributed system. In: Schmitt F, Worden F, eds: The Neurosciences Fourth Study Program. Cambridge: MIT Press, 1977:8, 21.

150. Naeser M, Gaddie A, Palumbo C, et al. Late recovery of auditory comprehension in global aphasia. Arch Neurol 1990;47:425–432.

151. Nathan P, Smith M. Effects of two unilateral cordotomies on the mobility of the lower limbs. Brain 1973;96:471–494.

152. Nathan P, Smith M, Deacon P. The corticospinal tracts in man. Brain 1990;113:303–324.

153. Nudo R, Jenkins W, Merzenich M, et al. Neurophysiological correlates of hand preference in primary motor cortex of adult squirrel monkeys. J Neurosci 1992;12:2918–2947.

154. Palmer E, Ashby P, Hajek V. Ipsilateral fast corticospinal pathways do not account for recovery in stroke. Ann Neurol 1992;32:519–525.

155. Pascual-Leone A, Cohen L, Hallet M, et al. Acquisition of fine motor skills in humans is associated with the modulation of cortical motor outputs. Neurology 1993;43(Suppl):A157.

156. Pascual-Leone A, Grafman J, Hallett M. Modulation of cortical output maps during development of implicit and explicit knowledge. Science 1994; 263:1287–1289.

157. Paus T, Petrides M, Evans A, et al. Role of the human cingulate cortex in the control of oculomotor, manual, and speech responses: A PET study. J Neurophysiol 1993;70:453–468.

158. Pavlides C, Miyashita E, Asanuma H. Projection from the sensory to the motor cortex is important in learning motor skills in the monkey. J Neurophysiol 1993;70:733–741.

159. Pearson K. Common principles of motor control in vertebrates and invertebrates. Annu Rev Neurosci 1993;16:265–297.

160. Perani D, Bressi S, Cappa F, et al. Evidence of multiple memory systems in the human brain: A PET metabolic study. Brain 1993;116:903–919.

161. Perrine K, Uysal S, Dogali M, et al. Functional mapping of memory and other nonlinguistic cognitive abilities in adults. In: Devinsky O, Beric A, Dogali M, eds: Electrical and Magnetic Stimulation of the Brain and Spinal Cord. New York: Raven Press, 1993:165–177.

162. Pette D, Staron R. Cellular and molecular diversities of mammalian skeletal muscle fibers. Rev Physiol Biochem Pharmacol 1990;116:1–76.

163. Pettit M, Schwark H. Receptive field reorganization in dorsal column nuclei during temporary denervation. Science 1993;262:2054–2056.

164. Pons T, Garraghty P, Ommaya A, et al. Massive cortical reorganization after sensory deafferentation in adult macaques. Science 1991;252:1857–1860.

165. Posner M. Seeing the mind. Science 1993; 262:673–674.

166. Posner M, Petersen S, Fox P, et al. Localization of cognitive operations in the human mind. Science 1988;240:1627–1631.

167. Qiu Y, Wada Y, Otomo E, et al. Morphometric study of cervical anterior horn cells and pyramidal tracts in medulla oblongata and the spinal cord in patients with cerebrovascular diseases. J Neurosci 1991;102:137–143.

168. Ramachandran V, Rogers-Ramachandran D, Stewart M. Perceptual correlates of massive cortical reorganization. Science 1992;258:1159–1160.

169. Rao S, Binder J, Bandettini P. Functional magnetic resonance imaging of complex human movements. Neurology 1993;43:2311–2318.

170. Recanzone G, Merzenich M, Jenkins W, et al. Topographic reorganization of the hand representation in cortical area 3b of owl monkeys trained in a frequency-discrimination task. J Neurophysiol 1992;67:1031–1056.

171. Recanzone G, Merzenich M, Schreiner C. Changes in the distributed temporal response properties of SI cortical neurons reflect improvements in performance on a temporally based tactile discrimination task. J Neurophysiol 1992; 5:1071–1091.

172. Remy P, Zilbovicius M, Leroy-Willig A, et al. Movement- and task-related activations of motor cortical areas: A positron emission tomographic study. Ann Neurol 1994;36:19–26.

173. Requejo P, Harkema S, Edgerton V, et al. Direct relationship between the level of weight bearing and EMG activity during treadmill stepping in control and spinally injured subjects. In: Twelfth Annual Meeting of the Society For Neurotrauma. Miami, 1994.

174. Riddoch G. The reflex functions of the completely divided spinal cord in man, compared with those associated with less severe lesions. Brain 1917;40:264–402.

175. Roby-Brami A, Bussel B. Long-latency spinal reflex in man after flexor afferent stimulation. Brain 1987;110:707–725.

176. Roland P. Cortical organization of voluntary behavior in man. Hum Neurobiol 1985;4:155–167.

177. Rossignol S, Barbeau H, Julien C. Locomotion of the adult chronic spinal cat and its modification by monaminergic agonists and antagonists. In: Goldberger M, Gorio A, Murray M, eds: Development and Plasticity of the Mammalian Spinal Cord. Padova: Liviana Press, 1986:323–345.

178. Roy R, Baldwin K, Edgerton V. The plasticity of skeletal muscle: Effects of neuromuscular activity. In: Holloszy J, ed: Exercise and Sports Reviews. Baltimore: Williams & Wilkins, 1991:269–312.

179. Sabatini U, Toni D, Pantano P, et al. Motor recovery after early brain damage. Stroke 1994; 25:514–517.

179a. Sanes JN, Donoghue J, Thangarai V, et al. Shared neural substrates controlling hand movements in human cortex. Science 1995;268:1775–1777.

180. Schieber M. How might the cortex individuate movements? Trends Neurosci 1990;13:440–445.

181. Schieber M, Hibbard L. How somatotopic is the motor cortex hand area? Science 1993;261:489–492.

182. Schoner G, Kelso J. Dynamic pattern generation in behavioral and neural systems. Science 1988; 239:1513–1520.

183. Schott G. Penfield's homunculus: A note on cerebral cartography. J Neurol Neurosurg Psychiatry 1993;56:329–333.

184. Schwartz A, Kettner R, Georgopoulous A. Primate motor cortex and free arm movements to visual targets in three-dimensional space. J Neurosci 1988;8:2913–2927.

185. Shimoyama I, Dauth G, Gilman S, et al. Thalamic, brainstem and cerebellar glucose metabolism in the hemiplegic monkey. Ann Neurol 1988; 24:718–726.

186. Signorile J, Banovac K, Gomez M, et al. Increased muscle strength in paralyzed patients after spinal cord injury: Effect of beta-2 adrenergic agonist. Arch Phys Med Rehabil 1995;76:55–58.

187. Silvestrini M, Caltagirone C, Cupini L, et al. Activation of healthy hemisphere in poststroke recovery: A transcranial Doppler study. Stroke 1993;24:1673–1677.

188. Smith J, Greer J, Liu G, et al. Neural mechanisms generating respiratory pattern in mammalian brainstem-spinal cord in vitro. J Neurophysiol 1990;64:1149–1169.

189. Sprague J. Interaction of cortex and superior colliculus in mediation of visually guided behavior in the cat. Science 1966;153:1544–1547.

190. Stein R. Reflex modulation during locomotion: functional significance. In: Patla A, ed: Adaptability of Human Gait. Amsterdam: Elsevier-North Holland, 1991:21–36.

191. Stein R, Yang J, Edamura M, et al. Reflex modulation during normal and pathological human locomotion. In: Shimamura M, Grillner S, Edgerton V, eds: Neurobiological Basis of Human Locomotion. Tokyo: Japan Scientific Societies Press, 1991:335–346.

192. Strick P. Anatomical organization of multiple motor areas in the frontal lobe. In: Waxman S, ed: Functional Recovery in Neurological Disease. New York: Raven Press, 1988:293–312.

193. Sutton R, Feeney D. Alpha-noradrenergic agonists and antagonists affect recovery and maintenance of beam walking ability after sensorimotor cortex ablation in the rat. Restorative Neurology and Neuroscience 1992;4:1–11.

194. Sutton R, Hovda D, Feeney D. Amphetamine accelerates recovery of locomotor function following bilateral frontal cortex ablation in cats. Behav Neurosci 1989;103:837–841.

195. Taga G, Yamaguchi Y, Shimizu H. Self-organized control of bipedal locomotion by neural oscillators in unpredictable environment. Biol Cybern 1991;65:147–159.

196. Taira M, Mine S, Georgopoulos A, et al. Parietal cortex neurones of the monkey related to the visual guidance of hand movement. Exp Brain Res 1990;80:351–364.

197. Taub E, Crago J, Burgio L, et al. An operant approach to rehabilitation medicine: Overcoming learned nonuse by shaping. J Exp Anal Behav 1994;61:287–318.

198. Topka H, Cohen L, Cole R, et al. Reorganization of corticospinal pathways following spinal cord injury. Neurology 1991;41:1276–1283.

199. Turner R. Magnetic resonance imaging of brain function. Ann Neurol 1994;35:637–638.

200. Vilensky J, Moore A, Eidelberg E, et al. Recovery of locomotion in monkeys with spinal cord lesions. J Mot Behav 1992;24:288–296.

201. Villablanca J, Burgess J, Olmstead C. Recovery of function after neonatal or adult hemispherectomy in cats: I. Time course, movement, posture and sensorimotor tests. Behav Brain Res 1986; 19:205–226.

202. Visintin M, Barbeau H. The effect of body weight support on the locomotor pattern of spastic paretic patients. Can J Neurol Sci 1989;16:315–325.

203. Vrobova G. The concept of neuromuscular plasticity. Journal of Neurologic Rehabilitation 1989; 3:1–6.

204. Wall J. Variable organization in cortical maps of the skin as an indication of the lifelong adaptive capacities of circuits in the mammalian brain. Trends Neurosci 1988;11:549–557.

205. Warabi T, Inoue K, Noda H, et al. Recovery of voluntary movement in hemiplegic patients. Brain 1990;113:177–189.

206. Wasserman E, Fuhr P, Cohen L, et al. Effects of

transcranial magnetic stimulation on ipsilateral muscles. Neurology 1991;41:1795–1799.

207. Waxman S, Ritchie J. Molecular dissection of the myelinated axon. Ann Neurol 1993;33:121–136.

208. Weder B, Herzog H, Seitz R, et al. Tactile exploration of shape after subcortical ischaemic infarction studied with PET. Brain 1994;117:593–605.

209. Weiller C, Chollet F, Friston K, et al. Functional reorganization of the brain in recovery from striatocapsular infarction in man. Ann Neurol 1992; 31:463–472.

210. Weiller C, Ramsay S, Wise R, et al. Individual patterns of functional reorganization in the human cerebral cortex after capsular infarction. Ann Neurol 1993;33:181–189.

211. Weimann J, Meyrand P, Marder E. Neurons that form multiple pattern generators. J Neurophysiol 1991;65:111–122.

212. Wernig A, Muller S. Laufband locomotion with body weight support improved walking in persons with severe spinal cord injuries. Paraplegia 1992; 30:229–238.

213. Whishaw I, Pellis S, Gorny B, et al. The impairments in reaching and the movements of compensation in rats with motor cortex lesions: An endpoint, videorecording and movement notation analysis. Behav Brain Res 1991;42:77–91.

214. Wickens J, Hyland B, Anson G. Cortical cell assemblies: A possible mechanism for motor programs. J Mot Behav 1994;26:66–82.

215. Willmes K, Poeck K. To what extent can aphasic syndromes be localized? Brain 1993;116:1527–1540.

216. Wilson M, McNaughton B. Reactivation of hippocampal ensemble memories during sleep. Science 1994;265:676–679.

217. Wolpaw J. Acquisition and maintenance of the simplest motor skill: Investigation of CNS mechanisms. Med Sci Sports Exerc 1994;26:1475–1479.

218. Wolpaw J, Carp J. Memory traces in spinal cord. Trends Neurosci 1990;13:137–142.

219. Wolpaw J, Schmidt J, Vaughan T, eds. Activity-driven CNS changes in learning and development. Ann NY Acad Sci;1991;627:399.

220. Yarasheski K, Zachwieja J. Growth hormone therapy for the elderly. JAMA 1993;270:1694.

221. Yue G, Cole K. Strength increases from the motor program: Comparison of training with maximal voluntary and imagined muscle contractions. J Neurophysiol 1992;67:1114–1123.

CHAPTER 2

BIOLOGIC MECHANISMS FOR RECOVERY

Experimental work in the neurosciences in developmental neurobiology, ischemic or hypoxic brain injury, and degenerative diseases offers the possibility that clinicians will one day have methods to protect injured neurons, to prevent retrograde and transsynaptic degeneration after neuronal damage, and to regenerate axons and manipulate their environment to guide them to targets.[23] A remarkable number of molecular signaling agents have been defined during development and may be useful for restorative neurobiology.[39] The controversial success of embryonic dopaminergic tissue transplants into patients with Parkinson's disease offers hope that transplants into clinically important regions after injury, perhaps with supportive trophic factors, may have relevance to restitution after brain damage. Most of the potentially useful biologic manipulations have been studied in experimental models, however. Important contributions to these studies increase monthly.

GENERAL MECHANISMS

The most commonly invoked processes that can follow injury to potentially enhance recovery are described in general terms. These mechanisms are then applied to the model of spinal cord injury (SCI).

Activity-Dependent Changes in Synaptic Strength

The storage of information in the brain and the development of neural circuits appear to depend on enduring, activity-dependent changes in the efficacy of synaptic transmission. Accumulating data point to the relationship between learning and memory and changes in synaptic strength induced by cellular mechanisms such as long-term potentiation (LTP) and long-term depression (LTD) in the hippocampus and other regions of the brain.[43] The neurotransmitter triggers and subsequent biochemical cascades of events that increase LTP and decrease LTD synaptic efficacy are complex and are still poorly understood. As knowledge grows, these mechanisms may come to be modulated by clinicians in ways that increase motor and cognitive learning within uninjured or partially injured cortical networks. Manipulations may require the combination of a training paradigm and the pharmacologic activation of a cascade or the genetic activation of the synthesis of proteins necessary for forming new associations and memories.

Synaptogenesis

Reactive synaptogenesis or collateral sprouting has been demonstrated in many mammalian cortical pathways. For example, in the hippocampal circuits of rodents, one response to partial cell loss is the collateral sprouting of fibers from the same or another converging population of neurons.[19] In other animal models, both dendritic overgrowth and subsequent pruning have been observed during recovery after sensorimotor cortical damage (Experimental Case Study 2–1). This phenomenon has also been observed in subcortical, brainstem, and spinal clusters of denervated neurons (Experimental Case Study 2–2). In patients with Parkinson's disease, autopsy studies suggest that the excitatory cholinergic terminals that contact nigral dopaminergic dendrites increase, as do the dendrites of surviving nigral neurons themselves.[2] Thus, even the elderly brain can reveal synaptic plasticity likely to have clinical effects.

A few generalizations can be made about the potential contribution of these mechanisms of plasticity in extremely young and adult mammals.[25] Partial damage to a system, such as a dorsal root injury at several levels, can elicit sprouting of inputs from

---

EXPERIMENTAL CASE STUDY 2–1
Behavioral Changes and Morphologic Plasticity

Studies in animal models offer suggestive relationships between plasticity and morphologic modifications such as axonal sprouting or dendritic spine proliferation in sensorimotor cortex. For example, normal motor learning can produce dendritic arborization and synaptogenesis in the cerebral and cerebellar cortex.[7,18]

Ongoing series of experiments have offered insights into relationships between neural structural changes and behavioral demand after an injury. After a unilateral injury to the forelimb sensorimotor cortex of adult rats, growth of neuronal dendrites in the sensorimotor cortex of the contralateral side was found within 18 days, followed by a partial reduction in dendritic branches 2 to 4 months later.[28] This plasticity was behaviorally associated with early disuse of the impaired forelimb and increased use of the normal forelimb, followed by more symmetric use of both. The increase in arborization was likely secondary to an increase in the compensatory activity of the normal limb. The partial elimination or pruning of processes probably reflected more symmetric limb activity and less need for branches. This change might also have followed the typical developmental scheme of growth in which processes are overproduced at first and then cut back. These possibilities were investigated further. When movements of the forelimb ipsilateral to the lesion were restricted by a cast during the period of dendritic overgrowth, the arborization process failed, and greater sensorimotor impairments resulted.[29] Immobilization of the impaired limb during pruning did not prevent pruning, so this process was not related only to recovery of more symmetric limb movements. Of additional interest for rehabilitation, early training of the affected limb, within 24 hours of the brain damage, led to greater neuronal injury. In this model of use-dependent proliferation of dendritic processes, early use of a glutaminergic–N-methyl-D-aspartate (NMDA) receptor antagonist allows proliferation, but it prevents pruning and impairs behavior.[35] Thus, although an early neuroprotective strategy for ischemic or hypoxic neurons with an NMDA receptor antagonist has facilitated early recovery, the same drug could have a detrimental effect during a later rehabilitative phase.

EXPERIMENTAL CASE STUDY 2–2
Behavioral Change and Axonal Regeneration

Villablanca and colleagues tried to relate anatomic reorganization to a range of behavioral changes, including locomotion and reaching. These investigators used a hemispherectomy model in the neonatal and adult cat.[59] When the lesion was induced in adult cats, some corticorubral fibers that descended from the intact hemisphere developed novel axons that crossed the midline to innervate the red nucleus on the side of the hemispherectomy. Moreover, rubral terminals from the cerebellum on the ablated side expanded from the ventral to the dorsal aspect of the red nucleus. When the lesion was induced in neonatal kittens, more extensive reinnervation was found in the red nucleus. In addition, corticospinal tracts from the intact side crossed to the thalamus on the ablated side, and novel fibers terminated in the ipsilateral dorsal column nuclei and cervical spinal cord. Thalamic degeneration on the ablated side was also attenuated in the kitten compared with the adult. The timing of the lesion in relation to normal development of these tracts is, therefore, important in determining the extent of recovery. Presumably, the immature nervous system still expresses the growth factors, adhesion molecules, and other substances that nurture and guide normal axonal growth. The synaptic sprouting and axonal growth in relation to the red nucleus raised the possibility that a change in the dominance of its control between cortical and cerebellar inputs altered the electrophysiologic properties of its output and was related to some of the behavioral recovery found in both adult cats and kittens.[14] Although these sprouts appeared to make functional synaptic connections, it was not established that they accounted for recovery of motor behaviors.

Primates may not exhibit even the limited degree of morphologic plasticity found within the cat's motor systems. For example, ablation studies of the motor or sensorimotor cortex of infant monkeys revealed little evidence of a change in the subcortical projections of the contralateral cortex to replace lost connections.[54] The fiber systems of the monkey's brain are presumably too mature at birth to develop robust compensatory sprouting or to leave behind any of the anomalous connections of the immature brain that ordinarily retract by the time of maturity. The remarkable recovery of motor function found in these infant monkeys was thought to be related to the bilaterality of its cortical motor and extrapyramidal projections. After a low thoracic hemicordectomy in the monkey, however, lateral corticospinal tract fibers appeared to recross to the spinal gray matter of the hemisected side through collateral fibers.[3] Sprouting of residual ipsilateral fibers and of any of the other descending contralateral pathway fibers may have contributed to the primate's motor improvement and recovery of locomotion, which arose over several months.

---

spared dorsal root afferents and from others at neighboring levels and can lead to the recovery of a motor behavior that is likely to be close to normal. Damage to a descending system that deafferents neurons can elicit sprouting from interneurons and other descending inputs. This synaptic remodeling would constitute a large change in organization that is less likely to correlate with partial restitution of function. New connections could be anomalous and detrimental. For example, after a corticorubral pathway injury, the sprouting of undamaged terminals onto partially deafferented red nucleus cells, such as GABAergic (γ-aminobutyric acid) in-

terneurons within the red nucleus or inputs from the cerebellum, could inhibit the rubrospinal pathway from expressing its potential to mediate recovery of motor function.

Denervation Supersensitivity

Following the loss of some inputs, the receptors of postsynaptic neurons can become more sensitive to residual inputs. Denervation supersensitivity, which has been demonstrated in many dopaminergic, serotonergic, and noradrenergic systems, may lead to increased responsiveness of a neuron to diminished input, which would improve or restore function after a partial loss of homogeneous inputs. If several types of inputs were damaged, an imbalanced drive by supersensitivity could worsen the function of the system. When combined with reactive synaptogenesis, a complicated reorganization would make predictions about benefits difficult.

Axon Regeneration

After an axon in the peripheral nervous system is lesioned, the cell body, such as a spinal motoneuron, does not degenerate. The axon regrows in what is usually a growth-promoting environment made fertile by activated Schwann cells and by a Schwann cell–derived matrix that includes collagen, laminin, and fibronectin. Monocytes and macrophages from the blood remove myelin and other debris to help clear away physical and chemical barriers to regeneration. During regrowth, the axon can recognize appropriate target cells and can make functional connections. The dogma of regeneration in the central nervous system (CNS) poses a sharp contrast. Many CNS neurons die after an axotomy. Attempts by survivors to regrow are quickly inhibited by reactive oligodendrocytes and astrocytes, microglia, fibroblasts, monocytes, and other cells, as well as myelin and cellular debris.

Vertebrate experiments, however, reveal the capacity of neurons in the adult central nervous system to have axon growth extending more than the usual 1 to 2 mm.[4] One of the most striking examples is the growth of retinal ganglia cells into the superior colliculus through the nonneuronal environment provided by a peripheral nerve bridging graft.[1] In the model of Aguayo and colleagues, about 10 to 20 percent of the retinal ganglia cells survive an induced injury. These cells regrow about 4 cm to make functional connections that permit a response to light. Indeed, several investigators have met the criteria for the reconstruction of this CNS circuit (Table 2–1) and have shown, in related work, that the neutralization of oligodendrocyte-associated neurite growth inhibitors improves penetration and the innervation pattern.[31,58]

Table 2–1. CRITERIA FOR EXPERIMENTAL REGENERATION OF A CENTRAL CIRCUIT

Survival and function of axotomized neurons
Axonal regeneration over a long distance
Penetration of the central nervous system
Formation of synapses with arbors and boutons
Synapses made with proper targets
Connections produce behavioral effects

Reactive astrocytes and glia in an area of a CNS injury are likely to block regeneration, however. Hypotheses to explain this natural barrier include the following:

1. A mechanical wall is formed by the density and geometry of glia.
2. The scar includes chemicals that stop a growth cone.
3. An excess of growth factors is within the area of gliosis, so axons are not attracted to pass beyond them.
4. Local cells make inhibitory molecules that repel a growth cone.

Agents that appear to inhibit growth include the myelin components produced by oligodendrocytes and the extracellular matrix molecules such as proteoglycans. Regeneration studies have emphasized ways to identify and neutralize these factors.

Neurotrophic Factors

A variety of protein growth factors act on neuronal precursors to mediate differentiation and proliferation. Later, they promote the survival of mature neurons. They are part of the complex give-and-take system of chemical messengers and receptors that tie cells together by the context of the situation. Their signaling pathway involves receptors for one of the three forms of the proto-oncogene tyrosine kinase (trk). These receptors are found in both the peripheral nervous system and the CNS on a variety of cells (Table 2–2).[44] In addition, a P75 low-affinity receptor for neurotrophins is found on spinal motoneurons. Thus, these receptors are poised throughout the nervous system to

Table 2–2. **LOCALIZATION OF A SAMPLE OF NEUROTROPHIC FACTORS**

Neurotrophic Factor	Receptor	Peripheral Nervous System Neurons	Central Nervous System Neurons
NGF	TrkA	Sympathetic, trigeminal, dorsal root ganglia	Cholinergic basal forebrain, medial septal, striatal
BDNF	TrkB	Vestibular, nodose	Most neurons of hippocampus, cortex, corpus striatum, spinal cord
NT-3	TrkC	Nodose, enteric, trigeminal	Most neurons of hippocampus, cortex, corpus striatum, spinal cord

NGF = nerve growth factor; BDNF = brain-derived growth factor; NT-3 = Neurotrophin-3; Trk = tyrosine kinase.

contribute to cell processes that may contribute to recovery.

Many reports point to the survival of injured neurons after treatment with the class of growth factors that includes nerve growth factor (NGF) and the related neurotrophins, NT-3 and NT-4/5, and brain-derived neurotrophic factor (BDNF). For example, NGF was infused into the lateral ventricles of adult rats that had received bilateral lesions of all cholinergic axons that project from the medial septum to the dorsal hippocampus, an important pathway for memory. A 350 percent increase in survival of the axotomized septal cholinergic neurons was found, presumably related to the effects of the NGF on the cells after it was taken up by NGF receptors and transported in retrograde fashion.[36] Intracerebral grafts of fibroblasts that were genetically engineered by a retroviral vector to express NGF also sustained axotomized cholinergic septal neurons and promoted axon regeneration and reinnervation.[32] Brain lesions can result in delayed degeneration of neurons remote from the site of injury, such as in the thalamus. Fibroblast growth factor, another class of growth factors, was infused in an animal model to prevent this degeneration.[63]

The story of these extraordinary molecules continues to unfold. Some of the neuronal properties that they help to regulate are listed in Table 2–3. Because CNS neurons have many inputs and targets, they are likely to acquire many neurotrophic factors.[45] In the peripheral nervous system, NGF helps to prevent the peripheral neuropathy induced by paclitaxel (Taxol), diabetes, and cisplatin and may increase the pain threshold. After a ventral rhizotomy, NGF receptors reappear on motoneurons after having disappeared early in the development of the motor unit; the receptors disappear when the axon rejoins its target. BDNF protects motoneurons after axotomy. Ciliary neurotrophic factor (CNTF), which is produced by Schwann and glial cells, and glial-cell-line–derived neurotrophic factor are other developmentally present substances that can rescue motoneurons.[27,53] CNTF may also protect oligodendrocytes from the effects of tumor necrosis factor and other cytokines that arise in the milieu of inflammation.[42] These effects may be an important feature of a demyelinating lesion in multiple sclerosis and possibly after ischemia and trauma, and they also point to the complex actions of these families of growth factors.

The pharmacologic use of these factors, whether induced by manipulation of the genes that govern them or by supplying the proteins through engineered cells, could as-

Table 2–3. **NEURONAL PROPERTIES AFFECTED BY NEUROTROPHIC FACTORS**

Proliferation and survival of precursors

Axon growth: cytoskeletal elements, collateral branching

Synapse: function, rearrangements

Voltage-gated ion channels

Calcium-binding proteins

Neurotransmitter enzymes

sist recovery of function. Ideally, rehabilitation specialists would have the means to turn neurotrophin-producing cells on and off to specific triggers, such as exogenous stimuli and changing neural signals or environmental conditions, to allow their targets to survive and to make proper connections.

CENTRAL NERVOUS SYSTEM GRAFTS

Intracerebral grafting is a powerful tool for exploring CNS development and regeneration. Grafts have restored a variety of motor, cognitive, and sensory abilities in animal models, but methodologies must take into account many factors (Table 2–4).[21] In addition to growing clinical data in Parkinson's disease that support transplants of fetal tissue containing dopaminergic cells,[22,56] the evidence for graft survival, fiber outgrowth, neurotransmitter activity, and positive clinical effects in parkinsonian monkeys enhances the rationale of this approach.[38] Preliminary reports have suggested that graft survival in animal models of induced Parkinson's disease increases when engineered fibroblasts that make basic fibroblast growth factor are added to the dopamine-producing neurons. Fetal cortex can also survive grafting into infarcted areas of adult rat neocortex and may make what appear to be functional connections.[26] These preliminary

Table 2–4. CONSIDERATIONS FOR SUCCESSFUL CENTRAL NERVOUS SYSTEM GRAFTING

Donor and host age

Vascularization of the implant

Immunologic protection

Ability of cells to migrate, if necessary

Ability of progenitor cells to differentiate, if
   necessary

Access to the target

Myelination

Substrate accommodation

Nerve growth factors

Growth inhibitory factors

advances increase the chance that tissue grafts or cells grown in tissue culture will one day replace a particularly needed cell line or trophic or neurotransmitter substance.

An emerging field especially relevant to rehabilitation is that of neural stem cell biology. The notion that neural cell differentiation has ceased in the adult brain needs some revision.[24] Multipotent cell lines from mice that can differentiate into neurons and glia have been genetically engineered to transport specific genes or cells into the nervous system.[55] These donor cell lines act as stem cells, much as they may during development. Neuronal precursors have been identified in most adult mammalian brains[41] and, recently, in human brains. Adult human temporal lobe tissue removed during surgery for epilepsy has, in tissue culture, revealed neuronal progenitor cells derived from the periventricular subependymal zone and adjacent white matter.[34] These cells may produce one or more phenotypes. Some may turn out to be multipotential stem cells capable, given the right signals, of allowing specific types of neurons to be replaced. Multipotent cells are potentially useful for repairs, as replacements, and for transporting genes for trophic factors, proteins, and neurotransmitters.[55] Genes can also be delivered directly into neurons by infecting them with a virus that carries the message for cells to produce a neurotransmitter, growth factor, or other substance.[37]

As in normal development, the growth and connectivity of implanted cells may depend in part on physiologic activity. In a rat model, for example, the volume and number of neocortical grafts placed into ablated somatosensory cortex was reduced by sensory deprivation, which also caused permanent morphologic and functional isolation.[10] This phenomenon is yet another example of the importance of activity-dependent plasticity. Grafts will likely require commensurate rehabilitation strategies if they are to have functional significance.

Grafting techniques are being refined rapidly in animal models, spurred by the introduction of gene-transfer technology. Replacements with neurotransmitter and growth factor–producing cells and other modulating and bridging tissues will reach human studies in the near future. The treatment of SCI may be one of the first clinical uses.

EXPERIMENTAL INTERVENTIONS AFTER SPINAL CORD INJURY

One can imagine how a combination of neurobiologic interventions might increase functional connections after injury. This research is especially applicable to SCI, in which some clinicopathologic studies show that less than 10 percent of residual supraspinal input is needed for the recovery of walking.[8,30] Similarly, to regain one more level of useful upper extremity function, even to go from a C-5 to a C-6 quadriplegia, would greatly improve the independence of a patient. What follows is a selection of highly controlled experimental manipulations in specific animal models. These manipulations include approaches that protect fibers that have not been directly injured and methods to fill in the spinal-lesioned gap or to change its milieu. These potential manipulations may soon find clinical application.

Prevention of Transsynaptic Degeneration

To try to enhance supraspinal input after SCI, spinal motoneurons at the level of and below the lesion may need protection from transsynaptic injury. Several neurotrophic factors, perhaps working in concert, seem able to perform this function.[45] If the mechanism of transneuronal death were by disinhibition from loss of a specific inhibitory neurotransmitter, infusion of a GABA agonist might be tried.[50] These methods might also protect the cell bodies of axotomized corticospinal and other sensorimotor tracts from retrograde dysfunction or death.

Increasing Axonal Regeneration

Protein growth factors and other signals for transcription could also increase the expression of genes that encode the structural and growth-associated substances needed for axonal regeneration. Within the gray and white matter, a strategy may be needed to increase the growth-promoting molecules expressed by glial cells after injury and to decrease inhibitory molecules on neuronal and glial surfaces.[48] Laminin, fibronectin, and collagen, for example, seem to promote axon elongation. Netrins are a class of axonal guidance proteins that are important at least in the embryonic CNS.[33] Tenascin and keratan sulfate proteoglycan inhibit growth in cell culture systems. Various surface molecules on oligodendrocytes cause growth cones to collapse on contact. Along with a permissive milieu, axonal guidance depends on the right gradients of attractive and repulsive proteins and axonal outgrowth promoting and suppressing proteins.[6]

Antibodies to specific myelin-associated inhibitors of neurite growth might be given to prevent the milieu's inhibition of axonal regeneration.[52] Schwab and colleagues implanted hybridomas of plasma cells after inducing hemicordectomy into the ventricular system of newborn rats. The hybridomas produced myelin-associated neurite inhibitors that increased axonal growth, although the fibers mostly skirted the surgical scar. NT-3, but not BDNF, injected into the lesioned rat spinal cord increased the regenerative sprouting of the transected corticospinal tract; neutralizing the myelin-associated neurite growth-inhibitory proteins resulted in regeneration of up to 20 mm.[51] The axons generally do not pass through the lesion. The functional consequences of this model for patients are uncertain, but the possibilities that could accompany the regrowth of supraspinal, propriospinal, and segmental axons are enormous.

Remyelination

Demyelination with intact axons has been observed in pathologic specimens in animal models[9] and in humans[13] after compressive SCI, along with regions of remyelination. When myelinated fibers are damaged, strategies to manipulate the molecular plasticity of demyelinated axons might restore the conduction of action potentials. Both upregulation and downregulation of the expression of ion channels by growth factors have been demonstrated.[60] Remyelination associated with the regeneration of oligodendrocyte precursors also appears to have a human signaling mechanism that might be activated.[47] Remyelination might also be accomplished by implanting glial precursor cells derived from adult human brains. Up to 3 percent of the cells taken from excised temporal lobe tissue during surgery for epilepsy have, in culture, differentiated into oligodendrocytes and type II astrocytes.[17,34] These progenitor cells have sent out processes around axons in culture as well, but the signals that cause them to myelinate the axons have not yet been determined.

Fostering Reconnections Across the Injury

Cultured Schwann cell or peripheral nerve bridge implants and embryonic spinal cord transplants can permit central axon regeneration across the cavity and scar at the site of an SCI.[49] Then, axon-guiding chemoattractants may be induced naturally or by manipulation to be expressed in the milieu and by target spinal neurons.[5]

Applying a direct-current electrical field may also preserve central axons and induce them to elongate through an injured segment of spinal cord.[12,20] Modulation of the levels of particular neurotransmitters or trophic factors within the spinal gray matter may assist in making reconnections.[40]

Transplantation

Transplantation of tissue into the damaged spinal cord has met with increasing success. Embryonic motoneurons have been implanted into the anterior horn.[16] Such motoneurons may one day replace damaged motoneurons. Transplantation of fetal noradrenergic neurons from the locus coeruleus has led to the recovery of stepping in adult rats after spinal cord transection, presumably by replacing lost noradrenergic projections.[62] Fetal spinal and cerebral tissue transplanted into a partially injured or transected spinal cord seemed to enhance loco-

motion in several newborn and adult animal species,[57,61] but clinicoanatomic correlations are still wanting.

When the thoracic spinal cord is more than hemisected in rats, spinal embryonic transplants have supported the regeneration of brainstem-spinal and segmental dorsal root projections and associated recovery of hindlimb placement and aspects of locomotion; this growth is enhanced by providing neutralizing antibodies to neurite inhibitors.[11] In this model, descending serotonergic, noradrenergic, and corticospinal fibers traverse the transplant only in neonates. In adults, the implant seems to serve as a relay rather than as a bridge. Propriospinal neurons send axons into the embryonic tissue, providing segmental and intersegmental input that may account for the partial recovery in the adult animals.

Unmyelinated monoaminergic and serotonergic axons seem more able to traverse a scar or implant, at least within the spinal cord.[46] Implants offer a means to increase the likelihood of the passage of myelinated axons as well, although neurons may differ in their capacity for regeneration, in their requirements for regrowth, and in their ongoing needs to maintain that regrowth.

The challenges for successful transplantation into the spinal cord are no less formidable than those for intracerebral grafts of CNS tissue. Cell lines, rather than fetal tissue, are more likely to be implanted. Technical factors, the effects of endogenous and exogenous neurotrophic factors, immunosuppression, and pharmacologic modulation of the expression of the graft will interact to affect graft survival and its physiologic and behavioral function.[15] Still, transplants and supportive manipulations after profound SCI offer the most promise as a means of permitting the development of some descending and intersegmental control of movement.

SUMMARY

The means to manipulate the promoters and inhibitors of neuroplasticity are still in early development. Although single (let alone multiple simultaneous) techniques for directing cells, their processes, the scaffolds in their milieu, their navigational methods, and the usefulness of the synapses they make are still only a vision, basic research will provide promising plasticity enhancers for clinical trials. As with the potential mechanisms for neurorestoration described in Chapter 1, the functional effectiveness of any biologic manipulation will depend in part on the training strategies developed by specialists in rehabilitation to optimally induce activity in neural circuits.

REFERENCES

1. Aguayo A, Rasminsky M, Bray G, et al. Degenerative and regenerative responses of injured neurons in the central nervous system of adult mammals. Philos Trans R Soc Lond Biol 1991;331:337–343.
2. Anglade P, Tsuji S, Agid Y, et al. Plasticity of nerve afferents to nigrostriatal neurons in Parkinson's disease. Ann Neurol 1995;37:265–272.
3. Aoki M, Fujito Y, Mizuguchi A, et al. Recovery of hindlimb movement after spinal hemisection and collateral sprouting from corticospinal fibers in monkeys. In: Shimamura M, Grillner, S, Edgerton V, eds: Neurobiological Basis of Human Locomotion. Tokyo: Japan Scientific Societies Press, 1991:401–405.
4. Bahr M, Bonhoeffer F. Perspectives on axonal regeneration in the mammalian CNS. Trends Neurosci 1994;17:473–479.
5. Baier H, Bonhoeffer F. Axon guidance by gradients of a target-derived component. Science 1992; 255:472–475.
6. Baier H, Bonhoeffer F. Attractive axon guidance molecules. Science 1994;265:1541–1542.
7. Black J, Isaacs K, Anderson B, et al. Learning causes synaptogenesis, whereas motor activity causes angiogenesis, in cerebellar cortex of adult rats. Proc Natl Acad Sci USA 1990;87:5568–5572.
8. Blight A. Cellular morphology of chronic spinal cord injury in the cat: Analysis of myelinated axons by line-sampling. Neuroscience 1983;10:521–543.
9. Blight A. Remyelination, revascularization, and recovery of function in experimental spinal cord injury. In: Seil F, ed: Spinal Cord Injury. New York: Raven Press, 1993:91–104.
10. Bragin A, Vinogradova O, Stafekhina V. Sensory deprivation prevents integration of neocortical grafts with the host brain. Restorative Neurology and Neuroscience 1992;4:279–283.
11. Bregman B, Reier P, Kunkel-Bagden E, et al. Recovery of function after spinal cord injury: Mechanisms underlying transplant-mediated recovery of function differ after spinal cord injury in newborn and adult rats. Exp Neurol 1993;123:3–16.
12. Brogens R, Blight A, Murphy D, et al. Transected dorsal column axons within the guinea pig spinal cord regenerate in the presence of an applied electrical field. J Comp Neurol 1986;250:168–180.
13. Bunge R, Puckett W, Becerra J, et al. Observations on the pathology of human spinal cord injury. In: Seil F, ed: Spinal Cord Injury. New York: Raven Press, 1993:75–89.
14. Burgess J, Villablanca J. Recovery of function after neonatal or adult hemispherectomy in cats: II. Limb bias and development, paw usage, locomotion and rehabilitative effects of exercise. Behav Brain Res 1986;20:1–18.
15. Cassel J, Kelche C, Majchrzak M, et al. Factors influencing structure and function of intracerebral grafts in the mammalian brain: A review. Restorative Neurology and Neuroscience 1992;4:65–96.
16. Clowry G, Sieradzan K, Vrbova G. Transplants of embryonic motoneurones to adult spinal cord: Survival and innervation abilities. Trends Neurosci 1991;14:355–357.
17. Compston A. Development, Injury, and Repair of CNS Glia. 119th Annual Meeting of the American Neurological Association, San Francisco, 1994.
18. Connor J, Diamond M. A comparison of dendritic spine number and type on pyramidal neurons of the visual cortex of old adult rats from social or isolated environments. J Comp Neurol 1982;210:99–106.
19. Cotman C, Anderson K. Synaptic plasticity and functional stabilization in the hippocampal formation: Possible role in Alzheimer's disease. In: Waxman S, ed: Functional Recovery in Neurological Disease. New York: Raven Press, 1988.
20. Fehlings M, Tator C. The effect of direct current field polarity on recovery after experimental spinal cord injury. Brain Res 1992;579:32–42.
21. Fisher LFG. Grafting in the mammalian central nervous system. Physiol Rev 1993;73:583–616.
22. Freed C, Breeze R, Mazziotta J, et al. Survival of implanted fetal dopamine cells and neurologic improvement 12 to 48 months after transplantation for Parkinson's disease. N Engl J Med 1992;327:1549–1555.
23. Freed W, de Medinaceli L, Wyatt R. Promoting functional plasticity in the damaged nervous system. Science 1985;227:1544–1552.
24. Gage F. Challenging an old dogma: Neurogenesis in the adult hippocampus. Journal of NIH Research 1994;6:53–56.
25. Goldberger M, Murray M. Patterns of sprouting and implications for recovery of function. In: Waxman S, ed: Functional Recovery in Neurological Disease. New York: Raven Press, 1988:361–385.
26. Grabowski M, Brundin P, Johansson B. Functional integration of cortical grafts in brain infarcts of rats. Ann Neurol 1993;34:362–368.
27. Henderson C, Phillips H, Pollock R, et al. GDNF: A potent survival factor for motoneurons present in peripheral nerve and muscle. Science 1994;266:1062–1064.
28. Jones T, Schallert T. Overgrowth and pruning of dendrites in adult rats recovering from neocortical damage. Brain Res 1992;581:156–160.
29. Jones T, Schallert T. Use-dependent growth of pyramidal neurons after neocortical damage. J Neurosci 1994;14:2140–2152.
30. Kaelan C, Jacobsen P, Morling P, et al. A quantitative study of motoneurons and corticospinal fibres related to function in human spinal cord injury (abstract). Paraplegia 1989;27:148–149.

31. Kapfhammer J, Schwab M, Schneider J. Antibody neutralization of neurite growth inhibitors from oligodendrocytes results in expanded pattern of postnatally sprouting retinocollicular axons. J Neurosci 1992;12:2112–2119.

32. Kawaya M, Rosenberg M, Yoshida K, et al. Somatic gene transfer of nerve growth factor promotes survival of axotomized septal neurons and the regeneration of their axons in adult rats. J Neurosci 1992; 12:2849–2864.

33. Kennedy T, Serafini T, de la Torre J, et al. Netrins are diffusible chemotropic factors for commissural axons in the embryonic spinal cord. Cell 1994; 78:425–430.

34. Kirschenbaum B, Nedergaard M, Goldman S, et al. In vitro neuronal and glial production by precursor cells derived from the adult human forebrain. Ann Neurol 1994;36:322–323.

35. Kozlowski D, Jones T, Schallert T. Pruning of dendrites and restoration of function after brain damage: Role of the NMDA receptor. Restorative Neurology and Neuroscience 1994;7:119–126.

36. Kromer L. Nerve growth factor treatment after brain injury prevents neuronal death. Science 1987; 235:214–216.

37. LeGal-LaSalle G, Robert J, Berrard S, et al. An adenovirus vector for gene transfer into neurons and glia in the brain. Science 1993;259:988–990.

38. Lindvall O, Sawle G, Widner H, et al. Evidence for long-term survival and function of dopaminergic grafts in progressive Parkinson's disease. Ann Neurol 1994;35:172–180.

39. Lipton S. Growth factors for neuronal survival and process regeneration. Ann Neurol 1989;46:1241–1248.

40. Lipton S, Kater S. Neurotransmitter regulation of neuronal outgrowth, plasticity and survival. Trends Neurosci 1989;12:265–270.

41. Lois C, Alvarez-Buylla A. Long-distance neuronal migration in the adult mammalian brain. Science 1994;264:1145–1148.

42. Louis J, Magal E, Takayama S, et al. CNTF protection of oligodendrocytes against natural and tumor necrosis factor–induced death. Science 1993; 259:689–692.

43. Malenka R. LTP and LTD: Dynamic and interactive processes of synaptic plasticity. The Neuroscientist 1995;1:35–42.

44. Mendell L. Neurotrophic factors and the specification of neural function. The Neuroscientist 1995; 1:26–34.

45. Nishi R. Neurotrophic factors: Two are better than one. Science 1994;265:1052–1053.

46. Peschanski M, Le Forestier N, Rapisardi S. Neuroplasticity as a basis for therapeutics in spinal cord injuries and diseases. Restorative Neurology and Neuroscience 1993;5:87–97.

47. Prineas J, Barnard R, Kon E, et al. Multiple sclerosis: Remyelination of nascent lesions. Ann Neurol 1993; 33:137–151.

48. Rudge J, Silver J. Inhibition of neurite outgrowth on astroglial scars in vitro. J Neurosci 1990;10:3594–3603.

49. Rutkowski J, Tennekoon G, McGillicuddy J. Selective culture of mitotically active human Schwann cells from adult sural nerves. Ann Neurol 1992; 31:580–586.

50. Saji M, Reis D. Delayed transneuronal death of substantia nigra neurons prevented by GABA agonist. Science 1987;235:66–69.

51. Schnell L, Schneider R, Schwab M, et al. Neurotrophin-3 enhances sprouting of corticospinal tract during development and after adult spinal cord lesion. Nature 1994;367:170–173.

52. Schnell L, Schwab M. Axonal regeneration in the rat spinal cord produced by an antibody against myelin-associated neurite growth inhibitors. Nature 1990;343:269–272.

53. Sendtner M, Kreutzberg G, Thoenen H. Ciliary neurotrophic factor prevents the degeneration of motor neurons after axotomy. Nature 1990;345:440–441.

54. Sloper J, Brodal P, Powell T. An anatomical study of the effects of unilateral removal of sensorimotor cortex in infant monkeys. Brain 1983;106:707–716.

55. Snyder E, Deltcher D, Walsh C, et al. Multipotent neural cell lines can engraft and participate in development of mouse cerebellum. Cell 1992;68:33–51.

56. Spencer D, Robbins R, Naftolin F, et al. Unilateral transplantation of human fetal mesencephalic tissue into the caudate nucleus of patients with Parkinson's disease. N Engl J Med 1992;327:1541–1548.

57. Tessler A. Intraspinal transplants. Ann Neurol 1991; 29:115–123.

58. Thanos S. Adult retinofugal axons regenerating through peripheral nerve grafts can restore the light-induced pupilloconstriction reflex. Eur J Neurosci 1992;4:691–699.

59. Villablanca J, Burgess J, Olmstead C. Recovery of function after neonatal or adult hemispherectomy in cats: I. Time course, movement, posture and sensorimotor tests. Behav Brain Res 1986;19:205–226.

60. Waxman S, Ritchie J. Molecular dissection of the myelinated axon. Ann Neurol 1993;33:121–136.

61. Wirth E, Theele D, Mareci T, et al. In vivo magnetic resonance imaging of fetal cat neural tissue transplants in the adult cat spinal cord. J Neurosurg 1992;76:261–274.

62. Yakovleff A, Roby-Brami A, Guezard B, et al. Locomotion in rats transplanted with noradrenergic neurons. Brain Res Bull 1989;22:115–121.

63. Yamada K, Kinoshita A, Kohmore E, et al. Basic fibroblast growth factor prevents thalamic degeneration after cortical infarction. J Cereb Blood Flow Metab 1991;11:472–478.

PART 2

Common Issues in Neurologic Disorders

CHAPTER 3

NEUROLOGIC REHABILITATION TEAM

The goals of therapy are so ambitious and the problems of impairment, disability, and handicap are so complex that services have come to be provided by a team of professionals from many disciplines who work in a variety of inpatient and outpatient settings.

THE TEAM APPROACH

The team approach takes many forms. In a *multidisciplinary* model, each member with specialty training treats particular disabili-

ties. In an *interdisciplinary* model, roles blend in the management of disabilities. This structure is oriented around problem solving to improve functional outcomes rather than being bound by disciplines. For example, taking an interdisciplinary approach, training procedures for motor and cognitive learning or behavioral modification are reinforced by all members, using an agreed-upon technique. Moreover, an interdisciplinary structure tends to set its goals with a view toward dealing with a patient's handicaps, the impediments to a return to the patient's usual role.[78]

These styles of interaction are not exclusive. Most teams move between the two models when they formally meet to discuss and to update the patient's progress and to adjust goals and treatments. The satisfaction and success of the team as a group and of its member specialists depend more on interpersonal and interprofessional skills than on a specific model of interaction. Skills and traits that serve the team process include dedication to enhancing the well-being of patients, humility, humor, perseverance, creative thinking, and hypothesis making and testing.

Most important to the team approach, patients and their families are considered clients. The team helps them to articulate and to achieve the short-term and long-term functional objectives that will enhance their quality of life. The family and significant others who serve as caregivers play a critical collaborative role in setting and revamping goals and in carrying out supportive and therapeutic strategies.

Of all the services and personal care provided by hospital and outpatient staff, patients express the highest level of dissatisfaction with the duration of therapy.[93] Most acutely disabled patients, especially in the first year after a stroke or an injury of the spinal cord or brain, want treatment to continue until they have recovered. These patients and families must come to understand the limitations of their therapists. The ethical challenge for the therapists is to come to an agreement with the client about realistic medical, functional, and quality-of-life goals. Such an agreement is especially important because the team, not the patient and family alone, makes the final determination about when formal therapy will end. This decision is often made under some pressure by the health care insurer to limit services. The team, the patient, and the family must be convinced that their decision is right. This consensus takes some leadership, which often derives from the physician.

The team approach to solving problems differs, then, from the medical model, which focuses on an acute illness or an exacerbation of symptoms from a chronic disease. In the medical model, the physician controls the action and nearly all communication. The patient passively awaits amelioration or cure. Allied health professionals play limited, transient roles. Issues of quality of life are growing in importance, but patients' preferences for their health care still take a back seat in most deliberations on acute medical care. Indeed, the goals for patient care by rehabilitation specialists overlap, but they are far broader than those goals inherent in the medical model.

The milieu created by the rehabilitation team also differs from the patients' experience during acute hospitalization. Rehabilitation services try to quell the anxieties associated with a sudden, debilitating illness and its threat of death or permanent loss of functional independence. The team can help patients to break this terrifying link by educating them and by sharing stories of their lives. Anecdotes from the past and the present can provide the insights about each other that bind the working relationship needed between a patient and every member of the team. These personal webs make an unfamiliar world acceptable to the patient and make a familiar world new for clinicians. The team must also monitor the way in which patients see themselves through the course of rehabilitation and the way in which spouses and other caregivers view them.

Some cheerleading by the team can be supportive, but therapists must be careful not to talk down to a patient or to offer therapeutic activities that come across as too simpleminded. The elderly and those patients used to taking charge may reject such therapy if they believe that they are being infantilized. The team can expend much effort juggling notions about what is best for the patient's well-being while, on the other hand, respecting the patient's choices and shying away from paternalism.[42] Indeed, this tension is inherent in rehabilitation efforts, because success depends so strongly on the patient's participation.

The comprehensive rehabilitation approach has come under little scrutiny.[61] A few studies of inpatient rehabilitation of stroke victims support this approach as an efficient organization of services,[58] but other studies do not. For other neurologic diseases, almost no such trials exist. Clinical trials of comprehensive, coordinated approaches that might refine the combination of features that best serve short-term functional goals and ongoing medical and rehabilitative care pose enormously complex problems in their design. Economic pressures will likely push service providers to develop less expensive, perhaps less integrated approaches. Such changes may include technicians and supervised aides who function across disciplines, group therapy, treatments done by protocol, less frequent medical monitoring, and less organized rehabilitation carried out in skilled nursing centers, transitional living settings, and day and home care settings. Hands-on care may not be delivered by the most highly skilled professionals in these situations. Therapy may be limited to a short list of quickly reached functional goals. The onus will be on practitioners to determine whether more limitations on the activities of the interprofessional team will affect the quality of care and the quality of life of their patients.

No matter how closely the team functions,

individual leadership must be taken to manage the medical, neurophysiologic, functional, cognitive, psychologic, social, educational, and vocational needs of the patient. Quality assurance and innovation spring from the creativity of the individuals who work from the theories that underlie their activities. This chapter describes the primary responsibilities, treatment strategies, and research opportunities of each member of a rehabilitation team.

PHYSICIANS

Physicians involved in neurologic rehabilitation come from a range of training backgrounds. In the United States, physiatrists and neurologists are most likely to participate in an inpatient team. Some orthopedists have run services for patients with spinal cord injury (SCI), and internists and rheumatologists have come to lead programs focusing on patients who have had a stroke and other neurologic disorders. Other specialists consult with the team on complications such as contractures, decubitus ulcers, depression, heart disease, and bladder dysfunction.

Responsibilities

Besides being responsible for anticipating and intervening in the medical care of their patients, rehabilitation physicians educate patients and families about the consequences and overall prognosis of the nervous system disease. Physicians specializing in rehabilitation should explain to both patient and primary care physician the indications for medications, measures for secondary prevention of complications, management of risk factors for recurrence of the disease, and type and duration of rehabilitative interventions. In a study of disagreements between physicians and patients about their encounters, the discrepancies were greatest when, in the patient's opinion, the physician paid little attention to psychosocial issues or drew a quick conclusion about the problem without helping the patient to understand the basis for the decision.[97]

Rehabilitation physicians also tend to be the facilitators of the team, especially on an inpatient service. To perform this function well, these physicians must help to build the team's infrastructure and must understand the practices of its disciplines. A physician leader mobilizes and motivates the patient, the family, and the team of therapists toward goals that they come to share.

Interventions

The history, examination, and review of laboratory and neuroimaging studies performed by the physician are critical to the team's formulation of the way in which the patient's impairments will affect the rehabilitation potential. For example, the history must include details about the patient's premorbid functional activities, physical fitness, mood, and lifestyle. These details affect the patient's rehabilitation care and goal setting. The examination must explore the patient's attention, memory, judgment, language, behavior, and other cognitive functions appropriate to the history. Strength should be assessed in terms of graded manual muscle testing, functional movements, and fatigability. Although neuroimaging studies cannot predict impairments and prognosis, tests such as computed tomography (CT) and magnetic resonance imaging (MRI) offer insights about impairments and prognosis for most diseases. For example, profound dysphagia may not be expected in a patient with a recent lacunar infarct in the left internal capsule, but an MRI scan that reveals an old, silent lacuna of the right basis pontis offers insight about the cause of the dysphagia.

The clinician superimposes the specific contributions of neurologic, musculoskeletal, cardiopulmonary, and other impairments on a map of the patient's functional abilities and disabilities. For example, does spasticity or palpably tender musculoligamentous tissue cause pain or limit movement? Does a medication or the presence of episodic orthostatic hypotension lessen attention span and endurance for exercise? Does a muscle group show increased paresis with a few repetitive contractions against resistance, suggesting fatigability that might impede repeated use of a limb? Are cognitive problems related only to the cerebral injury, or does a metabolic abnormality, a medication, or, in an older person, an underlying dementia augment the findings? The evaluation also emphasizes the patient's premorbid experience with disability and any present degree of disability. By gradually determining the patient's prior level of competence in physical, mental, and psychosocial functioning in light of new impairments and disability, the physician can put the mutual goals of patient, family, and rehabilitation team into perspective.

In addition, because of their background in general medicine, neuromedicine, neuroscience, mechanisms of plasticity, and scientific experimentation, rehabilitation physicians should also serve as clinician scientists. They can encourage therapists to weigh, formulate, and test strategies. Drawing on current literature and by collaboration with basic and clinical researchers, the neurologic rehabilitation specialist assesses and develops interventions. During ward rounds and team meetings, a good leader questions whether all of the team's practices reflect the best means of restoration for a patient. Access to a good database drawn from the literature, the institution's own cases, and national studies such as the Uniform Data System for Medical Rehabilitation[40] helps to put features of the recovery of impairments and disabilities into perspective. This information stimulates collective deliberations that may build a consensus toward alternative solutions and the design of a single-case study or larger clinical trial.

NURSES

Responsibilities

Inpatient rehabilitation nurses monitor the vexing medical complications that accompany neurologic disease and immobility. The nurses initiate passive range of motion of paretic limbs, follow through on preventive measures for deep vein thrombosis, and turn an immobile patient every 2 hours, along with taking other measures to prevent pressure ulcers over bony prominences. These nurses warn staff and visitors not to pull the patient across the bed and thereby

shear the skin, and they find ways to prevent or treat incontinence, so that moisture does not macerate the skin. They also educate ancillary hospital personnel not to tug and painfully sublux a paretic shoulder. Other responsibilities include assessments for sleep disorders, respiratory function, swallowing, nutrition, and bowel and bladder function; training in self-catheterization and self-medication; education about disease and about personal matters such as sexuality; and practice in self-care skills outside the formal therapy setting.

Interventions

Nurses are on the front line, where they must help to balance what a patient can reasonably do alone and what assistance a patient requires. By observing the patient and family in less structured activities, away from the formal therapy provided by other team members, nurses can provide unique insight into physical and emotional functioning. Nurses are also in an ideal position to help patients to comply with lifestyle changes for disease prevention. Rehabilitation nurses should be armed with information and handout materials about primary and secondary disease prevention. Along with the physician, the psychologist, and the social worker, nurses can initiate discussions about drug abuse with young patients who have had a traumatic brain injury (TBI) or SCI. Nurses can explain the dose-response relationship between cigarette use and atherosclerotic vascular disease. For new medication to be used after hospital discharge, nurses can develop cues and rituals with the patient and caregiver to reinforce compliance.[26]

PHYSICAL THERAPISTS

Responsibilities

Physical therapists, also known as physiotherapists, contribute especially to the rehabilitation of patients with disabilities associated with bed mobility, transfers to a chair or a toilet, ambulation, and fitness for exercise. The goals of physical therapists for neurologic rehabilitation aim more toward compensatory strategies for performing activities of daily living (ADLs) than toward interventions to lessen specific impairments. They also deal with musculoskeletal and radicular pain, contractures, spasticity, and deconditioning. The assessments of physical therapists emphasize measures of range of motion, strength, balance, fatigability, gait, and functional status.

Like other rehabilitationists, physical therapists have increasingly sought strategies to improve the accuracy and reproducibility of clinical evaluations and their applications.[81] Some common approaches to movement-related problems are listed in Table 3–1. Two broad categories of exercise programs, therapeutic exercise and the so-called neurophysiologic or neurodevelopmental approaches, have received the most attention in the past. Newer concepts related to neuroplasticity, motor control, and the way in which motor skills are learned are merging with these older categories.[72] Success in retraining during rehabilitation depends on diverse variables that include the characteristics of a task, reinforcements, motivation, attention, memory for carryover of what is taught, environmental distractions, anxiety, sleep deprivation, and family support. All can influence the way in which, for example, motor and cognitive programs are built, shaped, and refined as the patient acquires a new skill. The daily practices of most neurologic physical therapists reveal an eclectic, problem-oriented approach.

Interventions

COMPENSATORY EXERCISE

Traditional exercise programs vary greatly. They emphasize repetitive passive and active joint-by-joint exercises and resistance exercises in anatomic planes to optimize strength and range of motion.[5] These programs aim to prevent the complications of immobilization. Therapists train patients in residual motor skills, often of the uninvolved side, to compensate for impairments. The acquisition of self-care and of mobility skills takes precedence over the quality of movement, so long as patients are safe. Upper and lower extremity orthotics and assistive devices tend to be used early in therapy to speed functional compensation.

Therapists also use breathing and general conditioning exercises and energy conservation techniques when needed, particularly to reduce the energy cost of a pathologic gait.[122] Strengthening and conditioning are achievable within the context of almost any neurologic disease.[31] These interventions can be particularly important to the maintenance of functional activities in aging patients and to the prevention of complications related to disuse and overuse of weak muscles. In addition, cardiorespiratory fitness reduces the risk of coronary heart disease in a dose-response fashion.[64]

NEURODEVELOPMENTAL APPROACHES

Many schools of physical therapy have developed what their proponents call "neurophysiologic" or "neurodevelopmental" approaches that focus on enhancing the movement of paretic limbs affected by upper motoneuron lesions. Techniques are based mostly on interpretations of Sherrington's neurophysiologic studies. These approaches were first formulated from the founding advocate's observations of children with cerebral palsy and adults with hemiplegic stroke. The approaches involve hands-on interaction between the therapist and the patient.

Table 3–1. **PRACTICES IN PHYSICAL THERAPY**

Therapeutic exercise and compensatory
   functional training
Neurodevelopmental techniques
   Proprioceptive neuromuscular facilitation
   Bobath technique
   Brunnstrom's technique
   Rood's technique
Motor skills learning
Task-oriented practice
Biofeedback
Forced use
Musculoskeletal techniques
Orthotics and assistive devices

The interventions use sensory stimuli and re-flexes to facilitate or inhibit tone. They aim to elicit individual and whole limb muscle movements, but schools vary in whether they try to initially elicit mass flexor and extensor patterns of movement called *synergies.*

Most schools of physical therapy have emphasized a progression in the sequence of therapies reminiscent of the neurodevelopmental evolution from reflexive to more complex movements. Neurodevelopmental techniques (NDT) call for reproducing the developmental sequence shown by infants as they develop motor control. Based on hands-on trials with children with cerebral palsy, practitioners believe that normal movement requires normal postural responses, that abnormal motor behaviors are compensatory, and that the quality of motor experiences helps to train patients in normal movement. These practitioners emphasize normal postural alignment before any movement. The patient's mobility activities proceed in a developmental pattern from rolling onto the side with arm and leg flexion on the same side, to extension of the neck and legs while prone, to lying prone while supported by the elbows, and then to doing static and weight-shifting movements while crawling on all four extremities. These mat activities are followed by sitting, standing, and, finally, walking. Different schools vary in their attempts to activate or to minimize reflexive movements and to train functional movements in ordinary activities.

A potential problem with NDT is the delay of standing and walking until the patient has achieved relative control of proximal and distal muscles. This delay in weight bearing may lead to complications such as deep vein thrombosis in patients who have had an acute stroke.[13] This approach may also delay the patient's recovery of stepping, if one believes that task-oriented therapy for ambulation is most likely to provide the sensory feedback and learning stimuli that can modulate neural assemblies and step generators at several levels of the neuraxis.

Proprioceptive Neuromuscular Facilitation Technique. This empiric technique, initiated by Kabat and Knott, arose in part from observing smooth, coordinated, diagonal, and spiral movements in athletes at the peak of their physical efforts.[120] Proprioceptive neuromuscular facilitation (PNF) facilitates mass movement patterns against resistance in a spiral or diagonal motion during flexion and extension. It is based on the belief that, because anterior horn cells for synergistic muscles are near each other, an appropriate level of resistance brings about changes in muscle tone by overflow to these motoneurons. The therapist uses proprioceptive sensory stimuli and brainstem reflexes to facilitate the desired movement and to inhibit unwanted movements. For example, the therapist may place the patient's upper extremity in extension, abduction, and internal rotation. While the patient's arm is rotated and extended out from the side, it is moved into flexion, adduction, and external rotation. Specific techniques include repeated quick stretch, contraction, contraction and relaxation, and rhythmic stabilization in which the patient tries to hold the arm still as resistance is applied by the therapist in an opposite direction. PNF stretching techniques call for an isometric contraction of the muscle under stretch, such as the hamstrings, followed by a concentric contraction of the opposing quadriceps muscle during stretch of the hamstrings, designated as contract-relax agonist-contract (CRAC). This technique is thought to alter the responses of muscle spindles to increase the maximum range of motion, although it may also do so by stimulating an increase in the force produced by each muscle.[70] Numerous specific exercise patterns are described by the practitioners of PNF. Similar spiral and diagonal movement patterns are later used for functional activities and walking. PNF has been applied to diseases of the motor unit as well.

Bobath Technique. This NDT approach, popularized by the Bobaths, aims to give patients control of abnormal patterns of posture and movement associated with spasticity by inhibiting pathologic reflexes.[10] In this theory, abnormal motor tone and primitive postural reactions are the key factors that interfere with proper motor functioning. Abnormal movements provide abnormal sensory feedback, which reinforces limited, nonselective, abnormal movement. Methods continue to evolve.[119]

Physical therapists use *reflex inhibitory patterns* to reduce tone and abnormal postures, and they stimulate *advanced postural reactions* to enhance motor recovery. They use pressure or support on proximal key points of the patient's body to inhibit or facilitate movement. They avoid inducing associated reactions in a muscle group away from the body part that is active and overflow movements within the same limb. Bobath therapists especially avoid provoking mass flexor shoulder, elbow, and wrist synergies of the arm and extensor knee and plantarflexor ankle synergistic movements of the leg. For example, the patient with hemiplegia with flexor spasticity of an arm that rides up during walking is trained to bend forward in a chair with the arm hanging down. The patient swings the affected arm, then both arms. The patient slowly sits upright with the neck flexed while the arm hangs, then raises the head and stands. When the elbow starts to flex again, the patient repeats these steps. Strengthening exercises are generally not used. During the early stages of recovery, weight bearing, postural responses, and selective movements are emphasized. Ankle-foot orthoses are discouraged, because they are thought to facilitate abnormal tone. The Bobath approach is the most popular NDT used for rehabilitation of patients with hemiplegia. Indeed, this approach has become synonymous with the term NDT.

Johnstone's technique has similarities to Bobath in its developmental approach,[57] but it adds a pressure splint around the affected arm or leg. The inflatable splint provides even pressure across joints and allows weight bearing, for example, on the arm through the extended wrist. This technique is thought to increase sensory input and decrease hypertonicity, according to the detailed description for therapy provided by this British physiotherapist.

Brunnstrom's Technique. Brunnstrom's training procedures facilitate synergies by using cutaneous and proprioceptive sensations and tonic neck and labyrinthine reflexes.[16] In contrast to the Bobath approach, this technique initially promotes associated reactions, mass movement synergies, primitive postural reactions, and strengthening exercises. Specific techniques are recommended for each of six stages of recovery, as follows: (1) flaccidity, (2) limb synergies with onset of spasticity, (3) increased spasticity and some voluntary control of synergies, (4) control of movement out of synergy, (5) selective control over synergistic movement, and (6) near-normal control. In clinical practice, Brunnstrom's approach is mostly restricted to patients who have persistent hypotonia and plegia.

Rood's Technique. This approach emphasizes the use of specific sensory stimuli to facilitate tonic and then phasic muscle contractions.[113] High-threshold receptors are thought to increase tonic responses, and low-threshold receptors are believed to activate phasic responses. Sensory stimuli include fast brushing, light touch, stroking, icing, stretching, tapping, applying pressure and resistance, and truncal rocking and rolling. The patient's response to cutaneous and other sensory inputs is used to facilitate developmental patterns and then purposeful movement. One common technique is light brushing of the patient's lips to facilitate both flexion of the hemiplegic arm and a hand-to-mouth pattern of movement. Rood's approach has not been formalized as thoroughly as other NDT strategies.

Efficacy. The approaches of the pioneering schools of physical therapy were derived from clinical observations that drew upon narrow assumptions about motor control. These approaches use normal movement as their point of reference, view the nervous system as a hierarchic organization that can be approached at the level of reflex activity, and presume that recovery from brain and spinal injury follows a predictable sequence similar to infant development. None of these assumptions is obviously correct. For example, shifting weight onto the affected hemiparetic leg before stepping has been a maxim of the developmental approaches. Joint compression is considered to increase proprioceptive and cutaneous stimuli, to affect tone, and to help train the leg to participate in postural tasks. One study, however, has suggested that loading only accentuates the extensor synergy of the lower leg muscles, rather than facilitating normal postural responses.[30] Kinematic studies of the recovery of upper extremity movement for reaching also refute the developmental notion that movement within a synergistic pattern of flexion or extension of a whole limb precedes more selective movements outside the synergy.[117] Indeed, some synergistic movements can be eliminated simply by changing the context of the elicited movement. For example, the influential study of motor recovery after hemiplegia by Twitchell,[118] from which Brunnstrom's technique derives its stages, is often quoted as evidence of specific stages of recovery of the upper extremity. Flexion of the elbow and shoulder is said to usually precede movements in extension, but when the paretic arm is supported to allow free movements of the forearm in a horizontal plane just below shoulder level, flexion and extension of the elbow and shoulder often can be brought out independently. Many patients have extension of the elbow that comes in earlier and better than flexion.[125] The potential for recovery of some motor control must take into account the context of a movement, its starting position, the patient's goal, the way in which movement toward the goal is reinforced, and other perhaps less obvious issues.

The NDT schools of physical therapy disagree over the use of resisted muscle activity, compensatory movements, and overflow or associated reactions. Bobath teaches that these techniques increase abnormal movements, whereas Kabat encourages resistance exercises, and Brunnstrom uses associated reactions early in treatment. Some studies support the value of strengthening exercises to improve mobility in patients with upper motor neuron lesions.[11,53] Strengthening can also improve movements that are *speed sensitive,* in that they have strict timing requirements and require forces of varying intensity.[23] At least one Brunnstrom technique for eliciting associated reactions has received some support.[38] In patients with hemiplegia, resisting hip movements of the nonparetic leg increased the magnitude of the torque in an opposite direction in the muscle group of the paretic hip. This approach may both strengthen and improve the motor control of hip movements, particularly if resistance is applied to the unaffected leg during gait training.

Some of the neurophysiologic principles used by the schools of physical therapy appear reasonable. Predictable motor responses are elicited by reflex reactions, by vibration to stimulate a muscle contraction,[43] by cutaneous stimulation to facilitate

a voluntary contraction,[76] and by upper extremity weight bearing through the extended elbow and heel of the hand to normalize corticospinal facilitation of motoneuronal excitability.[14] Any carryover of responses into functional or volitional movement begins to stretch the imagination, however. Consider the tonic neck reflexes in a patient who has had a brain injury. Turning the head to the hemiplegic side can facilitate the triceps, whereas turning toward the unaffected side can induce flexion and abduction of the paretic shoulder. Neck extension can facilitate extension of the affected arm and flexion of the leg. Neck flexion tends to produce flexion of the arms and extension of the legs. Bilateral responses are most remarkable after diffuse TBI and incomplete cervical SCI. These reflexes can be used to position patients and to alter tone on a mat or in a chair. The manipulation of these reflexes has not been shown to enhance the recovery or quality of movement or the functional use of the limbs. Some of the other specific hands-on methods of the physical therapy schools may produce a good product, however, even if some of the theory is questionable.

The better-designed studies comparing these approaches have been performed in patients with stroke, with no advantages found for any particular study. A meta-analysis of 37 pediatric patients, mostly children with cerebral palsy, suggested a small positive treatment effect from NDT alone or NDT combined with another approach, compared with other approaches.[88] All of those trials have serious methodologic flaws.

Studies of the efficacy of particular schools of therapy have used outcome measures that emphasize independence in ADLs and not an outcome directly related to the primary focus of their technique of physical therapy, which is motor performance and patterns of movement.[3] Outcome measures probably need to be more appropriately linked to the type and purpose of the intervention to demonstrate differences among approaches, if any exist. Moreover, treatment can be efficacious for its intended proximal purpose, but it may not necessarily contribute to the goal of functional gains for the patient.

Studies of efficacy should concentrate on the best well-defined practice for an important goal that may, in theory, be modulated by the intervention. For example, instead of trying to assess an effect of the Bobath method on a standard test of mobility and self-care skills, the research design may assess an aspect of movement of the affected upper extremity that is treated by the method. Then, a change in impairment can be correlated with a functional use of the arm that requires the movement pattern. A study of one school of therapy over another is probably not feasible or worthwhile if the search is for the best physical therapy that will optimally improve ADLs and mobility. The methods of the schools are not likely to be reproducible in a reliable way for clinical research, and their philosophies are too far from any scientific underpinning to justify an exclusive emphasis of one over another.

Evidence from many studies of neuroplasticity (see Chapter 1) suggests that therapy structured around learning new sensorimotor relationships in the wake of altered motor control is more effective than methods aimed to foster a developmental sequence. The approach of task-oriented motor learning attempts to put this notion into practice.

TASK-ORIENTED MOTOR LEARNING

An evolving approach to therapy combines theories of motor control and principles of motor learning. *Motor control* subsumes studies of the neural, physical, and behavioral aspects of movement. *Motor learning* includes studies of the acquisition of skilled movements as a consequence of practice, drawn mostly from work in animal and human experimental psychology. This approach, task-oriented motor learning, includes many models of motor control, including pattern generation, distributed systems, and relationships between kinematic variables and functional movements (see Chapter 1).[52] It draws upon evolving theories that may account for the interdependency and reciprocity of neuronal networks and the distributed control of a movement throughout these systems.

In contrast to NDT, task-oriented motor learning emphasizes visual, verbal, and other sensory feedback to achieve task-specific movements, rather than relying on cutaneous, proprioceptive, and other sensory stim-

uli to elicit facilitation and inhibition of movement patterns. The therapist does not necessarily desire the patient to seek normal movement. For any particular task, the motor control model stresses methods of solving a motor problem, rather than methods of relearning a pattern of movement. Therapists use cognitive and sensory feedback to train the patient with an impaired nervous system to accomplish a relevant task in any of a variety of ways, but not necessarily by striving to train the patient in a particular pattern of muscle activation. The goal becomes error detection, which the physical therapist uses to help patients correct themselves during the practice of, say, reaching, standing, or moving across a variety of environmental conditions.

The task-oriented approach assumes that success after practice under one condition does not necessarily transfer to another related task. For example, in one study, weight-shift training in patients with hemiparesis while they were standing improved the symmetry of weight bearing and balance in stance, but the gains did not improve the symmetry during walking.[127] This finding is consistent with motor learning concepts. Practice at hitting a golf ball is not likely to improve a baseball player's batting average any more than static therapy can train a patient to perform dynamic activity. For gait, task-specific physical therapy has to include stepping, not weight shifting alone. A program of early locomotor training made possible by body weight–supported treadmill stepping fits into this conceptual model.[32,36,86]

The task-oriented approach emphasizes training in motor skills. It seeks to formalize techniques that everyone on the rehabilitation team should consider. In rehabilitation settings, little attention has been paid to whether typical training procedures—not what is taught but how it is taught—optimize gains in cognitive skills, motor functions, and self-care and community activities. The essence of therapy for any disability and, indeed, for acquiring any novel motor skill, is *practice*. One must reconsider, however, that a practice session can have a powerful, but only temporary, effect. The goal of practice should be a permanent effect. A learned behavior must carry over when practice conditions are no longer provided to the patient.

Physical therapists tend to use practice procedures and reinforcements that increase the speed or quality of a patient's performance during training. A more important rehabilitative outcome is to have patients practice in a way that enhances posttraining performance and transfers that training to related tasks under differing conditions in the patient's environment. At first, it may seem counterintuitive that any training procedure that speeds the rate of improvement or results in a more effective performance during therapy would do anything other than enhance learning and subsequent long-term performance. Research on the processes that lead to learning in healthy persons, however, suggests that retention and ability to generalize may depend heavily on the type of practice used, regardless of the learner's immediate success during the acquisition phase.[101]

Learning Paradigms. What are some of the variables that a rehabilitation team may manipulate to obtain permanent, rather than simply transitory, results during a therapy session? In healthy persons, variations on a few standard training conditions have slowed the rate of improvement or have lowered performance at the end of the acquisition phase, but, remarkably, these variations have enhanced posttraining performance.[102,126] Feedback has been provided during training by several means. Verbal or visual information in the following examples is related to the activity itself, called *knowledge of performance,* or to the consequences of the action, called *knowledge of results.*

Practice. Blocked practice, the mass repetition of drilling, improves performance during the acquisition phase. Random schedules of practice, when several motor or verbal tasks are given so no task is practiced on successive trials and repetition is widely spaced, degrade success during acquisition. Random schedules enhance retention over the long run, however, and they can improve performance in contexts other than those evident during training.[129] These findings suggest that, although random practice adds difficulty for the learner during acquisition, it prevents superficial rehearsal. Unlike blocked practice, random practice forces the learner to retrieve and to organize a different outcome for each trial.

Feedback. Practice at performing a task along a single dimension, such as tossing beanbags at one distance or moving at one speed, produces better accuracy during acquisition than variable practice in which the bags are tossed at different distances or various speeds. However, variable practice seems to force a change in behavior from trial to trial that improves performance on tests of long-term retention of the motor skill and the ability to generalize it.[102] Any schedule of feedback that is frequent and accurate and immediately modifies what the learner does increases learning during the acquisition phase, although retention has been better for learning a complex arm movement when feedback is provided after every 15 trials compared with after every trial.[103] In a name-learning experiment in which feedback about correctness was given 100% of the time or gradually withdrawn over the first few trials to 50%, learning was similar during the acquisition phase, but it was better in the 50% group as the retention interval increased.[128] The investigators suggested that too frequent feedback may interfere with information processing, response-induced kinesthetic feedback, effective error detection, or the evolution of a stabilized cognitive and motor representation that helps to sustain performance on later tests of retention.

Thus, in people without a brain injury, repetitious practice and continuous guidance improve performance during the training session, but the improvement tends not to carry over to a later time as well as when practice involves a random ordering of tasks and reinforcement is infrequent. However, several small studies of subjects with abnormal cognition point to the need for experimental assessments of these findings in the variety of patients who need neurologic rehabilitation. For example, block practice was superior to random practice in mentally retarded subjects.[44a] Also, in subjects with an acquired amnestic disorder from trauma, encephalitis, or stroke, learning strategies that lessened the likelihood that the patients would make mistakes while learning new information or a new skill led to enhanced learning and reduced forgetting compared with trial-and-error learning strategies.[124a] Thus, at least in patients with poor episodic memory (see Chapter 9) who cannot remember enough to eliminate their mistakes during training trials, errorless learning could be superior to errorful learning techniques. Other variables such as the age of a patient and the novelty of a motor task can lessen differences between the types of practice and feedback.[74a] Still, drill-sergeant therapists who try to stamp in retention of a skill with block practice and constant attention to the details of performance need to become suspicious of their results.

Techniques. One of the first formalized physical therapy techniques to draw upon the literature of motor behavior marks the transition from the neurodevelopmental to a task-oriented approach.[19] Carr and Shepherd use a model that trains functional actions in a task-specific and context-specific manner. Patients practice the action to be learned with many repetitions to strengthen muscles and to optimize learning of the target action. Their use of learning principles is less well developed.

Physical therapists are just beginning to develop interventional strategies around these notions, none of which has been adequately evaluated. Some potential practical limitations of a task-oriented model deserve mention. The physical therapist must assess and design interventions for a range of motor problems encountered during tasks. The patient must absorb cognitive information about goals and reinforcements. Training for tasks should occur in many natural or simulated settings. Changing the context of the task should allow the patient to develop better problem-solving skills, it should act as a better reinforcer, and it should lead to greater ability to generalize when the patient attempts a similar task in another setting. This technique challenges the creativity of the therapist, as well as the residual cognitive skills of the patient with brain injury. Moreover, practice takes considerable time and expense. Those who pay for rehabilitation may prefer a more cost-effective strategy based on compensatory behavior.

Paradigms must be defined, and controlled trials must be initiated to find optimal schedules for practice and for feedback during rehabilitative training. The type, frequency, intensity, and delay in providing knowledge of results or knowledge of performance require a systematic study. The practice variables in healthy persons that affect the learning of movements subserving motor functions may differ among individual patients who suffer from the spectrum of brain injuries. For the physical therapist, speech pathologist, and occupational therapist, however, any information about variations of verbal and kinesthetic feedback that may optimize their efforts is invaluable. From the point of view of neuroplasticity, rewarded, goal-directed, task-specific practice enlarges motor maps (see Chapter 1). One training paradigm may be more effective than another in altering cortical representational remodeling, however. Activation studies with functional MRI or positron emission tomography (PET) may be used to help predict whether a particular learning paradigm incorporates the neural networks that must be included to optimize the acquisition of a skill or behavior.

ELECTROMYOGRAPHIC BIOFEEDBACK

Biofeedback (BFB) includes a variety of instrumented techniques that make subjects aware of physiologic information with the goal of learning to regulate the monitored function. In the rehabilitation setting, BFB has been used especially to reduce pain and anxiety and to improve postural balance and motor performance. Electromyographic (EMG) BFB to improve upper and lower extremity muscle activity, to decrease co-contraction of muscles, and to increase functional movements has been tried in patients with many diseases, including stroke, SCI, TBI, multiple sclerosis, neuropathies, and cerebral palsy.[4] For the most part, support for this approach derives more from the enthusiasm of a case series than from controlled studies. The poor design of most clinical trials limits any conclusions about efficacy, but the evidence does not favor the general use of EMG BFB.

The link between surface EMG changes during BFB and motor control is not simple, so the rationale for using the technique has inherent scientific limitations. EMG activity and isometric muscle force in normal subjects have a linear relationship. Such is not necessarily true in spastic, paretic muscle, which has great variability in the ease of recruitment of motor units. Other confounding relationships between muscle activity and function include the velocity of movement, the muscle length when a contraction is initiated, the duration of contraction, the instructions given to perform a movement, the intent of the movement, the spontaneous strategy used, and the resulting kinematics. For example, in a study of the recovery of reaching, the peak velocity of the required movement has increased and the time to carry out the reach toward a target has decreased without an increase in the force or change in the level of surface EMG activity in associated muscles.[117]

EMG BFB is often conceptualized as a means to help the patient learn motor control. Many studies of the use of this technique for the upper extremity suggest that it can improve performance during training, but not necessarily when visual or auditory guidance is stopped. In a single training session of pursuit tracking movements in 16 patients with hemiparesis, continuous EMG BFB from the spastic elbow flexors did not improve tracking any more than in the control group. Indeed, this technique negatively affected the transfer of gains in speed and accuracy when BFB was discontinued.[7] These findings raise the issue of whether EMG feedback is likely to be more or less useful than, say, kinematic or kinetic feedback. Moreover, perhaps an intermittent, rather than a continuous, feedback schedule should be considered to increase the likelihood of transfer of the training to the condition in which it is no longer used.

EMG BFB does focus attention on and isolate a muscle for contraction or relaxation. This focus can coordinate the neural activation of paretic muscles that are under limited supraspinal control; however, the movement practiced with BFB does not obviously enable one to generalize to another, more functional movement. Given an optimal motor learning paradigm, however, BFB should help to shape a central representation during movement training. Specific uses of BFB and of functional electrical stimulation are reviewed in Chapters 7 and 8.

THERAPEUTIC MODALITIES

Musculoskeletal and radicular pain often evolve during rehabilitation and aftercare in patients with neurologic disorders. Contractures, strains, and overuse of muscles are common sequelae of limited mobility and attempts at compensation. Deep palpation for tender areas and trigger points that produce radiation of pain can help to localize the source of pain. Physical agents such as hot or cold packs, ultrasound, transcutaneous electrical nerve stimulation, and a variety of techniques of massage, acupressure, traction, and manipulation are used by physical therapists and other health care practitioners. Therapeutic effectiveness is mostly anecdotal, but few practitioners deny that these methods can contribute psychologic and physical benefits.

TRAINING AMBULATION

Gait training conventionally begins once the patient has adequate endurance and stability to stand in the parallel bars or at a hemibar. The therapist may have to block or help control a paretic leg. The therapist concentrates on the most prominent deviations from normal during the gait cycle (see Chapter 4). Instrumented analyses of gait provide the most detailed description of events during the stance and swing phases of the gait cycle. Because quantification of EMG, joint angle, kinetic forces, and temporal measures are not in general use, physical therapists rely on systematic observations to train patients in stepping. In addition, the therapy team may intervene to strengthen and coordinate muscles, to diminish hypertonicity with inhibitory exercises and antispasticity medications, and to apply orthotics and functional electrical stimulation.

Outpatient therapy tends to concentrate on improving stride length, swing and stance symmetry of the legs, speed, stair climbing, balance on uneven ground, and confidence in moving about in the community. Energy consumption is higher in patients with a limp than in those with a normal gait pattern and rises faster with an increase in speed. The therapist helps the patient find a functional compromise among speed, safety, and energy demand. Task-specific therapy for gait, including treadmill training, has been used in several small trials and shows promise in improving the quality and speed of overground ambulation.[32,37,96,123]

Assistive Devices for Gait. These devices include orthotics, canes and walkers, and wheelchairs.

Orthotics. As a result of shortened inpatient stays, ankle-foot orthoses (AFOs) tend to be used early to achieve ambulation in patients with a central or peripheral lesion. Observation of gait is usually enough to determine the need for a trial with an orthosis. Often, clinicians can judge the likelihood that the device will control the ankle and knee if they can manually stabilize the affected leg when the patient stands and bears weight on it. The physical therapist and the orthotic specialist usually determine what

type of AFO will best benefit the patient, however.

Most patients with stroke or neuropathy can be managed with a thermoplastic orthosis (Fig. 3–1). This device fits into a shoe secured by laces or Velcro straps. A metal double-upright brace (Fig. 3–2) offers greater rigidity for mediolateral instability and allows more versatility in adjustments for the amount of plantarflexion and dorsiflexion, but it tends to be more expensive, heavy, and cosmetically unappealing to the patient with hemiplegia. Metal bracing systems find more use in selected patients with paraplegia from SCI and in those with poliomyelitis.

Indications for an AFO include inadequate dorsiflexion for initial heel contact or for toe clearance during midswing, excessive hip hiking during swing, mediolateral subtalar instability during stance, tibial instability during stance, uncontrolled foot place-

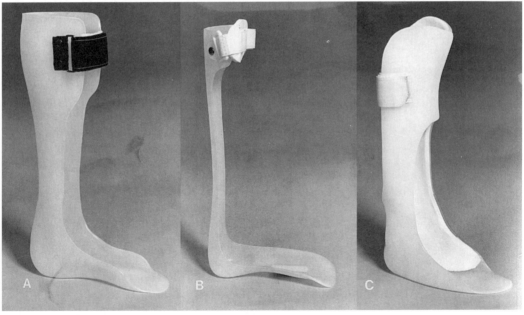

Figure 3–1. Solid ankle, thermoplastic, molded ankle-foot orthoses (AFOs) that fit into a shoe. (*A*) This lightweight, cosmetically acceptable design can help control the motion of the ankle in the sagittal plane, thus aiding heel strike and toe clearance and limiting knee flexion or extension, depending upon the angle at which the ankle joint is set. Greater stability for varus and valgus control is achieved by extending the mediolateral flanges at the distal leg and around the foot and by using straps with Velcro closures across the front of the ankle. (*B*) This leaf-spring variation in design offers little mediolateral control but permits flexibility at the ankle during the phases of stance, while preventing foot drop during swing. (*C*) The padded anterior solid portion of this ankle-foot orthosis (AFO) encourages knee extension when it presses against the proximal tibia during late stance. (*Courtesy of NovaCare Orthotics, Los Angeles, CA.*)

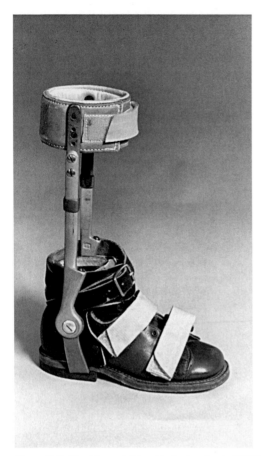

siflexion increases walking speed, increases the duration of heel strike and midstance, and improves the knee flexion moment in midstance.[68]

An articulated AFO with a posterior stop (Fig. 3–3) prevents plantarflexion due to hypertonicity, but it permits dorsiflexion and makes standing up easier because of the give at the ankle. In patients with greater spasticity, the plastic may be extended toward the forefoot and higher up the tibia. A pad under the distal metatarsal can reduce clawing of the toes. The lateral flanges can be extended for varus and valgus control of the ankle. Padding helps to protect the skin. Clinicians must monitor the patient for signs of pressure over the skin, especially over the

Figure 3–2. Double upright ankle-foot orthosis (AFO) for a child offers greater rigidity for control than the design in Figure 3–1A. The shoe stirrup of this metal alloy brace articulates with joints at the ankle that connect the vertical bars, which terminate at a rigid calf band fastened by Velcro closures. The design permits sagittal adjustments to the motion of the ankle and limits eversion and inversion of the foot. For example, the ankle joint can allow slight movement in the sagittal plane to provide dorsiflexion assistance or can be set to hold the foot in slight plantarflexion or dorsiflexion as needed as the gait pattern evolves. (*Courtesy of NovaCare Orthotics, Los Angeles, CA.*)

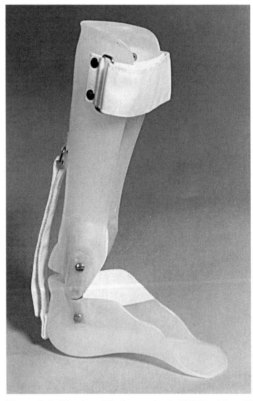

Figure 3–3. Plastic ankle-foot orthosis (AFO) with ankle articulation provides mediolateral stability and allows less superimposed control of the ankle as the patient's motor control improves. The articulation permits the tibia to flex over the foot upon standing up. This design includes a dorsiflexion strap stop. (*Courtesy of NovaCare Orthotics, Los Angeles, CA.*)

ment due to sensory loss, and an operative heel cord lengthening. If the knee of a patient with hemiplegia buckles during stance, angling the AFO in slight plantarflexion will extend the knee earlier. Dorsiflexing the AFO decreases knee hyperextension and helps prevent the snapping back that causes instability and pain in midstance. In patients with hemiplegia, an AFO in 5 degrees of dor-

malleoli. Velcro straps allow one-handed closure of the brace and can help to hold the heel in place. As the patient regains greater leg control, remodeling can include changing the angle or cutting away the medial and lateral flanges or the tibial portion to give the AFO greater flexibility.

Lightweight plastic knee-ankle-foot orthoses (KAFOs) with locking metal knee joints can assist patients with profound polyneuropathy, muscular dystrophy, myelomeningocele, and SCI. Orthotic systems with wire cables that link flexion of one hip to extension of the opposite hip for patients with paraplegia are described in Chapter 8 on SCI.

Canes and Walkers. These devices improve stability through a lever arm that handles a modest force, generates a moment to assist the hip abductor muscles and to reduce loading on the knee, and shares the body's weight between the leg and the device. The metabolic energy expenditure of various forms of assisted gait varies with the device, with the impairment, with the patient's cardiovascular status, and especially with the patient's upper limb strength.[28]

Walking aids fall into several categories, although many models exist for each. Clinicians can obtain some sense of what may help most by walking beside and slightly behind the patient while gently holding onto a safety belt. Clinicians can also let the patient use the clinician's forearms as a walker and test for the force exerted on their arms, while observing the patient's balance. Placing a hand under the patient's grip on a cane or walker provides a sense of how much weight the patient needs to transfer to the device. Rolling walkers allow a step-through gait pattern, whereas a pick-up walker tends to foster a step-to pattern. Single-point canes offer the narrowest base of support and vary in whether forces are distributed directly beneath or in front of the tip. Quadcanes and hemiwalkers offer a wider base for stability. A cane held opposite the paretic leg helps to keep the pelvis level during stance on the weak leg. The cane should swing forward with the involved limb and should bear the most weight during stance on that leg. Handgrips are usually set at a height that allows about 20 to 30 degrees of elbow flexion.

For patients with ataxia, heavy walkers with brakes and wheels are best.

Wheelchairs. Wheelchair prescriptions must take into account many factors, particularly for the highly mobile patient with paraplegia or the patient with quadriparesis who needs an electric wheelchair system.[39] A prescription specifies the dimensions and components listed in Table 3–2. Many models of different weights and materials are available from vendors. Wheelchair clinics have been created in many rehabilitation facilities to bring in representatives of manufacturers to match the patient's needs. Considerations include safety, comfort, trunk and thigh support, skin and pressure-point protection, type of transfers into the chair, ease of propulsion, transportability, use for recreation or on uneven terrain, special accommodations for work, control systems,

Table 3–2. WHEELCHAIR PRESCRIPTION PARAMETERS

Frame
  Material
  Weight
Seat
  Height, width, depth, angle
  Sling or cushioned; inserts
  Cushion: foam, air, fluid, gel, gelfoam
Back
  Height; fixed or reclining; head rest
  Flexible, custom molded; foam or gel inserts
Arms
  Height: fixed or adjustable
  Fixed, removable, swingaway
  Arm troughs; clear plastic lap board; power
    controls
Leg and footrest
  Height; adjustment from edge of seat
  Fixed, removable, swingaway; straps
Wheels
  Materials: alloys, plastic
  Tires: width, tread; pneumatic or solid
  Angulation
  Handrims
Front casters
Brakes: locking, backsliding
Antitip bars
Power supply; control system

barriers such as narrow doorways, and anticipation of changes related to progression of impairments. For example, the patient with hemiplegia may require a seat set low enough to allow one leg to help propel the chair. A powered wheelchair run by a joystick, a sip-and-puff device, the patient's chin, or voice-command controller may be ideal for a patient with quadriparesis who has cerebral palsy or a cervical SCI, but would be hazardous for a patient with hemi-inattention or poor judgment.

Motorized scooters with three or four wheels are convenient for community mobility for patients who are limited to home ambulation. Some patients with paraparesis, particularly those with multiple sclerosis or diseases of the motor unit such as polio, find that scooters allow them efficient mobility. These patients must be able to transfer themselves to the scooter easily, and they must have good trunk and upper extremity motor control. A portable telephone in the home and a cellular telephone for the community provide great convenience and a measure of safety to the patient confined to a wheelchair or scooter. Ongoing studies in ergonomics, engineering, computerized safety and control devices, and materials for seating systems, wheels, and frames should continue to refine the wheelchair.

OCCUPATIONAL THERAPISTS

Responsibilities

The philosophic foundation of occupational therapy is that purposeful activity helps prevent and remediate dysfunction and elicits maximal adaptation.[59] These goal-oriented tasks are meant to be culturally meaningful and important to the needs of clients and their families. Activities include exercise, recreation, crafts, and daily life and work skills.

Occupational therapists bring expertise to the rehabilitation team in enhancing the independence and personal satisfaction of patients in their ADLs, community and leisure activities, social integration, and work performance. They tend to manage the training of an affected upper extremity and assess the need for slings, splints, and orthotics for the shoulder and hand. For patients with stroke and brain injury, therapists work closely with the neuropsychologist to address visuospatial inattention, memory loss, apraxia, difficulties in problem solving, and the skills needed to return these patients to school or employment. Many occupational therapists evaluate and manage dysphagia. They establish the need for a range of assistive devices. In the patient's home and workplace, therapists provide grab bars, rails, ramps, environmental controls, architectural changes such as widening of doorways to allow wheelchair access, and emergency remote-control calling systems. For the working person with a disability, the therapist can design a work-hardening program to prevent back injuries or pain from overuse of a joint or muscle.

Interventions

For neurologic rehabilitation, theories about assessment and intervention by the occupational therapist are perhaps less developed than for the physical therapist.[109] The approaches of occupational therapists rely on behavioral and educational techniques that combine skill training, compensation, and environmental adaptation. These techniques emphasize verbal, visual, or manual patterning of the patient through parts of a task, then through the entire task, with frequent positive feedback. Some therapists use NDT and EMG BFB techniques for the upper extremity.

Task-oriented and motor learning strategies are beginning to gain attention.[75,91] Using this approach, the occupational therapist presents activities in a way that elicits the retention and transfer of particular skills for use in a functional setting.[55] For example, upper extremity reaching by patients with spasticity after TBI improves the arm's range of motion significantly more during game playing than during rote exercise.[106] Neurodevelopmental handling and positioning techniques can provide cues for postural alignment during functional movement activities. However, training of postural adjustments may improve with active planning, initiation, execution, and termination of the motor sequence through open-ended tasks and random practice on several tasks in the same training session that require postural adjustments.[98] These approaches to skills training are especially appropriate to achieving what may be considered the primary goal of the occupational therapist, which is to help patients become competent problem solvers for a variety of functional tasks and in different performance contexts.

A behavioral approach that can be considered a corollary to the task-oriented motor learning concept has shown promise in patients with hemiparesis who have at least 20 degrees of wrist extension and 10 degrees of finger extension. The strategy calls for forced use of the affected upper extremity and gradual shaping of a variety of functional movements to overcome what is theorized to be learned nonuse of the limb.[115] Learned nonuse may derive from unsuccessful early attempts to use the affected limb after a stroke or, in studies of monkeys, after deafferentation.[63] This failure leads to behavioral suppression and masks any subsequent ability to use the limb. Positive reinforcement comes from successful use of the unaffected limb, which leads to the permanent compensatory behavior for nonuse of the paretic hand. Restraining the unaffected arm and engaging the affected arm in the practice of functional tasks has improved the strength, frequency, and quality of daily arm use in a 2-week trial.[116] The addition of a shaping paradigm of reinforcement to elicit functional movements appears to have a longer-lasting effect than conditioned-response training.[115] In the shaping paradigm, the patient may obtain feedback during the steps it takes to improve from a rudimentary early training response, such as slow extension of the elbow, to a more complex response, such as using the proximal arm to push a shuffleboard puck to a target. The shaped movement is complex, has functional significance to the person, and takes considerable training to achieve, so it seems likely to carry over into daily activities, thereby ending the period of nonuse. As discussed earlier, therapy structured around learning new sensorimotor relationships in the wake of altered motor control seems more likely to be effective than methods that foster only a developmental sequence.

ORTHOTICS

Upper extremity orthoses are frequently used for patients with upper and lower motoneuron impairments. These devices can stabilize a joint in a chosen position, produce stretch and prevent contracture, assist the function of nearby muscles that would otherwise be at a biomechanical disadvantage, provide an attachment for an assistive device, and, perhaps, reduce hypertonicity. Static orthoses allow no motion of the primary joint. Dynamic orthoses use elastic, wire, or powered levers that compensate for weakness or an imbalance in strength and allow some controlled movement. Devices for prehension are finger or wrist driven.

Shoulder slings and resting hand splints may improve function when they are used early, when they influence tone, or when they limit contracture and pain, but the supporting data are scanty.[85] Dorsal and volar resting splints that extend up the forearm and across the wrist have been found in some small studies to reduce tone in adults and children.[34,79] Dorsal splints that provide a Bobath reflex-inhibiting pattern and splints that partially supinate the forearm and abduct the thumb and fingers are also said to be effective.[20] Therapists have used an inflatable splint around the patient's whole forearm and hand with fingers in abduction to produce a similar inhibitory effect, although the technique was not found to be efficacious as a resting splint in one trial.[92] The daily amount of wear, length of time of use, and lasting effect after removal vary considerably in these studies. Thus, the choice of a splint often depends more on personal experience than on objective data. Cost effectiveness is uncertain.

The hemicuff and Bobath slings are often used to reduce shoulder subluxation as a prophylactic measure to avoid pain. Adjustable fabric shoulder straps pull the cloth cuff around the patient's elbow and forearm and lift the humerus toward the glenoid fossa. The Bobath sling raises the humeral head by means of a foam rubber roll under the axilla. Other than serving as a warning not to yank the patient's arm, however, these slings have not been shown to prevent a painful shoulder.

ADAPTIVE AIDS

Adaptive aids are assistive devices that extend capabilities for home, work, and leisure. Recent designs for items from wheelchairs to utensils create a positive, even a sporty image. Clever industrial designs, lightweight materials, computers, and electronics offer a growing list of ways to diminish disabilities. Computer manufacturers, including Apple and IBM, have developed programs for people with special needs. Table 3–3 lists some especially functional, off-the-shelf items. Other simple or highly engineered items can contribute to independent living.[33,108]

Many different portable communication devices are available commercially for the patient who cannot speak and has little or no limb movement. Some software can "learn" to predict the next word and can list words and word endings often chosen by the user. These packages include speech synthesizers. Portable computers can be controlled with small, one-handed keyboards or microswitches that move a cursor with a flicker of the user's residual motion, even if that motion is only a twitch of the frontalis muscle. Patients can operate on-screen keyboards by using a mouse under ultrasonic or infrared head control, by blowing into a straw, and by voice recognition. With additional interfaces, these controls can access telephones, lights, alarms, intercoms, and other electronic equipment at home and at work. These devices are of particular value to the patient with quadriparesis from SCI, amyotrophic lateral sclerosis, or stroke. The Applied Science and Engineering Laboratories at the University of Delaware's A. I. duPont Institute regularly publish an evaluation of computer devices and software for communication.

More remarkable tools for the disabled will be available soon. These include robotic manipulators,[51] mobile robots,[95] manipulations of a virtual reality environment, and neural prostheses.[74] Already, interfaces that can convert a muscle motion or an eye movement or a cerebral biosignal into a control signal for a computer are available (e.g., BioControl Systems, Inc., Palo Alto, CA). For the profoundly immobile patient, electroencephalographic rhythms, ready potentials such as the P300, and evoked potentials such as the visual-evoked response are being developed to control a cursor and to command a computer that interfaces with the person's environment.[77,114] As aids become more sophisticated, designers and manufacturers will have to consider the varied needs of the disabled person, or clever products in search of a use will result.[6]

SPEECH AND LANGUAGE THERAPISTS

At least one in three early survivors of an acute stroke or serious TBI has dysarthric

Table 3–3. ADAPTIVE AIDS FOR DAILY LIVING

Feeding
  Utensil: thickened or palm handle; cuff holder
  Dish: scoop; food guard; suction holder
  Cup: no-spill covers; holders; straws

Bathing
  Shower seat, transfer bench
  Washing: mitt, long-handle scrub brush, hose
  Safety: grab bars; tub rails

Dressing
  Velcro closure: shoes, pants
  Button hook, zipper pull
  Low closet rods

Toileting
  Toilet safety rails; raised seat
  Commode

Mobility
  Prefabricated ramps
  Stair lifts
  Transfer devices and ceiling-mounted track lifts
  Automobile: lifts; hand controls

Computer workstation
  Environmental controls
  Communication: printing; voice synthesis
  Interface adaptations: keyboard, microswitch, voice activation

Miscellaneous
  One-handed jar opener
  Doorknob extension
  Book holder, page turner
  Holder for cutting with loop scissor or knife
  Long-reach grabbers

speech or aphasia. Dementias, brain tumors, meningoencephalitides, and other neurologic diseases also affect language. The prevalence of aphasia is uncertain, but given the frequency of these entities, an annual incidence of 200,000 cases seems likely. Articulatory disorders and oropharyngeal dysphagia are even more common, in both acute and chronic or degenerative neurologic diseases. Speech therapists generally take the lead in assessing and managing these problems. Because neurogenic dysphagia has significant medical consequences, its assessment and management are covered in Chapter 6.

Responsibilities

DYSARTHIA

Dysarthria arises from injury to the neural pathways for articulation, the shaping of sounds within the mouth. Weakness, slowness, and incoordination can be appreciated in a patient's phonation, respiratory support for speech, resonance, and prosody. Therapists also characterize the patient's vocal quality, pitch, and loudness, particularly for sounds made with the vocal cords abducted (voiceless sounds such as "f" and "s") or adducted and vibrating (voiced sounds such as "v" and "z"). Laryngoscopy and pulmonary function tests, such as forced expiratory volume measurements, can help to localize associated impairments. Acoustic analysis provides an objective measure of the dysphonic voice and can guide therapy.[62]

A few syndromes are common. Bilateral cerebral lesions produce pseudobulbar palsy with spastic dysarthia. This effortful articulation is hyponasal, harsh, and strained. The flaccid dysarthia from lower motoneuron and motor unit dysfunction is characterized by breathy, hypernasal, imprecise articulation in short phrases. Other categories include the monotonous, soft rushes of Parkinson's hypokinetic dysarthia, the distortions associated with dystonias, and the dysrhythmic pitch and prosody of ataxic dysarthia.

APHASIA

The speech and language therapist must determine whether a patient has a disorder of language and, if so, the way in which it relates to overall cognitive function. Formal and informal testing leads to a classification of the problem. Many formal tests of the components of speech and language have come into common use by therapists and for clinical studies. Table 3–4 lists some useful standardized tests.

Table 3–5 lists the most common clinico-anatomic classification of the aphasias. As locations on a map of brain and language, this schematic is highly simplified. For example, Broca's aphasia involves several regions of the left hemisphere in addition to the frontal operculum and usually evolves from incomplete recovery of a more severe aphasia.[83] The presence or absence of the pathways for activational, semantic, motor planning, and articulatory aspects of language determines the kind of function that may follow this anterior injury.

From 20 to 50 percent of patients with aphasia do not easily fit into a classic category.[104] Many have partial features or mixed syndromes with an emphasis on components of language that are associated with anterior, posterior, or subcortical lesions. Some studies have found so little correlation between the traditional aphasia subtype classification and anatomic localization that they question its usefulness.[124] For rehabilitation therapy,

Table 3–4. DIAGNOSTIC TESTS FOR APHASIA

General[2]
  Porch Index of Communicative Ability (PICA)
  Boston Diagnostic Aphasia Examination
    (BDAE)
    Aphasia Severity Rating Scale
    Rating Scale Profile of Speech
      Characteristics
  Neurosensory Center Comprehensive
    Examination for Aphasia (NCCEA)
  Western Aphasia Battery (WAB)
  Communication Abilities in Daily Living
    (CADL)
  Functional Communication Profile (FCP)
Specialized
  Token Test
  Boston Naming Test
  Boston Assessment of Severe Aphasia
    (BASA)[50]

Table 3–5. **TRADITIONAL APHASIA SYNDROMES**

Type	Expression	Comprehension	Repetition	Brodmann's Area Injured	Adjunct Therapy
Broca's	Effortful, nonfluent, agrammatic Anomia: proper and common nouns Proper nouns	Mostly intact	Impaired; best for nouns and action verbs	44, 45; ± nearby 6, 8, 9, 10, 46, subcortex 20, 21 38	MIT; VCIU; manual signing; HELPSS; RET; MIPT; bromocriptine
Wernicke's	Melodic, fluent, phoneme and word choice errors	Impaired; reading better	Impaired	22; ± 37, 39, 40	SLAC
Global	Nonfluent; expletives; facial and intonation expression	Poor; best for personally relevant material	Absent	Above combined	VAT; symbols; computerized systems
Conduction	Fluent; letter and word substitutions	Mostly intact	Poor for sentences and multisyllabic words	40, 41, 42 subinsula	PACE
Transcortical Motor	Decreased fluency	Mostly intact	Mostly intact	Anterosuperior to Broca's	Bromocriptine
Sensory	Fluent; substitutions	Impaired	Mostly intact	Posteroinferior to Wernicke's	
Subcortical Basal ganglia	Transient mutism; decreased fluency or dysarthria	Mildly impaired	Intact or mildly impaired	Caudate head, anterior limb of internal capsule	
Thalamus	Fluent; neologisms	Mildly impaired	Intact	Anterolateral	
Right hemisphere	Impaired prosody and organization of a narrative	Impaired recognition of emotional tone	Impaired attention	Parallels with Broca's and Wernicke's areas	

HELPSS, Helm Elicited Language Program for Syntax Stimulation; MIPT, Multiple Input Phoneme Therapy; MIT, Melodic Intonation Therapy; PACE, Promoting Aphasics' Communicative Effectiveness; RET, Response Elaboration Training; SLAC, Sentence Level Auditory Comprehension; VAT, Visual Action Therapy; VCIU, Voluntary Control of Involuntary Utterance.

the broadly defined features used to classify patients often do not address in enough detail the underlying disturbances of aphasic language. Thus, traditional pigeonholes may not direct treatment optimally.

Interventions

DYSARTHRIA

Therapies aim to improve the patient's intelligibility, volume, and fluidity by means of exercises for the affected muscles. Patients may slow their articulation, use shorter sentences, extend the jaw's motion, or exaggerate articulatory movements. Behavioral retraining methods include pacing and delayed auditory feedback. Some patients benefit from oral prosthetic devices when weakness of muscles around the velopharyngeal port impairs resonance. Apraxia of oromotor function, which refers to the inability to perform volitional movements with the articulators, is managed by methods that overlap those used to treat dysarthria.

APHASIA

Treatment for aphasia is based on the clinical evaluation of the patient's cognitive and linguistic assets and deficits. This treatment is refined by standardized language and neuropsychologic tests, knowledge of the cortical and subcortical structures that are damaged, and the ongoing response to specific therapies. The patient's casual interactions with the family and the rehabilitation team often broaden the therapist's analysis of the patient's linguistic and nonlinguistic strengths and weaknesses for communication. The speech therapist must assist the team, as well as the patient, to understand the processes and strategies that the patient uses to communicate. Successful treatment approaches depend on the profile of impaired and spared abilities and build upon the patient's residual problem-solving strategies. Language therapists usually use an idiosyncratic combination of techniques. The overall efficacy of aphasia therapy after stroke is discussed in Chapter 7.

General Strategies. In a general sense, speech therapists attempt to find ways to circumvent, deblock, or help the patient compensate for defective language behaviors. For patients with impaired expression and comprehension of language, finding a way to obtain reliable verbal or gestural "yes-no" responses quickly is essential. Otherwise, these patients may feel isolated and withdraw from persons around them. Initial treatments for aphasia often deal with tasks that relate to self-care, the immediate environment, and emotionally positive experiences. As specific syndromes of impairments become apparent during assessment and treatment, a variety of specific techniques can be applied. The most common interventions use visual and verbal cueing techniques, which include picture-matching and sentence-completion tasks, along with frequent repetition and positive reinforcement as the patient approaches the desired responses (Table 3–6). One note of caution. Some patients become upset and withdraw from therapists and from family or friends whom they perceive to be talking down to

Table 3–6. SOME TRADITIONAL THERAPY TASKS IN APHASIA

Body part identification

Word discrimination

Word-to-picture matching

Yes-no response reliability

Auditory processing at the phrase level, then at the sentence level

Reading at the word level, phrase level, and then sentence level

Gestural expression and pointing

Oral-motor imitation

Phoneme repetition, then word repetition

Verbal cueing for words and sentence completion

Contextual cueing

Phonemic and semantic word retrieval strategies

Priming for responses

Melodic stimulation

Graphic tasks: tracing, copying, word completions

Calculations

Pragmatic linguistic and nonlinguistic conversational skills

Psychosocial supports

them. Nothing turns these patients away from therapy more than seemingly irrelevant, simple, repetitive tasks.

Pragmatics refers to the use of language in a social context. Along with the attentional and memory deficits and other cognitive problems of the patient after TBI, this aspect of communication is most often impaired. The Communication Abilities in Daily Living (CADLs) and the Pragmatic Protocol are useful assessment tools.[94] Behavioral techniques tend to be used to improve skills in eye contact, body posture, initiating and staying on a topic of conversation, turn-taking during conversation, adapting to the needs of the listener, and using speech to warn, assert, request, acknowledge, or comment.

Therapies for Specific Syndromes. A few techniques have been designed and evaluated for specific aphasia syndromes and neurolinguistic impairments.[18,46,65] The evidence for efficacy of these structured approaches to difficulties in expression and comprehension rests on small group and case studies. Table 3–5 lists the most thoroughly evaluated adjunct techniques that include a well-documented procedure for the intervention.

Melodic intonation therapy (MIT) is one of the few interventions that can be defined and applied consistently enough to make it applicable for research.[87] In MIT, therapist and patient melodically intone multisyllabic words and commonly used short phrases while the therapist taps the patient's left hand to mark each syllable.[48,110] Gradually, the continuous voicing and tapping are withdrawn. MIT works best in patients with Broca's aphasia with sparse or stereotyped nonsense speech and good auditory comprehension. Short-term, qualitative benefits have resulted from this demanding approach.

When a single sound, word, or phrase overwhelms any other attempted output, the Voluntary Control of Involuntary Utterance (VCIU) program can help the patient gain control over perseverative intrusions.[45]

The agrammatism of Broca's aphasia has been treated with the Helm Elicited Language Program for Syntax Stimulation (HELPSS),[49] which uses a series of drawings that picture common activities. The therapist provides a brief verbal description that ends with a question about the story and contains a target sentence. When the patient responds with the target words, the patient is then asked to complete the story without benefit of having heard the target sentence. Each probe seeks a target response that requires an increasingly more difficult syntactic construction.

Some patients with little or only stereotyped output, even patients with impaired comprehension, have responded to multiple input phoneme therapy (MIPT).[112] This 22-step hierarchic program aims to build from an analysis of phonemes produced by the patient to eliciting a target phoneme to achieving consonant blends, multisyllabic words, and eventually sentence production.

Response elaboration training (RET) shapes and chains the responses patients give to their descriptions of familiar activities in line drawings.[60] This technique reinforces informational content, rather than linguistic form.

Some patients with mute or nonfluent aphasia can acquire a limited but useful repertoire of gestures using, for example, American Indian sign language.[41]

Attempts to improve comprehension in patients with global and Wernicke's aphasia have taken many forms. The Sentence Level Auditory Comprehension (SLAC) program trains patients to discriminate consonant-vowel-consonant words that are the same or that differ by only one phoneme (e.g., bill, pill, fill).[84] Patients then try to associate the word sounds with the written word and later try to identify the target word embedded in a sentence. Gains in some patients have generalized to improve scores on the Token Test for comprehension.

For patients with global aphasia, nonverbal communication with pantomime through a technique called Visual Action Therapy (VAT) has decreased limb apraxia and has improved auditory comprehension.[47] The technique called Promoting Aphasics' Communicative Effectiveness (PACE) emphasizes ideas to be conveyed in face-to-face interactions, rather than linguistic accuracy.[27] This technique aims to develop any modality that can be used to transmit a message, such as limited speech, limb or facial gestures, and drawing. The success of these techniques suggests that the left hemisphere has a linguistic, rather than a general, symbolic specialization for the components of language. It produces sign and spoken language, whereas both hemispheres are capable of producing the nonlinguistic gestures of pantomime.[24]

One study of writing to dictation with the right arm attached to a skateboard prosthesis and a penholder suggests that the observed success in writing single words may come from the activation of preprocessing levels of language in association with older, proximal motor systems.[15] Use of the proximal arm for pointing to pictured objects can also improve simultaneous vocal naming.[44]

Programmed instruction techniques have been combined with operant conditioning.[71] Efficacy is unclear.

Some preliminary studies suggest that priming techniques (see Chapter 9) may improve certain language functions. Priming is a phenomenon found even in patients with amnesia in whom cues and prompts result in the recall of previously provided information. A patient with poor comprehension of spoken words had normal levels of priming on two auditory priming tasks, even though the patient had not comprehended the studied items.[100] Auditory perceptual priming may, then, depend upon access to a presemantic auditory word-form system. Related techniques that expose patients with aphasia to target items may also improve their performance by using implicit or nonconscious memory. Implicit reading strategies can also be used to help the patient with alexia to read. A task that asks the patient with alexia to name a written word tends to produce a letter-by-letter reading strategy.[25] When instructed to make a lexical decision or a semantic judgment about rapidly presented words, some patients use a whole-word strategy.

Some of the foregoing strategies, such as the SLAC program,[17] investigate and treat aphasia from the approach of the neurolinguist's understanding of phonemic, syntactic, and lexical deviations. Impairments and their treatment are defined in terms of multicomponent information processors that activate the major classes of linguistic representations of the code for language. Within a conceptual model, a patient can be diagnosed with any number of language processing impairments, instead of with a specific syndrome of aphasia. The aim of the neurolinguistic assessment of aphasia is to specify the types of representations or units of language, such as simple words, word formations, sentences, and discourse, that are abnormally processed during speech, auditory comprehension, reading, and writing.[18] For each unit, the therapist ascertains the way in which the disturbance affects linguistic forms, such as phonemes, syntactic structures, and semantic meanings. Some of these distinctions are made by a speech therapist's traditional evaluation. For example, the therapist may assess differences in the patient's ability to express or understand words that are familiar or novel, regular or irregular, and concrete or abstract. A traditional analysis often is not as detailed as a neurolinguistic study, however. Perhaps greater clarification of the nature of patients' impairments will produce additional therapeutic strategies,[17,82] based on the real architecture of language processing.

Iconic Language. After extensive training, some patients benefit from learning alternative languages. These include the Blisssymbol lexicon,[56] which includes 100 icons for concrete objects and concepts, and computerized visual communication systems,[111] which use symbols to create a syntax and vocabulary. Lingraphica (Tolfa Corporation, Mountain View, CA) is a commercially available language prosthesis that combines spoken and printed words with about 2000 concept images with storyboards. Microcomputer-based therapies have been suggested for a hierarchic approach to aphasic neurolinguistic impairments. These techniques have been successful in treating specific problems, such as to improve the ability to name an item presented visually.[29]

Pharmacotherapy. Pharmacotherapy is another potential adjunctive treatment for aphasia.[107] Several small group and case studies suggest that bromocriptine, in an average dose of 30 mg, or with carbidopa and levodopa, can improve the fluency of moderately affected patients with chronic Broca's and transcortical motor aphasia.[1,99] However, a placebo-controlled trial using 15 mg of bromocriptine in 20 patients with chronic nonfluent aphasia reported no change in speech, language, or cognitive skills.[80] Hemidystonia on the paretic side, sometimes with painful spasms, developed in 5 of 7 patients with chronic nonfluent aphasia who were given 30 to 60 mg of bromocriptine daily.[69] Speech therapy has also been paired with 10 mg to 15 mg of *d*-amphetamine in acute cases. Purported improvements were found in an uncontrolled protocol.[121]

The reported decrease in hesitations and the improvement in word finding may be related to a drug-induced increase in activity in dopaminergic and noradrenergic pathways for arousal, attention, and intention after interruption of projections from the ventral tegmental tract and from diffuse frontal projections. These drugs can alter mood as well. Pharmacotherapy given to patients during language therapy appears to hold some promise, although the proof of this benefit will require carefully designed trials. As pharmacotherapeutic adjuncts are tried in single-case study designs, rehabilitationists must also consider whether other drugs that affect the central nervous system may modulate neurotransmitter and receptor function in a way that negatively affects recovery.

Therapeutic strategies in the future are likely to encompass the combined analytic approaches of speech pathology, neurolinguistics, neuropsychology, neuroimaging, pharmacology, and computer sciences. This combined approach should lead to theory-based treatments that will define the short-term and long-term benefits of a specific intervention on a particular aspect of language. Single-case studies and clinical trials should also address the optimal intensity, duration, and learning paradigm for a treatment.

NEUROPSYCHOLOGISTS

Neuropsychologists with skills in clinical psychology help to define and manage cognitive impairments and mood and behavioral disorders. Their responsibilities range from counseling the patient, the rehabilitation team, and the patient's family on managing these problems to interpreting formal neuropsychologic tests in relation to the patient's functional needs. Neuropsychologists

who specialize in TBI may set up a token reward-based economy to reinforce appropriate social interactions or develop learning paradigms for patients with disorders of memory. Neuropsychologists specializing in patients with stroke may help the team work through patients' visuoperceptual and hemi-inattentional impairments and may identify brain and behavior abnormalities. Although neuropsychologists can administer many neuropsychologic tools, no single battery of tests has won the approval of these clinicians (see Chapter 5). With their background in biostatistics and the design of experimental studies, these professionals can contribute to the assessment of interventions.

The neuropsychologist can also aid the team in identifying a posttraumatic stress disorder (PTSD) in patients or in family members who witnessed the anxiety-provoking onset of a stroke, SCI, or TBI. Although little is yet known about the risk in a rehabilitation population, the rate of PTSD among young urban adults is 24%, and the lifetime prevalence is 9%.[12] Symptom criteria include emotional numbness or constriction and avoidance, the phenomenon of re-experiencing aspects of the traumatic event, and hyperarousal. The neuropsychologist may need to undertake considerable detective work to identify environmental events that symbolize or resemble the traumatic event and produce the equivalent of a startle response. Posttraumatic amnesia and other memory, cognitive, and behavioral disorders may mask or delay the onset of PTSD in patients. The National Center for PTSD Clinician-Administered PTSD Scale helps to evaluate the frequency and intensity of symptoms and their impact.[9]

SOCIAL WORKERS

Social workers identify financial, family, and community resources that allow optimal continuity of care and disposition from inpatient rehabilitation. The psychosocial training of these workers puts them in the best position to provide family caregivers with a realistic assessment of the physical and emotional burden that will follow discharge from an inpatient facility. Social workers often address familial conflicts and emotional

Table 3–7. GENERAL INSTRUMENTS THAT MEASURE PSYCHOSOCIAL ADJUSTMENT

General Health Questionnaire-60
Millon Behavioral Health Inventory
Psychosocial Adjustment to Illness Scale
Sickness Index Profile
Acceptance of Loss Scale

issues with a short course of crisis intervention. Along with the psychologist, social workers are the most likely team members to recognize substance abuse, PTSD, suicidal thoughts, and psychopathologic processes that may interfere with inpatient and outpatient care.

Adjustment to neurologic disability involves a gradual process of psychologic assimilation to changes in body image, self-concept, and ability to interact with the environment.[73] Social workers can be aided in the assessment and management of patients' psychosocial adjustment by some standard measures (Table 3–7). These scales have considerable weaknesses, however.[73]

Social workers use a variety of interventions. Traditional psychotherapeutic theories and strategies draw upon concepts of personality and self-awareness. Behavioral therapy tries to eliminate maladaptive behaviors to disability and to condition acceptable behaviors. Educational approaches provide accurate information that aims to reduce anxiety and misconceptions about impairments and disability. Patients can also learn coping skills and methods to help solve problems. Social workers often develop support groups that exchange ideas.

The mechanisms and outcomes of psychosocial supports and other adaptations for coping with a sudden or chronic neurologic disability require more research.[21,67]

RECREATIONAL THERAPISTS

Recreational therapists involve patients in an inpatient facility in group games, crafts, and other activities to help them socialize and enjoy the physical and emotional value of recreation. This therapy sets the tone for outpatient activities for fitness and recreation that foster socialization.

An adequate level of fitness may reduce the long-term risk of mortality from cardiovascular disease and cancer.[8] Even low-intensity exercise, the equivalent of brisk walking to increase heart rate to the range of 120 to 140 beats per minute, done three times a week for 20 minutes, achieves this level of fitness. The Centers For Disease Control and Prevention has recommended 30 minutes or more of moderate-intensity physical activity at least 5 days a week.[90] In wheelchair-bound outpatients with paraplegia, participation in sports and recreation can produce a more rapid increase in upper body strength than can routine physical therapy alone. This activity also more fully reintegrates these patients into the community and enhances self-esteem.[54] Depression has been associated with low levels of physical and recreational activity in nondisabled women.[35] Little activity may be an even more important risk factor in the disabled population.

An increase in physical activity, whether through a fitness program, recreation, or competitive sports, seems likely to improve the disabled person's quality of life.[105] Many opportunities are available to people with physical disabilities. For example, advances in equipment design for wheelchairs make racing, basketball, and tennis possible. The same holds for snow skiing.[22,66] Over 200 local, national, and international organizations have developed rules and equipment for at least 50 sports and recreational activities that take into account a range of functional abilities.[31,89] Self-esteem and problem-solving skills can grow as one learns a martial art or follows outdoor experiential educational pursuits that, for example, use ropes courses.

More research is needed to design exercise and recreational programs for young and older persons with neurologic diseases. These studies should assess both useful and possibly injurious effects. Outcome measures may include changes in medical morbidity, ADLs, leisure-time physical activity, and quality of life, with follow-up through middle and late life. Sports and exercise activities can easily be incorporated into subacute and chronic neurologic rehabilitation programs to enhance and maintain functional recovery and to build self-esteem.

OTHER TEAM MEMBERS

The rehabilitation team consults many other professionals, including case managers who act as ombudsmen for patients, nutritionists, vocational counselors, bioengineers, orthotists, and, increasingly, clinical researchers and statisticians. The ethicist may become an even more valued team member. Ethical dilemmas are bound to increase as society sets limits on who receives what treatment and for what amount of time. Will we no longer accept elderly inpatients who are not candidates for cardiopulmonary resuscitation? Will we no longer provide rehabilitation if it is less expensive for patients to remain disabled? Will we be able to apply group studies of cost-effective interventions to individual patients?

Staying current within their areas of expertise has become an increasingly challenging task for the rehabilitation team. Computerized publication services or regular downloading from library databases can make updating more efficient. Scores of basic science, general clinical, and specialized clinical publications contain information relevant to practitioners of neurologic rehabilitation.

SUMMARY

An interdisciplinary team approach to issues of medical care, mobility, self-care and community skills, cognition and language, and psychosocial needs by physicians, nurses, therapists, social workers, psychologists, and others embodies what is peculiar to the culture of a neurologic rehabilitation service. This culture concerns itself as much with the experience of illness and disability of the patient and family as with the details of a particular disease. Each team member has particular key responsibilities for the team, and each brings a point of view about the basis and style for assessments and interventions. Most physical and cognitive interventions require practice in a learning par-

adigm that can modulate neural networks. Every approach can be challenged. Every challenge deserves thought about how to better understand a behavioral phenomenon and its neural correlates and how to best manage its consequences on patients with impairment and disability.

REFERENCES

1. Albert M, Bachman D, Morgan A, et al. Pharmacotherapy for aphasia. Neurology 1988;38:877–879.
2. Albert M, Helm-Estabrooks N. Diagnosis and treatment of aphasia. JAMA 1988;259:1043–1047, 1205–1210.
3. Ashburn A, Partridge C, De Souza L. Physiotherapy in the rehabilitation of stroke: A review. Clin Rehabil 1993;7:337–345.
4. Basmajian J. Biofeedback for neuromuscular rehabilitation. Crit Rev Phys Rehabil Med 1989;1:37–58.
5. Basmajian J, Wolf S. Therapeutic Exercise. Baltimore: Williams & Wilkins, 1990:460.
6. Batavia A, Hammer G. Toward the development of consumer-based criteria for the evaluation of assistive devices. J Rehabil Res Dev 1990;27:425–436.
7. Bate P, Matyas T. Negative transfer of training following brief practice of elbow tracking movements with electromyographic feedback from spastic antagonists. Arch Phys Med Rehabil 1992;73:1050–1058.
8. Blair S, Kohl H, Paffenbarger R. Physical fitness and all-cause mortality. JAMA 1989;262:2395–2401.
9. Blake D, Weathers F, Nagy L, et al. A clinician rating scale for assessing current and lifetime PTSD: The CAPS-1. Behavioral Therapist 1990;13:187–188.
10. Bobath B. Adult Hemiplegia. Oxford: Heinemann, 1990:190.
11. Bohannon R. Relevance of muscle strength to gait performance in patients with neurologic disability. Journal of Neurologic Rehabilitation 1989;3:97–100.
12. Breslau N. Traumatic events and posttraumatic stress disorder in an urban population of young adults. Arch Gen Psychiatry 1991;48:216–222.
13. Bromfield E, Reding M. Relative risk of deep vein thrombosis or pulmonary embolism post stroke based on ambulatory status. Journal of Neurologic Rehabilitation 1988;2:51–57.
14. Brouwer B, Ambury P. Upper extremity weight-bearing effect on corticospinal excitability following stroke. Arch Phys Med Rehabil 1994;75:861–866.
15. Brown J, Leader B. Hemiplegic writing in severe aphasia. Brain Lang 1983;19:204–215.
16. Brunnstrom S. Movement Therapy in Hemiplegia. Philadelphia: Harper & Row, 1970:190.
17. Byung S. Sentence processing deficits: Theory

and therapy. Cognitive Neuropsychology 1988; 5:629–676.

18. Caplan D. Toward a psycholinguistic approach to acquired neurogenic language disorders. American Journal of Speech Language Pathology 1993; 9:59–83.

19. Carr J, Shepherd R. A Motor Relearning Programme for Stroke. London: Heinemann, 1987.

20. Casey C, Kratz E. Soft splinting with neoprene: The thumb abduction supinator splint. Am J Occup Ther 1988;42:395–399.

21. Cohen S, Syme S. Social Support and Health. New York: Academic Press, 1985.

22. Cooper R. Wheelchair racing sports science: A review. J Rehabil Res Dev 1990;27:295–312.

23. Corcos D. Strategies underlying the control of disordered movement. Phys Ther 1991;71:25–32.

24. Corina D, Vaid J, Bellugi U. The linguistic basis of left hemisphere specialization. Science 1992; 255:1258–1260.

25. Coslett H, Saffran E, Greenbaum S, et al. Reading in pure alexia: The effect of strategy. Brain 1993; 116:21–37.

26. Cramer J. Identifying and improving compliance patterns: A composite plan for health care providers. In: Cramer J, Spilker B, eds: Patient Compliance in Medical Practice and Clinical Trials. New York: Raven Press, 1991:387–392.

27. Davis G, Wilcox M. Adult Aphasia Rehabilitation: Applied Pragmatics. San Diego: College-Hill Press, 1985.

28. Deathe A, Hayes K, Winter D. The biomechanics of canes, crutches, and walkers. Crit Rev Phys Rehabil Med 1993;5:15–29.

29. Deloche G, Ferrand I, Dordain M, et al. Confrontation naming rehabilitation in aphasics: A computerised written technique. Neuropsycholog Rehabil 1992;2:117–124.

30. Dickstein R, Edmonstone M, Stivens K. Therapeutic weight shift in hemiparetic patients: Surface electromyographic activity of lower extremity muscles during postural tasks. Journal of Neurologic Rehabilitation 1990;4:17–25.

31. Dobkin B. Exercise fitness and sports for individuals with neurologic disability. In: Gordon S, Gonzalez-Mestre X, Garrett W, eds: Sports and Exercise in Midlife. Rosemont, IL: American Academy of Orthopaedic Surgeons, 1993:235–252.

32. Dobkin B, Fowler E, Gregor R. A strategy to train locomotion in patients with chronic hemiplegic stroke. Ann Neurol 1991;30:278.

33. Enders A, Hall M, eds. Assistive Technology Sourcebook. Washington, DC: RESNA Press, 1990:576.

34. Exner C, Bondere B. Comparative effects of three hand splints on bilateral hand use, grasp and arm-hand posture in hemiplegic children. Occupational Therapy Journal of Research 1983;3:75–81.

35. Farmer M. Physical activity and depressive symptoms: The NHANES 1 epidemiologic follow-up study. American Journal of Epidemiology 1988; 128:1340–1351.

36. Finch L, Barbeau H. Hemiplegic gait: New treatment strategies. Physiotherapy Canada 1986; 38:36–41.

37. Finch L, Barbeau H, Arsenault B. Influence of body weight support on normal human gait. Phys Ther 1991;71:842–856.

38. Gauthier J, Bourbonnais D, Filiatrault J, et al. Characterization of contralateral torques during static hip efforts in healthy subjects and subjects with hemiparesis. Brain 1992;115:1193–1207.

39. Giannini M. Choosing a wheelchair system. J Rehabil Res Dev 1990;(Suppl 2):1–118.

40. Granger C, Hamilton B. The Uniform Data System for Medical Rehabilitation report of first admissions for 1992. Am J Phys Med Rehabil 1994; 73:51–55.

41. Guilford A, Scheurele J, Sherik P. Manual communication skills in aphasia. Arch Phys Med Rehabil 1982;63:601–604.

42. Haas J, Mackenzie C. The role of ethics in rehabilitation medicine. Am J Phys Med Rehabil 1993; 72:48–51.

43. Hagbarth K-E, Eklund G. The effects of muscle vibration in spasticity, rigidity, and cerebellar disorders. J Neurol Neurosurg Psychiatry 1968; 31:207–213.

44. Hanlon R, Brown J. Enhancement of naming in nonfluent aphasia through gesture. Brain Lang 1990;38:298–314.

44a. Heitman RJ, Gilley W. Effects of blocked versus random practice by mentally retarded subjects on learning a novel skill. Percept Mot Skills 1989; 69:443–447.

45. Helm N, Barresi B. Voluntary control of involuntary utterances. In: Brookshire R, ed: Clinical Aphasiology. Minneapolis: BRK Publishers, 1980: 308–315.

46. Helm-Estabrooks N, Albert M. Manual of Aphasia Therapy. Austin, TX: Pro-Ed, 1991.

47. Helm-Estabrooks N, Fitzpatrick P, Barresi B. Visual action therapy for global aphasia. Journal of Speech and Hearing Disorders 1982;47:385–389.

48. Helm-Estabrooks N, Nicholas M, Morgan A. Melodic Intonation Therapy Program. San Antonio: Special Press, 1989.

49. Helm-Estabrooks N, Ramsberger G. Treatment of agrammatism in long-term Broca's aphasia. British Journal of Disorders of Communication 1986; 21:39–45.

50. Helm-Estabrooks N, Ramsberger G, Morgan A, et al. Boston Assessment of Severe Aphasia. Chicago: Riverside, 1989.

51. Hillman M. Rehabilitation robotics. Crit Rev Phys Rehabil Med 1992;4:79–103.

52. Horak F. Assumptions underlying motor control for neurologic rehabilitation. In: Lister M, ed: Contemporary Management of Motor Control Problems: Proceedings of the II Step Conference. Alexandria, VA: Foundation for Physical Therapy, 1991:11–27.

53. Inuba M, Edberg E, Montgomery J, et al. Effectiveness of functional training, active exercise and resistive exercise for patients with hemiplegia. Phys Ther 1973;53:28–35.

54. Jackson R, Davis G. The value of sports and recreation for the physically disabled. Orthop Clin North Am 1983;14:301–315.

55. Jarus T. Motor learning and occupational ther-

apy: The organization of practice. Am J Occup Ther 1994;48:810–816.

56. Johannsen-Horback H, Cegla B, Mager U, et al. Treatment of chronic global aphasia with a non-verbal communication system. Brain Lang 1985; 24:74–82.

57. Johnstone M. Restoration of Motor Function in the Stroke Patient. London: Churchill Livingstone, 1978:187.

58. Kalra L. The influence of stroke unit rehabilitation on functional recovery from stroke. Stroke 1994;25:821–825.

59. Katz N, Marcus S, Weiss P. Purposeful activity in physical rehabilitation. Crit Rev Phys Rehabil Med 1994;6:199–218.

60. Kearns K. Broca's aphasia. In: LaPointe L, ed: Aphasia and Related Neurogenic Language Disorders. New York: Thieme, 1990.

61. Keith R. The comprehensive treatment team in rehabilitation. Arch Phys Med Rehabil 1991; 72:269–274.

62. Kempler D. Speech pathology: Evaluation and treatment of speech, language, cognitive, and swallowing disorders. In: Meyerhoff W, Rice D, eds: Otolaryngology—Head and Neck Surgery. Philadelphia: WB Saunders, 1992:128–151.

63. Knapp H, Taub E, Berman A. Movements in monkeys with deafferented limbs. Exp Neurol 1963; 7:305–315.

64. Lakka T, Venalainen J, Salonen J, et al. Relation of leisure-time physical activity and cardiorespiratory fitness to the risk of acute myocardial infarction in men. N Engl J Med 1994;330:1549–1554.

65. LaPointe L. Aphasia and Related Neurogenic Language Disorders. New York: Thieme, 1990:238.

66. Laskowski E. Snow skiing for the physically disabled. Mayo Clin Proc 1991;66:160–172.

67. Lazarus R, Folkman S. Stress, Appraisal and Coping. New York: Springer, 1984.

68. Lehmann J, Condon S, Price R, et al. Gait abnormalities in hemiplegia: Their correction by ankle-foot orthoses. Arch Phys Med Rehabil 1987; 68:763–771.

69. Leiguarda R, Merello M, Sabe L, et al. Bromocriptine-induced dystonia in patients with aphasia and hemiparesis. Neurology 1993;43:2319–2322.

70. Liebesman J, Cafarelli E. Physiology of range of motion in human joints: A critical review. Crit Rev Phys Rehabil Med 1994;6:131–160.

71. Lincoln N, Pickersgill M. The effectiveness of programmed instruction with operant training in the language rehabilitation of severely aphasic patients. Behavioral Psychotherapy 1984;12:237–248.

72. Lister M, ed. Contemporary Management of Motor Control Problems: Proceedings of the II Step Conference. Alexandria, VA: Foundation for Physical Therapy, 1991:278.

73. Livneh H, Antonak R. Psychosocial reactions to disability: A review and critique of the literature. Crit Rev Phys Rehabil Med 1994;6:1–100.

74. Loeb G. Neural prosthetic interfaces with the nervous system. Trends Neurosci 1989;12:195–201.

74a. Magill RA, Hall K. A review of the contextual interference effect in motor skill acquisition. Human Movement Science 1990;9:241–289.

75. Mathiowetz V, Haugen J. Motor behavior research: Implications for therapeutic approaches to central nervous system dysfunction. Am J Occup Ther 1994;48:733–745.

76. Matyas T, Galea M, Spicer S. Facilitation of the maximum voluntary contraction in hemiplegia by concomitant cutaneous stimulation. Am J Phys Med Rehabil 1986;65:125–134.

77. McFarland D, Neat G, Read R, et al. An EEG-based method for graded cursor control. Psychobiology 1993;21:77–81.

78. McGrath J, Davis A. Rehabilitation: Where are we going and how do we get there? Clin Rehabil 1992;6:225–235.

79. McPherson J, Kreimeyer D, Aalderks M, et al. A comparison of dorsal and volar resting hand splints in the reduction of hypertonus. Am J Occup Ther 1982;36:664–670.

80. Micoch A, Gupta S, Scolaro C, et al. Bromocriptine treatment of nonfluent aphasia. Annual Meeting of the American Speech and Hearing Association, abstracts, 1994.

81. Mitchell R. The quality of evaluation in physical therapy. Crit Rev Phys Rehabil Med 1992;4:61–77.

82. Mitchum C. Traditional and contemporary views of aphasia: Implications for clinical management. Topics in Stroke Rehabilitation 1994;1:14–36.

83. Mohr J, Pessin M, Finkelstein S, et al. Broca's aphasia: Pathologic and clinical findings. Neurology 1978;28:311–324.

84. Naeser M, Haas G, Mazurski P, et al. Sentence level auditory comprehension treatment program for aphasic adults. Arch Phys Med Rehabil 1986;67:393–399.

85. Naganuma G, Billingsley F. The use of hand splints with the neurologically involved child. Crit Rev Phys Rehabil Med 1990;2:87–100.

86. Nativ A. Kinesiological issues in motor training following brain trauma. Crit Rev Phys Rehabil Med 1993;5:227–246.

87. Neurology Technology Assessment Committee, American Academy of Neurology. Melodic intonation therapy. Neurology 1994;44:566–568.

88. Ottenbacher K, Biocca R, DeCremer O, et al. Quantitative analysis of the effectiveness of pediatric therapy. Phys Ther 1986;66:1095–1101.

89. Paciorek M, Jones J. Sports and Recreation for the Disabled: A Resource Handbook. Indianapolis: Benchmark Press, 1989.

90. Pate R, Pratt M, Blair S, et al. Physical activity and public health. JAMA 1995;273:402–407.

91. Poole J. Application of motor learning principles in occupational therapy. Am J Occup Ther 1991; 45:531–539.

92. Poole J, Whitney S, Hangeland N, et al. The effectiveness of inflatable pressure splints on motor function in stroke patients. Occupational Therapy Journal of Research 1990;10:360–366.

93. Pound P, Gompertz P, Ebrahim S. Patients' satisfaction with stroke services. Clinical Rehabilitation 1994;8:7–17.

94. Prutting C, Kirchner D. A clinical appraisal of the pragmatic aspects of language. J Speech Hear Disord 1987;52:105–119.

95. Regalbuto M, Krouskop T, Cheatham J. Toward a practical robotic aid system for people with severe physical disabilities. J Rehabil Res Dev 1992; 29:19–26.

96. Richards C, Malouin F, Wood-Dauphinee S, et al. Task-specific physical therapy for optimization of gait recovery in acute stroke patients. Arch Phys Med Rehabil 1993;74:612–620.

97. Rohrbaugh M, Rogers J. What did the doctor do? When physicians and patients disagree. Arch Fam Med 1994;3:125–129.

98. Sabari J. Motor learning concepts applied to activity-based intervention with adults with hemiplegia. Am J Occup Ther 1991;45:523–530.

99. Sabe L, Leiguarda R, Starkstein S. An open-label trial of bromocriptine in nonfluent aphasia. Neurology 1992;42:1637–1638.

100. Schacter D, McGlynn S, Milberg W, et al. Spared priming despite impaired comprehension: Implicit memory in a case of word meaning deafness. Neuropsychology 1993;7:107–118.

101. Schmidt R. Motor Control and Learning. Champaign, IL: Human Kinetics, 1988.

102. Schmidt R. Motor learning principles for physical therapy. In: Lister M, ed: Contemporary Management of Motor Control Problems. Alexandria, VA: Foundation for Physical Therapy, 1991:49–63.

103. Schmidt R, Lange C, Young D. Optimizing summary knowledge of results for skill learning. Human Movement Science 1990;9:325–348.

104. Schwartz M. What the classical aphasia categories can't do for us, and why. Brain Lang 1984;21:3–8.

105. Shepard R. Benefit of sport and physical activity for the disabled: Implications for the individual and for society. Scand J Rehabil Med 1991; 23:233–241.

106. Sietsema J, Nelson D, Mulder R, et al. The use of a game to promote arm reach in persons with traumatic brain injury. Am J Occup Ther 1993; 47:19–24.

107. Small S. Pharmacotherapy of aphasia. Stroke 1994;25:1282–1289.

108. Smith R, Leslie J, eds. Rehabilitation Engineering. Boca Raton, FL: CRC Press, 1990:548.

109. Soderback I, Ekholm J. Occupational therapy in brain damage rehabilitation. Crit Rev Phys Rehabil Med 1993;5:315–355.

110. Sparks R, Helm N, Albert M. Aphasia rehabilitation resulting from melodic intonation therapy. Cortex 1974;10:303–316.

111. Steele R, Kleczewska M, Carlson G, et al. Computers in the rehabilitation of chronic, severe aphasia: C-VIC cross modal studies. Aphasiology 1992;6:185–194.

112. Stevens E. Efficacy of multiple input phoneme therapy in the treatment of severe expressive aphasia and apraxia of speech. Phys Med Rehabil: State of the Art Reviews 1989;3:194–199.

113. Stockmeyer S. An interpretation of the approach

114. of Rood to the treatment of neuromuscular dysfunction. Am J Phys Med 1967;46:900–956.

114. Sutter E. The brain response interface: Communication through visually induced electrical brain responses. Journal of Microcomputer Applications 1992;15:31–45.

115. Taub E, Crago J, Burgio L, et al. An operant approach to rehabilitation medicine: Overcoming learned nonuse by shaping. J Exp Anal Behav 1994;61:287–318.

116. Taub E, Miller N, Novack T, et al. Technique to improve chronic motor deficit after stroke. Arch Phys Med Rehabil 1993;74:347–354.

117. Trombly C. Observations of improvement of reaching in five subjects with left hemiparesis. J Neurol Neurosurg Psychiatry 1993;56:40–45.

118. Twitchell T. The restoration of motor function following hemiplegia in man. Brain 1951;74:443–480.

119. Valvano J, Long T. Neurodevelopmental treatment: A review of the writings of the Bobaths. Pediatric Physical Therapy 1991:125–129.

120. Voss D, Ionta M, Myers B. Proprioceptive Neuromuscular Facilitation. Philadelphia: Harper & Row, 1985:370.

121. Walker-Batson D, Unwin H, Curtis S, et al. Use of amphetamine in the treatment of aphasia. Restorative Neurology and Neuroscience 1992;4:47–50.

122. Waters R, Yakura J. The energy expenditure of normal and pathological gait. Crit Rev Phys Rehabil Med 1989;1:183–209.

123. Wernig A, Muller S. Laufband locomotion with body weight support improved walking in persons with severe spinal cord injuries. Paraplegia 1992; 30:229–238.

124. Willmes K, Poeck K. To what extent can aphasic syndromes be localized? Brain 1993;116:1527–1540.

124a. Wilson BA, Baddeley A, Evans J, Shiel A. Errorless learning in the rehabilitation of memory impaired people. Neuropsychological Rehabilitation 1994;4:307–326.

125. Wing A, Lough S, Turton A, et al. Recovery of elbow function in voluntary positioning of the hand following hemiplegia due to stroke. J Neurol Neurosurg Psychiatry 1990;53:126–134.

126. Winstein C. Knowledge of results and motor learning: Implications for physical therapy. Phys Ther 1991;71:140–149.

127. Winstein C, Gardner E, McNeal D. Standing balance training: Effect on balance and locomotion in hemiparetic adults. Arch Phys Med Rehab 1989;70:755–762.

128. Winstein C, Schmidt R. Reduced frequency of knowledge of results enhances motor skill learning. J Exp Psychol 1990;16:677–691.

129. Wulf C, Schmidt R. Variability in practice: Facilitation in retention and transfer through schema formation or context effects? J Mot Behav 1988; 20:133–149.

CHAPTER 4

ASSESSMENT OF GAIT DEVIATIONS

The neurorehabilitation team makes a great effort toward achieving the most independent and the safest level of ambulation possible for the patient. For assessment, the team relies on observational analysis, trial-and-error approaches, and, sometimes, formal gait analysis. This chapter bridges portions of the preceding and the next chapters by describing the common gait deviations dealt with by physical therapists and orthotists and then by looking at measures of gait that quantify assessments and outcomes.

NORMAL GAIT

Mechanisms of postural and locomotor control are described in Chapter 1. Observational and quantitative methods that evaluate human locomotion assess the cyclic movements occurring between successive contacts with the heel of the same foot. During the normal gait cycle, each muscle fires briefly. It acts either as a shock absorber for deceleration, through a lengthening or eccentric contraction, or as an accelerator, by a shortening or concentric contraction. This action permits fine control of forward progression during stepping and maintains a stable upright posture. Properly timed changes in the joint angles at the hip, knee, and ankle help to minimize the energy expended as ambulators shift their center of gravity. For the stance and swing phases of the step cycle (Fig. 4–1), these changes include the following:

1. Early in the stance phase, the knee flexes about 15 degrees.
2. During the first part of stance, controlled plantarflexion allows the transfer of weight from the heel to the flat foot.
3. The knee flexes about 30 to 40 degrees near the end of stance.
4. The pelvis is displaced toward the stance limb.
5. In the swing phase, the pelvis rotates, so that the swinging hip moves forward faster than the hip that is in stance.
6. The pelvis tilts down on the side of the swinging hip, under the control of the opposite hip abductor muscles.

Healthy elderly people walk more slowly and have a shorter stride length than young adults. Hemiplegia, paraplegia, disorders of the motor unit, extrapyramidal disorders,

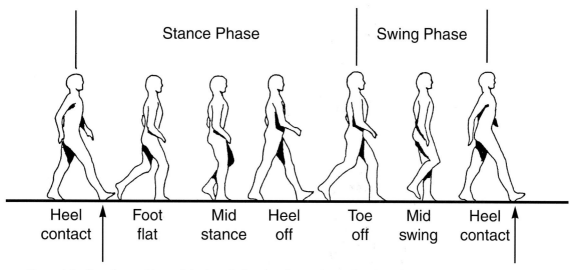

Figure 4–1. Changing positions of the legs during the phases of a single gait cycle from right heel contact to the next right heel contact. (Adapted from Norkin, C, and Levangie, P, Joint Structure and Function: A Comprehensive Analysis, ed. 2. F.A. Davis, Philadelphia, 1992, p 451.)

ataxias, and hydrocephalus all cause changes in the temporal and kinematic variables of the gait cycle.

HEMIPLEGIC GAIT

The Rancho Los Amigos charting system provides a systematic observational method for gait analysis.[2,11] This system incorporates 32 of the most common gait deviations that can affect the trunk, pelvis, hip, knee, ankle, foot, and toes during swing and stance. These observable deviations are listed in Tables 4–1 and 4–2.[2,8] Observational methods for assessing gait and for measuring the outcomes of rehabilitative interventions are probably not reliable in the hands of any but the most experienced clinicians, however.[5] Moreover, data from healthy walkers are not necessarily appropriate for comparing and correcting the characteristics of hemiplegic gait. Patients should be trained to achieve an adaptive, functional gait, not necessarily one that is typical of able-bodied persons.

After an upper motoneuron injury, myriad combinations of problems can interfere with the gait pattern. These problems include weakness, impaired activation of mus-

cles, coactivation of muscle groups, hypertonicity, leg length asymmetries of more than about an inch, laxity of ligaments, joint and soft tissue stiffness, contractures, and pain. Therapists make their adjustments to deviations that occur during the six most easily separable events of the gait cycle (see Fig. 4–1), as described in the following paragraphs:

1. *Initial contact with heel strike:* Normally, work at the knee flexors is mostly eccentric during weight acceptance in stance. This phenomenon prevents hyperextension of the knee. The tibialis anterior muscle contracts eccentrically to touch, rather than slap, the foot to the ground. The patient with hemiplegia can lose heel strike and the heel rocker action that increases step length and adds forward propulsion. The patient often lands on the forefoot because of poor ankle dorsiflexion and knee extension. Poor dorsiflexion can arise from a heel cord contracture, from sustained or early activation of the triceps surae muscles, and from a synergistic pattern that prevents the combination of hip flexion, ankle dorsiflexion, and knee extension.

Table 4–1. **OBSERVATIONAL ANALYSIS OF COMMON HEMIPARETIC GAIT DEVIATIONS IN THE STANCE PHASE**

Deviations	Causes	Consequences
Hip adduction	Increased adductor activity Inadequate strength of abductors	Narrow base of support Loss of balance
Contralateral pelvic drop	Weakness or inadequate control of hip abductors	Decreased stance stability
Inadequate hip extension	Inadequate quadriceps Hip flexion contracture Increased activity of hip flexors Excessive knee flexion posture	Increased energy demand Decreased forward progression and velocity
Inadequate knee extension	Inadequate quadriceps strength and control Knee flexion contracture Increased hamstring or gastrocnemius activity Inadequate hip extension or excessive dorsiflexion	Increased energy demand Decreased stance time Decreased forward progression and velocity
Knee extensor thrust	Inadequate quadriceps control Increased quadriceps or plantarflexion activity Ankle instability Plantarflexion contracture	Loss of loading response at knee Decreased forward progression and velocity Joint pain
Excessive plantarflexion	Increased plantarflexion activity Inadequate plantarflexion strength and control Plantarflexion contracture	Decreased forward progression and velocity Compensatory postures Increased energy demand Shortened stance time
Excessive dorsiflexion	Accommodation for knee flexion contracture Plantarflexion paresis	Stance instability Decreased stance time Compensatory hip and knee flexion requiring increased energy Decreased forward progression and velocity
No heel-off	Inadequate plantarflexion strength and control Restricted ankle or metatarsal motion	Decreased preswing knee flexion Decreased forward progression and velocity
Excess varus	Increased invertor muscle activity	Unstable base of support Decreased forward progression and velocity
Clawed toes	Increased toe flexor muscle activity or weak intrinsic foot muscles Exaggerated compensation for poor balance Toe flexion contracture	Pain from skin pressure and weight bearing on toes Decreased forward progression and velocity

Source: Adapted from Gillis M.[2]

Table 4–2. **OBSERVATIONAL ANALYSIS OF COMMON HEMIPARETIC GAIT DEVIATIONS IN THE SWING PHASE**

Deviations	Causes	Consequences
Impaired hip flexion	Increased extensor activity at knee and ankle Inadequate control of hip flexors	Decreased forward progression and velocity Shortened step length Increased energy demand
Impaired knee flexion	Inadequate preswing knee flexion Increased knee extensor activity Contracture Hamstring paresis	Toe drag at initial swing
Inadequate knee extension at end of swing	Knee flexion contracture Flexor synergy or withdrawal preventing knee extension during hip flexion Increased knee flexor activity	Shortened step length Decreased forward progression and velocity
Hip adduction	Increased adductor activity Excessive flexor or extensor synergy	Swing limb abutting stance limb or unsafely narrowing base of support Decreased forward progression
Excessive plantarflexion at midswing to end swing	Inadequate dorsiflexion strength Contracture Increased plantarflexor activity or extensor synergy	Toe drag Initial contact with foot flat or toes first Loss of loading response at ankle

Source: Adapted from Gillis M.[2]

2. *Foot flat or load acceptance:* Normally, rapid passive plantarflexion is restrained by the tibialis anterior and toe extensor muscles and by flexion of the knee, which occurs when the tibia moves forward faster than the thigh. These actions prevent the vertical force at load acceptance from rapidly building up at impact. The initial rocker action at the ankle and foot also reduces this impact. In the patient with hemiplegia who loads the forefoot, the tibia is forced back and the knee is thrust into extension, thereby impeding forward momentum. The foot turns in varus and becomes an unstable weight-bearing surface. The quadriceps may give way or the knee may hyperextend.

3. *Midstance:* At this time, the leg in swing passes the stance leg, and the feet come next to each other. The body slows its forward velocity as it progresses over the stance leg. The trunk is at its highest point, creating the potential energy of height, and is displaced to a maximum toward the stance leg. The hip extends. The quadriceps muscle stops contracting, and the soleus contracts to slow the forward motion of the tibia. The ground reaction force moves forward along the foot as the ankle rotates from about 15 degrees of plantarflexion to 10 degrees of dorsiflexion. The gluteus muscles contract on the opposite side to maintain pelvic alignment. In the patient with hemiplegia, the inability to dorsiflex the ankle about 5 degrees may hyperextend the knee or lean the trunk forward, a situation that slows momentum and causes a shorter step by the opposite leg. If the soleus contraction is inadequate, the quadriceps muscle continues to fire to compensate for the dorsiflexed ankle. If it cannot, the patient must avoid stance phase flexion and maintain extension from the swing phase.

4. *Terminal stance or heel-off:* This event occurs just before heel contact by the opposite leg. The trunk loses vertical height, the iliopsoas muscle contracts eccentrically to resist the hip as it con-

tinues to extend, the knee peaks in its extension and begins to flex, and the gastrocnemius joins the soleus contraction to oppose dorsiflexion. In the patient with hemiplegia, toe clawing, contracture, or excessive muscle activity may prevent weight from advancing to the forefoot. The opposite side of the pelvis may drop from impaired hip abductor activity.

5. *Preswing and initial swing or toe-off:* Stance ends and swing begins at the end of the second double-limb support phase. Gravity, the rectus femoris muscle, and the hip adductor muscles flex the hip. The rectus femoris muscle also controls knee flexion by an eccentric contraction. Muscles that act across the ankle stabilize the foot as the triceps surae muscles contract. The ground reaction force rapidly dissipates through the metatarsal heads. Work at the ankle is mostly concentric and is highest at push-off. The patient with hemiplegia often misses this phase because of sustained knee extension from excessive quadriceps activity or because of compensation for poor calf control. Patients also compensate for toe drag by circumducting the leg or by vaulting off or leaning toward the unaffected leg.

6. *Midswing:* About 40 percent of the normal gait cycle is for swing. The timing of midswing corresponds to midstance for the other leg. Swing has an initial acceleration at the hip from the iliopsoas and other flexor muscles and a deceleration phase controlled by contraction of the hamstrings. The knee flexes like a pendulum, powered by hip flexion. At the end of swing, the hamstrings prevent knee hyperextension. The toe clears the ground by less than 3 cm as a result of contraction of the tibialis anterior muscle, putting the ankle into a neutral position, and as a result of shortening of the leg by knee flexion. The patient with hemiplegia often cannot flex at the hip and ankle while extending the knee. The leg becomes functionally too long. Hip hiking by the paraspinal and abdominal muscles is one energy-taxing compensatory strategy when the hamstrings are

weak. The knee extends prematurely, so the leg is too long near the end of swing. Circumduction, vaulting off the foot of the stance leg, and excessive hip and knee flexion in the presence of a prominent footdrop are other voluntary techniques.

In summary, the hemiplegic gait is prone to the following:

1. A shorter step length with the unaffected leg
2. Longer stance duration, mostly from longer double-limb support time with shorter time on the paretic limb
3. Shorter duration of swing
4. Greater flexion at the hip during midstance, which, by moving the center of mass forward, is associated with an increased knee extension moment
5. Decreased lateral shift to the paretic side during single-limb support
6. Less knee flexion and ankle dorsiflexion during swing, which is associated with circumduction

Casual walking speed in hemiplegic gait is about half of casual walking speed in unaffected persons. Speed is a good reflection of the overall gait pattern. Normal casual walking speed for older adults is about 90 cm per second (2 mph).[15] Healthy geriatric patients can increase their speed to walk 50 feet in 12 seconds (130 cm per second or 2.9 mph).[12] Mean ranges for gait speed in several studies of recovery from hemiplegic stroke are 25 to 50 cm per second.[13] Although patients experience no increase in the rate of energy expenditure, mostly because of their slower gait, their energy demand is higher because it takes longer to cover a distance.[17]

PARAPLEGIC GAIT

The observational gait of patients with spastic paraparesis reveals a variety of compensatory mechanisms used to achieve locomotion. Hip and knee flexion can be prominent in swing and stance. Heel contact may be absent, replaced by a plantarflexed or flat initial floor contact. The plantarflexors perform 80 percent of the positive work of gait. Excess plantarflexion in early stance prevents the ankle from dorsiflexing into a position where the plantarflexors can contribute to forward impulse by an active push-off.[19] Poor proprioception at a knee and ankle joint can contribute to pathologic deviations. Electromyographic (EMG) analysis often shows a prolonged duration of EMG activation with premature recruitment and delayed relaxation compared with healthy persons. The EMG bursts tend to be flat, with decreased-to-absent peaks. The rectus femoris and gastrocnemius muscles often show reduced activity over the whole step cycle, whereas the tibialis anterior muscle may show increased activity during early swing. Prolonged bursts can accompany passive muscle lengthening.

GAIT IN PATIENTS WITH PERIPHERAL NEUROPATHY

A single nerve injury can cause considerable deviation and secondary compensations in gait. For example, paralysis of the tibialis anterior muscle decreases velocity by several mechanisms. Step length decreases, mostly on the nonparalyzed side. On the paralyzed side, one can find a decrease in ankle dorsiflexion moment at the end of stance, a decrease in vertical ground reaction force, a decrease in weight transfer to the forward part of the foot, a decrease in knee extension range and torque at stance, an increase in ankle dorsiflexion range at stance, and increased work.[6] Peroneal palsy causes somewhat greater gait changes. Step length decreases on the nonparalyzed side. On the paralyzed side, vertical forces on push-off decrease, the knee extension moment with stance decreases, the plantarflexion moment with early stance decreases, and the dorsiflexion moment with late stance decreases. Ankle inversion occurs at heel strike. To ensure foot clearance, hip and knee flexion must increase during swing.[7]

GAIT IN PATIENTS WITH POLIOMYELITIS

Anterior trunk flexion with knee hyperextension is a common compensation for severe quadriceps muscle weakness resulting from poliomyelitis. This paresis can cause degenerative disease of the knee joint. Weakness of other muscle groups, such as the paraspinal muscles and the muscles controlling hip and ankle movements, yields a variety of gait deviations.

QUANTITATIVE GAIT ANALYSIS

Biomechanics, kinesiology, electrophysiology, and computer modeling have contributed to research into the mechanisms and evaluation of normal and pathologic gait. Quantitative methods of gait analysis draw from these disciplines. They reveal information about normal[20] and abnormal[9] motor control and can lead to therapeutic interventions and to assessments that monitor change reliably. Some practical techniques for gait analysis are listed in Table 4–3.

Temporal Measures

The least complicated and least expensive instrumented techniques use footswitches under the heel, under the heads of the first

Table 4–3. TECHNIQUES FOR GAIT ANALYSIS

Observational description
Time-distance variables
    Footswitch stride analyzer
    Footprint analysis
    Conductive or pressure-sensitive walkway
Kinematics
    Electrogoniometers
    Computerized video analysis with joint markers
Dynamic electromyography
    Surface and fine wire electrodes
Kinetics
    Force plate in walkway
    Piezoelectric and load cell force transducers under feet
Metabolic energy expenditure
    Oxygen consumption by respirometry

and fifth metatarsal, and under the great toe. While in contact with the ground, each small transducer's circuit closes and produces a voltage signal on a strip chart or computer. From this signal, temporal and distance measures are obtained, including speed, cadence (step frequency), stride length (the distance between two consecutive heel strikes by the same foot), step length (the distance between left and right heel strikes), and the percentage of the gait cycle spent in single-limb (swing phase) and double-limb (stance phase) support. Figure 4–2 defines the phases of the normal step cycle. Retest reliability is good, but random and systematic errors and the inherent variability of overground velocity can make serial measures difficult to interpret.[4]

Footswitch techniques reveal asymmetries between the limbs, such as reduced stance time on a hemiparetic leg. These techniques can enable one to measure improvement in the symmetry of the swing phase and in the stance-to-swing ratio that is associated with motor recovery after stroke.[1] They cannot, alone, enable one to assess dysfunctions in gait or compensatory strategies.

Kinematics

Whole limb motion can be recorded with electrogoniometers placed across each joint. Movement in one plane or, for more sophis-

ticated devices, in three planes produces a change in resistance and a recordable voltage that reveals the change in joint angles. Motion-analysis systems increasingly use front and side cameras that videotape the movements of accurately placed reflective markers or light-emitting diodes.[3] By a variety of techniques, the data are digitized to make a moving stick figure. Changes in the angle of a single joint can be derived across the gait cycle.

The bottom of Figure 4–3 shows the sagittal plane of the hip, the knee, and the ankle during a normal step cycle. Figure 4–4 shows the joint angles of a 70-year-old man with a left hemiparesis due to a right internal capsule infarction who walks with a cane at his preferred cadence without an ankle-foot orthosis. Hip, knee, and ankle flexion are much less than in a healthy person. On a coronal view, one would appreciate a modest amount of leg circumduction to help clear the foot. Plots of one joint angle versus another during the step cycle provide a more dynamic view of gait.[18]

Electromyography

EMG recordings during gait reveal the onset, duration, and amplitude of muscle bursts in relation to the step cycle (see Fig. 4–3A). Dedicated recording and signal processing systems have defined EMG patterns

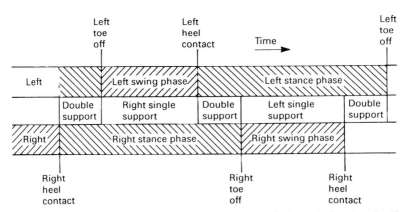

Figure 4–2. Average temporal features of single and double limb support during a single gait cycle. About 60 percent of the cycle is in stance during walking at the casual speed of 2.5 mph. This timing is the same in Figures 4–3 and 4–4. (From Whittle, MW: Gait Analysis: An Introduction. Butterworth Heinemann, Oxford, 1991, p 54, with permission.)

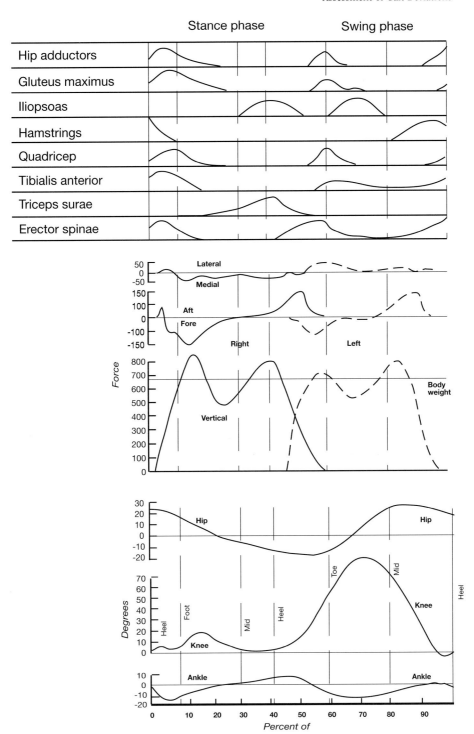

Figure 4–3. (*A*) Linear envelopes of the average timing of electromyographic bursts of the major muscle groups during one gait cycle. (*B*) Lateral, fore-aft, and vertical components of the ground reaction force in newtons for the right foot (solid line) and the left foot (dashed line). (*C*) Kinematics of a single gait cycle. Average joint angles made at the hip (flexion is a positive angle), knee (flexion positive), and ankle (dorsiflexion positive). (Adapted from Whittle, MW: Gait Analysis: An Introduction. Butterworth Heinemann, Oxford, 1991).

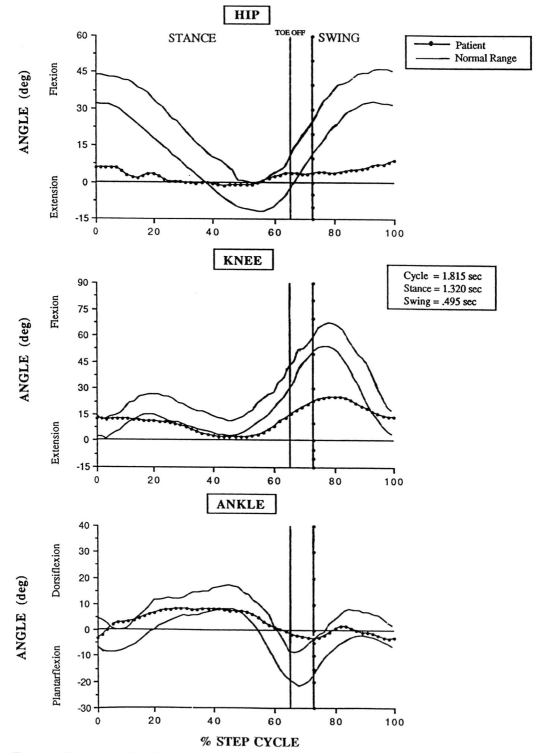

Figure 4–4. Kinematics of the affected leg in a patient with a chronic hemiplegic gait (dotted lines) compared with the average range of joint angles (solid lines). The patient's excursions are flatter, with little hip and knee flexion in swing. (From the UCLA Functional Assessment Laboratory, Los Angeles, CA.)

in relation to footswitch signals.[10] Surface and fine wire electrodes can be attached to cable and telemetry systems. The raw EMG signal is usually processed by full wave rectification, which reflects the absolute value of the signal's amplitude. Further low-pass filtering gives a linear envelope or moving average signal.

Recordings show when the muscle is active or when it changes its activity, but they tell nothing about strength, voluntary control, or type of muscle contraction. Muscle timing errors during gait have been defined as premature, prolonged, continuous, curtailed, delayed, absent, and out of phase.[3] This categorization provides information related to motor control and has led to strategies such as tendon releases and transfers. The timing of bursts among muscle groups in individual patients with pathologic gaits can be compared over time. Amplitude changes in paretic muscles that are reassessed at different times are difficult to interpret unless they are normalized to a maximal contraction with reproducible electrode placement.

Kinetics

Vertical, horizontal, and medial ground reaction forces during the stance phase reveal changes in limb loading caused by a pathologic gait (see Fig. 4–3B). Laboratories have used pressure-sensitive insole systems and in-ground force plates with strain gauge or piezoelectric transducers. For example, a force plate mounted in the ground rapidly measures changes in force and in the center of pressure under the foot to give the maximum vertical impulse in relation to body weight. The plate has to be camouflaged so that patients do not target their steps unnaturally. Normally, the vertical load peaks at about 110 percent of body weight. This vertical load curve can be unreliable, however, because it is sensitive to motion and displacements of any body segment and to changes in cadence.[3]

Energy Expenditure

The energy cost during normal and pathologic gait is measured by having patients walk at a casual or maximum speed while they breathe into a Douglas collecting bag or a mobile gas analyzer until a steady state is reached. The oxygen and carbon dioxide contents are analyzed to allow the calculation of the maximum oxygen consumption ($\dot{V}O_2$max), the $\dot{V}O_2$ for a given level of work, the anaerobic threshold, and related measures of the efficiency of walking.[17] The technique has been applied to help determine the usefulness of an orthotic or an assistive device. In a simpler fashion, the cardiovascular efficiency of walking in adults can be estimated by comparing the heart rate before and after 3 minutes of walking.[16] Over a wide range of walking speeds, healthy children and those with cerebral palsy also show a linear relationship between heart rate and oxygen uptake.[14]

SUMMARY

Gait analysis allows relative comparisons and quantitative observations about stepping that reflect the adaptability of the controls for locomotion. Laboratory studies of the gait cycle are rarely needed for clinical care, except perhaps preoperatively for surgical interventions to improve stepping and for drug injections for dysfunctional muscle firing. Analyses of velocity, cadence, and leg symmetries in stride length and swing and stance times are useful for serial comparisons of the effectiveness of physical and drug therapies for ambulation. EMG, kinematic, and kinetic studies are likely to be limited to research protocols that investigate aspects of basic mechanisms of locomotion and outcomes of invasive procedures, such as dorsal rhizotomy for spasticity in diplegic cerebral palsy.

REFERENCES

1. Brandstater M, deBruin H, Gowland C, et al. Hemiplegic gait: Analysis of temporal variables. Arch Phys Med Rehabil 1983;64:583–587.
2. Gillis M. Observational gait analysis. In: Scully R, Barnes M, eds: Physical Therapy. Philadelphia: JB Lippincott, 1989:670–695.
3. Harris G, Wertsch J. Procedures for gait analysis. Arch Phys Med Rehabil 1994;75:216–225.
4. Hill K, Goldie P, Baker P, et al. Retest reliability of the temporal and distance characteristics of hemi-

plegic gait using a footswitch system. Arch Phys Med Rehabil 1994;75:577–583.

5. Krebs D, Edelstein J, Fishman S. Reliability of observational kinematic gait analysis. Phys Ther 1985; 65:1027–1034.

6. Lehmann J, Condon S, deLateur B, et al. Gait abnormalities in tibial nerve paralysis. Arch Phys Med Rehabil 1985;66:80–85.

7. Lehmann J, Condon S, deLateur B, et al. Gait abnormalities in peroneal nerve paralysis and their corrections by orthoses. Arch Phys Med Rehabil 1986;67:380–386.

8. Lehmann J, de Lateur B, Price R. Biomechanics of abnormal gait. Physical Medicine Rehabilitation Clinics of North America 1992;3:125–138.

9. Perry J. Gait Analysis. Thorofare, NJ: Slack, 1992:524.

10. Perry J, Bontrager E, Bogey R, et al. The Rancho EMG analyzer: A computerized system for gait analysis. J Biomed Eng 1993;15:487–496.

11. Rancho Professional Staff Association. Normal and Pathological Gait Syllabus. Downey, CA: Rancho Los Amigos Hospital, 1981.

12. Reuben D, Siu A. An objective measure of physical function of elderly outpatients. J Am Geriatr Soc 1990;38:1105–1112.

13. Richards C, Malouin F, Wood-Dauphinee S, et al. Task-specific physical therapy for optimization of gait recovery in acute stroke patients. Arch Phys Med Rehabil 1993;74:612–620.

14. Rose J, Gamble J, Burgos A, et al. Energy expenditure index of walking for normal children and for children with cerebral palsy. Dev Med Child Neurol 1990;32:333–340.

15. Smidt G, ed. Gait in Rehabilitation. New York: Churchill Livingstone, 1990:329.

16. Waters R, Hislop HJP. Energetics: Application to the study and management of locomotor disabilities. Orthop Clin North Am 1978;9:351–377.

17. Waters R, Yakura J. The energy expenditure of normal and pathological gait. Critical Reviews in Physical Rehabilitation Medicine 1989;1:183–209.

18. Winstein C, Garfinkel A. Qualitative dynamics of disordered human locomotion: A preliminary study. J Mot Behav 1989;21:373–391.

19. Winter D. Energy generation and absorption at the ankle and knee during fast, natural, and slow cadences. Clin Orthop 1983;175:147–154.

20. Winter D. The Biomechanics and Motor Control of Human Gait. Waterloo, Ontario, Canada: Waterloo University Press, 1987.

CHAPTER 5

ASSESSMENT AND OUTCOME MEASURES

Research on the effectiveness and appropriateness of medical interventions will increasingly affect the practices of health care professionals.[121] To study the best ways to lessen impairments, disabilities, and handicaps in patients with neurologic diseases, rehabilitation specialists need reliable and valid measurement instruments that are sensitive to important changes. Those who pay for health care, along with the rehabilitation team, also require meaningful measures gathered for internal program evaluations, individual patient monitoring, quality assurance, quality improvement, and determination of the cost-effectiveness of procedures.

No absolute scales or measures exist in neurologic rehabilitation, so researchers and practitioners must consider what each measure purports to offer and how best to make use of it.[77] Clinical researchers in Europe and North America are making real progress in the conceptualization and measurement of physical and cognitive impairments, of functional status, and of the domains that fall within the notion of quality of life (QOL), however. Creative designs for tool development, clinical trials, and statistical analyses have been proposed in the literature. This chapter looks at some of the existing measures that have been most successfully used in studies and at other methods that are evolving in their importance for use in single-subject and group experimental designs.

PRINCIPLES OF MEASUREMENT

The vocabulary of measures and scales is not necessarily familiar to rehabilitation specialists. The choice of measures and statistical methods to assess outcomes requires a general grasp of measurement principles.

99

Types of Measurements

Nominal measures are simply classifications into categories that have no particular ordered relation to one another. Only those patients who fall within a group are counted, such as males and females or patients with a stroke who have left hemiplegia versus right hemiplegia versus no weakness.

With an *interval* scale, the numeric differences between measured points are interpretable. The distance between a joint angle of 10 degrees and one of 18 degrees is the same as the difference between an angle of 25 degrees and one of 33 degrees. The same holds for temperature. Some instrumentation is needed to quantify these measures. Measures that use an interval scale with magnitude and an absolute zero, such as the force exerted by a concentric muscle contraction in Newton-meters or the time in seconds to walk 50 m, are also *ratio* scales. Temperature is not a ratio scale because, for example, 38°C is not twice as hot as 19°, although it is 19° warmer.

Ordinal scales measure magnitude by a predetermined order among possible responses in a classification, but they do not possess equal intervals and may not have an absolute zero. Most rehabilitation measures have magnitude, but they do not possess equal intervals or an absolute zero. These ordinal scales can be viewed as having numerically ordered ranks. The British Medical Council Scale for strength—from 0 equals no movement to 5 equals full resistance—is ordinal, as are any of the functional assessment scales in which 0 means dependence, 1 means assistance is needed, and 2 means independence. The lack of linearity of these scales can be a problem in rehabilitation outcomes when a gain from 0 to 1 is not the equivalent of a gain from 1 to 2, however. Separate items on scales such as the Functional Independence Measure and Barthel Index can be summed, so that higher scores indicate greater independence. A change from a score on the Barthel Index of 30 to 60 may then be correlated with a patient's capacity to live at home after a stroke, but rehabilitation has not made the patient twice as independent. Sometimes, however, methods of analysis developed for interval or ratio measures can be usefully applied to ordinal data that, for example, approximate a continuous underlying measure of functionality. Moreover, hierarchic ordinal scales for a specific function, such as mobility, that are set up in their order of difficulty (for example, wheelchair transfers, wheelchair mobility, room ambulation, stairs, and community ambulation) can be given a coefficient of scalability and reproducibility using the Guttman scaling procedure.

The Rasch analysis is a sophisticated approach for transforming ordinal data into interval data to create a more linear measure in scales used for functional assessment.[131] The underlying concept is that each item or test has a certain level of difficulty. Each person has a certain level of ability. Success and failure rates on test items are a function of both parameters. Data items are positioned along the measurement continuum according to their level of difficulty for patients. Patients are positioned by their ability to perform the test items. In this model, the log odds of an individual item, which are the successes of the patient on an item divided by the failures of the patient on the same item, are equal to the independence of the patient, which is the log of successes, minus the difficulty of the item, the log of failures. An iterative procedure using a Rasch analysis software program computes estimates of item difficulty, associated errors of measurement, and each item's fit into the measurement model. An estimate of each item's difficulty, expressed in logits, locates each item on a continuous and additive scale, so that a change of, say, 3 points on the scale has equal value at any level. New ordinal scales may need to be designed to take full advantage of this evolving technique.

Statistical Analyses

The distinctions among nominal, ordinal, interval, and ratio measures are particularly important when one considers which conventional statistical analyses can be applied to collected data. The choice of analysis must be a part of any research design. For rehabilitation research, a biostatistician becomes an important team resource. Numerous books[7,8,20,43] and reviews[9,19,42,80,112,113] that emphasize principles and methods of statistics in medicine and rehabilitation are available for the beginner as well as for the advanced student.

Statistical tests are conducted to determine whether the null hypothesis, which states that no difference exists between the comparison groups or conditions in a clinical trial, should be rejected. When statistical testing determines that the null hypothesis can be rejected at a chosen level of statistical significance, the clinician must keep in mind that this positive result for one intervention over another is not necessarily an indicator of the magnitude or clinical importance of the result or a sign of its reproducibility. Thus, statistical test significance is not synonymous with clinical significance. Rehabilitation practices are affected by repeated studies of practical interventions shown to have statistical significance and functional importance for large enough populations of subjects that resemble a clinician's own patients.

Table 5–1 lists some of the tests of statistical significance most commonly used in rehabilitation studies. The variety of tests is related to the need for different mathematical approaches to handle differing types of data, as well as to the different assumptions incorporated into each statistical method. For example, when an investigator wants to compare the Barthel Index scores between two groups of patients with stroke who were randomized to different interventions, an appropriate test for ordinal data that compares two independent samples is the Mann-Whitney U test. If a researcher wants to compare 12 consecutive elderly men with stroke and left hemi-inattention with 14 women with the same impairment 2 weeks after the stroke to study the proportion of male and female subjects who returned home, Fisher's Exact test will be appropriate for these categoric data that compare two independent samples. When walking speed before and after an intervention such as treadmill training is studied in patients with Parkinson's disease who are matched pairs or the same patients, the paired t test allows a comparison of two related samples with interval data. An unpaired t test allows a comparison of treat-

Table 5–1. STATISTICAL APPLICATIONS

Comparison	Nominal	Ordinal	Interval/Ratio
Group description	Frequencies; proportions; mode	Median; range	Mean (arithmetic/ geometric); variance; coefficient of variation
Two independent samples	Fisher's Exact for n < 30; Chi-square (1 df) for large samples and expected cell frequencies > 5	Mann-Whitney	Unpaired t test if sample variances are similar by F ratio
Two related samples	Chi-square for changes with continuity correction; Fisher's for small sample	Sign test for change of better/same/ worse; Wilcoxon for changes ranked in order of size	Paired t test
Multiple (k) independent samples	Chi-square (k-1 df)	Kruskal-Wallis	One-way analysis of variance (ANOVA)
Multiple related samples	Cochran's Q	Friedman two-way ANOVA by ranks	Two-way ANOVA

Source: Adapted from Barer D. Choice of statistical methods. Clin Rehabil 1992;6:1–6.

ment effects on two groups when the individuals are not paired and are different people. This method is commonly used in clinical trials that compare a treated group with a placebo group, each of which meets entry criteria. The *t* test requires that each group have a normal distribution, meaning that their measures fall within a bell-shaped curve characterized by a mean and a standard deviation. A two-tailed *t* test allows testing the hypothesis that a treatment is significantly more or less effective than a placebo, whereas the one-tailed test allows only a test of the null hypothesis, which states that no difference exists between the treated group and the placebo group in one direction of change. The two-tailed test is more conservative and is used most often. As a final example, if a therapist compared k = 3 different modalities in different orders to increase the range of motion at the hip in the same children with cerebral palsy, a two-way analysis of variance (ANOVA) would be a starting point for the analysis of this randomized block design with interval data. ANOVA allows the comparison of more than two groups at once or of more than one intervention at the same time. This form of analysis is used often in rehabilitation studies.

A few other examples show the flexibility of statistical methods. The Kendall rank correlation coefficient measures the degree of association between two variables such as degree of independence in toileting and length of inpatient stay. The Kendall partial rank correlation coefficient allows one to control for the effect of a third ordinal variable, such as attention, to see if the relation between toileting and length of stay persists. Whether parametric statistical procedures, which require normal distributions around a mean, should be applied to nonparametric ordinal data is controversial. However, calculations of the mean and standard deviation and reliability using Pearson correlation coefficients, which are usually reserved for interval and ratio data, are sometimes reported in rehabilitation studies that use ordinal scales. Several other strategies have been proposed to assess reproducibility and responsiveness to change when using health status instruments.[32] In many situations, the conclusions from parametric and nonparametric analyses are similar. Thus, the appli-cation of a less appropriate method does not automatically lead to an invalid conclusion.

Reliability and Validity

For research and clinical applications, measurement tools must be reliable and valid. *Reliability* is the extent to which the measure yields the same number or score when no true change in what is measured has occurred. This concept is not unlike a measure's signal-to-noise ratio. Reliability takes into account the random aspect of error in measurement, as well as a bias or a systemic error. *Validity* is the degree to which a measure reflects what it is meant to measure. A measure may always yield the same score for a patient, but it may not be a measure of its intended purpose. Neither of these attributes is all or nothing.

Reliability measures take several forms. *Interrater reliability* is needed for measures that require a rating by someone other than the patient. The statistics most commonly used to indicate reliability include Pearson correlations, Kappa correlations, and the intraclass correlation coefficient, which is specifically designed to address the degree to which scores from the same rater resemble one another more closely than do scores from other raters. For example, a good standard interobserver agreement for measures of a group is 0.70 and for an individual is 0.90, using the Kappa statistic for nominal and ordinal data. *Test-retest reliability* compares measures at two points in time, close enough so that no true change should have occurred. For functional assessments, the fewer the steps in a scale, the higher the level of agreement, but sensitivity to change and the ability to discriminate between two populations tend to fall. Reliability of scales with many items is often assessed by Cronbach's reliability coefficient, which measures internal consistency of the items. This analysis detects the relatedness of items that can be correctly added together.

An assessment measure becomes validated by an accumulation of validity analyses. *Content validity* is usually subjectively decided by, say, a panel of experts who suggest whether items and their measure are appropriate and cover the domain of interest. Choices must be made about which items are most common and important to the population studied. This face validity, the logic of a measure, is especially important. The clinician, not the statistician, draws from knowledge and experience to determine what is relevant and practical about a scale. In rehabilitation, one must especially consider whether an instrument is valid for the purpose at hand. *Construct validity* is the degree to which a tool behaves as hypothesized. This concept requires measures tied to a theory about the construct. If, for example, functional independence after a stroke is the disability construct, then validity comes from the pattern of younger patients who walk longer distances than elderly patients, the greater success of younger patients at reintegrating into the community, and the absence of confounding relationships. *Criterion validity* assesses whether a measure can be related to some standard external to it. In functional assessments and QOL measures, no absolute standards exist. A group of measures may have predictive validity, however. A set of cognitive measures that reveals poor scores has criterion validity if the measures correctly predict some event outside of themselves, such as a low success rate at subsequent employment. In tests for *concurrent validity*, two assessment tools that supposedly measure the same domains can be compared in the same group to see whether they do, indeed, correlate.

Choosing Measurement Tools

Available assessment and outcome measures for neurologic rehabilitation vary considerably, not only in their reliability and validity, but also in their purpose, content, and depth of detail, in the way questions are posed, and in the time and ancillary equipment needed to complete the instrument. Researchers and program evaluators are often tempted to design their own instrument for a specific population, such as the elderly, or for a particular disease. Great care must be taken to construct a clinically relevant, reliable, and valid tool.[62,136] Before choosing an existing instrument for research or patient care, researchers may consider the following questions[15,40,100]:

1. Based on its prior use, is the instrument likely to be appropriate for the population you intend to study? Has it been validated in patients with the same disease, of similar age and health characteristics, culture, education, language, stage of recovery (acute inpatients or subacute and chronic outpatients), and type and degree of disability? Are normative data available? Is the format for the instrument's administration practical for your population and resources?

2. Does the instrument have a conceptual basis consistent with its intended use? For an interventional trial, will it include the important expected outcomes and their magnitude within the time frame of the trial?

3. Are items asked and scaled in a sensible way? Do they take into account how much personal effort, motivation, and outside help is needed, for example, to complete a 50-foot timed walk or a self-care task? Can the scale discriminate change over time within or across patients? Do questions or statements include a transition index to help one measure change? Comparative categories between two administrations of a scale may include ''much better,'' ''somewhat better,'' ''same,'' ''somewhat worse,'' and ''much worse.''

4. Is the patient asked about the capacity to perform or about the actual performance of tasks? Is the patient actually performing the tasks under the eye of a trained examiner? Does the measure focus on the patient's preferences about the relative importance of the disabilities?

5. Are all the different variables aggregated into one summation score? If so, the same score can be reached by many variations in scoring the components. Can a hierarchy of the scale's components, ranked by their importance to the patient or to expected positive and negative outcomes, be used to group and score items? Can items be grouped into separate dimensions, such as physical, cognitive, and psychosocial functions, that are scored individually?

REHABILITATION STUDY DESIGNS

Designs for research in rehabilitation have received much attention in professional journals and symposia, particularly among physiatrists and physical therapists.[16,31] Former tendencies not to foster the notion of the clinical scientist in rehabilitation settings and training programs and to view rigorous research designs such as the randomized controlled trial as difficult, impractical, or unethical[119] have led to the problem that clinical research and the application of basic research have been less productive in this field, compared with most other fields of medicine. The National Center for Medical Rehabilitation Research has targeted this problem in its agenda for training.[21] Clinical practices should be based on sound evidence for their efficacy. This burden of all rehabilitation specialists must also be their calling.

Confounding Issues

The design of a clinical trial in neurologic rehabilitation must take into account many potentially confounding problems. Rehabilitation trials are not as straightforward as trials of a drug or surgical procedure for a well-defined medical problem that uses cure, death, or onset of a major illness as a readily recognizable end point. Even in medical trials, recruitment of an adequately homogeneous population that has the identifiable problem, complies with the treatment, and completes the trial takes great motivation and work on the part of subjects and investigators.

In rehabilitation trials of physical and cognitive interventions, pathologies with a resulting range of impairments are associated with disabilities and handicaps that are equally heterogeneous. All four variables are subject to potentially unforeseen interactions. In addition, the focus of a rehabilitation trial may be at the level of pathologic process, impairment, disability, or handicap, and the outcome measures may also fall within any one or more of these levels. If these 4 sites of a treatment intervention are the rows and the same 4 sites of outcome assessment are the columns, 16 possible

strategies for rehabilitation research are apparent.[158] For example, an intervention at the level of an impairment such as leg weakness in a patient with hemiparesis may alter the outcome at the level of impairment (improved strength) or disability (faster walking) or handicap (new ability to walk up stairs, so no further need for an elevator). If an intervention only alters an impairment, such as improving leg strength, but it does not lessen disability (walking was still assisted or very slow), the intervention will be of little interest to rehabilitation specialists. Of course, an intervention can simultaneously be at more than one level or may affect more than one level of outcome measurement. Taking into account all of these potential relationships can produce enough wobble in a trial to flaw all but the best designs.

Noise may also arise from the style of a therapist's approach and from the fact, derived from many uncontrolled trials, that any acceptable therapy and the overall amount of time spent in therapy lead to some gains in patients at almost any time after the onset of the impairment. The placebo effect is present in up to one-third of patients who serve as controls in a drug trial. With any hands-on intervention, the control group should receive some defined level of attention from the therapists who treat the experimental group. A large enough sample size works around the placebo effect, as well as the variations in any population sample. Without a large enough sample size, tests of statistical significance can lead to a conclusion that an intervention does not work, when it really does, a phenomenon known as a type II error. This situation is in contrast to the more frequent concern of erroneous rejection of a true null hypothesis by statistical methods, the finding that the intervention works when it really does not, a phenomenon called a type I error.

Statistical power is an important concept. It is the ability of a statistical test to find a significant difference that really does exist. In statistical significance testing, power is the probability that a test will lead to the rejection of the null hypothesis when the null hypothesis should be rejected because it is false. Low statistical power to detect small, medium, and large treatment effects has been shown to be due partly to small sample sizes in a group of clinical trials of stroke rehabilitation.[98] Larger sample sizes, more observations, and the greater treatment effects of one intervention over another reduce the risks of a type II error.

Stratification of subjects into groups that take into account a potentially confounding variable can help, but this method may also require a larger sample size. For example, in a trial of a new locomotor intervention compared with a conventional intervention for hemiplegic stroke that starts by 2 weeks after onset, the investigator may want to stratify groups into patients who had only a motor impairment and those who had both sensorimotor and hemianopic impairments, because most of the first group tend to become independent in gait by 12 weeks after onset of the disorders, and relatively few of the second group reach an unassisted level of mobility. At 12 weeks, the new treatment may appear to have no benefit if most subjects for each arm of the study had only a motor impairment and the intervention has appeared not to improve upon the good natural history of recovery, at least by the chosen measure of functional independence. Perhaps the data on the more impaired subjects are drowned out by the data of their peers, however. If each of the two impairment subgroups had been randomized to each of the two therapy arms of the study, the new intervention may have revealed a benefit for the more severely impaired group.

Other aspects of the research design can dramatically moderate the results of an intervention. For example, in a review of 124 trials in stroke rehabilitation with a meta-analysis (see later) of 36, Ottenbacher and Jannell found that the type of research design affected the values for the mean effect size of the intervention.[114] In nonrandomized trials, failure to have blinded recording of outcome measures led to smaller differences in outcomes, compared with designs that included blinding. In randomized or controlled trials, the mean effect was not affected by whether researchers who performed the outcome measures were blinded.

Small sample sizes and other problems in the design of completed individual clinical trials have led to the use of a meta-analysis across neurologic rehabilitation studies. This statistical technique integrates the results of a pool of similar studies that meet certain minimal criteria, such as including

randomization, to look at the efficacy of a type of intervention. The technique seems to work well, for example, when used to study all antiplatelet trials that assess the outcome variables of stroke, myocardial infarction, and vascular death in studies of patients with any form of vascular disease.[5] The utility of this technique in rehabilitation trials is uncertain, however. These studies may compare and aggregate patients who vary widely in their characteristics and may then use different outcome parameters that vary in the reliability of their measurement. The technique wraps together small trials of uncertain quality and is biased by the likelihood that negative trials tend not to be published. A meta-analysis may be better interpreted if it includes a calculation of the number of negative results needed to overturn a significant-seeming result. Although care in the selection of studies and complicated statistical methods is said to help account for these and other biases,[114,126] the results of meta-analyses are best used to justify better designed investigations that directly address a hypothesis.

Clinical Trial Designs

Table 5–2 lists some of the designs that have been used in a clinical neurologic rehabilitation setting for interventional studies. Specific designs have been explained in texts and articles.[72,102,111] Unfortunately, too much emphasis has fallen on descriptive designs, often with retrospectively gathered data. These designs generate no more than pilot information. Quasi-experimental designs do not randomize patients. Indeed, most use no control or comparison group, or they rely on historical controls. Their conclusions, like those of experimental designs, are strengthened by blind testing and treatment and by care, for example, to allow equal intervals of time to pass between serial outcome measures.

The randomized, double-blind controlled trial is the most acceptable design to determine statistically significant differences between two interventions, one of which can be a placebo. This method allows the investigator to reach a conclusion, or an inference, in the statistician's terms, about the relative merits of an intervention in the face

Table 5–2. CLINICAL RESEARCH STUDY DESIGNS FOR INTERVENTIONS

Descriptive
  Case study
  Cross-sectional survey
  Cohort study
  One experimental group: treat and test
  One experimental group: treat and test versus
    test nonrandomized control group
  One experimental group: test, treat, retest

Inferential
  Quasi-experimental
    Multiple treated cohort groups versus
      multiple untreated control cohort groups
    Experimental group: test, treat, test versus
      nonrandomized control group test, no
      treatment, test
    Experimental group: test, test, treat, test,
      test, remove treatment or use placebo,
      test
    Experimental group: test, test, treat, test,
      remove treatment or use placebo, test,
      treat, test
    Single-subject designs
      N-of-1 randomized, blinded trial
      Single time series with repeated baselines
      Time series with repeated introduction of
        intervention
  Experimental
    Randomized, blinded experimental versus
      control group
    Randomized, blinded matched pairs
    Randomized, blinded block design
    Randomized, blinded crossover design

of variation and bias. One of the more confounding problems of using a group-comparison approach is that most facilities do not have a sufficient number of homogeneous patients who meet entry criteria and are willing to participate. This approach lends itself to multicenter trials, unless the impact of the treatment is so large that its probability of detection is high even with a relatively small population.

Single-subject or N-of-1 randomized controlled trials have been advocated to establish a definite clinical and sometimes a statistical answer to the question of whether a drug intervention alters a symptom for a particular patient.[63] For example, a patient with spinal injury who has frequent, distressing flexor and extensor spasms may be placed into a trial of clonidine versus a placebo. A pharmacist, with the patient's consent, can prepare the medications in unidentifiable capsules. The patient and physician are blinded to which agent the patient has been randomized for each 2-week study period. Each day, the patient grades symptoms on a 7-point scale: (1) a very great deal of trouble or distress; (2) a great deal of distress; (3) a good deal of distress; (4) a moderate amount of distress; (5) some distress; (6) very little distress; and (7) no trouble or distress. The two treatments are then graphed against each other for visual inspection. The mean difference in symptom score per question between active and placebo periods can be submitted to a paired t test. Other drugs or different dosages may be added in more trials. Additional symptoms or interval measures can serve as outcomes. This approach is especially useful when the clinician tries to manage a new symptom or wants to determine whether continued use of a drug is warranted. This approach also formalizes what physicians and patients already do when they experiment with a medication. Results, of course, are not generalizable to other patients as they might be in a large, randomized, controlled drug trial.

Other single-case, quasi-experimental designs in which a placebo cannot be used in a blinded fashion have come into increased use in neurologic rehabilitation services.[24,161] These designs enable the investigator to learn whether an intervention in a particular patient alters an outcome. Pretreatment baseline measures serve as the comparison for posttreatment outcomes. Multiple baseline measures must show little variability. At least 25 points in time should be measured.[82] If a treatment is expected to have an immediate effect and its withdrawal is expected to alter that effect in the opposite direction toward the baseline measure, then the design is improved by repeated introduction and withdrawal of the treatment over equal intervals. This circumstance requires fewer measurement points.

In a multiple time series design, groups of patients, whether assigned randomly or not, are assessed before, sometimes during, and after the intervention. If the trends for each group are similar before implementation and change abruptly once treatment begins, the change can be attributed to the intervention. Several visual analyses of data and statistical approaches can evaluate trends over time to assess whether the interventional program alters outcomes.[113,141]

MEASURES OF IMPAIRMENT

Impairments from brain dysfunction are commonly related to size and location of the pathology and, by physiologic means, are visualized by computed tomography, magnetic resonance imaging (MRI), computed electroencephalographic mapping, nerve conduction studies and electromyography, evoked potentials, cortical magnetic stimulation, positron or single-photon emission computed tomography, magnetic resonance spectroscopy, and functional MRI. The quantitative approaches to neurologic impairment of potential use in rehabilitation most often include neuropsychologic tests, rating scales, and mechanical and computerized measures across a range of domains (Table 5–3).[28,69,76,107] Quantitative measures of neurologic impairments, whether performed with a hands-on examination or with gadgetry connected to a microcomputer, can vary greatly in their interexaminer and intraexaminer reliability,[41] and they should not be relied upon until the limits of reproducibility are established by the rehabilitation specialist. What has been done with technology and what can be done are functions of the sophistication and cost of hardware and software.

Table 5–3. SOME STANDARD MEASURES OF NEUROLOGIC IMPAIRMENT

Consciousness
  Glasgow Coma Scale
  Rancho Los Amigos Level of Cognitive
    Function
  Coma Recovery Scale[50]
  Galveston Orientation and Amnesia Test

Cognition
  General
    WAIS-R
    Raven's Progressive Matrices
    Mini-Mental State Examination (MMSE)
    Neurobehavioral Cognitive Status
      Examination (NCSE)
  Memory, Learning
    Wechsler Memory Scale
    Rivermead Behavioral Memory Test[162]
    Selective Reminding Test
    Rey Auditory Verbal Learning Test
    California Verbal Learning Test
    Benton Visual Retention Test
    Rey-Osterietth visual learning complex
  Attention/Concentration
    Trail Making Test
    Wechsler Digit Span
    Paced Auditory Serial Addition Test
    Cancellation Test for visual neglect
    Visual Recovery Neglect Index[140]
  Perception
    Hooper Visual Organization Test
    Line Bisection
  Executive Functions
    Wisconsin Card Sorting Test
    Stroop

Sensorimotor Scales
  Ashworth Score of spasticity
  Fugl-Meyer
  Motor Assessment Scale
  Motricity Index
  National Institutes of Health Stroke Scale
  Kurtzke Functional System (FS) and
    Expanded Disability Status Scale (EDSS)
  United Parkinson's Disease Rating Scale
    (UPDRS)
  ASIA Neurological and Functional
    Classification for SCI
  Tufts Quantitative Neuromuscular
    Examination (TQNE)
Timed performance
  Physical Performance Test (PPT)
  Tufts Assessment of Motor Performance
    (TAMP)
  Timed walk
  Reaction time
  Purdue grooved pegboard
Instrumented evaluations
  Gait analysis
  Strength: dynamometry
  Balance: center of pressure on force plate
  Range of motion: goniometry
  Metabolic energy expenditure
  Instrumented neurologic examination

Consciousness

Scales that measure the level of responsiveness have mostly been developed for traumatic brain injury (TBI), subarachnoid hemorrhage, stroke, and hypoxic or ischemic brain injury. The most widely used tool is the Glascow Coma Scale (GCS).[74] The total score for the best eye opening, motor response, and verbal response ranges from 3 to 15 (Table 5–4). Scores in patients with mild TBI are 13 to 15, scores in patients with moderate TBI are 9 to 12, and scores in patients with severe TBI are 8 or less. The scale has considerable prognostic utility (see Chapter 9). Some coma and minimal responsiveness scales add details about responses to stimuli such as sound, visual threat, touch, and olfaction. They include the Coma Recovery Scale,[50] the Rappaport Coma–Near Coma Scale,[117] the Western Neurosensory Stimulation Profile,[4] and the Sensory Stimulation Assessment Measure.[38] Studies in patients with TBI have also shown the prognostic significance of measures of posttraumatic amnesia measured by the Galveston Orientation and Amnesia Test (Table 5–5; see Chapter 9).

Cognition

A standard battery of neuropsychologic assessments is usually put together by a psychologist and by speech and occupational therapists at a particular institution. The most frequently used measures are listed in Table 5–3. For a specific neurologic disease or a particular range of impairments, a battery of core tests helps to describe patient populations across facilities and provides some common measures across interventional studies, especially in patients with stroke and brain injury. For example, the Consortium to Establish a Registry for Alzheimer's Disease (CERAD) combined nine standard tests to monitor the course of patients with this dementia.[105] Across institutions, the test battery was found to be reliable, sensitive to change, and easily administered. Validity has been supported by clinicopathologic correlations.

Table 5–4. **GLASGOW COMA SCALE**

	Examiner's Test	Patient's Response	Assigned Score
Eye opening	Spontaneous	Opens eyes on own	4
	speech	Opens eyes when asked in a loud voice	3
	Pain	Opens eyes to pressure	2
	Pain	Does not open eyes	1
Best motor response	Commands	Follows simple commands	6
	Pain	Pulls examiner's hand away to pressure	5
	Pain	Pulls a part of body away with pressure	4
	Pain	Decorticate posturing	3
	Pain	Decerebrate posturing	2
	Pain	No motor response to pressure	1
Verbal response	Speech	Converses and states where he or she is, who he or she is, the month and year	5
	Speech	Confused or disoriented	4
	Speech	Talks so examiner can understand but makes no sense	3
	Speech	Makes sounds, not understood	2
	Speech	Makes no noise	1

Table 5–5. GALVESTON ORIENTATION AND AMNESIA TEST (GOAT)

1. What is your name? (2) ___ When were you born? (4) ___ Where do you live? (4) ___
2. Where are you now? (5) City ___ (5) Hospital ___ (unnecessary to state name of hospital)
3. On what date were you admitted to this hospital? (5) ___ How did you get here? (5) ___
4. What is the first event you can remember *after* the injury? (5) ___ Can you describe in detail (e.g., date, time, companions) the first event you can recall *after* the injury? (5) ___
5. What is the last event you recall *before* the injury? (5) ___ Can you describe in detail (e.g., date, time, companions) the last event you can recall *before* the injury? (5) ___
6. What time is it now? ___ (−1 for each half-hour removed from correct time to maximum of −5)
7. What day of the week is it? ___ (−1 for each day removed from correct one)
8. What day of the month is it? ___ (−1 for each day removed from correct date to maximum of −5)
9. What is the month? ___ (−5 for each month removed from correct one to maximum of −15)
10. What is the year? ___ (−10 for each year removed from correct one to maximum of −30)

Total GOAT Score (100 − total error points) ___

The Mini-Mental State Examination (MMSE) is perhaps the most frequently used cognitive screening test, but it has limited sensitivity in detecting language dysfunction[39] and in determining the cognitive basis for disability in the neurorehabilitation population. Scoring must be considered within educational and age-adjusted norms.[26,146] The Neurobehavioral Cognitive Status Examination is more sensitive to cognitive impairments than is the MMSE.[83] It uses a graded series of tasks within domains such as orientation, attention, constructions, memory, language (including comprehension, naming, and repetition), abstractions, and social judgment. Scores have correlated with stroke rehabilitation outcomes on the Barthel Index.[108] Other batteries of fre-

quently used and lesser known tests that extract greater information about a patient include assessments for impairment in sensorimotor integration[78] and in perceptual function.[132] Attempts have also been made to develop disease-specific test batteries, especially for patients with stroke and cerebral trauma.[51]

Impairment Scales

STRENGTH

Strength is most commonly measured by the 5 grades of the British Medical Council Scale. This scale is least sensitive to change at grade 4 of 5, which represents movement against less than full resistance. Handheld dynamometry can be performed in most muscles in a sensitive and reliable way,[128,159] but limb positioning and rater experience are critical. Many devices measure grip and pinch strength, although the reproducibility and validity for any specific purpose are often unclear.[96] Grip strength, tested by a Jamar dynamometer with the patient's elbow extended, is often used for monitoring diseases of the motor unit and correlates with overall strength in the elderly. The Tufts Quantitative Neuromuscular Examination[2] battery uses an inexpensive, nonportable strain gauge to quantitate maximal voluntary isometric contraction of many muscles, along with pulmonary function tests that reflect strength. This system has been successfully used in longitudinal studies and in a randomized trial with ciliary neurotrophic factor in patients with amyotrophic lateral sclerosis.

The most objective, reliable, and sensitive, but expensive and cumbersome, instruments are the isokinetic dynamometers such as the Cybex II (Cybex, Division of Lumex, Ronkonkoma, NY) and Kin-Com (Chattex, Hixson, TN). These devices measure torque throughout the range of motion as the limb moves at a constant velocity. Their computer programs provide data on the pattern of force generation, on the effect of speed in the development of force, on the work performed, and on fatigability.[152] Eccentric and concentric contractions can be evaluated. Computerized dynamometry, along with the Ashworth Score, pendulum test, and other methods can also be used to study spasticity (see Chapter 6).

MOTOR PERFORMANCE

Several reliable and valid measures of sensorimotor impairment are a bridge to tests of disability. They assess the performance of a patient's affected limbs within the context of the motor components of activities of daily living (ADLs). The Fugl-Meyer assessment,[46] developed for the evaluation of hemiplegia, is cumbersome. It scores defined actions at each limb joint based on whether they are accomplished by selective muscular contractions or by an abnormal synergistic pattern. Thus, an isolated biceps contraction with resistance is scored as better than the same resistance produced by a flexor synergy response by the arm. This distinction is important in measuring a change in motor control in patients with upper motoneuron impairment. The upper extremity and lower extremity motor function score components (maximum of 66 and 34, respectively) can be converted into percentages of the total possible score for that extremity, to compare changes in the percentage of recovery over time.[35] Total motor scores can help to stratify patients for outcome studies in stroke (0 to 35, severe; 36 to 55, moderately severe; 56 to 79, moderate; and more than 79, mild).[36]

The Motricity Index[22] has been used in several outcome studies of patients with stroke (see Chapter 7), but it should be valid for patients with any upper motoneuron disease. Weighted scores are given for levels of ability for a thumb and forefinger pinch grip and for power at the elbow flexors, shoulder abductors, hip and ankle flexors, and knee extensors. The Modified Motor Assessment Scale uses a 6-point scoring system to grade the following: supine position to side-lying; supine position to sitting over the side of the bed; balanced sitting; sitting to standing; walking; upper arm selective movements; hand movement; and finer arm and hand activities.[149] Scores correlate with the Barthel Index after stroke.[92]

Many other ordinal and quantitative tests of sensorimotor and oculobulbar function are in common use or have been instrumented.[28,107] Disease-specific ordinal measures with good reliability include the National Institutes of Health (NIH) Stroke Scale,[18] the Kurtzke Functional System[86] for multiple sclerosis, and most portions of the United Parkinson's Disease Rating Scale (UPDRS).[87] The Canadian Neurological Stroke Scale and the NIH Stroke Scale use differing four-part grades that, along with the rest of their components, are reliable and valid as measures of impairment for patients with acute and chronic stroke. The two scales are not reliably interconverted, however.[106] These and other commonly used scales of stroke impairment underestimate functional outcomes for disability and psychosocial functioning.[30]

Instrumented approaches have been attempted for studies of multiple sclerosis[147] and Parkinson's disease.[87] Mechanical goniometry is adequate for static range of motion measures in neurologic diseases, but electrogoniometers are important in dynamic studies, particularly in gait analysis. Fiberoptic technology and software programming, initially applied to make the DataGlove[164] and a suit for whole body virtual reality experiments, offer a potential method to assess limb positioning and joint range across joints and in three dimensions.

TIMED TASKS

Direct observation of a patient's physical functioning requires more staff time, training, and effort than a self-report or proxy report by a family member. Direct observation built upon a set of rules for task completion generally provides a more objective serial measure, however. From the perspective of measurement, a timed performance task is even more attractive. Timed self-care tasks, the time needed to walk a particular distance in the range of 25 to 300 feet, and the distance walked within a given time, usually ranging from 2 to 15 minutes, all potentially add to the reproducibility and sensitivity to change of repeated measures. Tests of walking endurance, such as the distance covered in a 2-minute walk, are reliable indicators and can be more sensitive to change during stroke rehabilitation than the walking subscore of the Functional Independence Measure or speed of ambulation over 50 feet.[125,149]

Some of the tests described previously may be considered measures of disability. They can be measures of impairment, however, if the scale is not one of level of dependence and if a factor analysis performed on patients who carry out the tasks reveals loading on specified impairments. Distinctions can blur. For example, the test with Standard Practical Equipment uses four levels of dependence to grade 12 observed household tasks, such as inserting an electric plug into a socket and using a key to open a lock.[91] Factors that explain most of the variance of the 12 tasks are mobility and balance, cognition, and coordination and hand function. If the well-defined lock-opening task were timed, it would not be any less a measure of impairment of upper extremity sensorimotor function and dexterity than, say, the timed Purdue Grooved Pegboard or the Nine Hole Peg Test.[97]

The Physical Performance Test (PPT)[120] was devised as a quick screen of elderly patients to measure common domains of function, including upper body strength and dexterity, mobility, and stamina in tasks that simulate ADLs (Table 5–6). Although its set of tasks and the range of scores derived from reliability and validity studies are unlikely to apply to rehabilitation inpatients with severe impairments, we have found it useful in the setting of outpatient neurologic rehabilitation. Further development of similar quantitative approaches would aid in decision making about whether a patient is becoming more or less functional. For example, if an outpatient with a stroke takes longer to walk 50 feet and to climb steps, as measured by serial testing, the physician may then order a brief period of physical therapy, if no medical complication accounts for the decline in function.

The Tufts Assessment of Motor Performance (TAMP)[48] was designed for the neurologically impaired, with the notion that any functional activity requires at least several distinct gross and fine motor performance capabilities. It defines 32 motor tasks that encompass the domains of mobility, ADLs, and physical aspects of communication. It goes beyond any other impairment or disability instrument by creating five measures by which to evaluate each task: time to completion, a 5-point scale of assistance needed, dichotomous scales to indicate the normality of the approach used and to rate the normality of specific gross and fine movements, and a 3-point proficiency scale to rate movement control and accuracy of the task. A factor analysis of these measurement dimensions reduced the large set of variables to seven factors that included tasks associated with mat mobility, dynamic balance, ambulation, working fasteners, gross and fine manipulation, grasp and release, and typing.[64] Although the TAMP, as it exists, is daunting, continued psychometric analyses may eliminate redundant items, determine unidimensional variables, identify the way in which motor performances change after an impairment and during rehabilitation, and establish the most sensitive measures of change. This methodology is no different from the challenge posed in the construction of meaningful measures of disability and quality of life.[62]

BALANCE

Measures of balance and mobility can be acquired with and without instrumentation. Elderly patients have been graded on the following: rising from and sitting down in a chair; withstanding a nudge to the sternum; reaching up and bending over; standing with head turning and eyes closed; and initiating ambulation as step height, step symmetry, path deviation, and turning are observed.[145] An accelerometer attached to the patient's leg or waist can measure the number of steps and the amount of time a patient spends ambulating. Balance and mobility interact with other measures. For example, walking speed and symmetry of the swing phase in patients with hemiplegia correlate best with the Brunnstrom stage of motor recovery and the Fugl-Meyer score.[17] Gait velocity, cadence, degree of independence, and appearance show significant correlations with muscle strength of hemiparetic lower extremity groups.[13] Although self-selected velocity and maximal speed are cumulative quality scores of the patient's ability and confidence in walking, a formal gait analysis allows for the evaluation of drug regimens and surgical interventions (see Chapter 4).

Balance has been measured by ordinal scales (0 = unable to stand with feet apart to 6 = able to stand on one leg for 60 seconds), by timed efforts,[14] by balance beam walking, and by the distance along a yard-

Table 5–6. **PHYSICAL PERFORMANCE TEST**

	Time	Scoring	Score
1. Write a sentence (Whales live in the blue ocean.)	___sec	$\leq$ 10 sec = 4 10.5–15 sec = 3 15.5–20 sec = 2 > 20 sec = 1 Unable = 0	___
2. Simulate eating	___sec	< 10 sec = 4 10.5–15 sec = 3 15.5–20 sec = 2 > 20 sec = 1 Unable = 0	___
3. Lift a book and put it on a shelf	___sec	$\leq$ 2 sec = 4 2.5–4 sec = 3 4.5–6 sec = 2 > 6 sec = 1 Unable = 0	___
4. Put on and remove a jacket	___sec	$\leq$ 10 sec = 4 10.5–15 sec = 3 15.5–20 sec = 2 > 20 sec = 1 Unable = 0	___
5. Pick up penny from floor	___sec	< 2 sec = 4 2.5–4 sec = 3 4.5–6 sec = 2 > 6 sec = 1 Unable = 0	___
6. Turn 360 degrees		Discontinuous steps 0 Continuous steps 2 Unsteady (grabs, staggers) 0 Steady 2	___
7. Perform 50-foot walk test	___sec	$\leq$ 15 sec = 4 15.5–20 sec = 3 20.5–25 sec = 2 > 25 sec = 1 Unable = 0	___
8. Climb one flight of stairs	___sec	< 5 sec = 4 5.5–10 sec = 3 10.5–15 sec = 2 > 15 sec = 1 Unable = 0	___
9. Climb stairs		Number of flights of stairs up and down (maximum 4)	___
TOTAL SCORE (maximum 36 for 9-item score, 28 for 7-item score)			___9-item score ___7-item score

stick that a patient can reach while sitting or standing in place.[37] Single-limb balance has limited usefulness in many neurologically impaired patients, especially inpatients. Instrumented techniques include force plate studies of sway, tests of the ability to maintain the body's center of gravity or center of pressure, and assessments of symmetry of weight bearing on each leg.[89,163] Other measures of balance include kinematic analysis during attempts at maintaining balance, the pattern and latencies of leg muscle EMG responses after perturbing a standing patient, and computerized moving platform posturography. Dynamic posturography has been somewhat useful in detecting elderly patients who may be at risk for falls[165] and patients with vestibular disorders.[109] The technique includes recording force plate measured responses to small, brief rotational and translational movements of the plate and to combinations of visual and somatosensory inputs. The reliability of this method and its validity for other neurologic impairments are unproved.[47]

BEHAVIORAL MEASURES

The rehabilitation team often seeks to alter a patient's behavior. An increasingly popular approach is to assess a targeted behavior over time with an interval measure (Table 5–7).[111] For example, a male patient with a frontotemporoparietal infarction and hemi-inattention to his left side is instructed to shave his entire face with an electric razor in front of a mirror. The therapist records the number of verbal cues required to remind

Table 5–7. STRATEGY FOR BEHAVIORAL MEASUREMENTS OF CHANGE

1. Specify a discrete target behavior and associated conditions.
2. Define an observable or measurable action that makes the behavior functional.
3. Sample the behavior by a chosen measure, such as frequency or duration of the behavior in a given time.

the patient that he had not yet finished whenever he stopped. In addition, the therapist may tally the number of times the patient discontinued the task, the amount of facial area shaved after a given time, and the total time to completion with cues as needed. The targeted behavior is monitored daily during morning self-care activities. This approach is especially useful in assessing behavioral modification paradigms in patients with TBI.

In another variation, the therapist may set the goal of no choking during six feedings in a day for a patient with stroke and dysphagia who coughs if liquids are swallowed quickly. The patient must remember to limit intake to one sip at a time with a straw and to properly position the head before each swallow. The number of times that the correct technique is used independently for the first dozen swallows is graphed over each of the six feedings.

When performed carefully, this measure also lends itself to single-case study designs for testing an intervention. If the behavioral measurement is to be used for many patients or to evaluate an intervention for statistical purposes, the investigator must assess for interrater reliability and must use one of the graphing techniques described under clinical trials.

Some modest technology has been used to create behavioral measures. For example, a pressure sensor on a wheelchair seat can record the patient's attempts at pressure relief and can also signal the patient to do so.[61] A computerized system was designed to quantify defined communicative behaviors and to measure changes in the conversational speech between patients with aphasia and their therapists.[103] The investigators hoped to improve feedback to patient and therapist about gains within and between treatments, to assess variability in function, to promote changes in strategies when appropriate, and to create a measure of outcome.

MEASURES OF DISABILITY

Thoughtful descriptions and comparisons of instruments that measure disability have been published.[76,100,134,149] A minority of functional assessment scales were specifically developed for the neurologically disabled or for a rehabilitation setting.[144] Many instruments used pediatric or geriatric populations[6] for reliability and validity studies. Other instruments aimed at specific diseases, such as cancer, mental illness, and arthritis.

Much effort has been devoted to broadly applicable scales that emphasize self-care–related ADLs and instrumental ADLs (IADLs), which are tasks commonly carried out in the community. Table 5–8 lists some of the scales useful in neurologic rehabilitation studies. Most scales include three, four, or seven levels for the degree of dependency for each item. When a scale exceeds the levels of "independent," "needs assistance," and "dependent," guidelines are needed to reliably rate the patient's performance during a formal screening by a trained observer. The sensitivity of existing scales to clinically meaningful change during acute and outpatient therapy is controversial. The Barthel Index (BI) has a relatively long history in North America, Great Britain, and Australia, and the Functional Independence Measure (FIM) has gained a strong foothold in the United States over the past 5 years. In the spirit of achieving the goal of greater standardization of disability scales,[10] these assessments are emphasized.

Table 5–8. MEASURES OF FUNCTIONAL DISABILITY

General

Barthel Index
Functional Independence Measure
Program Evaluation Conference System
Katz Index of ADLs
Klein-Bell ADL Scale
Rivermead ADL Index
Frenchay Activities Index
OPCS Disability Scales

Global

Rankin Disability Scale
Glasgow Outcome Scale
Karnofsky Scale
Disability Rating Scale

The FIM and BI are designed around the issue of dependency, which translates into the burden of care. Less often, scales such as the OPCS (Office Population Censuses Surveys) reflect more about the severity and dimensions of disability.

In the future, functional assessment tools may undergo the previously described Rasch analysis so they can be linked together. For example, a study has demonstrated the feasibility of using the admission and discharge motor skills items of the FIM and the Patient Evaluation Conference System and creating scale values for all items in the same measurement units.[44] Ratings from each scale can then be interconverted in terms of the "rehabit," the rehabilitation functional assessment measuring unit.

Functional Independence Measure

The Task Force to Develop a Uniform Data System for Medical Rehabilitation (UDS) introduced the FIM in 1986.[59] Subsequently, a WeeFIM was developed for pediatric patients. The FIM has 18 items graded on 4-level and 7-level ordinal scales (Table 5–9). The lowest score is 18; 126 is the highest independent level of function. The popularity of this system arises in part from the remarkable support provided for users by the UDS Data Management Service at the State University of New York at Buffalo. A manual, videotape, training workshop, newsletter (with ongoing examples of how to rate a particular level of activity) (Tables 5–10 and 5–11), and computer software accompany a subscription. Users must pass a credentialing test. Data are aggregated at the central office. An institution can compare the scores of its patients with those of all facilities in any of over 20 categories of disease or impairment. Data such as length of inpatient stay, discharge placement, age, mean admission and discharge total scores and subscores for self-care, sphincter control, mobility, locomotion, communication, and social cognition provide valuable insights into important descriptors of neurorehabilitation.

Interrater reliability for the 4-level and 7-level scales is good.[65] The FIM, particularly

Table 5–9. FUNCTIONAL INDEPENDENCE MEASURE (FIM) ITEMS

Bladder management

Bowel management

Social interaction

Problem solving

Memory

Comprehension

Bed-to-chair and wheelchair-to-chair transfer

Toilet transfer

Tub and shower transfer

Locomotion (walking or wheelchair)

Climbing stairs

Eating

Grooming

Bathing

Dressing (upper body)

Dressing (lower body)

Toileting

Burden of Care

7. Complete independence (in a timely manner, safely)

6. Modified independence (device)

5. Supervision

4. Minimal assistance (subject = 75%+)

3. Moderate assistance (subject = 50%+)

2. Maximal assistance (subject = 25%+)

1. Total assistance (subject = 0%+)

its mobility and ADL subscales, also correlates with the BI.[122] A Rasch analysis of 27,000 inpatients across 13 impairment groups has shown that the FIM reflects a 13-item motor and a 5-item cognitive measure of function. This study also supports the FIM's construct validity and suggests that FIM could be scaled as an interval measure.[68] As expected, raw scores are not linear, so they are not appropriate for parametric statistical analyses.

The FIM detects the severity of disability among patients with neurologic disorders, correlates with the burden of care required, and broadly demonstrates responsiveness.[34] Across neurologic diseases, the scale's motor and cognitive functions are important predictors of function; functional status at ad-

Table 5–10. DESCRIPTION OF FUNCTIONAL INDEPENDENCE MEASURE (FIM) LEVELS OF FUNCTION

INDEPENDENT (ANOTHER PERSON IS NOT REQUIRED FOR THE ACTIVITY [NO HELPER])

7. Complete independence—All of the tasks described as making up the activity are typically performed safely without modification, assistive devices, or aids and within a reasonable time.

6. Modified independence—The activity involves any one or more of the following: An assistive device is required, more than a reasonable time is needed, or safety (risk) considerations exist.

DEPENDENT (ANOTHER PERSON IS REQUIRED FOR EITHER SUPERVISION OR PHYSICAL ASSISTANCE FOR THE ACTIVITY TO BE PERFORMED, OR IT IS NOT PERFORMED [REQUIRES HELPER])

Modified Dependence—Patient expends half (50 percent) or more of the effort; The levels of assistance required are the following:

5. Supervision or setup—The patient requires no more help than standby assistance, cueing, or coaxing, without physical contact, or the helper sets up needed items or applies orthoses.

4. Minimal contact assistance—With physical contact, the patient requires no more help than touching and expends 75 percent or more of the effort.

3. Moderate assistance—The patient requires no more help than touching or expends half (50 percent) or more (up to 75 percent) of the effort.

Complete Dependence—Patient expends *less* than 50 percent of the effort; maximal or total assistance is required, or the activity is not performed; levels of assistance required are the following:

2. Maximal assistance—The patient expends less than 50 percent of the effort, but at least 25 percent.

1. Total assistance—The patient expends less than 25 percent of the effort.

Source: Granger C, Hamilton B, Sherwin F. Guide for Use of the Uniform Data Set for Medical Rehabilitation. Buffalo, NY: Buffalo General Hospital, 1986.

Table 5–11. DEFINITIONS FOR AMBULATION FOR THE FUNCTIONAL INDEPENDENCE MEASURE (FIM)*

NO HELPER

---

7. Independent: Patient can be left alone to walk a minimum of 150 feet safely, within a reasonable length of time and without assistive devices.
6. Independent with equipment: Patient walks a minimum of 150 feet but uses a brace (orthosis) or prosthesis on the leg, or special adaptive shoes, cane, crutches, or walker, or takes more than a reasonable time.

HELPER

---

5. Needs supervision: Patient may need verbal cueing, demonstration, ''hands-off'' guarding, or standby assistance; patient cannot be left alone to perform the activity safely but does not require physical assistance or contact to perform the activity; patient walks at least 50 feet.
4. Needs minimal physical assistance: Patient performs 75 percent or more of the task; patient may require ''hands-on'' or contact guarding; patient walks at least 50 feet.
3. Needs moderate physical assistance: Patient performs 25 to 50 percent of the task; only one person is required for physical assistance; patient walks at least 50 feet.
2. Needs maximum physical assistance: Patient performs 25 to 50 percent of the task; only one person is required for physical assistance; patient walks at least 50 feet.
1. Dependent: Patient requires total assistance and performs less than 25 percent of the task; one or more persons may be required to help the patient perform the activity.

---

*Defined as the ability to walk on a level surface indoors once in a standing position (not in parallel bars) and to negotiate barriers.

mission to a facility is the best predictor of function at discharge.[67] For a given FIM admission score, normative standards can be calculated for average expected gains within a FIM impairment group.[93] These findings lend support to including the FIM when one develops rehabilitation resource use models. The FIM also predicts the burden of care at home for patients with stroke[56] and multiple sclerosis.[55] A change of one point in total FIM score corresponds to about 3.5 minutes of help required from another person each day. The FIM does not predict the hours of supervision required.[33]

The FIM is not an ideal instrument. FIM scores during inpatient rehabilitation could be considered an estimate of the patient's safety and need for help more than of real-life functionality in carrying out ADLs. For example, the patient can be so slow walking 150 feet that even home ambulation is not practical, but the patient is graded a 6 on the FIM. The cognitive scale is too midrange to adequately describe patients with stroke and TBI. The social cognition and communication subscales show a ceiling effect compared with neuropsychologic testing.[27] The motor scale does not reflect fine motor function, ease of completion of a task, quality of execution of the task, and use of an affected limb. UDS plans to add an impairment scale that may partially mitigate this deficiency. Moreover, FIM data analyses include a calculation of the length of stay efficiency—the mean change in FIM score per day of inpatient rehabilitation.[57] That the instrument is a measure of progress related to a rehabilitation program and, thus, to program quality is not clear, although the temptation will be great for programs to use their data to compare themselves with the aggregate.

The FIM will likely become the most commonly used broad-based scale measure in the United States. It has already been incorporated into another measure for brain injury, the Functional Assessment Measure, which may increase the sensitivity of the FIM, but it needs much more study.[124] In addition, the whole FIM score or its motor and cognitive subscores, combined with a patient's UDS impairment group and age, is said to characterize the expected length of inpatient rehabilitation stay. This FIM-Functional Related Groups (FIM-FRG) classification has been proposed as a payment scheme, like that of the Diagnostic Related Groups for acute hospital care.[138,139] A FIM-FRG may not reflect the costs of inpatient rehabilitation and hospital length of stay without allowing for modifiers that take into account the severity of impairments, the management of medical complications, and comorbidities, all of which can retard progress over the short run.

Barthel Index

The BI is a weighted scale of 10 activities, with maximum independence equal to a score of 100 (Table 5–12).[95] Items considered more important for independence are weighted more heavily. Patients who score 100 on the BI are continent and feed, bathe, and dress themselves; get up out of bed and chairs; walk at least a block; and ascend and

Table 5–12. **BARTHEL INDEX**

	Help	Independent
1. Feeding (Food needing to be cut up = help)	5	10
2. Moving from wheelchair to bed and return (including sitting up in bed)	5–10	15
3. Performing personal toilet (washing face, combing hair, shaving, cleaning teeth)	0	5
4. Transferring on and off toilet (handling clothes, wiping, flushing)	5	10
5. Bathing self	0	5
6. Walking on level surface (or, if unable to walk, propelling wheelchair) (*score only if unable to walk)	10 0*	15 5*
7. Ascending and descending stairs	5	10
8. Dressing (including tying shoes, fastening fasteners)	5	10
9. Controlling bowels	5	10
10. Controlling bladder	5	10

descend stairs. This score does not mean that these patients can cook, keep house, live alone, and meet the public, but they can survive without attendant care. Scores below 61 on hospital discharge after a stroke predict a level of dependence that makes discharge to home less likely.[54,58] The BI and the FIM have been used for patient self-reports.[60] Although a correlation exists between the trained observer's findings and the patient's perception, well-defined disability assessments are best left to a trained therapist who takes the patient through the tasks.

No other scale to date has been used as much in studies of neurologic disease and for rehabilitation. The BI has been used in epidemiologic studies such as the Framingham Study to assess patients over time after stroke and to complement impairment measures in multicenter trials of acute interventions for stroke, TBI, and spinal cord injury. The BI has also been subject to modifications to increase its sensitivity to changes in disability. A scoring modification with five, rather than three, levels of dependence has been recommended by one study.[130] The Modified BI measures the functional ability to perform 15 tasks.[88] This variation includes a limited independence score for bowel and bladder continence, divides upper and lower body dressing, and adds brace placement and care of the perineum. European studies have used the same 10 categories for their version of the BI, but they score different items from 0 to 1 up to 0 to 3, for a total maximum score of 20.[151]

The BI has its limitations and weaknesses. As with most functional assessments, a change by a given number of points does not mean an equivalent change in disability across different activities. The BI has no language or cognitive measure, so another scale must be added. The BI, however, is the scale to which new measures will be compared.

Other Scales

The Patient Evaluation Conference System (PECS) has 115 items in a 6-step ordinal scale ranging from independence to dependence for motor, self-care, cognitive, and common neurologic impairments.[66] It is designed to reveal progress in rehabilitation for specific goals. PECS data can be transformed into interval, unidimensional measures that may lead to improvement in the items and their measurement properties.[131]

The Katz Index rates six ADLs with a three-level scale, then grades the cumulative level of independence.[81] Although widely used across many neurologic diseases, this scale does not include a dimension for ambulation. The scale lacks evidence of reliability and validity and may be sensitive to change only at an early stage of inpatient rehabilitation. The Klein-Bell scale is a weighted scale with good test-retest reliability and seems about as responsive as the BI.[85] The Rivermead ADL Index[90] covers a greater range than any of the foregoing assessments. It includes 16 self-care skills (but excludes incontinence) and 15 household and community tasks scored as "independent" or "needs help." An earlier version had a middle grade of "needs verbal assistance." This method uses operational definitions that improve reliability.

The Frenchay Activities Index (FAI) was developed for chronic stroke,[71] but it may be of value for assessment of an adult population of patients with neurologic disorders. It covers IADL and some aspects of handicap. Reliability and construct validity appear good when the test is used to discriminate between prestroke and poststroke function in domestic and outdoor activities.[127] One of its 15 questions, walking outside more than 15 minutes with a choice of "never," "1 to 2 times in the past 3 months," "3 to 12 times," or "at least weekly," has been a sensitive measure of outcome in a trial of patients with chronic stroke who are undergoing long-term rehabilitation, although it is not as sensitive as the time required to walk 10 m.[150] Studies of another predominantly IADL scale, the Extended ADL Scale (EADL), have shown content and construct validity and good reliability for outpatients with stroke.[53] The EADL's scores for important home activities correlate with measures of disability, perceived health, mood, and satisfaction. IADL scales can be sensitive to gender, racial, cultural, and social class differences, however, so care must be taken when using them as outcome tools.

The OPCS (Office Population Census Surveys) Scale[149] is an even more inclusive set of disabilities that are operationally defined, weighted, and scored as "done" or "not accomplished." This scale includes dimensions related to locomotion, reaching needed for dressing, dexterity with common objects, and to self-care, continence, vision, audition, communication, feeding, and cognitive function that, in general, have face validity for neurologic patients. Although the scale is designed for a British survey of disability, its statements about functioning have a hierarchic quality that may show responsiveness to change if studied more. For example, the OPCS scales measure levels of disability in neurologically impaired patients over time that are beyond the ceiling effect of the BI and are more sensitive to change in severely disabled patients.[101]

The National Highway Traffic Safety Administration has proposed the adoption of its Functional Capacity Index.[12] This index uses three to six levels to grade eating, excretory function, sexual function, ambulation, hand and arm function, bending and lifting, vision and audition, speech, and cognition. This method does not appear to be compromised by the floor and ceiling effects of most scales and requires patients to use the affected upper extremity.

Other disability scales are frequently used for a particular disease. The Karnofsky Performance Status Scale was developed in the 1950s for oncology clinical trials and has been used in occasional studies of patients with head injury and brain tumor. The scale ranges from normal without disease, to symptoms and signs of disease, to levels of required assistance, to death. The Glasgow Outcome Scale (Table 5–13) has been incorporated into studies of head injury, whereas the Rankin Disability Scale (Table 5–14) has a special niche in trials of stroke. The high interrater reliability of these scales makes them especially useful in multicenter studies. They mix disability and impairment, however, and serve as rather insensitive measures best used for large population studies that require a simple assessment.

Some scales are useful for specific diseases. The Disability Rating Scale is an impairment and disability measure in TBI with prognostic value for the patient's return to employability.[118] The United Parkinson's

Table 5–13. GLASGOW OUTCOME SCALE

Score	Outcome
1	Death
2	Vegetative state: unresponsive and speechless
3	Severe disability: depends on others for all or part of care or supervision because of mental or physical disability
4	Moderate disability: disabled, but independent in ADLs and in the community
5	Good recovery: resumes normal life; may have minor neurologic or psychologic deficits

Disease Rating Scale (UPDRS) and the Extended Disability Status Scale (EDSS) for multiple sclerosis also mix the concepts of impairment and disability. The EDSS is heavily weighted for mobility. Reliability studies suggest the need for a 2-step change in this 20-step scale to mean significant change.[45,110] The EDSS is not sensitive to clinical exacerbations of multiple sclerosis.

Scales for depression and personality profiles such as the Minnesota Multiphasic Personality Inventory can augment the assessment of neurologic symptoms that cause disability. The more frequently used self-rating depression scales are the Geriatric De-

Table 5–14. RANKIN DISABILITY SCALE

Score	Outcome
1	No disability
2	Slight disability: unable to carry out some previous activities, but looks after own affairs without assistance
3	Moderate disability: requires some help, but walks without assistance
4	Moderately severe disability: unable to walk and do bodily care without help
5	Severe disability: bedridden, incontinent, needs constant nursing care

pression Scale, the Zung Scale, and the Center for Epidemiologic Studies Depression Scale. Examiner rating scales include the Hamilton Rating Scale, the Cornell Scale, and the Comprehensive Psychopathological Rating Scale–Depression. In a study of depression in geriatric patients with stroke, the Zung Scale had the highest predictive value.[1] These scales have also been used in studies of disability that is caused by dizziness,[167] headache, and chronic pain.[104,160]

HEALTH-RELATED QUALITY OF LIFE

Quality of life (QOL) measures use the patient's perspective to assess domains that include physical, mental, social, and general health.[134] These measures are meant to evaluate the overall impact of a disease and its treatment. A well-designed instrument for rehabilitation can determine areas that patients believe are important to work on and areas in need of additional support. Indeed, some investigators suggest that QOL can be measured only by determining patients' opinions and, less so, by supplementing with instruments developed by experts.[52]

Scales differ widely in the number of items included for the dimensions of each domain (Table 5–15). Some studies lend themselves to a battery of scales. Although the conceptualization, reliability, and validity of QOL instruments need continued research, these scales have already made their impact on oncologic and medical studies.[143,156] These instruments should have a natural home in patient-oriented rehabilitation. For example, these measures have shown that the strongest predictor of life satisfaction among disabled adults is satisfaction with leisure activities.[84] In another study, a battery of instruments has revealed that patients who have had a stroke have greater depression, cause more stress for their relatives, and are less socially active than a control group.[3] In a study of multiple sclerosis, a QOL instrument showed the impact of the disease in meaningful ways that the EDSS did not.[123]

A patient's cognitive and communicative impairments can limit the utility of QOL tools. In one study, proxy agreement was

Table 5–15. COMPONENTS OF QUALITY-OF-LIFE (QOL) DOMAINS

Physical Health
   Mobility and self-care
   Level of physical activity
   Pain
   Role limitations with family and work

Mental Health
   Psychologic and emotional well-being and
     distress
   Cognitive functioning and distress
   Role limitations

Social Well-Being
   Social supports
   Home and social roles
   Sexuality
   Participation in work, hobbies
   Social contacts and interactions
   Role limitations

General Health
   Medical symptoms
   Energy, fatigue
   Sleep difficulty
   Changes in health
   Life satisfaction
   Health perceptions and distresses
   Overall perception of QOL

poor for the Health Status Questionnaire (see later) in patients with stroke and cognitive impairment, whereas it was good between patient and caregiver for the FIM and the Frenchay Activities Index.[129] Even for patients with chronic diseases and no serious cognitive dysfunction, the observations of physicians and caregivers are generally not a substitute for the patient's own perception of most QOL domains.[135]

Instruments

A University of California-Rand Interest Group on Quality of Life studied existing instruments. In 1992, these researchers found an average of 18 tools that can enable one to assess, with varying reliability and validity for a neurologic population, at least some of the dimensions of each domain, along with 20 measures of global QOL (unpublished data, 1992). No instrument appears likely to serve as either a generic measure for neurorehabilitation or as a singular tool for any particular disease or level of disability, however. The instruments in Table 5–16 offer comprehensiveness and ease of administration. They are representative of the range of ways that questions have been asked and scored.

The Sickness Index Profile (SIP)[11] (the Functional Limitations Profile is a British version) provides 136 statements grouped into 12 categories weighted for scoring in a way that reflects dependence, distress, and social isolation. The subject chooses those categories that apply. This instrument has been used in studies of stroke, TBI, and other neurologic diseases. It may be more responsive to group changes than to individual changes.[29,100,133] In a similar format, the Nottingham Health Profile[100] asks about emotions more directly than does the SIP.

The Health Status Questionnaire[73] has grown out of the Medical Outcomes Study (MOS) Questionnaire, and another study by the Rand Corporation aimed at constructing scales sensitive to changes in functioning associated with changing health. This health-related QOL survey has taken the form of 20,[137] 36, and 74 questions that cover all domains with a progressively greater number of dimensions.[154] The Short Form (SF-36) version (a 39-item version includes three items that screen for depression) has received much support for its ability to enable one to distinguish between ill and well people, among different illnesses, and the severity of illness.[49,153] This instrument is likely to appear in more rehabilitation studies. For

Table 5–16. GLOBAL HEALTH-RELATED QUALITY-OF-LIFE MEASURES

Sickness Impact Profile
Health Status Questionnaire/Medical Outcomes
   Study Health Status Questionnaire
Functional Status Questionnaire
Nottingham Health Profile
Quality of Well-Being Scale

example, the SF-36 is the core measure within the well-designed Epilepsy Surgery Inventory, which evaluates 11 health-related QOL concepts.[148]

The Functional Status Questionnaire (FSQ)[75] has many similarities to the SF-36 in its format of 34 items. It has been applied to general practice and to a geriatric population.

The Quality of Well-Being is a utility scale that may find increasing use in cost-effectiveness analyses.[79] This scale is based on a household survey that asks people to rate different states of health ranging from perfect health ("drove a car or used a bus or train without help; walked without physical problems and did work, schoolwork, or housework and other activities") to "in special care unit, in bed or chair, had help with self-care." Then it weights each combination of symptoms and problems. Perfect health is weighted 1.000, and death is 0.000. This concept has been used to rank the degree of health care that would be provided to Medicaid recipients in Oregon.

Many individual scales of social adjustment,[155] social support,[99] mood, and other components of QOL exist.[134] The Katz Social Adjustment Scale[70] includes 127 questions filled out by a relative about a patient with TBI. The Hamilton, Zung, and Beck Depression Scales appear with some regularity in studies related to neurologic rehabilitation.

Style of Questions

The way in which QOL questions are phrased is critical. Along with rating a specific domain in a semiquantitative way, patients should rate the importance of the domain to their QOL. This rating helps to ensure that the questions take into account the patient's values, not the examiner's biases about response to disability. To be QOL questions, they must reflect the patient's experience and personal perception. Otherwise, the questions merely rate health status, much like a disability measure.

The Functional Status Questionnaire's psychologic and emotional functioning questions offer six choices for answers, such as "Have you felt downhearted and blue (1)

all of the time, (2) most of the time, (3) a good bit of the time, (4) some of the time, (5) a little bit of the time, (6) none of the time?" The physical functioning scale in the HSQ asks how much the subject is limited (a lot, a little, not at all), with the lowest level for mobility "walking one block." The HSQ includes questions about difficulty in the past month in "moving in and out of a bed or chair" and "walking indoors," with possible responses of "(0) usually did not do for other reasons, (1) usually did not do because of health, (2) usually did with much difficulty, (3) usually did with some difficulty, (4) usually did with no difficulty."

For acute inpatient use, the physical well-being dimensions may not provide a meaningful inquiry about physical functioning. These dimensions do not strike within the ranges of function of such patients. The sensitivity of typical QOL questions to change with outpatient rehabilitation has not been established. Sensitivity to change may be increased with an additional patient-specific transition index.[94] One asks patients at baseline about their maximum physical activity, the mental activity that takes the most concentration, and their most stressful or emotionally difficult problem. At follow-up, the transition index asks whether and how these elements have changed. For example, are they much better, slightly better, the same, slightly worse or much worse?

Visual analog scales can also be helpful, at least as far as a single global measure can provide information. Patients may mark their level of QOL from the worst to the best on a 7-step or 10-step ladder, or they may circle one of the faces on a row that gradually changes from a frown to a smile.[100] This approach can serve as a helpful screen for the clinician who wants to learn how the patient perceives life with disabilities. Some investigators strongly recommend a single global rating, because it can reflect the disparate values and preferences of individual patients.[52]

MEASURES OF HANDICAP

Handicap related to neurologic disease has received less attention than impairments and disabilities.

The World Health Organization Handicap Scale[166] uses eight graded categories to describe the difference between an individual's performance or status and what that person expects of himself or herself or of those in a similar situation. The domains assessed are orientation and interaction with surroundings, physical independence in ADLs, mobility, occupation, social integration, and economic self-sufficiency. Although this scale includes some guidelines for rating patients, its reliability is uncertain.

The Craig Handicap Assessment and Reporting Technique (CHART)[157] uses the same dimensions without directly making the orientation component operational, but it defines the dimensions in measurable, behavioral terms. For example, mobility is measured by the hours per day spent out of bed and is multiplied by 2, plus the days per week spent out of bed and multiplied by 5. Another 20 points are given for spending nights away from home and for independence in transportation. The answers to the 27 questions are weighted so that each of the 5 dimensions is worth 100 points when answers reflect no handicap. Reliability and validity appear good when the CHART measure is applied to able-bodied persons and patients with chronic spinal injury.[157] A Rasch analysis defined 11 statistically distinct handicap strata and a linearity consistent with interval data.

Many test batteries and a few individual measures have been used to assess patients for vocational rehabilitation,[25] but a more uniform measure for ability to return to work is needed.[23]

SUMMARY

The development of clinically relevant measures of complex, integrated functional performance has been a great challenge for rehabilitation specialists. Issues of measurement, designs of clinical trials, and statistical methods are conceptually and practically demanding. The rehabilitation team seeks links, in the example of youngsters with Duchenne muscular dystrophy who receive therapy for mobility, between a readily measured marker of pathology (the serum aldolase level), an impairment (strength mea-

sured by manual muscle testing or, more precisely, by dynamometry), a disability (inability to walk more than 10 feet), and a handicap (inability to visit a friend's home because of limited mobility).

No single, general-purpose measure is likely to meet all the needs of clinical investigators, particularly if the investigators want to identify small but clinically important changes after a specified intervention.[116] Available assessments of impairment, disability, and QOL that have already shown clinical relevance, reliability, and validity in pilot studies of a similar population can be combined in a battery for meaningful program evaluation, for comparisons across facilities or diseases, and for research interventions. Insights into the factors that may account for particular and global outcomes, both successes and failures, can begin to be derived from this three-pronged approach. Increasingly, this strategy has been used by investigators in therapeutic clinical trials of patients with neurologic diseases.[115]

Methods are still under development that incorporate functional assessment and QOL measures and identify the morbidity associated with particular interventions. Before health policies, payment rules, and practice guidelines based on these instruments are embraced for rehabilitation care, we must know that they accomplish their intended task. For example, before the FIM becomes a national standard, studies should show its validity for a variety of purposes. Clinicians should be wary about the use of FIM scores or any other disability measures as predictors of outcome when scores are used to determine eligibility for rehabilitation services. For any set of data, even one likely to be more complete than the FIM, more than one equation can be used to fit the data. An extrapolation from models that are still evolving and have uncertain accuracy or are statistical inferences based on data trends can lead to unscientific conclusions and may thereby produce health care policies derived from a false premise.

One should also keep in mind the possible limitations of aggregate studies in neurorehabilitation. As in the rest of medical practice, we cannot easily transpose a clinical research finding to a particular patient.[142] Individuals present complex medical challenges with their inherent biologic uncertainty. This factor is amplified by psychosocial and other personal and societal issues. What happens to a particular patient can, of course, differ considerably from what may have been predicted from a multicenter study of 500 patients, especially if the intervention and population studied were ill-defined.

On the other hand, well-designed trials with an adequate sample size are more likely to serve individual patient decision making well. Neurologic rehabilitation clinicians must continue to expand their borders of care by trying to answer the following question: "Do we know that what we do works for our patient?"

REFERENCES

1. Agrell B, Dehlin O. Comparison of six depression rating scales in geriatric stroke patients. Stroke 1989;20:1190–1194.
2. Andres P, Hedlund W, Finison L, et al. Quantitative motor assessment in amyotrophic lateral sclerosis. Neurology 1986;36:937–941.
3. Angeleri F, Angereri V, Foschi N, et al. The influence of depression, social activity, and family stress on functional outcome after stroke. Stroke 1993;24:1478–1483.
4. Ansell B, Keenan J. The Western Neurosensory Stimulation Profile: A tool for assessing slow to recover head-injured patients. Arch Phys Med Rehabil 1989;70:104–108.
5. Antiplatelet Trialists' Collaboration. Collaborative overview of randomised trials of antiplatelet therapy. Br Med J 1994;308:81–106.
6. Applegate W, Blass J, Williams T. Instruments for the functional assessment of older patients. N Engl J Med 1990;322:1207–1214.
7. Armitage P, Berry G. Statistical Methods in Medical Research. Oxford: Blackwell, 1987.
8. Bailar J, Mosteller F. Medical Uses of Statistics. Waltham, MA: NEJM Books, 1992.
9. Barer D. Choice of statistical methods. Clinical Rehabilitation 1992;6:1–6.
10. Barer D, Nouri F. Measurement of activities of daily living. Clinical Rehabilitation 1989;3:179–187.
11. Bergner M, Bobbitt R, Carter W, et al. The Sickness Impact Profile: Development and final revision of a health status measure. Medical Care 1981;19:787–805.
12. Bischoff D. NHTSA Functional Capacity Index. Federal Register 1992;57:13157–13165.
13. Bohannon R. Relevance of muscle strength to gait performance in patients with neurologic disability. Journal of Neurologic Rehabilitation 1989;3:97–100.
14. Bohannon R, Walsh S, Joseph M. Ordinal and

15. Bombardier C, Tugwell P. Methodological considerations in functional assessment. J Rheumatol 1987;14(Suppl 15):6–14.
16. Braddom R. Why is physiatric research important? Am J Phys Med Rehabil 1991;70(Suppl):S2–S3.
17. Brandstater M, deBruin H, Gowland C, et al. Hemiplegic gait: Analysis of temporal variables. Arch Phys Med Rehabil 1983;64:583–587.
18. Brott T, Adams H, Olinger C, et al. Measurements of acute cerebral infarction: A clinical examination scale. Stroke 1989;20:864–870.
19. Buchner D, Findley T. Research in physical medicine and rehabilitation. VIII: Preliminary data analysis. Am J Phys Med Rehabil 1991;70(Suppl 1):S68–S93.
20. Cohen J. Statistical power analysis for the behavioral sciences. Hillsdale, NJ: Lawrence Erlbaum, 1988.
21. Cole T, Edgerton V. Report of the Task Force on Medical Rehabilitation Research. Bethesda, MD: National Institutes of Health, 1990.
22. Collen C, Wade D. Assessing motor impairment after stroke: A pilot reliability study. J Neurol Neurosurg Psychiatry 1990;53:576–579.
23. Cornes P, Roy C. Vocational Rehabilitation Index assessment of rehabilitation medicine service patients. International Disability Studies 1991;13:5–8.
24. Crabtree B, Ray S, Schmidt P, et al. The individual over time: Time series applications in health care research. J Clin Epidemiol 1990;43:241–260.
25. Crewe N, Athelstan G. Functional assessment in vocational rehabilitation: Systemic approach to diagnosis and goal setting. Arch Phys Med Rehabil 1981;62:299–305.
26. Crum R, Anthony J, Bassett S, et al. Population-based norms for the Mini-Mental State Examination by age and educational level. JAMA 1993;269:2386–2391.
27. Davidoff G, Roth E, Haughton J, et al. Cognitive dysfunction in spinal cord injury patients: Sensitivity of the FIM subscales vs neuropsychologic assessment. Arch Phys Med Rehabil 1990;71:326–329.
28. Davis R, Kondraske G, Tourtellotte W, et al, eds. Quantifying Neurologic Performance. Philadelphia: Hanley & Belfus, 1989.
29. De Haan R, Aaronson N, Limburg M, et al. Measuring quality of life in stroke. Stroke 1993;24:320–327.
30. De Haan R, Horn J, Limburg M, et al. A comparison of five stroke scales with measures of disability, handicap, and quality of life. Stroke 1993;24:1178–1181.
31. DeLisa J, Jain S, McCutcheon P. Current status of chairpersons in physical medicine and rehabilitation. Am J Phys Med Rehabil 1992;71:258–262.
32. Deyo R, Diehr P, Patrick D. Reproducibility and responsiveness of health status measures: Statistics and strategies for evaluation. Controlled Clin Trials 1991;12:142S–158S.
33. Disler P, Roy C, Smith B. Predicting hours of care needed. Arch Phys Med Rehabil 1993;74:139–143.

34. Dodds T, Martin D, Stolov W, et al. A validation of the Functional Independence Measurement and its performance among rehabilitation inpatients. Arch Phys Med Rehabil 1993;74:531–536.

35. Duncan P, Goldstein L, Horner R, et al. Similar motor recovery of upper and lower extremities after stroke. Stroke 1994;25:1181–1188.

36. Duncan P, Goldstein L, Matchar D, et al. Measurement of motor recovery after stroke: Outcome assessment and sample size requirements. Stroke 1992;23:1084–1089.

37. Duncan P, Weiner D, Chandler J, et al. Functional reach: a new clinical measure of balance. J Gerontol 1990;45:192–197.

38. Ellis D, Rader R. Structured sensory stimulation. In: Sandel M, Ellis D, eds: The Coma-Emerging Patient. Philadelphia: Hanley & Belfus, 1990:465–477.

39. Feher E, Mahurin R, Doody R, et al. Establishing the limits of the Mini-Mental State: Examination of "subtests." Arch Neurol 1992;49:87–92.

40. Feinstein A, Josephy B, Wells C. Scientific and clinical problems in indexes of functional disability. Ann Intern Med 1986;105:413–420.

41. Fillyaw M, Badger G, Bradley W. Quantitative measures of neurological function in chronic neuromuscular diseases and ataxia. J Neurol Sci 1989;92:17–36.

42. Findley T. Research in physical medicine and rehabilitation. IX: Primary data analysis. Am J Phys Med Rehabil 1990;69:209–218.

43. Finkelstein M. Statistics at Your Fingertips. Belmont, CA: Wadsworth Publishing, 1985:312.

44. Fisher W, Harvey R, Taylor P, et al. Rehabits: A common language of functional assessment. Arch Phys Med Rehabil 1995;76:113–122.

45. Francis D, Bain P, Swan A, et al. An assessment of disability rating scales used in multiple sclerosis. Arch Neurol 1991;48:299–301.

46. Fugl-Meyer A, Jaasko L. The post stroke hemiplegic patient: A method of evaluation of physical performance. Scand J Rehabil Med 1975;7:13–31.

47. Furman J, Baloh R, Barin K, et al. Therapeutics and Technology Assessment Subcommittee, American Academy of Neurology: Posturography. Neurology 1993;43:1261–1264.

48. Gans B, Haley S, Hallenberg S, et al. Description and interobserver reliability of the Tufts Assessment of Motor Performance. Am J Phys Med Rehabil 1988;67:202–210.

49. Garratt A, Rutta D, Abdulla M, et al. The SF36 health survey questionnaire: An outcome measure suitable for routine use within the NHS? Br Med J 1993;306:1440–1444.

50. Giacino J, Kezmarsky M, DeLuca J, et al. Monitoring rate of recovery to predict outcome in minimally responsive patients. Arch Phys Med Rehabil 1991;72:897–901.

51. Gibson L, MacLennan W, Gray C, et al. Evaluation of a comprehensive assessment battery for stroke patients. Int J Rehabil Res 1991;14:93–100.

52. Gill T, Feinstein A. A critical appraisal of the quality of quality-of-life measurements. JAMA 1994;272:619–626.

53. Gompertz P, Pound P, Ebrahim S. Validity of the extended activities of daily living scale. Clinical Rehabilitation 1994;8:275–280.

54. Granger C, Albrecht G, Hamilton B. Outcome of comprehensive rehabilitation: Measurement by PULSES and Barthel Index. Arch Phys Med Rehabil 1979;60:145–154.

55. Granger C, Cotter A, Hamilton B, et al. Functional assessment scales: A study of persons with multiple sclerosis. Arch Phys Med Rehabil 1990;71:870–875.

56. Granger C, Cotter A, Hamilton B, et al. Functional assessment scales: A study of persons after stroke. Arch Phys Med Rehabil 1993;74:133–138.

57. Granger C, Hamilton B. The Uniform Data System for Medical Rehabilitation report of first admissions for 1991. Am J Phys Med Rehabil 1993;72:33–38.

58. Granger C, Hamilton B, Gresham G. The stroke rehabilitation outcome study. Part 1: General description. Arch Phys Med Rehabil 1988;69:506–509.

59. Granger C, Hamilton B, Sherwin F. Guide for Use of the Uniform Data Set for Medical Rehabilitation. Buffalo, NY: Buffalo General Hospital, 1986.

60. Grey N, Kennedy P. The Functional Independence Measure: A comparative study of clinician and self ratings. Paraplegia 1993;31:457–461.

61. Grip J, Merbitz C. Wheelchair based mobile measurement of behavior for pressure sore prevention. Journal of Computer Methods for Progress in Biomedicine 1986;22:137–144.

62. Guyatt G, Bombardier C, Tugwell P. Measuring disease-specific quality of life in clinical trials. Can Med Assoc J 1986;134:889–895.

63. Guyatt G, Keller J, Jaeschke R, et al. The n-of-1 randomized controlled trial: Clinical usefulness. Ann Intern Med 1990;112:293–299.

64. Haley S, Ludlow L, Gans B, et al. Tufts Assessment of Motor Performance: An empirical approach to identifying motor performance categories. Arch Phys Med Rehabil 1991;72:358–366.

65. Hamilton B, Laughlin J, Granger C, et al. Interrater agreement of the seven level FIM (abstract). Arch Phys Med Rehabil 1991;72:790.

66. Harvey R, Jellinek H. Functional performance assessment: A program approach. Arch Phys Med Rehabil 1981;62:456–461.

67. Heinemann A, Linacre J, Hamilton B, et al. Prediction of rehabilitation outcomes with disability measures. Arch Phys Med Rehabil 1994;75:133–143.

68. Heinemann A, Linacre J, Wright B, et al. Relationship between impairment and physical disability as measured by the FIM. Arch Phys Med Rehabil 1993;74:566–573.

69. Hinderer S, Hinderer K. Quantitative methods of evaluation. In: DeLisa J, ed: Rehabilitation Medicine: Principles and Practice. Philadelphia: JB Lippincott, 1993:96–121.

70. Hogarty G, Katz M. Norms of adjustment and social behavior. Arch Gen Psychiatry 1971;25:470–480.

71. Holbrook M, Skilbeck C. An activities index for use with stroke patients. Age Ageing 1983;12:166–170.

72. Hulley S, Cummings, S. Designing Clinical Research. Baltimore: Williams & Wilkins, 1988.

73. Institute For Health Outcomes. Health Status

Questionnaire (HSQ): 2.0 User Guide. Bloomington, MN: Institute for Health Outcomes, 1993.

74. Jennett B, Bond M. Assessment of outcome after severe head injury: A practical scale. Lancet 1975; 1:480–484.

75. Jette A, Davies A, Rubenstein L, et al. The Functional Status Questionnaire: Reliability and validity when used in primary care. J Gen Intern Med 1986;1:143–149.

76. Johnston M, Findley T, DeLuca J, et al. Research in physical medicine and rehabilitation. XII: Measurement tools with application to brain injury. Am J Phys Med Rehabil 1991;70:40–56.

77. Johnston M, Keith R, Hinderer S. Measurement standards for interdisciplinary medical rehabilitation. Arch Phys Med Rehabil 1992;73(Suppl 12):S1–S23.

78. Jongbloed L, Collins J, Jones W. A sensorimotor integration test battery for CVA clients: Preliminary evidence of reliability and validity. Occupational Therapy Journal of Research 1986;6:131–150.

79. Kaplan R, Bush J, Berry C. Health status: Types of validity and the Index of Well-Being. Health Serv Res 1976;11:478–507.

80. Katz R, Campagnolo D, Goldberg G, et al. Critical evaluation of clinical research. Arch Phys Med Rehabil 1995;76:82–93.

81. Katz R, Downs T, Cash H, et al. Progress in development of the index of ADL. Gerontologist 1970; 10:20–25.

82. Kazdin A. Single-case research designs. New York: Oxford University Press, 1982.

83. Kiernan R, Mueller J, Langston J, et al. The Neurobehavioral Cognitive Status Examination. Ann Intern Med 1987;107:481–491.

84. Kinney W, Boyle C. Predicting life satisfaction among adults with physical disabilities. Arch Phys Med Rehabil 1992;73:863–869.

85. Klein R, Bell B. Self-care skills: Behavioral measurement with the Klein-Bell ADL Scale. Arch Phys Med Rehabil 1982;63:335–338.

86. Kurtzke J. Rating neurologic impairment in multiple sclerosis: An expanded disability status scale. Neurology 1983;33:1444–1452.

87. Lang A, Fahn S. Assessment of Parkinson's Disease. In: Munsat T, ed: Quantification of Neurologic Deficit. Stoneham, MA: Butterworth, 1989: 285–309.

88. Lazar R, Yarkony G, Ortolano D, et al. Prediction of functional outcome by motor capability after spinal cord injury. Arch Phys Med Rehabil 1989; 70:819–822.

89. Lehmann J, Boswell S, Price R, et al. Quantitative evaluation of sway as an indicator of functional balance in post-traumatic brain injury. Arch Phys Med Rehabil 1990;71:955–962.

90. Lincoln N, Edmans J. A re-validation of the Rivermead ADL scale for elderly patients with stroke. Age Ageing 1990;19:9–24.

91. Lindmark B, Hamrin E, Tornquist K. Testing daily functions post-stroke with Standardized Practical Equipment. Scand J Rehabil Med 1990;22:9–14.

92. Loewen S, Anderson B. Predictors of stroke outcome using objective measurement scales. Stroke 1990;21:78–81.

93. Long W, Sacco W, Coombes S, et al. Determining normative standards for Functional Independence Measure transitions in rehabilitation. Arch Phys Med Rehabil 1994;75:144–148.

94. MacKenzie C, Charlson M, DiGioia D, et al. A patient-specific measure of change in maximal function. Arch Intern Med 1986;146:1325–1329.

95. Mahoney F, Barthel D. Functional evaluation: The Barthel Index. Maryland State Med J 1965;14:61–65.

96. Mathiowetz V. Reliability and validity of grip and pinch strength measurements. Crit Rev Phys Rehabil Med 1991;2:201–212.

97. Mathiowetz V, Weber K, Kashman N, et al. Adult norms for the nine-hole peg test of finger dexterity. Occupational Therapy Journal of Research 1985;5:24–37.

98. Matyas T, Ottenbacher K. Confounds of insensitivity and blind luck: Statistical conclusion validity in stroke rehabilitation. Arch Phys Med Rehabil 1993; 74:559–565.

99. McColl M, Skinner H. Concepts and measurement of social support in a rehabilitation setting. Canadian Journal of Rehabilitation 1988;2:93–107.

100. McDowell I, Newell C. Measuring Health: A Guide to Rating Scales and Questionnaires. New York: Oxford University Press, 1987:342.

101. McPherson K, Sloan R, Hunter J, et al. Validation studies of the OPCS scale: More useful than the Barthel Index? Clin Rehabil 1993;7:105–112.

102. Meinert C. Clinical Trials: Design, Conduct, and Analysis. New York: Oxford University Press, 1986.

103. Merbitz C, Grip J, Halper A, et al. The Communication Analysis System. Arch Phys Med Rehabil 1989;70:118–123.

104. Millard R. The Functional Assessment Screening Questionnaire: Application for evaluating pain-related disability. Arch Phys Med Rehabil 1989; 70:303–307.

105. Morris J, Heyman A, Mohs R, et al. The Consortium to Establish a Registry for Alzheimer's Disease (CERAD). Neurology 1989;39:1159–1165.

106. Muir K, Grosset D, Lees K. Interconversion of stroke scales. Stroke 1994;25:1366–1370.

107. Munsat T, ed. Quantification of Neurologic Deficit. Stoneham, MA: Butterworth, 1989:357.

108. Mysiw W, Beegan J, Gatens P. Prospective cognitive assessment of stroke patients before inpatient rehabilitation. Am J Phys Med Rehabil 1989;68:168–171.

109. Nashner L, Peters J. Dynamic posturography in the diagnosis and management of dizziness and balance disorders. Neurol Clin 1990;8:331–349.

110. Noseworthy J, Vandervoort M, Wong C, et al. Interrater variability with the EDSS and FS in a multiple sclerosis clinical trial. Neurology 1990; 40:971–975.

111. Ottenbacher K. Evaluating Clinical Change: Strategies for Occupational and Physical Therapists. Baltimore: Williams & Wilkins, 1986.

112. Ottenbacher K. Statistical conclusion validity: Multiple inferences in rehabilitation research. Am J Phys Med Rehabil 1991;70:317–322.

113. Ottenbacher K. Analysis of data in idiographic research. Am J Phys Med Rehabil 1992;71:202–208.

114. Ottenbacher K, Jannell S. The results of clinical

trials in stroke rehabilitation research. Arch Neurol 1993;50:37–44.

115. Parkinson Study Group. DATATOP: A multicenter controlled clinical trial in early Parkinson's disease. Arch Neurol 1989;46:1052–1060.

116. Patrick D, Deyo R. Generic and disease-specific measures in assessing health status and quality of life. Med Care 1989;27(Suppl 3):S217–S232.

117. Rappaport M, Dougherty A, Kelting D. Evaluation of coma and vegetative states. Arch Phys Med Rehabil 1992;73:628–634.

118. Rappaport M, Herrero-Backe C, Rappaport M, et al. Head injury outcome up to ten years later. Arch Phys Med Rehabil 1989;70:885–892.

119. Reilly R, Findley T. Research in physical medicine and rehabilitation. IV: Some practical designs in applied research. Am J Phys Med Rehabil 1989; 70(Suppl):S31–S36.

120. Reuben D, Siu A. An objective measure of physical function of elderly outpatients. J AM Geriatr Soc 1990;38:1105–1112.

121. Roper W, Winkenwerder W, Hackbarth G, et al. Effectiveness in health care. N Engl J Med 1988; 319:1197–1202.

122. Roth E, Davidoff G, Haughton J, et al. Functional assessment in spinal cord injury: A comparison of the Modified Barthel Index and the "adapted" Functional Independence Measure. Clin Rehabil 1990;4:277–285.

123. Rudick R, Miller D, Clough J, et al. Quality of life in multiple sclerosis. Arch Neurol 1992;49:1237–1242.

124. Santa Clara Valley Medical Center. Functional Assessment Measure. San Jose, CA: Department of Rehabilitation, 1990.

125. Satta N, Benson S, Reding M, et al. Walking endurance is better than speed or FIM walking subscore for documenting ambulation recovery after stroke. Stroke 1995;26:157.

126. Schleenbaker R, Mainous A. Electromyographic biofeedback for the neuromuscular reeducation of the hemiplegic stroke patient: A meta-analysis. Arch Phys Med Rehabil 1993;74:1301–1304.

127. Schuling J, de Haan R, Limburg M, et al. The Frenchay Activities Index. Stroke 1993;24:1173–1177.

128. Schwartz S, Cohen M, Herbison G, et al. Relationship between two measures of upper extremity strength: Manual muscle test compared to handheld myometry. Arch Phys Med Rehabil 1992; 73:1063–1068.

129. Segal M, Schall R. Determining functional/health status and its relation to disability in stroke survivors. Stroke 1994;25:2391–2397.

130. Shah S, Vanclay F, Cooper B. Improving the sensitivity of the Barthel Index for stroke rehabilitation. J Clin Epidemiol 1989;42:703–709.

131. Silverstein B, Fisher W, Kilgore K, et al. Applying psychometric criteria to functional assessment. II: Defining interval measures. Arch Phys Med Rehabil 1992;73:507–518.

132. Sloan R, Downie C, Hornby J, et al. Routine screening of brain-damaged patients: A comparison of the Rivermead Perceptual Assessment Battery and the Chessington Occupational Therapy Neurological Assessment Battery. Clin Rehabil 1991;5:265–272.

133. Smith H. Head injury follow-up: Is the Sickness Impact Profile a useful clinical tool? Clin Rehabil 1992;6:31–39.

134. Spilker B, ed. Quality of Life Assessments in Clinical Trials. New York: Raven Press, 1990:470.

135. Sprangers M, Aaronson N. The role of health care providers and significant others in evaluating the quality of life of patients with chronic disease. J Clin Epidemiol 1992;45:743–760.

136. Stewart A, Hays R, Ware J. The MOS short-form general health survey. Med Care 1988;26:724–735.

137. Stewart AL, Ware JE, Greenfield S, et al. Functional status and well-being of patients with chronic conditions: Results from the Medical Outcomes Study. JAMA 1989;262:907–919.

138. Stineman M, Escarce J, Granger C, et al. A case mix classification system for medical rehabilitation. Med Care 1994;32:60–67.

139. Stineman M, Hamilton B, Granger C, et al. Four methods for characterizing disability in the formation of function related groups. Arch Phys Med Rehabil 1994;75:1277–1283.

140. Stone S, Patel P, Greenwood R, et al. Measuring visual neglect in acute stroke and predicting its recovery: The Visual Neglect Recovery Index. J Neurol Neurosurg Psychiatry 1992;55:431–436.

141. Sunderland A. Single-case experiments in neurological rehabilitation. Clin Rehabil 1990;4:181–192.

142. Tanenbaum S. Sounding Board: What physicians know. N Engl J Med 1993;329:1268–1271.

143. Tchekmedyian N, Cella D. Quality of life in current oncology practice and research. Oncology 1990;4:11–233.

144. terSteeg A, Lankhorst G. Screening instruments for disability. Crit Rev Phys Rehabil Med 1994; 6:101–112.

145. Tinetti M, Speechley M. Prevention of falls among the elderly. N Engl J Med 1989;320:1055–1059.

146. Tombaugh T, McIntyre N. The Mini-Mental State Examination: A comprehensive review. J Am Geriatr Soc 1992;40:922–935.

147. Tourtelotte W, Syndulko K. Quantifying the neurologic examination. In: Munsat T, ed: Quantification of Neurologic Deficit. Stoneham, MA: Butterworth, 1989:7–48.

148. Vickrey B, Hays R, Graber J, et al. A health-related quality of life instrument for patients evaluated for epilepsy surgery. Med Care 1992;30:299–319.

149. Wade D. Measurement in Neurological Rehabilitation. New York: Oxford University Press, 1992: 388.

150. Wade D, Collen F, Robb G, et al. Physiotherapy intervention late after stroke and mobility. Br Med J 1992;304:609–613.

151. Wade D, Collin C. The Barthel ADL index: A standard measure of physical disability? International Disability Studies 1988;11:64–67.

152. Walmsley R, Pentland W. An overview of isokinetic dynamometry with specific reference to the upper limb. Clin Rehabil 1993;7:239–247.

153. Ware J. Measuring patients' views: The optimum outcome measure. Br Med J 1993;306:1429–1430.

154. Ware J, Sherbourne C. The MOS 36-item Short-Form Health Survey (SF-36): Conceptual frame-

work and item selection. Med Care 1992;30:473–483.

155. Weissman M. The assessment of social adjustment: An update. Arch Gen Psychiatry 1981;38:1250–1258.

156. Wells K, Stewart A, Hays R, et al. The functioning and well-being of depressed patients. JAMA 1989;282:914–919.

157. Whiteneck G, Charlifue S, Gerhart K, et al. Quantifying handicap: A new measure of long-term rehabilitation outcomes. Arch Phys Med Rehabil 1992;73:519–526.

158. Whyte J. Toward a methodology for rehabilitation research. Am J Phys Med Rehabil 1994;73:428–435.

159. Wiles C, Karni Y. The measurement of strength in patients with peripheral neuromuscular disorders. J Neurol Neurosurg Psychiatry 1983;46:1006–1013.

160. Williams R. Toward a set of reliable and valid measures for chronic pain assessment and outcome research. Pain 1988;35:239–251.

161. Wilson B. Single-case experimental designs in neuropsychological rehabilitation. J Clin Exp Neuropsychol 1987;9:527–544.

162. Wilson B, Cockburn J, Baddeley A, et al. The development and validation of a test battery for detecting and monitoring everyday memory problems. J Clin Exp Neuropsychol 1989;11:855–870.

163. Winstein C, Gardner E, McNeal D. Standing balance training: Effect on balance and locomotion in hemiparetic adults. Arch Phys Med Rehab 1989;70:755–762.

164. Wise S, Gardner W, Sabelman E, et al. Evaluation of a fiber optic glove for semi-automated goniometric measurements. Journal of Rehabilitation Research 1990;27:411–424.

165. Wolfson L, Whipple R, Derby C, et al. A dynamic posturography study of balance in healthy elderly. Neurology 1992;42:2069–2075.

166. World Health Organization. WHO International Classification of Impairments, Disabilities and Handicaps: A Manual of Classification Relating to the Consequences of Disease. Geneva: World Health Organization, 1980.

167. Yardley L, Putnam J. Quantitative analysis of factors contributing to handicap and distress in vertiginous patients: A questionnaire study. Clin Otolaryngol 1992;17:231–236.

CHAPTER 6

PROBLEMS OF MEDICAL MANAGEMENT

A handful of medical issues come up repeatedly during the chronic rehabilitation management of patients with neurologic diseases. This chapter reviews the mechanisms of and treatment for spasticity, contractures, neurogenic bowel and bladder, pressure sores, and dysphagia.

SPASTICITY

The upper motoneuron (UMN) syndrome that arises from a chronic injury along the corticofugal pathways often includes the sequela of spasticity. Spasticity is clinically characterized by combinations of brisk tendon reflexes, exaggerated cutaneous and autonomic reflexes, involuntary flexor and extensor spasms, clonus, Babinski's sign, and hypertonicity with a velocity-dependent increase in tonic stretch reflexes. A flexor posture of the arm and an extensor posture of the leg can follow hemiplegic stroke, whereas flexion and adduction of the legs often follow severe paraplegia from a myelopathy. Chronic spasticity is sometimes accompanied by dystonic postures, rigidity, and contractures. These signs, however, are generally less important to functional recovery than the accompanying UMN decrement in motor control associated with dyssynergic patterns of muscle activation, with coactivation of agonist and antagonist groups during movements, with the degree of paresis and the loss of dexterity, and with fatigability.[69] The linkage among residual muscle strength, synergistic movements, and spasticity is not well defined.

Spasticity can be assessed by clinical, biomechanical, and electrophysiologic measures, although these measures indicate little about the degree to which the increased tone affects motor performance or contributes to disability. Because spasticity is the one sign of the UMN syndrome that is likely to respond to drug therapy, it is commonly treated. With the exception of painful or disruptive spasms and dystonic postures, however, these interventions generally do not decrease impairments or lessen disabilities.

The great clinical spectrum of spasticity can be understood within the context of its diverse pathophysiologic features.

Pathophysiology

In general, more than the pyramidal tracts must be lesioned to produce spasticity, but just which additional cortical, subcortical, or spinal pathways must be included to induce it is uncertain. Incomplete spinal lesions in humans are associated with the most clinically evident and most commonly treated manifestations of hypertonicity and spasms (see Chapter 8). The likely common denominator for altered tone during both passive and active movements is the combination of an abnormal net modulation by residual descending and propriospinal excitatory and inhibitory inputs and by the range of segmental peripheral sensory inputs that converge on spinal interneurons. The loss of inhibitory control appears especially likely to cause hyperexcitability of the spinal motor pools and also leads to the loss of the orderly recruitment of motor units and of the modulation of the rate of a unit's action potential discharges.[58] The clinical manifestations include high fatigability and a lack of smoothness during movements.

As a point of convergence, the interneuronal pools provide much greater flexibility for motor control than that provided by simple spinal reflexes on motoneurons. Along with the mechanical properties of muscle and connective tissue, these pools contribute to normally flexible responses to active and passive muscle stretch.[28] The loss of descending pathways can lead to a variety of adaptations within the motoneuron and interneuron pools. These modifications include altered neurotransmitter release, membrane potential alterations, sprouting with new synapses, and increased activity within previously ineffective synapses (see Chapter 1 on reflex spinal pathways). One possible clinical example of activity-induced changes is the rapid development of the dystonic flexor posture of the arm in patients with hemiparesis who regularly perform strenuous resistive exercises. The neural circuitry that induces this spasticity is presumably reinforced, perhaps by residual supraspinal drive on motoneurons and interneurons.[33]

In patients with spasticity, electrophysiologic studies have begun to detail some of the changes that arise within the spinal cord. Table 6–1, drawn from many investigators, summarizes some relevant experimental work on possible mechanisms.[107,144] The variations in results are consistent with the amount of residual supraspinal input and the plasticity of the spinal cord. These studies are of interest to rehabilitation specialists

Table 6–1. SPINAL MECHANISMS THAT MAY CONTRIBUTE TO SPASTICITY AND HYPERREFLEXIA

Mechanism	Activity	Neurotransmitter
Alpha motoneuron excitability	Increase	—
Gamma motoneuron excitability	No change	—
Excitatory interneuron		
Ia excitability	Increase	Glutamate
Flexor reflex afferents	Increase	NE,* 5HT*
Inhibitory interneuron		
Presynaptic Ia inhibition	Decrease	GABA*
Recurrent Renshaw cell inhibition	Increase or decrease	Glycine
Nonreciprocal Ib inhibition	Decrease	—
Reciprocal Ia inhibition	Decrease	Glycine
Group II inhibition	No change	—
Renshaw cell inhibition	No change	—

*NE = norepinephrine, 5-HT = 5-hydroxytryptamine, GABA = γ-aminobutyric acid.

because they provide insight into the way in which drugs and noxious inputs may affect spinal mechanisms. Hyperexcitability of alpha motoneurons, perhaps related to changes in their membrane properties from fewer or abnormal synaptic inputs, may contribute to spasticity. In addition, decreased presynaptic inhibition of Ia primary muscle spindle endings, decreased reciprocal inhibition of antagonist motoneuron pools by Ia terminals, and decreased nonreciprocal inhibition are suggested contributors. Not believed involved is an increased sensitivity of muscle spindle Ia endings or any other pathologic increase of peripheral input to the spinal cord, nor has a decrease in Renshaw cell and group II afferent inhibition been shown.

Responses of these circuits vary widely in human studies. For example, some experiments using the conditioned H-reflex technique in patients with hemiplegia and hereditary spastic paraparesis suggested reduced or no recurrent inhibition and sometimes increased inhibition during voluntary movement, whereas another study of patients after spinal cord injuries (SCI) above T-4 consistently pointed to increased recurrent inhibition at rest.[122] How may spasticity arise from an increase in the inhibitory activity of a pathway that inhibits alpha motoneuron output? The investigators suggested that another Renshaw cell connection, an inhibitory synapse on Ia interneurons, may lead to a stronger reciprocal facilitation of the motoneuron.

Responses may also vary for different manifestations of the UMN syndrome. For example, a study found facilitation or reduced nonreciprocal Ib inhibition in patients with spastic paresis who also had spastic dystonia.[144] Patients who had hyperreflexia without dystonia had normal inhibition.

All of these potential mechanisms of spasticity would be complicated, especially after SCI, by what remained of the noradrenergic projections from the locus coeruleus that tonically inhibit Renshaw cells and directly excite motoneurons. The loss of tonic inhibition of the Renshaw cell may explain the way in which alpha-2–adrenergic agonists such as clonidine reduce spasticity.

Clinicians tend to define spasticity in terms of a few manifestations of the neurologic examination. Muscle stretch reflex excitability is most commonly assessed by the briskness of the tendon jerk. This monosynaptic and oligosynaptic pathway does not reflect an alteration as well as the more naturally elicited stretch reflex response derived from limb displacement, however.[44] In patients with spasticity, faster movements of an affected muscle evoke a reflex response that increases in proportion to the velocity of the stretch. EMG activity persists throughout the movement, but it ceases at whatever angle is reached, even when the stretch is maintained. The reflex contraction that opposes stretch is carried by the rapidly conducting Ia afferents from primary spindle endings into homonymous and synergistic motoneurons and interneurons.

Reflex irradiation produces hyperreflexia. This phenomenon arises from spread of the percussion wave or of a vibration along bone and muscle to the spindle endings of multiple muscle groups. The clasp-knife catch and giveway phenomenon appear to arise from disinhibition of interneurons that receive flexor reflex afferents (FRA).[17] Flexor and extensor spasms, particularly from cutaneous and nociceptive inputs, also seem to involve the short-latency FRA pathways normally inhibited by the dorsal reticular and the noradrenergic-mediated and serotonergic-mediated reticulospinal systems. The corticospinal and rubrospinal pathways facilitate these cells. In patients with paraparesis, electrical stimulation over the foot can generate a flexor response of the hip and knee by the FRAs strong enough to be of use during functional electrical stimulation–assisted gait. The interneuronal organization of the FRAs also plays a role in the generation of locomotor movements by the lumbar motor pools (see Chapter 1).

Spasticity is also the consequence of interactions between central and peripheral factors. The mechanical resistance to a passive change in the angle of a joint results from the elastic and viscous properties of muscle, tendons, and connective tissue, as well as from reflexively mediated stiffness. During active contraction, the contractile properties of the muscle add to its mechanical impedance. Some investigators have proposed that secondary changes in spastic muscle, such as an increase in connective tissue and a loss of muscle fibers or a change in their properties, explain at least some of the increased stiffness in patients.[36,50] For example, myosin crossbridges to actin filaments may increase after a muscle contraction and may produce stiffness.[19] Excessive fatigability and exaggerated metabolic responses similar to those seen in disuse atrophy have been elicited by tetanic stimulation of the tibialis anterior muscle in patients with spastic paresis,[93] a finding that supports the hypothesis that structural changes can contribute to resistance to movement in this muscle.[63]

Measures

In patients, clinical scales and instrumented measures of spasticity have been developed to reveal the effects of interventions on tone and to provide insight into mechanisms.

CLINICAL SCALES

The history of how and when hypertonicity interferes with a patient's activities is the most useful way to determine whether an intervention is needed. Bouts of clonus and flexor and extensor spasms during ambulation, driving, wheelchair push-up pressure releases, transfers, reclining, bed mobility, sleep, sexual function, and self-care activities can be counted over the course of a day or a week.

Commonly used clinical scales of spasticity are listed in Table 6–2. The Ashworth Scale[5,77] has good interrater reliability and reproducibility if it is measured under the same conditions, such as similar positioning of the patient. Associated reactions are another potential measure. An involuntary movement of the spastic limb can often be elicited by a forceful movement in another part of the body. For example, the hemiparetic arm may flex when the patient stands. Such movements can be counted or the change in angle of a joint can be measured.[40] The relationship between changes in the Ashworth score or in associated reactions to changes in functional activities is moot.

Table 6–2. CLINICAL SCALES OF SPASTICITY

Ashworth Scale Score:

  0 No increase in tone
  1 Slight increase, producing a catch when joint is moved in flexion or extension
  2 More marked increase in tone, but joint easily flexed
  3 Considerable increase, and passive movement difficult
  4 Affected part rigid in flexion or extension

Spasm Score[91]:

  0 No spasms
  1 Mild spasms induced by stimulation
  2 Spasms occurring less than 1/h
  3 Spasms occurring more than 1/h
  4 Spasms occurring more than 10/h

Reflex Score

  0 (absent) to 5 (sustained clonus)

BIOMECHANICAL TECHNIQUES

Biomechanical techniques evaluate changes in the phasic and tonic reflex activity of the muscles across a joint.[69,110]

For the Wartenberg's pendulum or "drop" test, the patient is supine or propped up 45 degrees with the legs dangling over the edge of a table. The tester lifts a relaxed leg to the horizontal and releases it so the leg swings by gravity alone. In patients with spasticity of the quadriceps and hamstrings, the initial swing from full extension usually does not reach the vertical, whereas an unaffected leg tends to flex beyond that point to about 70 degrees. The maximum angular velocity, the knee angle in flexion, and the number of swings tend to decrease with hypertonicity. Commercially available isokinetic exercise equipment, an electrogoniometer that records the changing knee joint angle, or computerized video equipment for studying leg kinematics can be used to quantitate this practical, although perhaps theoretically flawed measure of hypertonicity.[130] The drop test has provided more detailed and observer-independent measurements than the Ashworth score in studies of patients with chronic hemiplegia after stroke[68] and of patients with multiple sclerosis,[80] and it has correlated with the Ashworth score in a study of tizanidine in patients with spastic paraparesis and SCI.[97] The antispasticity effects of clonidine, cyproheptadine, and baclofen were revealed by a video motion analysis of the pendulum test in patients with spastic SCI.[96]

Other devices can quantitate the torque or amount of force elicited by motorically moving the elbow, wrist, knee, or ankle over a particular angle at a specified velocity. These devices can also quantitate the threshold angle at which the torque or EMG starts to increase in an initially passive muscle. Although the findings emulate the clinician's qualitative tests, results from different laboratories are often inconsistent. Differences may be related to idiosyncracies in equipment and technique, in the joint tested, and in the patient population studied. For example, biomechanical evidence has been used to support the opposing hypotheses that spastic hypertonia at the elbow results primarily from the following:

1. A decrease in stretch reflex threshold and preserved reflex gain implies that the motoneurons activated at smaller joint angles and lower angular velocities start out more depolarized.[109]
2. A pathologic increase in stretch reflex gain implies that the response is mediated by a late polysynaptic pathway, probably from muscle spindle afferents.[134]
3. Responses differ under passive and active movements; for example, during active flexion, a change is more apparent in reflex gain than in reflex threshold, but a change in the mechanical properties of the muscle is also important.[64]

Whether studies of stretch-evoked EMG and torque signals or of other biomechanical methods[78] will provide reproducible measures and insights into mechanisms of hypertonicity or demonstrate the effects of interventions is not yet clear. Many of these strategies were compared in a study of 10 patients with chronic hemiplegia.[68] The Ashworth and Fugl-Meyer scores correlated with torque and EMG measurements during ramp-and-hold angular displacements about the elbow and with a pendulum test of the affected leg. The results were reproducible over several weeks. The H/M ratio showed a wide intrasubject variation and did not correlate with the clinical picture. However, correlations among these methods point more to the fair reliability than to the validity of these measures for functionally important conditions.

ELECTROPHYSIOLOGIC TECHNIQUES

Hoffmann's reflex (H-reflex) has been used in clinical settings[30,32] (Table 6–3). The amplitude of the H response compared with that of the motor response (H_{max}/M_{max} ratio) measures the excitability of the soleus motoneurons that respond to supramaximal stimulation of the sciatic nerve. When the patient is tested at rest, the ratio tends to increase with spasticity, but studies have not shown it to correlate with the intensity of spasticity. The ratio and H-reflex amplitude have been shown to increase significantly about 3 months after a clinically complete SCI.[83] The hyperactive H-reflex is not con-

Table 6–3. INSTRUMENTED CLINICAL TECHNIQUES TO MEASURE SPASTICITY

Mechanical Methods
  Pendulum drop with relaxation index
  Manual stretch with electromyographic (EMG) response
  Ramp, sinusoidal, or random
    Controlled displacement with torque or EMG response
    Controlled torque with displacement or EMG response

Neurophysiologic Methods
  H-reflex
    H_{max}/M_{max}
    H-reflex suppression by vibration
    H-reflex recovery after conditioning stimulus train
    Audiospinal modulated H-reflex[37]
  Dynamic integrated EMG recruitment periods
    Bicycle ergometry[11]
    Treadmill walking
  Joint probability density amplitudes
  Kinematic gait studies with angle-angle plots

sistently modulated during ambulation in patients with spastic paresis, unlike healthy persons, so the usefulness of this reflex as a measure of reflex abnormality may be limited.[140] The gain of the H-reflex in some patients with spasticity may already be so high that the response cannot rise with stimulation.

The $H_{max\ vibration}/H_{max\ control}$ ratio decreases in patients with spasticity. This ratio measures the inhibition of the soleus monosynaptic reflex by vibration at 100 Hz over the Achilles tendon. It is due to presynaptic inhibition of Ia fibers exerted through interneurons that make γ-aminobutyric acid (GABA)ergic connections with the terminal arborizations of Ia fibers. Spasticity is also associated with brief facilitation of the H-reflex recovery curve, rather than the normal suppression, after it is conditioned by a train of four 300-Hz shocks applied to the posterior tibial nerve at the ankle. This phenomenon presumably reflects the hyperexcitability of motoneurons. Several of these electrophysiologic tests have been used in spastic patients in an attempt to detect and to best treat the predominant pathophysiologic features underlying their hypertonicity and hyperreflexia.[31] Diazepam, and tizanidine to some degree, have increased vibratory inhibition of the H-reflex. Baclofen has facilitated the H-reflex recovery curve. The drugs have not affected the H_{max}/M_{max} ratio.

ELECTROMYOGRAPHIC AND KINEMATIC METHODS

Abnormal coactivation of antagonistic muscle groups, as well as inappropriate timing of muscle activity, can interfere with walking in patients with a UMN syndrome. This activity can be partially quantified during formal gait analysis with surface EMG and kinematic studies. Such dynamic studies open up the possibility that measures of spasticity, a type of disordered motor control, can be made during a clinically relevant activity such as ambulation.

In one technique, the EMG from each muscle from initial foot contact with the floor to the next ipsilateral foot contact is integrated and normalized to 100 percent of the step cycle. The patient's EMG data are then divided into windows that identify when each muscle is active or inactive compared with the timing of the activity of normal controls. An index is defined as the ratio of integrated EMG area in ordinarily "off" windows to that in the "on" windows. If the timing of muscle activity in a patient is similar to that of healthy persons, then the index is a small fraction. For patients with significant spasticity or disordered motor control, muscles are on when they would be off in controls, so the ratio is greater than 1.[47] The analysis provides a dynamic within-step quantification of inappropriate activity with respect to the step cycle for each muscle studied. Drawbacks include the complexity of obtaining the data, performing the analysis, and accounting for the great variation in the EMG bursts of healthy persons who serve as controls and of patients with spasticity during ambulation.

The EMG amplitudes of an agonist-antagonist pair can also be simultaneously plotted using a statistical technique called *joint probability density distribution,* which reflects the likelihood of coactivation of the pair.[29] Kinematically derived diagrams of the angles made at one joint compared with the angles of the joint above or below as the gait cycle proceeds also provide insight into motor control and spasticity.[139]

Quantitative measures of spasticity or of disordered motor control that are sensitive to functionally important actions of the arm and leg need further development for a clinical setting. Single-joint movements are of less importance to rehabilitation specialists than are the dynamic, more complex, movement-evoked responses of the motor system.

Management

Hypertonicity has potential value. It may decrease muscle atrophy and bone demineralization, and it may increase venous return from the legs. An extensor thrust can provide the rigidity for weight-bearing stance. Learning to induce an extensor spasm can assist a patient with paraplegia in making transfers. FRAs can be modulated to assist in stepping. Trying to reduce spasticity is worthwhile, however, when the spasticity interferes with nursing care and perineal hygiene, contributes to contractures and pressure sores, and jogs the patient with painful or disconcerting flexor or extensor spasms during transfers, intermittent self-catheterization, or modest cutaneous stimulation.

Treatment of spasticity also is potentially useful when co-contraction of agonist and antagonist muscle groups appears to restrain voluntary upper or lower limb movements. The neurodevelopmental schools of physical therapy often attribute poor muscle use to the action of spastic antagonists, but interventions that reduce tone in the antagonist generally do not improve the strength and control of the agonist. For example, at the elbow of patients with hemiparesis after stroke, the positive contribution of agonist muscle strength to movement appears to be more important than any negative contribution of antagonistic muscle tone.[14] Overactivity of an antagonist elbow extensor may play a role in disturbing a flexion-extension movement made at low velocity or during a perturbation of movement that induces a reflex contraction. Antagonist activity during movement made against a load, however, which is a more normal circumstance than simply testing spasticity at various elbow angular velocities, appears to be low or normal, even in patients with long-term sequelae of stroke who have severe passive muscle hypertonia.[45] During locomotion, exaggerated reflexes generally contribute little to impairment of movement.[35] Again, agonist muscle paresis, not antagonist hypertonia, is most important in interfering with voluntary movement.

Different therapeutic approaches might arise if one could separate the reflexive from the passive tissue components that increase joint impedance. For example, electrical stimulation, passive range of motion, and loading of joints as soon as possible after onset of UMN lesions may limit certain negative changes in muscle and connective tissue that add to the manifestations of spasticity. An overall approach to hypertonicity includes reversing any noxious stimulus as a cause, using simple physical interventions before adding drug trials, and reserving more invasive techniques such as nerve blocks and orthopedic or neurosurgical procedures for selected patients with recalcitrant cases.

PHYSICAL MODALITIES

Patients should be educated about the way in which slow movements and daily passive range of motion stretches reduce motion-sensitive symptoms of spasticity. Nociception can exacerbate hypertonicity and can trigger flexor and extensor spasms. Even an ordinarily innocuous stimulus, such as tight clothing or a sunburn, can abruptly increase tone, much as it can cause autonomic dysreflexia in the patient with a cervicothoracic SCI. Treatable noxious sources include bowel and bladder distention, urinary tract infection, epididymitis, joint pain especially on range of motion, fractures, pressure sores, ingrown toenails, and deep venous thrombosis.

Static stretching with splints and serial casting can reduce stretch reflex activity and contractures. For example, tonic toe flexion, which is a plantar grasp reflex, is reduced by using a toe spreader. This correction can significantly increase gait velocity and cadence.[115] Muscle cooling with an ice pack for 20 minutes decreases spasticity for about an hour,[111] so cryotherapy is commonly used to prepare for other modalities such as stretching, range of motion, and gait. Tendon vibration, reflex-inhibiting postures and bed positioning, and EMG biofeedback can complement a stretching program during the activity, but formal studies of the use of these techniques are too limited to judge any added benefit. Patients with spastic paraplegia who have multiple sclerosis (MS) and SCI often report that standing in a support frame for as little as half an hour a day reduces spasms. The effect may be related to a modulation by afferent inputs from prolonged stretching and from loading of the joints. Formal studies of standing in nonambulatory patients have not clearly demonstrated the efficacy of this technique on clinical measures of hypertonicity or on limiting of contractures and osteoporosis.[73]

ELECTRICAL STIMULATION

Electrical stimulation of motor and sensory nerves, muscles, and dermatomes by a variety of paradigms has, in general, reduced spasticity at the ankle and knee.[130] A single stimulation session decreases resistance and clonus for a few hours. Studies of long-term use show a range of responses that, in part, result from variations in patient characteristics, outcome measures, location of the stimulation, and parameters of the electrical stimuli. For example, after twice-daily 20-minute stimulations of the quadriceps for 4 weeks, an increase in spasticity has been found, based on the leg relaxation time after a pendulum drop test, especially in patients with incomplete paraplegia and quadriplegia who were more spastic before the stimulation program.[114] Stimulation over the surface of the tibialis anterior muscle for 20 minutes has decreased the viscoelastic stiffness in patients with TBI and SCI for up to 24 hours, although a functional benefit has been found only in the patients with SCI who had ankle clonus.[119] One study of patients with chronic stroke spastic hemiparesis who had showed that 15 daily, low-intensity, high-frequency, transcutaneous electrical nerve stimulation (TENS) applications for 1 hour over the proximal common peroneal nerve decreased a clinical measure of spasticity, increased vibratory inhibition of the H-reflex of the soleus muscle, improved voluntary dorsiflexion force, and reduced the magnitude of the stretch reflex in the affected ankle.[81] Enhanced presynaptic inhibition was considered a contributing mechanism.

Stimulation of FRAs by peroneal and sural nerve stimulation has also been suggested as the cause of similar positive results in patients with myelopathies.[104,105] Electrostimulation for 5 to 10 minutes by a rectal probe to elicit ejaculation had the added effect of reducing muscle spasms and tone in 10 of 14 patients for about 9 hours.[55]

Changes in muscle tone have not been systematically reported during functional electrical stimulation (FES) studies of muscle in which the primary aim is to increase muscle mass, improve conditioning, or assist ambulation, but some patients with SCI report less spasticity. Electrical stimulation of the forearm muscles can at least transiently reduce flexor tone in the hand. Moreover, a chain-link glove that conducts electrical impulses has decreased finger flexor postures in the hemiplegic upper extremity in some patients. The subjective measures of spasticity, the variations in stimulation techniques, and the lack of a control therapy during trials make the clinical usefulness of neuromuscular stimulation equivocal until more research is completed.

Stimulation of the spinal cord, using techniques similar to those tried for pain control, has been of equivocal value in reports and seems like an extraordinary measure even for the management of disabling flexor and extensor spasms that are refractory to oral medications. Intrathecal baclofen administration is a better option.

PHARMACOTHERAPY

Drug approaches to spasticity generally aim to alter spinal or muscular mechanisms associated with hypertonicity and spasms. When small, controlled trials have been completed to measure benefits, the target symptoms and their assessments have varied, only a particular neurologic disease has been considered, and many patients did not tolerate the side effects of a drug, so they dropped out of the study before an individualized approach to dosing was undertaken. Dose-response studies for individuals within a trial allow a more practical assessment of potential benefits, but this approach was rarely taken before the mid 1980s. In addition, measurable functional gains related to locomotion and upper limb use are often not significant. The impact of a purported benefit should be weighed. For example, if an intervention diminishes extensor spasms by 50 percent over placebo, but spasms still thrust a patient out of the wheelchair three times a day and make every transfer dangerous, the reduction in spasms does not achieve a critical goal.

The mechanisms of action and the uses of these agents have been reviewed in texts[52] and journals.[27,145] The range of average dosages is shown in Table 6–4. Whenever a drug appears to be useful for an individual, it is worth tapering the dose down from time to time so that the patient can help to judge the presence of continued benefits.

Dantrolene. This medication competitively blocks the release of calcium from the sarcoplasmic reticulum in a dose-response fashion. This effect decreases the force produced by electrical excitation—muscle contraction coupling. Dantrolene acts on both intrafusal and extrafusal fibers. Its half-life is

Table 6–4. INITIAL AND MAXIMUM DOSAGES OF MEDICATIONS FOR SPASTICITY

General First-Line Use
   Diazepam: 2 mg bid to 15 mg qid
   Dantrolene: 25 mg bid to 100 mg qid
   Baclofen: 5 mg bid to 40 mg qid

For Spasms
   Clonidine: 0.05 mg qid to 0.2 mg tid
   Tizanidine: 2 mg bid to 12 mg tid

Second-Line or Supplementary Use
   Phenytoin: serum concentration 10 to 20 mg/
      dL
   Phenobarbital: serum concentration 10 to 30
      mg/dL
   Threonine: 500 mg to 2.5 g tid
   Cyproheptadine: 4 mg bid to 8 mg qid
   Chlorpromazine: 10 mg qd to 50 mg tid
   Cannabinoids: 5 mg THC qd to 10 mg tid

9 hours. Adverse reactions include lethargy, nausea, diarrhea, lightheadedness, and paresthesias. In early trials, a reversible hepatotoxicity developed in 1.8 percent of patients, with fatalities in 0.3 percent. A surveillance study of reports uncovered by the manufacturer estimated 9 asymptomatic and symptomatic cases of hepatotoxicity per 100,000 prescriptions, with 0.8 fatal hepatic reactions.[20] Biochemical tests of liver function should be monitored monthly for the first few months and at 3-month intervals, especially if the daily dose is more than 200 mg.

Small clinical trials of patients with chronic myelopathies,[8,87] stroke,[70] MS,[135] and cerebral palsy (CP)[56] show that dantrolene can decrease passive resistance, clonus, and spasms, but at any dose it can cause weakness that impairs mobility. Studies have not been designed to reveal effects on ADLs and ambulation. A 14-week, placebo-controlled crossover study of 31 patients with hemiparesis and no initial spasticity who entered the study early after the onset of stroke rehabilitation revealed no change in functional assessment and no reduction in muscle tone by clinical or mechanical measures after reaching doses of 200 mg per day, but

the investigators found a reduction in the maximal torque developed by the unaffected arm and leg.[67] Thus, even prophylactic use of the drug can weaken paretic and normal muscle.

Dantrolene is most commonly used for spasticity resulting from a cerebral injury, especially for dystonic flexed upper limbs or extended lower limbs in patients with hemiplegia. The drug's induction of paresis assists hygiene and nursing care in immobile patients with severe arm or leg adduction.

Baclofen. This GABA-B agonist restricts the influx of calcium into presynaptic terminals. It acts on monosynaptic and polysynaptic reflexes and gamma efferents by the presynaptic inhibition of the release of excitatory neurotransmitters, including those released from nociceptive afferents from the periphery that cause flexor and extensor muscle spasms. Baclofen may also have a glycine-mediated postsynaptic action for reciprocal inhibition.[26] Its half-life is 4 hours. Side effects of administration by any route include fatigue, drowsiness, nausea, dizziness, paresthesia, and weakness. Abrupt withdrawal can cause hallucinations, confusion, and generalized seizures. Seizures are avoided by tapering half the dose every 3 days. Physostigmine may partially antagonize an intrathecal overdose.

The drug is most effective in reducing involuntary flexor and extensor spasms, clonus, and the resistance to passive movements associated with myelopathies from SCI and MS.[39,43,89] Baclofen has not been shown to quantitatively reduce the viscous and elastic stiffness produced by the reflexive response to sinusoidal motion of the ankle joint in patients with moderate spasticity and SCI, however.[60] When combined with a modest stretching program, baclofen has improved scores on the Ashworth Scale and on a quantitative measure of quadriceps hypertonicity, but it has not altered ADLs.[15] The benefits of this drug in patients with hemiparesis from stroke and head trauma and in patients with CP are uncertain.

Baclofen has also been used intrathecally in patients with SCI, MS, and CP when oral therapy has failed.[3,86,90,103] It presumably penetrates the substantia gelatinosa. Continuous infusion by a programmable pump with a catheter in the lumbar subarachnoid space avoids the fluxes in CSF concentration caused by boluses. This continuous administration also allows patients to use larger doses when needed, such as during sleep, when a spasm would awaken them. The peak effect of a bolus occurs about 4 hours after injection, and maximum activity during continuous infusion is found at 24 to 48 hours.

Intrathecal baclofen administration has significantly decreased the Ashworth score and the frequency of spasms in a randomized double-blind crossover study of 20 subjects with severe spasticity from SCI or MS.[103] Their spasticity had interfered with their ADLs when they took 60 to 200 mg of oral baclofen. When these patients received daily doses ranging from 60 to 750 µg infused by a programmable implanted lumbar pump, their lower scores persisted for 19 months of follow-up. In many of these patients, wheelchair transfers and self-care improved.

In a study of three patients with progressive hereditary spastic paraparesis who had no response to oral baclofen, intrathecal baclofen, infused at 50 to 100 µg per day and increased over 3 months to as much as 264 µg, caused subjective, but not objective weakness.[91] It significantly decreased muscle tone on the Ashworth Scale by 1 to 2 points at all joints and reduced the frequency of spasms. In addition, the drug improved the patients' rigid, scissoring gait with toe strike at the onset of stance. These patients became able to ascend stairs and walk with either no devices or a single-point cane. Two patients returned to the workforce.

Tolerance develops to intrathecal baclofen, probably because of downregulation of the number of neuronal receptors or because of a change from high-affinity to low-affinity receptors brought on by the high local concentrations of drug. Interference with flow from the catheter tip may also decrease effectiveness. Higher infusion rates, often doubling in the first year, reportedly maintain the effect on spasms, however. In a follow-up study of 100 patients with MS and SCI treated for up to 6 years, spontaneous spasms and muscle tone continued to be decreased in 95 patients, and 23 of 41 previously bedridden patients became able to use a wheelchair.[99] Twenty patients required a catheter revision, 3 had a wound infection, and 3 suffered a drug overdose.

Benzodiazepines. This family of agents augments the postsynaptic actions of GABA by increasing the affinity of GABA to GABA-A receptors. Activation of the receptor site initiates the opening of the chloride channel for presynaptic inhibition of the release of excitatory neurotransmitters from spinal afferents, as well as inhibition of polysynaptic descending brainstem facilitatory inputs.[26]

Although adverse effects vary within the family of drugs, all these agents can produce sedation, depression, weakness, fatigue, psychomotor slowing, antegrade amnesia, lightheadedness, and imbalance. No specific reason exists not to try a shorter-acting benzodiazepine, especially for nighttime relief of spasms, although untapered withdrawal after long-term use is more likely to cause self-limited symptoms of anxiety and insomnia. These drugs are commonly used in patients with anxiety disorders, which have a 1-year prevalence in the United States of 5 to 15 percent, and in panic disorders, with a 1 to 2 percent prevalence.[120] These disorders have an average age of onset of 18 to 45 years, so one may expect that the younger disabled population with spasticity, under added emotional distress, may prefer a benzodiazepine alone or as an addition to other agents.

Small, less than optimal clinical studies suggest that diazepam can modestly decrease spasms and the resistance to passive movement in patients with SCI, MS, stroke, and CP, but when specifically evaluated, diazepam does not improve upper limb function or ambulation. Alprazolam, clorazepate,[85] ketazolam, and clonazepam are other benzodiazepines with long, intermediate, and short half-lives that have been used in small groups of patients. Benefits seem similar to those of diazepam, but the studies are not easily compared, and plasma concentrations are usually not reported.

GABA receptors are downregulated with benzodiazepines and are modulated by barbiturates. Benzodiazepines open the chloride channel more often, and barbiturates help keep it open longer. The combination may be useful in immobile patients with uncontrolled spasms. Progabide, another GABA agonist, reduces spasms and passive resistance in patients with MS.[118] Daily doses range from 1000 to 3000 mg (up to 45 mg/

kg). This drug does not improve functional measures, and 25 percent of patients studied have developed reversibly elevated liver function test results. Other new drugs designed for the management of epilepsy that affect the GABA receptor may be useful in patients with spasticity.

Clonidine. The monoamines, serotonin (5-HT) and norepinephrine, have an inhibitory effect on spinal interneurons. Their facilitatory effect on motoneurons is by particular 5-HT receptors and, in the case of norepinephrine, via alpha-1 receptors.[58] Thus, specific monoamines have selective actions that could serve therapeutic strategies. Clonidine is a presynaptic and postsynaptic alpha-2 adrenergic receptor agonist that is active in the locus coeruleus and within the substantia gelatinosa of the dorsal horns at nociceptive sites. It decreases motoneuron excitability, perhaps especially by enhancing alpha-2–mediated presynaptic inhibition of sensory afferents.[9] Thus, clonidine would be expected to have a modulating influence on peripheral pain inputs and on noxious and nonnoxious sensory inputs that cause spasms, especially in patients with a myelopathy.

Oral use led to subjective improvement in hypertonicity in approximately half of a group of 55 SCI subjects when used as an adjunct to baclofen.[38] Baclofen and clonidine are especially useful in reducing clonus and extensor spasms due to a myelopathy, probably by their effects on inhibiting the excitatory influences of sensory inputs on motoneurons. The transdermal clonidine patch also seems effective, starting with a daily dose of 0.1 mg.

Tizanidine. This alpha-2 receptor agonist is similar to clonidine in its structure and mechanisms of action. It appears to have greater muscle relaxant properties, acting upon spinal polysynaptic reflexes.[24] The drug peaks in serum concentration in approximately 2 hours and is detectable for about 6 hours. In some studies, tizanidine is comparable to or is better than baclofen in clinical and functional measures in patients with SCI and MS,[62] and it is better than diazepam in patients with spastic hemiplegia.[12] Tizanidine significantly decreased the number of spasms in placebo-controlled trials of patients with MS[125] and SCI.[97] Hypotension,

lightheadedness, fatigue, dry mouth, and sedation, but not weakness, are occasional adverse reactions of both agonist agents.

Glycine. This agent crosses the blood-brain barrier and acts on receptors of motoneurons and interneurons of the brainstem and the spinal cord. Glycine hyperpolarizes neuronal membranes to decrease cell firing and to dampen reflex excitability. This action occurs when glycine is released by spinal inhibitory interneurons and Renshaw cells. Oral doses of up to 1 g qid have been used in small series and case reports with favorable clinical results but without good measures of outcome.[132] Threonine has been used to try to increase levels of glycine. In a crossover trial of 24 ambulatory patients with MS whose flexor spasms or spasticity was felt to interfere with ADLs, the amino acid had no effect on the Ashworth score or on electrophysiologic measures of spasticity, gait, and symptoms, but the agent reduced clinical signs of spasticity.[57] Plasma and CSF concentrations of glycine were not raised by threonine treatment.

Other Agents. Other medications have been tried to manage spasticity. Cyproheptadine, a serotonin antagonist, decreased clonus and spasms and enhanced gait in a small group of well-studied patients with MS and SCI.[137] The action of this drug on 5-hydroxytryptamine receptors may give it an adjunctive role with the alpha-2 agonists on the spinal motor pools.

The anticonvulsants phenytoin and carbamazepine have multiple effects, including presynaptic inhibition of afferent fibers that may affect spinal cord function. Presumably by inhibiting spinal polysynaptic pathways, oral cannabinoids have reduced spasms in patients with MS.[106] Marijuana has altered spasticity in some patients with paraplegia after SCI. Epidural and intrathecal opioids have also reduced spasms, presumably by acting on lumbar multisynaptic reflexes mediated by A-delta and C-fibers.[42] The phenothiazines have been tried, based on the assumption that inhibition of the discharge of fusimotor fibers in models of decerebrate rigidity is a mechanism that can also reduce spasticity. Any effects on hypertonicity seem to occur above the spinal cord, at dopaminergic sites, and in the brainstem reticular formation, however.[26] Benefits in reducing tone and spasms have been reported,[23] but sedation is common, and movement disorders may arise. Finally, the muscle relaxants carisoprodol, methocarbamol, and cyclobenzaprine have had minimal clinical effects in small studies.

To limit drug-induced lethargy, confusion, weakness, hypotension, and other side effects, dosages of all of these medications must be titrated from very low starting points and increased, in general, no more often than once a week. A diary of the number of episodes of spasms, clonus, or unwanted involuntary movements is most helpful in deciding whether a drug is efficacious at a particular dose. To measure the benefit for other goals of antispasticity therapy, such as improving ambulation or upper extremity function, is more difficult, but efforts should be made to use some objective assessment. A change in walking speed over a distance of 50 feet or in the range of motion, reach, or speed of a functional arm movement helps in making drug adjustments. Even higher dosages than listed in Table 6–4 have been used, especially for patients with intractable flexor and extensor spasms. Combinations of drugs, such as baclofen with clonidine or cyproheptadine, sometimes also help in that setting. When disabling spasms persist, intrathecal drug therapy with baclofen should be considered.

CHEMICAL BLOCKS

Chemical agents can be injected into a nerve, a motor point, or a muscle to reduce localized clonus, inappropriate muscle activity, velocity-dependent tone, and, sometimes, dystonic postures.[124] Blocks are usually not as useful in diminishing non–velocity-dependent tone, rigidity, and flexor or extensor spasms. Because motor point blocks can partially spare voluntary movement and can reduce reciprocal inhibition when they are given to an antagonist muscle, they may improve some aspects of motor control. The short-term effects of chemical agents can also allow physical therapies and oral medications to have a greater ancillary effect.

Phenol. Blocks with phenol as a 2 to 10 percent solution and with ethyl alcohol have been used for over 30 years.[54] The nerve or motor point is most often located by percutaneous electrical stimulation through a hypodermic needle cathode, but an intraneural injection by an open procedure is sometimes advocated.[48] An initial injection of a long-acting local anesthetic such as bupivacaine helps to predict the efficacy of a subsequent phenol block. The most commonly injected nerves include the following: posterior tibial, to decrease equinovarus positioning of the feet and to decrease clonus; the obturator nerve, to reduce adductor scissoring with gait and to improve skin care; and the sciatic nerve, to allow better positioning of a patient with spasticity and paralysis. In the upper extremity, blocks of the musculocutaneous, median, or ulnar nerves may improve resting position of the arm and hand. Painful dysesthesias can follow a nerve trunk injection. The effect of a block persists for 6 to 12 months, and repeat injections can be given, although the percutaneous localization becomes more difficult.[51] Intrathecal and epidural phenol blocks are rarely used today.

Intramuscular infiltrative injections of 50 percent ethanol have reduced spasticity for up to 6 weeks. Motor point blocks have been administered most often in the tibialis posterior, triceps surae, hamstrings, subscapularis, and the flexors of the wrist and fingers. The hip flexors can be blocked with localization by ultrasound, rather than by resorting to a lumbar nerve block.[72]

Botulinum Toxin. Botulinum toxin A (BTX) is one of seven serotypes and appears to be increasingly popular in the management of the local effects of spasticity. The toxin exerts its paralytic action within a few hours by binding to presynaptic cholinergic nerve terminals.[65] The muscle becomes functionally denervated and atrophies, but axon terminals quickly sprout to make new synaptic connections to neighboring muscle fibers. Retrograde transport probably puts some of the drug into spinal segments, where it can block recurrent inhibition mediated by Renshaw cells. The onset of the drug's effect takes up to 72 hours. Side effects include malaise, local discomfort, and weakening of the affected muscles and, if diffusion occurs, of neighboring muscles.

The drug is supplied in the United States as BOTOX in vials in which 100 mouse units equal 400 ng of type A toxin, diluted to 10 U per 0.1 mL or less. The lethal parenteral dose in primates is 39 U/kg.[22] In adults, up to 400 U have been given safely in one or more muscles at one visit. The optimal dose is uncertain. As in its use for movement disorders, the quantity, usually in increments of 40 U, depends upon the mass of the target muscle. Needle EMG studies that identify the region of the muscle's motor end plate localize injections to the areas of greatest efficacy.

Clinical trials of BTX for spasticity suggest some practical uses. Injected into the leg adductors in a divided dose of 200 U, BTX improved manual abduction and perineal hygiene for up to 3 months.[127] In 25 patients with stroke and TBI, injections into single muscles of the arm or leg reduced spasticity in 80 percent and led to functional improvements in 68 percent, with gains in range of motion, brace tolerance, and pain relief.[108] An injection of 400 U by EMG guidance into the soleus, tibialis anterior, and both heads of the gastrocnemius reduced plantarflexor spasticity in patients with hemiplegia for at least 8 weeks.[59] Gait improved in velocity, stride length, loading on the foot, and push-off in many of these patients. In several small, controlled trials of children with CP, injection into a variety of spastic paretic leg muscles improved aspects of their gait for 6 weeks to 4 months.[22,71] Larger randomized, placebo-controlled trials of children with spastic diplegia are in progress.

SURGICAL INTERVENTIONS

Ablative neurosurgical procedures and orthopedic operations that correct deformities and improve function by a tendon lengthening, tenotomy, or tendon transfer can decrease hypertonicity or some of its consequences. Along with the obvious mechanisms of action of a procedure, altering the action of a tendon or muscle may decrease sensory inputs that increase reflexive spasms. Surgery seems to work best when followed by physical therapy. Patients with CP, stroke, SCI, or TBI are occasionally surgical candidates. A gait analysis with EMG helps to determine which procedure may aid mobility.

Various interventions have been used based on the patient's age, amount of strength and sensation, and disabilities. Both an obturator neurectomy and an adductor tenotomy relieve severe spasms in the hip adductor muscles. Tendon transfers and lengthenings preserve some function, whereas ablative procedures tend to eliminate any residual motor control. For example, a hamstring tendon release, transfer, or lengthening improves a spastic knee flexion deformity or contracture. An Achilles tendon lengthening can decrease an equinus deformity. A tibialis posterior transfer can reduce a varus deformity of the foot.

Spinal Cord Approaches. Microsurgical lesions at the dorsal root entry zone have been reported to reduce spasticity in 75 percent and to reduce pain in 90 percent of 47 patients with paraplegia who had these problems.[123] Joint range of motion and positioning especially improved in the most severely handicapped patients with spasticity, so they could sit and lie in comfort. Minor and more serious complications, however, affected half of these patients, and 5 died. A longitudinal myelotomy that divides the spinal cord into anterior and posterior halves from T-12 to S-1 preserves some function, unlike a cordotomy, and usually eliminates spasticity over the long run.[112]

Posterior Rhizotomy. Dorsal rhizotomy for reduction of spasticity was first introduced in 1913 and has been modified to improve its safety and efficacy. Selective division of posterior nerve rootlets of the second lumbar to first or second sacral level is based on intraoperative EMG responses of lower extremity muscles to posterior nerve rootlet stimulation.[136] Those rootlets associated with hyperactive responses deemed to be abnormal are divided, whereas those associated with more normal responses are spared. Abnormal reactions have been characterized by incremental, multiphasic, or clonic responses to a steady 1-second train of stimuli. Additional abnormalities include spread of the response to muscle groups that are not innervated by the root being tested, as well as sustained responses that continue beyond the 1-second stimulus interval. Some of these responses may be valid criteria of an abnormality,[131] but this concept is controversial.

Depending on the severity of the spasticity, approximately 25 to 50 percent of the posterior nerve rootlets are cut. By dividing only selected posterior nerve rootlets, the influence of excitatory (primarily Ia) afferents on the alpha motoneuron pools can be diminished while preserving sensory function.

Practitioners state that appropriate selection of patients is vital to the success of the selective posterior rhizotomy procedure. Patients with the most dramatic functional improvements have been bright and motivated ambulatory youngsters with spastic diplegia; minimal, fixed contractures; and good strength.[102] Children with selective control of movement and freedom from synergistic movement patterns are more likely to improve their movement patterns following rhizotomy.

Some critics of the procedure argue that this population would do well with any supportive intervention.[74] Moreover, electrical stimulation of rootlets has no clear electrophysiologic rationale and only prolongs the surgical procedure. The claims for a positive effect have been supported by H-reflex studies, EMG assessment, and measures of resistance to passive motion using a force transducer. In addition, gait analyses of children with CP who underwent rhizotomy reveal greater range of motion at the hip, knee, and ankle with accompanying increases in stride length and speed of walking, as well as more normal relationships between movement of limb segments during gait.[18,102] A randomized trial would help settle the controversy over this procedure.[116] Indeed, clinical trials with outcome measures of frequency of spasms and functional assessments of ADLs, hygiene, and mobility would lead to guidelines about when a particular ablative surgery is better than a noninvasive approach.

CONTRACTURES

Impaired range of motion of a joint associated with UMN disorders can develop from spasticity and from pathologic changes in the joint and surrounding connective tissue and muscle. Immobilization produces degenerative changes within a joint. Eventu-

ally, the cartilage thins, hyaluronate and other components decrease, vessels proliferate, and fibrous adhesions form.[2] Collagen fibers around the joint shorten when they are not passively loaded or stretched. They stiffen by increasing their crosslinks. Collagen within muscle can also change, along with a reduction in the number and length of sarcomeres in muscle across the shortened position of a joint.[10]

In one study,[142] 15 percent of patients with SCI admitted for rehabilitation and, in another,[143] 84 percent admitted after TBI had lost more than 15 percent of the normal range of motion of at least one joint. Patients with hemiparesis and stroke fall between these extremes. Contractures are found especially in the lower extremities in patients with neuromuscular diseases, affecting at least 70 percent of outpatients with Duchenne muscular dystrophy.[66] Contractures can limit functional use of a limb and impair hygiene, mobility, and self-care. Serious contractures can cause pressure sores, pain, and, especially in youngsters, emotional distress when odd postures distort the body.

Certain strategies have been tried to manage contractures (Table 6–5). A local anesthetic motor point block can help separate the effects of spasticity from a contracture fixed by bone and soft tissue disorders. If the joint's range of motion greatly improves after a motor point block, any of the therapies for spasticity can be applied. Some of these interventions may have to be added to manual stretching performed for at least half an hour a day, followed by appropriate joint positioning. Ultrasound applied to the joint capsule and musculotendinous junction can make stretching more effective. Serial splinting or casting when the contracture is fixed can gradually stretch tissue under a low load, but this treatment must be monitored to prevent pressure sores, compression neuropathies, and connective tissue injury. Casts are usually reapplied every 2 to 5 days for plantarflexion and for knee and elbow flexion contractures.[79]

Various surgical procedures and chemical blocks have been described to reduce contractures at most joints (see Table 6–5).[10] EMG and temporary nerve blocks are used to better define which muscles are inappro-

Table 6–5. **THERAPIES FOR JOINT CONTRACTURES USUALLY ASSOCIATED WITH SPASTICITY**

Joint	Range of Motion Exercise	Splints and Orthotics	Chemical Blocks	Surgerical Procedures
Shoulder	Abduction and external rotation; manipulation under anesthesia	Adjustable hemi-sling	Pectoralis major; teres major	Tendon transection
Elbow	Continuous passive range of motion	Low-load dynamic splint; turnbuckle orthotic; serial casting	Musculocutaneous nerve; brachioradialis motor point	Brachioradialis muscle release; biceps tendon lengthening; aponeurotic section of brachialis; anterior capsulotomy
Forearm	Supination and pronation		Pronator teres	Pronator teres release or tendon transfer for supination
Wrist and hand	Extension, rotation, sliding fingers; elastic gloves, massage, elevation for edema	Air splint for entire upper extremity	Differential temporary median, radial, ulnar nerve blocks; percutaneous phenol nerve blocks	Release of individual muscles or elevation of all forearm muscles from bone and interosseous membranes; tendon transfers or lengthening for thumb function
Hip	Assessment for subluxation; hip extension and abduction	Foam wedge to separate thighs	Temporary or phenol blocks of obturator nerve, L-2–L-3 roots, sciatic nerve or branches, quadriceps motor points	Iliopsoas, tensor fasciae latae, rectus femoris release; adductor longus and gracilis tenotomy or transfer to ischial tuberosity; adductor myotomy; neurectomy of obturator nerve branches
Knee	Hamstring stretch	Serial casting; plastic ankle-foot orthosis	Phenol block of femoral nerve	Hamstrings lengthening; femoral or tibial osteotomies; rectus femoris transfer

Table 6–5. **THERAPIES FOR JOINT CONTRACTURES USUALLY ASSOCIATED WITH SPASTICITY** (*Continued*)

Joint	Range of Motion Exercise	Splints and Orthotics	Chemical Blocks	Surgerical Procedures
Ankle and foot	Ambulation; gastrocnemius stretch	Ankle-foot orthosis: double upright versus molded with lateral flare for varus tilt; metatarsal arch support; serial casting for severe equinovarus posture	Temporary or phenol blocks of tibial nerve or motor points of gastrocnemius, soleus, tibialis posterior, flexor digitorum longus, flexor hallucis longus	Achilles tendon lengthening; split anterior tibial tendon transfer; release or transfer of long toe flexors; arthrodeses

priately active. EMG studies of a partially functioning hand and, in an ambulatory patient, during formal gait analysis are mandatory before attempting an invasive intervention. Otherwise, selection of the optimal procedure for the right muscle is guesswork and can lead to iatrogenic complications. For example, if the hip adductors are used for stepping, an obturator neurectomy for an adductor contracture can prevent the subject from ambulating. Surgery of the leg must also take into account that muscles such as the hamstrings and rectus femoris cross both the hip and knee, and the gastrocnemius crosses the knee and ankle. For instance, if the long head of the biceps femoris is lengthened too much for a knee contracture, the hip may not be stable. Overcorrection of an equinovarus foot by heel cord lengthening can cause a calcaneovalgus foot deformity and may require heel stabilization. Surgery and blocks are followed by vigorous physical therapy for ranging, strengthening, and improving functional activities.

Preventing contractures is far better than treating them once they have occurred. Success depends upon manual stretching of joints twice a day when active ranging and strengthening exercises cannot be done, proper bed and wheelchair positioning, early weight bearing, and adequate treatment of limb pain. The optimal physical methods of maintaining the range of motion of a joint in healthy persons and in patients

with spasticity or paresis has yet to be clarified.[82]

Lower limb orthoses can decrease muscle tone in response to cutaneous and postural reflexes. Static splints for the hand and wrist are most commonly used when muscle tone increases (Table 6–6). These splints aim to prevent contractures and pain by stretching elastic tissues and by maintaining the normal adaptation of muscle to elongation. They are also said to lessen spasticity, particularly by inhibiting flexor reflexes by cutaneous stimulation. Many small clinical trials of various diseases suggest subjective value for the use of almost every variation of hand orthotic.[76] Dynamic splints for the hands and continuous passive motion devices for the arm or leg are more expensive. Schedules for wearing time of any device vary from 2 to 24 hours a day. The optimum time has not been established. Any approach that lengthens the affected tissues is worth a try. Unfortunately, no particular approach has been put to a good clinical trial.

Table 6–6. **HAND SPLINTS TO REDUCE SPASTICITY AND CONTRACTURES**

Volar and dorsal wrist and forearm splint
Foam finger spreader
Inflatable pressure splint (Johnson)
Firm cone in palm

NEUROGENIC BLADDER

Incontinence, urine retention, and a combination of both result from lesions at a variety of levels of the nervous system. Serious consequences include urinary tract infections, pyelonephritis, hydronephrosis, renal and bladder calculi, breakdown of skin, and social embarrassment.

Pathophysiology

The anatomy and pharmacology of the controls for micturition provide insight into evaluation and management of dysfunction.[13,49] Conscious cortical control modulates the micturition center of the pontine reticular formation and the pudendal nerve to the striated external sphincter. The micturition center coordinates bladder and sphincter activity by means of inputs to the sacral spinal cord. The net effect of frontal lobe and reticulospinal control is inhibition of bladder wall detrusor neurons. Parasympathetic fibers from S-2 to S-4 provide motor control to the bladder detrusor muscle, as well as to the proximal urethra and the external sphincter. Parasympathetic afferents carry the sensation for bladder filling back to the sacral nuclei. Sympathetic fibers from T-11 to L-1 relax the detrusor muscle, contract the bladder neck and proximal urethra, and inhibit parasympathetic flow. Activation leads to continence and the storage of urine. The usual bladder capacity is up to 500 mL, and the sensation of filling is perceived at about 125 mL.

Insight into the mechanism of urinary tract dysfunction comes from finding a postvoid residual of more than 50 mL by catheterization. During inpatient rehabilitation, nurses are increasingly using ultrasonography equipment that automatically calculates the volume of urine in the bladder. This technique eliminates the urethral trauma and risk of infection with repeated catheterizations for residual urine volumes. A urodynamic study by cystometrography (CMG) shows whether the problem is primarily a failure to store or to empty urine as a result of bladder or urethral dysfunction. The CMG allows characterization of the bladder volume when the patient first senses the urge to void, records uninhibited detrusor contractions, measures bladder compliance, reveals external sphincter activity during filling and emptying, and measures urine flow rate. The results classify micturition as follows: (1) normal; (2) detrusor hyperreflexia, if involuntary contractions cannot be suppressed; (3) detrusor areflexia, if contractions are poor; and (4) detrusor-sphincter dyssynergia, if the urethra fails to contract or to relax during a detrusor contraction.[133] In older men, the test also helps to evaluate the contribution of bladder outlet obstruction from prostatic hypertrophy. In diabetic cystopathy, urodynamic studies often reveal impaired bladder sensation, decreased detrusor contractility, large bladder capacity, and impaired urine flow, generally in association with a peripheral neuropathy.

In a general way, clinicians may anticipate the type of bladder dysfunction from the location of a lesion. For example, a frontal lobe TBI can cause urgency and incontinence because of loss of cortical inhibitory control. Indeed, detrusor hyperreflexia, which also occurs in patients with stroke, MS, and Parkinson's disease, is the most common cause of a neurogenic bladder. Postvoid residuals are usually not high. Detrusor-sphincter dyssynergia, with either the internal or external sphincter affected, can occur in patients with brainstem injury or MS, but it most often follows SCI above the conus.

Management

Therapy takes many forms. The first step is to treat an intercurrent urinary tract infection. Systemic antimicrobial drugs for prophylaxis, such as trimethoprim, and acidifying and alkalinizing agents do not clearly reduce the incidence of infection over the long run.[95] Of interest, 300 mL of cranberry juice did reduce the frequency of bacteriuria with pyuria in elderly women,[6] so prophylaxis may be tried after, say, a stroke in older patients.

Behavioral techniques can be used to maintain continence in cognitively and behaviorally impaired patients, especially after a TBI. Patients with myelopathies are often trained to perform intermittent catheterization of the bladder three to five times a day. Catheters can be washed, stored in a plastic bag, and reused.

Many drugs have been tried, based on their potential effects on the alpha-adrenergic and beta-adrenergic and nicotinic and muscarinic cholinergic receptors within the micturition reflex (Table 6–7). Patients with frequency and urgency whose postvoid residual is greater than 100 mL often benefit from the combination of an anticholinergic drug and self-intermittent catheterization. Desmopressin nasal spray taken at night has reduced overnight urine volumes enough to help relieve nocturia in patients with SCI and MS.[21] The antidiuretic effect of this drug only occasionally causes hyponatremia. Detrusor hyperreflexia with a low storage capacity is usually treated with a gradually increasing dose of an anticholinergic drug such as oxybutynin or a tricyclic antidepres-

Table 6–7. PHARMACOLOGIC MANIPULATION OF BLADDER DYSFUNCTION

Medication	Indication	Mechanisms of Action	Dose
Bethanechol	Facilitation of emptying	Increase of detrusor contraction	25 mg bid–50 mg qid
Clonidine	Facilitation of emptying; internal sphincter dyssynergia	Decrease of urethral tone	0.1–0.2 mg bid
Prazosin Terazosin	Facilitation of emptying; outlet obstruction	Alpha blockade of external sphincter to decrease tone	1–2 mg bid 1–5 mg bid
Diazepam Baclofen Dantrolene	Facilitation of emptying; outlet obstruction	Decrease of external sphincter tone	2–5 mg tid 10–20 mg tid 25 mg qid
Imipramine or other tricyclic antidepressant	Facilitation of storage; urge incontinence; enuresis	Increase of internal sphincter tone; decrease of detrusor contractions	25–100 mg hs
Verapamil	Facilitation of storage	Relaxation of detrusor; decrease of bladder contractility	40–80 mg qd, intravesically
Indomethacin	Facilitation of storage	Prostaglandin inhibition of detrusor	25–50 mg tid
Oxybutynin Hyoscyamine	Facilitation of storage; urge incontinence; frequency	Relaxation of detrusor; increase of internal sphincter tone	5 mg hs–5 mg qid 0.125 mg bid–0.25 mg qid
Pseudoephedrine	Facilitation of storage	Contraction of bladder neck	30–60 mg bid or qid
Desmopressin (DDAVP)	Nocturia	Antidiuretic effect	10 μg hs, intranasally

sant such as imipramine. Imipramine, when used to decrease bladder contractility and to increase outlet resistance, can accentuate dysautonomia, as can the alpha-adrenoceptor blockers terazosin, doxazosin, and prazosin, which are sometimes used to decrease bladder outlet resistance. The alpha-adrenergic antagonists also decrease bladder neck and urethral resistance in men with prostatic hypertrophy.

Neurostimulation techniques and surgical procedures, such as augmentation cystoplasty and other urinary diversions, are used mostly for patients with myelopathies from SCI and MS who cannot maintain a low-pressure detrusor with intermittent catheterization. These patients run the risk of recurrent urinary infection, vesicoureteral reflux, and stone formation. The bladder can be enlarged by anastomosing a piece of bowel to a resected patch of its wall. Augmentation cystoplasty has mostly replaced the sphincterotomies and other urinary diversions performed more than 10 years ago. Infants and children with a meningomyelocele often require surgical diversionary methods.

Parasympathetic stimulation by electrodes placed intradurally on the anterior roots of S-2 to S-4 can reduce urine residual volumes, increase bladder capacity, and reduce fecal impaction and constipation.[16] This stimulation requires a laminectomy, posterior rhizotomy, and implantation of a radio receiver. The S-3 nerve root is most critical for bladder control. Percutaneous methods of stimulation that lead to implanting electrodes at the neural foramina are in trial as a less invasive means for electrical neuromodulation. Stimulation is sometimes effective at other sites, including the bladder wall, pelvic floor, vaginal or anal sphincter, and over pudendal and tibial nerves.[138]

Nonroutine management options are best discussed with a urologist who knows the patient and who can evaluate surgical procedures and unusual pharmacologic interventions, such as the treatment of dyssynergia with BTX[41] and intravesical instillations of capsaicin.[46] Long-term management of the bladder tends to be dictated by the individual's physical, vocational, and psychosocial needs.

BOWEL DYSFUNCTION

Incontinence, constipation, loose stools, fecal impaction, and abdominal distention are common problems in patients with acute and chronic neurologic diseases. The prevalence of fecal incontinence from all causes in hospitalized elderly patients, with and without a normal pelvic floor, is 13 to 47 percent.[88]

Pathophysiology

Abnormal function at any level of the nervous system can cause incontinence.[129] Motor innervation to the rectum and the internal and external sphincters arises from sacral roots S-2, S-3, and S-4. The internal sphincter is supplied by the hypogastric nerve and by the parasympathetic nerves. The pudendal nerve without parasympathetic input controls the external sphincter.

Certain symptoms are associated with lesions at particular levels of the neuraxis. Patients with uninhibited neurogenic bowel incontinence have a sudden urge to defecate, or their awareness can be distorted so that defecation happens without any urge. Lesions are cortical or subcortical. Reflex neurogenic incontinence occurs abruptly without warning or is part of a mass reflex. The lesion is within the spinal cord, above the conus medullaris. High spinal lesions cause incontinence that is more easily managed than lesions that involve the conus medullaris. A conus or cauda equina lesion produces an autonomous neurogenic bowel. Incontinence can occur with increased abdominal pressure, or it may be continuous. An autonomic or sensory neuropathy from diabetes that is superimposed upon a hemispheric stroke may produce incontinence when either lesion alone would not.

Management

Alert patients must be involved in their program to achieve continence without obstipation. Constipation and impaction are common complications of inactivity, limited fluid and fiber intake, anticholinergic medication, and depression. Episodes of incontinence should be related to time of day, frequency, stool consistency, diet (fiber content, gas-forming foods such as berries, constipating items such as cheese and rice), fluid intake, physical activity, history of laxative abuse, and medications. Stool softeners, colonic stimulants, contact irritants, and bulk formers help in management. The use of these agents takes art and patience. Digital stimulation of the anal sphincter often aids elimination in the patient with SCI. Diarrhea that is not caused by an impaction or tube feedings is sometimes the residual effect of antibiotics. Live yogurt cultures can replace bowel flora and improve control. A gastrointestinal infection, particularly by *Clostridium fecalis,* is assessed by culture of the loose stool. Persistent bowel incontinence can indicate diffuse brain injury or the inability to express the need to defecate and move to a toilet. A toileting schedule or specific communication to signal need can solve the problem. A rectal bag fastened around the anus can keep the severely disabled patient clean.

PRESSURE SORES

The incidence and prevalence of pressure ulcers is high in immobile patients with a neurologic disorder and in residents of nursing homes. In 1987, over 2.2 million Medicare hospital days went to the care of decubitus ulcers.[128]

Pathophysiology

Pressure sores develop primarily over bony prominences such as the occiput, heels, coccyx and sacrum, and greater trochanter. In addition to immobility, major risk factors include incontinence, poor nutrition, altered consciousness and poor cognition, exposure to friction and shearing forces on the skin, aged skin, anemia, and prior skin wounds and healed ulcers. Some of these mechanisms have been studied.[4] For example, pulling a patient across a bed sheet can cause intraepidermal blisters and super-

ficial erosions. Moisture increases the friction between two surfaces and produces maceration. Shearing forces are generated when a seated person slides across a surface. Such force can stretch and angulate tissue and blood vessels; the effect is reduced blood flow, especially in elderly persons and patients with paraplegia, who tend to have compromised circulation in general. Both high focal pressure and lower pressures for a longer duration, as little as 60 mm Hg, compromise capillaries, produce erythema, and, if not relieved, lead to irreversible cellular damage. This finding is the basis for surface interventions that aim to distribute and relieve pressure.

The most frequently used classification of pressure sores was proposed by the National Pressure Ulcer Advisory Panel in 1989 (Table 6–8). In addition to the ulcer stage, cli-

Table 6–8. **PRESSURE ULCER CLASSIFICATION**

Stage I
Nonblanchable erythema of intact skin, heralding lesion of skin ulceration (Note: Reactive hyperemia can normally be expected to be present for one-half to three-fourths as long as the pressure-occluded blood flow to the area; it should not be confused with a stage I pressure ulcer.)

Stage II
Partial-thickness skin loss involving epidermis or dermis; superficial ulcer clinically apparent as an abrasion, blister, or shallow crater

Stage III
Full-thickness skin loss involving damage or necrosis of subcutaneous tissue that may extend down to, but not through, underlying fascia; ulcer clinically manifests as a deep crater with or without undermining of adjacent tissue

Stage IV
Full-thickness skin loss with extensive destruction, tissue necrosis, or damage to muscle, bone, or supporting structures (for example, tendon or joint capsule) (Note: Undermining and sinus tracts may also be associated with stage IV pressure ulcers.)

nicians should describe the location, size, depth, edges, exudate, necrotic tissue, eschar, surrounding skin, and signs of healing. Ulcers are photographed for serial evaluation.

Management

Clinical practice guidelines have been offered by the Agency for Health Care Policy and Research.[1] Prevention involves dealing with the foregoing risk factors. For example, skin should be cleansed without irritating or drying it out. Lubricants such as cornstarch, protective film dressings, padding, and protective dressings such as hydrocolloids can minimize friction and shear injuries when positioning and turning techniques may compromise the patient. Pillows and wedges protect bony prominences. The patient's heels are best lifted off the bed with pillows under the calves. Pressure-reducing devices that include foam, static air, alternating air, gel, and water mattresses, as well as similar materials for wheelchair seats, can lower the risk of sores. Costly, high-technology beds can cause dehydration and can limit mobility, and they are difficult to adjust to for some patients. These beds do not eliminate the need for turning or for pressure relief. Immobile patients should be turned at least every 2 hours.

No single approach can be recommended for the treatment of a pressure ulcer.[141] Table 6–9 lists the categories of products that are most often used.[42a] Many concoctions have been smeared on reddened skin. Iodine and hydrogen peroxide should be avoided. Polyurethane films and gauze can damage new epithelium when they are removed. Debridement by one of many methods and the administration of topical antibiotics are most important for a stage 3 or stage 4 ulcer. The clinical evaluation of osteomyelitis that has developed beneath a pressure sore is less accurate than a percutaneous needle biopsy of bone taken for aerobic and anaerobic cultures.[25] Growth factors may be of value in promoting healing. Myocutaneous and other types of protective flaps must be accompanied by education of the patient and family about flap care and pressure sore prevention.

DYSPHAGIA

Oropharyngeal dysphagia is usually treated by occupational or speech therapists and is supported by nurses and caregivers. *Neurogenic dysphagia* means dysfunction in the mechanisms that deliver a food or liquid bolus into the esophagus. Aspiration, respiratory compromise, malnutrition, and dehydration are the serious consequences. In-

Table 6–9. **PRODUCTS FOR PRESSURE ULCER CARE**

Description	Indications	Comments
Damp cotton gauze	Wound covered by eschar; infected large wounds	Can dehydrate or adhere to wound; must change often and cover
Gas-permeable polyurethane film	Stage I ulcer	Can use for 7 days
Semipermeable polyurethane foam	Stage I or II uninfected ulcer	Cushions wound; absorbs exudate
Self-adhesive hydrocolloid	State II or III uninfected small wound	Can use for 7 days
Hydrogels	State II or IV ulcer with moderate exudate	Absorbent but readily dry out; must cover
Alginates	Stage III or IV ulcer with copious drainage	Can dessicate wound; must cover
Topical antibiotics and antiseptics	Generally not recommended	Can impair healing

deed, dysphagia is the potential cause of a pulmonary infection in any patient with stroke, TBI, motoneuron disease, MS, advanced Parkinson's disease, cervicomedullary disorders such as a syrinx, Guillain-Barré syndrome, myasthenia gravis, and most neuromuscular diseases. Details about prevalence and natural history follow in later chapters.

Pathophysiology

Relevant pathologic features can be found at several levels of the nervous system (Table 6–10). The interactions of these structures are complex. A brainstem neural network for swallowing, related to the functionally associated network for respiration,[126] probably has the features of a pattern generator that initiates and organizes the motor sequence for automatic swallow and distributes impulses for deglutition. Stimulation of the oropharyngeal and laryngeal region or of the superior laryngeal and glossopharyngeal nerves is the most powerful way to lower the threshold for swallowing.[92] Higher command centers for initiation exist, of course, in the cortex.

Lesions in these areas interfere with the oral, oral preparatory, and reflex or pharyngeal phases of deglutition. In the first phase, chewed food particles and liquids are held in a bolus against the palate by the tongue. Bolus volume affects the timing of laryngeal and cricopharyngeal actions. During the oral phase of deglutition, the tongue propels the bolus posteriorly through the pillars of the anterior fauces. A labial seal and tension in the buccal muscles prevent loss of the bolus. The reflexive swallow starts the pharyngeal phase. Velopharyngeal closure excludes the bolus from the nasophayrnx. Pharyngeal peristalsis, closure of the larynx, and the pumping action of the tongue sweep the bolus through the cricopharyngeal sphincter. Aspiration is prevented by elevation and anterior movement of the larynx under the root of the tongue, noted clinically by the superior and anterior motion of the thyroid cartilage. In addition, the epiglottis diverts a bolus into the valleculae, and the aryepiglottic folds, false vocal cords, and true vocal cords approximate to prevent aspiration. The motion of the larynx also helps to open the cricopharyngeal sphincter to let the bolus pass into the esophagus. This action triggers a peristaltic wave.

Assessment

Clinical symptoms and signs, bedside tests, and procedures can enable one to identify patients with dysphagia who are at risk of aspiration. A wet-hoarse voice, drooling, and cough shortly after deglutition suggest dysphagia. The presence or absence of palatal, gag, and pharyngeal reflexes does not necessarily predict the safety of swallowing. Swallowing water at less than 10 mL per second[98] or coughing or a wet-hoarse quality to the voice within 1 minute of continuously swallowing 90 mL of water points to the risk of aspiration.[34] Silent aspiration, however, especially during sleep, may occur in the absence of these signs.

The modified barium swallow (MBS) during videofluoroscopy helps to reveal laryngeal penetration, as well as mechanisms of dysphagia. This evaluation usually includes attempts at swallowing 5 mL of thin and thick liquid barium, 5 mL of a barium-impregnated gel or pudding, a piece of a cookie coated with barium paste, 20 mL of thin barium liquid, and successive swallows of about 30 mL of thin barium liquid.

Table 6–10. **LOCALIZATION OF PATHOLOGIC PROCESSES CAUSING NEUROGENIC DYSPHAGIA**

Cortex
   Inferior precentral and posterior inferior
     frontal gyrus
   Bilateral corticobulbar pathway interruption
Basal ganglia and cerebellum
Brainstem
   Solitary tract and adjacent reticular formation
   Lateral reticular formation near nucleus
     ambiguous
Cranial nerves V, VII, IX, and X
Neuromuscular junction
Bulbar muscles

The rate of false-positive and false-negative results in various diseases and the relation of these results to the risk of clinically significant aspiration are uncertain.[53] In a study of 114 inpatients undergoing stroke rehabilitation, the MBS revealed the relative risk of developing pneumonia.[61] This risk was about 7 times higher in patients who aspirated than in those who did not, about 5.5 times higher for silent aspirators, and 8 times higher for those who aspirated 10 percent or more on one or more barium swallows. Dehydration and death were not associated with MBS findings. Ultrasound, manometry, EMG, and biomechanical assessments[113] have been used less often in the clinical setting. Fiberoptic endoscopic examination of swallowing appears especially promising for repeated examinations without radiation exposure, if the procedure is tolerated by the patient.[75] The interpretation of tests is discussed with regard to stroke in Chapter 7.

Treatment

Lesions that may not ordinarily cause symptoms may do so in patients with depressed consciousness or attention, a weak cough, loose dentures, oral candidiasis, laryngeal trauma from intubation, poor head control, reduced saliva from anticholinergic medications, tracheostomy or nasopharyngeal feeding tube, and esophageal motility disorders or reflux esophagitis. When possible, these superimposed problems should be managed.

Specific treatments for neurogenic dysphagia depend in part on the impairment at each stage of swallowing.[84,100] Good motivation and cognition are necessary for successful therapy. Table 6–11 outlines some of the most commonly used techniques. Controlled trials are few, although the efficacy of several techniques is borne out during MBS.[94] The need for controlled trials of any invasive or expensive therapeutic program is especially appropriate, because the natural history of dysphagia after stroke and TBI is for most patients to recover.

Thickening and altering the size of the bolus affect each stage of swallowing. For example, the patient who drools and does not move liquids in the oral preparatory and oral

Table 6–11. GENERAL THERAPY FOR DYSPHAGIA

Compensation
Head positioning
　Chin tuck
　Head rotation to weak pharyngeal side
Altered consistency of food
Thickening of liquids
Altered volume of food
Altered pace of intake
Compensatory maneuvers
　Double swallow
　Supraglottic swallow
　Laryngeal elevation

Sensorimotor Exercises
Oral sensory stimulation
　Thermal
　Vibration
Resistance and placement exercises of tongue
　and jaw
Chewing
Oral manipulation of bolus
Laryngeal adduction
Biofeedback

Direct Interventions
Palatal prosthesis
Surgery
　Cricopharyngeal myotomy
　Epiglottopexy

phases may note an improvement with liquids thickened by a gel or added to foods such as mashed potatoes. Oral exercises, postural changes with the head turned or chin down, and thermal stimulation of the anterior faucial pillars are often used, although responses of patients differ widely.[117,121] Cricopharyngeal myotomy[7] followed by swallowing therapy can improve deglutition when hypopharyngeal pooling and failure of the sphincter to relax are evident, especially in patients with motoneuron disease and after a pontomedullary stroke.

When dysphagia persists to the end of inpatient rehabilitation, or when it develops in a chronic or progressive neurologic disorder, gastrostomy has usually been more effective than nasogastric tube (NGT) feeding. Neither method prevents aspiration of saliva or of gastric contents.[101] The NGT often dislodges. Even small-bore NGTs are associated with nasal irritation and bleeding, esophagitis, pulmonary intubation, traumatic pneumothorax, and aspiration pneumonia. Percutaneous endoscopic gastrostomy has been complicated by gastric perforation, hemorrhage, fistula formation, and stomal infection. Rarely, jejunostomy, esophagostomy, or pharyngostomy is better suited for the patient with neurologic dysfunction and prior gastrointestinal disease or surgery.

SUMMARY

Acute and long-term prevention and management of neuromedical complications fall to physicians and other members of the neurorehabilitation team. Approaches to the care of some frequent management issues are described. Better methods for surveillance and for physical and pharmacologic intervention are still needed. The measurement and treatment of spasticity in a clinically important manner remain particularly vexing.

When patients are discharged from inpatient rehabilitation facilities, physicians must especially be proactive in ensuring that their patients are routinely monitored for risk factors for complications and for recurrent illness, as well as for disabilities that may be lessened by a brief, goal-specific trial of a rehabilitation therapy. The rehabilitation team works toward ways to gain the compliance of patients and their families so that serious complications can be avoided. If these measures are successful, the quality of life for patients is less likely to be unnecessarily compromised by bedsores, contractures, infections, poor nutrition, and pain.

REFERENCES

1. Agency for Health Care Policy and Research. Pressure ulcers in adults: Prediction and prevention. Washington, DC: US Department of Health and Human Services, 1992.
2. Akeson W, Amiel D, Abel M, et al. Effects of immobilization on joints. Clin Orthop 1985;219:28–39.
3. Albright A, Cervi A, Singletary J. Intrathecal baclofen for spasticity in cerebral palsy. JAMA 1991;265:1418–1422.
4. Allman R. Pressure sores among the elderly. N Engl J Med 1989;320:850–853.
5. Ashworth B. Carisoprodol in multiple sclerosis. Practitioner 1964;192:540–542.
6. Avorn J, Monane M, Gurwitz J, et al. Reduction of bacteriuria and pyuria after ingestion of cranberry juice. JAMA 1994;271:751–754.
7. Baredes S. Surgical management of swallowing disorders. Otolaryngol Clin North Am 1988;21:711–720.
8. Basmajian J, Super G. Dantrolene sodium in the treatment of spasticity. Arch Phys Med Rehabil 1973;54:60–64.
9. Bedard P, Tremblay L, Barbeau H, et al. Action of 5-hydroxytryptamine, substance P, thyrotropin-releasing hormone and clonidine on motoneurone excitability. Can J Neurol Sci 1987;14:506–509.
10. Bell K, Halar E. Contractures: Prevention and management. Crit Rev Phys Rehabil Med 1990;1(4):231–246.
11. Benecke R, Conrad B, Meinck H, et al. Electromyographic analysis of bicycling on an ergometer for evaluation of spasticity of lower limbs in man. In: Desmedt J, ed: Motor Control Mechanisms in Health and Disease. New York: Raven Press, 1983.
12. Bes A, Eysette M, Pierrot-Deseilligny E. A multicentre, double-blind trial of tizanidine in spasticity associated with hemiplegia. Curr Med Res Opin 1988;10:709–718.
13. Blaivas J. Bladder function in the SCI patient. Journal of Neurologic Rehabilitation 1994;8:47–53.
14. Bohannon R. Relationship between active range of motion deficits and muscle strength and tone at the elbow in patients with hemiparesis. Clinical Rehabilitation 1991;5:219–224.
15. Brar S, Smith M, Nelson L, et al. Evaluation of treatment protocols on minimal to moderate spasticity in multiple sclerosis. Arch Phys Med Rehabil 1991;72:186–189.
16. Brindley G, Rushton D. Long term follow-up of patients with sacral anterior root stimulator implants. Paraplegia 1990;28:469–475.
17. Burke D. Spasticity as an adaptation to pyramidal tract injury. In: Waxman S, ed: Functional Recovery in Neurological Disease. New York: Raven Press, 1988:401–423.
18. Cahan L, Asams J, Perry J, et al. Instrumented gait analysis after selective dorsal rhizotomy. Dev Med Child Neurol 1990;32:1037–1043.
19. Carey J, Burghardt T. Movement dysfunction following central nervous system lesions: A problem of neurologic or muscular impairment? Phys Ther 1993;73:538–547.
20. Chan C. Dantrolene sodium and hepatic injury. Neurology 1990;40:1427–1432.
21. Chancellor M, Rivas D, Staas W. DDAVP in the urological management of the difficult neurogenic bladder in spinal cord injury. J Am Paraplegia Soc 1994;17:165–167.
22. Chutorian A, Root L. Management of spasticity in children with botulinum-A toxin. International Pediatrics 1994;9:35–43.
23. Cohan S, Raines A, Panagakos J, et al. Phenytoin and chlorpromazine in the treatment of spasticity. Arch Neurol 1980;37:360–364.
24. Coward D. Tizanidine: Neuropharmacology and mechanism of action. Neurology 1994;44(Suppl 9):S6–S11.
25. Darouiche R. Osteomyelitis associated with pressure sores. Arch Intern Med 1994;154:753–758.
26. Davidoff R. Antispasticity drugs: Mechanisms of action. Ann Neurol 1985;17:107–116.

27. Davidoff R. Mode of action of antispasticity drugs. Neurosurgery: State of the Art Reviews 1989; 4:315–324.

28. Davidoff R. Skeletal muscle tone and the misunderstood stretch reflex. Neurology 1992;42:951–963.

29. deGuzman C, Roy R, Hodgson J, et al. Coordination of motor pools controlling the ankle musculature in adult spinal cats during treadmill walking. Brain Res 1991;555:202–214.

30. Delwaide P. Contribution of human reflex studies to the understanding and management of the pyramidal syndrome. In: Shahani B, ed: Electromyography in CNS Disorders: Central EMG. Boston: Butterworth, 1984:77–109.

31. Delwaide P. Electrophysiological analysis of the mode of action of muscle relaxants in spasticity. Ann Neurol 1985;17:90–95.

32. Delwaide P, Pennisi G. Tizanidine and electrophysiologic analysis of spinal control mechanisms in humans with spasticity. Neurology 1994; 44(Suppl 9):S21–S28.

33. Denny-Brown D. The Cerebral Control of Movement. Liverpool: Liverpool University Press, 1966.

34. DePippo K, Holas M, Reding M. Validation of the 3-oz water swallow test for aspiration following stroke. Arch Neurol 1992;49:1259–1261.

35. Dietz V. Human neuronal control of automatic functional movements: Interaction between central programs and afferent input. Physiol Rev 1992; 72:33–69.

36. Dietz V, Quintern J, Berger W. Electrophysiological studies of gait in spasticity and rigidity. Brain 1981;104:431–449.

37. Dobkin B, Taly A, Su G. Use of the audiospinal reflex to test for completeness of spinal cord injury. Journal of Neurologic Rehabilitation 1994; 8:187–191.

38. Donovan W, Carter R, Rossi C, et al. Clonidine effect on spasticity: A clinical trial. Arch Phys Med Rehabil 1988;69:193–194.

39. Duncan G, Shahani B, Young R. An evaluation of baclofen treatment for certain symptoms in patients with spinal cord lesions. Neurology 1976; 26:441–446.

40. Dvir Z, Panturin E. Measurement of spasticity and associated reactions in stroke patients before and after physiotherapeutic intervention. Clin Rehabil 1993;7:15–21.

41. Dyskstra D, Sidi A. Treatment of detrusor-sphincter dyssynergia with botulinum A toxin: A double blind study. Arch Phys Med Rehabil 1990;71:24–26.

42. Erickson D, Blacklock J, Michaelson M, et al. Control of spasticity by implantable continuous flow morphine pump. Neurosurgery 1985;16:215–217.

42a. Evans JM, Andrews K, Chutka D, et al. Pressure ulcers: Prevention and management. Mayo Clin Proc 1995;70:789–799.

43. Feldman R, Kelly-Hayes M, Conomy J, et al. Baclofen for spasticity in multiple sclerosis: Double blind crossover and three-year study. Neurology 1978;28:1094–1098.

44. Fellows S, Ross H, Thilmann A. The limitations of the tendon jerk as a marker of pathological stretch reflex activity in human spasticity. J Neurol Neurosurg Psychiatry 1993;56:531–537.

45. Fellows S, Kaus C, Thilmann A. Voluntary movement at the elbow in spastic hemiparesis. Ann Neurol 1994;36:397–407.

46. Fowler C, Jewkes D, McDonald W, et al. Intravesical capsaicin for neurogenic bladder dysfunction. Lancet 1992;339:1239–1240.

47. Fung J, Barbeau H. A dynamic EMG profile index to quantify muscular activation disorder in spastic paretic gait. Electroencephalogr Clin Neurophysiol 1989;73:233–244.

48. Garland D, Lucie R, Walters R. Current uses of open phenol nerve block for adult acquired spasticity. Clin Orthop 1982;165:217–222.

49. Gelber D. Bladder dysfunction. In: Good D, Couch J, eds: Handbook of Neurorehabilitation. New York: Marcel Dekker, 1994:373–402.

50. Given J, Dewald J, McGuire J, et al. Mechanical properties of spastic muscle in hemiparetic stroke. Proceedings of the Second North American Congress on Biomechanics. Chicago, 1992:573–574.

51. Glenn M. Nerve blocks. In: Glenn M, Whyte J, eds: The Practical Management of Spasticity in Children and Adults. Philadelphia: Lea & Febiger, 1990.

52. Glenn M, Whyte J, eds. The Practical Management of Spasticity in Children and Adults. Philadelphia: Lea & Febiger, 1990.

53. Grober M. The detection of aspiration and videofluoroscopy. Dysphagia 1994;9:147–148.

54. Halpern D, Meelhuysen F. Phenol motor point block in the management of muscular hypertonia. Arch Phys Med Rehabil 1966;47:659–664.

55. Halstead L, Seager S. The effects of rectal probe electrostimulation on SCI spasticity. Paraplegia 1991;29:43–47.

56. Haslam R, Walcher J, Lietman P. Dantrolene sodium in children with spasticity. Arch Phys Med Rehabil 1974;55:384–388.

57. Hauser S, Doolittle T, Lopez-Bresnahan M, et al. An antispasticity effect of threonine in multiple sclerosis. Arch Neurol 1992;49:923–926.

58. Heckman C. Alterations in synaptic input to motoneurons during partial spinal cord injury. Med Sci Sports Exerc 1994;26:1480–1490.

59. Hesse S, Lucke D, Malezic M, et al. Botulinum toxin treatment for lower limb extensor spasticity in chronic hemiparetic patients. J Neurol Neurosurg Psychiatry 1994;57:1321–1324.

60. Hinderer S, Lehmann J, Price R, et al. Spasticity in spinal cord injured persons: Quantitative effects of baclofen and placebo treatments. Am J Phys Med Rehabil 1990;69:311–317.

61. Holas M, DePippo K, Reding M. Aspiration and relative risk of medical complications following stroke. Arch Neurol 1994;51:1051–1053.

62. Hoogstraten M, van der Ploeg R, Van der Berg W, et al. Tizanidine versus baclofen in the treatment of multiple sclerosis patients. Acta Neurol Scand 1988;77:224–230.

63. Hufschmidt A, Mauritz K. Chronic transformation of muscle in spasticity: A peripheral contribution to increased tone. J Neurol Neurosurg Psychiatry 1985;48:676–685.

64. Ibrahim I, Berger W, Trippel M, et al. Stretch-induced electromyographic activity and torque in spastic elbow muscles. Brain 1993;116:971–989.

65. Jankovic J, Brin M. Therapeutic uses of botulinum toxin. N Engl J Med 1991;324:1186–1194.
66. Johnson E, Fowler W, Lieberman J. Contractures in neuromuscular disease. Arch Phys Med Rehabil 1992;73:807–810.
67. Katrak P, Cole A, Poulos C, et al. Objective assessment of spasticity, strength, and function with early administration of dantrolene sodium after cerebrovascular accident: A randomized double-blind study. Arch Phys Med Rehabil 1992;73:4–9.
68. Katz R, Rovai G, Brait C, et al. Objective quantification of spastic hypertonia: Correlation with clinical findings. Arch Phys Med Rehabil 1992;73:339–347.
69. Katz R, Rymer W. Spastic hypertonia: Mechanisms and measurement. Arch Phys Med Rehabil 1989; 70:144–155.
70. Ketel W, Kolb M. Long term treatment with dantrolene sodium of stroke patients with spasticity limiting the return of function. Curr Med Res Opin 1984;9:161–169.
71. Koman L, Mooney J, Smith B, et al. Management of spasticity in cerebral palsy with botulinum-A toxin. J Pediatr Orthop 1994;14:299–303.
72. Koyama H, Murakami K, Suzuki T, et al. Phenol block for hip muscle spasticity under ultrasonic monitoring. Arch Phys Med Rehabil 1992;73: 1040–1043.
73. Kunkel C, Scremin E, Eisenberg B, et al. Effect of "standing" on spasticity, contracture, and osteoporosis in paralyzed males. Arch Phys Med Rehabil 1993;74:73–78.
74. Landau W, Hunt C. Dorsal rhizotomy, a treatment of unproven efficacy. J Child Neurol 1990;5:174–178.
75. Langmore S, Schatz K, Olson N. Endoscopic and videofluoroscopic evaluation of swallowing and aspiration. Ann Otol Rhinol Laryngol 1991;100:678–681.
76. Langlois S, MacKinnon J. Hand splints and cerebral spasticity: A review of the literature. Canadian Journal of Occupational Therapy 1989;56:113–119.
77. Lee K, Carson L, Kinnin E, et al. The Ashworth Scale: A reliable and reproducible method of measuring spasticity. Journal of Neurologic Rehabilitation 1989;3:205–209.
78. Lehmann J, Price R, deLateur B, et al. Spasticity: Quantitative measurements as a basis for assessing effectiveness of therapeutic intervention. Arch Phys Med Rehabil 1989;70:6–15.
79. Lehmkuhl L, Thoi L, Bontke C, et al. Multimodality treatment of joint contractures in patients with severe brain injury: Cost, effectiveness, and integration of therapies in the application of serial/inhibitive casts. Journal of Head Trauma Rehabilitation 1990;5:25–42.
80. Leslie G, Muir C, Part N, et al. A comparison of the assessment of spasticity by the Wartenberg pendulum test and the Ashworth grading scale in patients with multiple sclerosis. Clinical Rehabilitation 1992;6:41–48.
81. Levin M, Hui-Chan C. Relief of hemiparetic spasticity by TENS is associated with improvement in reflex and voluntary motor functions. Electroencephalogr Clin Neurophysiol 1992;85:131–142.
82. Liebesman J, Cafarelli E. Physiology of range of

motion in human joints: A critical review. Crit Rev Phys Rehabil Med 1994;6:131–160.
83. Little J, Halar E. H-reflex changes following spinal cord injury. Arch Phys Med Rehabil 1985;66:19–22.
84. Logemann J. Approaches to the management of disordered swallowing. Clin Gastroenterol 1991; 5:269–280.
85. Lossius R, Dietrichson P, Lunde P. Effects of clorazepate in spasticity and rigidity: A quantitative study of reflexes and plasma concentrations. Acta Neurol Scand 1985;71:190–194.
86. Loubser P, Narayan R, Sandin K, et al. Continuous infusion of intrathecal baclofen: Long-term effects on spasticity in spinal cord injury. Paraplegia 1991; 29:48–64.
87. Luisto M, Moller K, Nuutila A. Dantrolene sodium in chronic spasticity of varying etiology. Acta Neurol Scand 1982;65:355–362.
88. Madoff R, Williams J, Caushaj P. Fecal incontinence. N Engl J Med 1992;326:1002–1007.
89. McLellan D. Co-contraction and stretch reflexes in spasticity during treatment with baclofen. J Neurol Neurosurg Psychiatry 1977;40:30–38.
90. Meythaler J, Steers W, Tuel S, et al. Continuous intrathecal baclofen in spinal cord spasticity. Am J Phys Med Rehabil 1992;71:321–327.
91. Meythaler J, Steers W, Tuel S, et al. Intrathecal baclofen in hereditary spastic paraparesis. Arch Phys Med Rehabil 1992;73:794–797.
92. Miller A. Neurophysiological basis of swallowing. Dysphagia 1986;1:91–100.
93. Miller R, Green A, Moussavi R, et al. Excessive muscular fatigue in patients with spastic paraparesis. Neurology 1990;40:1271–1274.
94. Miller R, Langmore S. Treatment efficacy for adults with oropharyngeal dysphagia. Arch Phys Med Rehabil 1994;75:1256–1262.
95. Mohler J, Cowen D, Flanigan R. Suppression and treatment of urinary tract infection in patients with intermittently catheterized neurogenic bladder. J Urol 1987;138:336–341.
96. Nance P. A comparison of clonidine, cyproheptadine and baclofen in spastic spinal cord injured patients. J Am Paraplegia Soc 1994;17:150–156.
97. Nance P, Bugaresti J, Shellenberger K, et al. Efficacy and safety of tizanidine in the treatment of spasticity in patients with spinal cord injury. Neurology 1994;44(Suppl 9):S44–S52.
98. Nathadwarawala K, Nicklin J, Wiles C. A timed test of swallowing capacity for neurological patients. J Neurol Neurosurg Psychiatry 1993;55:822–825.
99. Ochs G, Delhaas E. Aspects of long-term treatment with intrathecal baclofen for severe spasticity (abstract). Neurology 1992;42(Suppl 3):466.
100. Park C, O'Neill P. Management of neurological dysphagia. Clin Rehabil 1994;8:166–174.
101. Park R, Allison M, Lang J, et al. Randomised comparison of percutaneous endoscopic gastrostomy and nasogastric tube feeding in patients with persisting neurological dysphagia. Br Med J 1992; 304:1406–1409.
102. Peacock W, Staudt L. Functional outcomes following selective posterior rhizotomy in children with cerebral palsy. J Neurosurg 1991;74:380–385.
103. Penn R, Savoy S, Corcos D, et al. Intrathecal baclo-

fen for severe spinal spasticity. N Engl J Med 1989; 320:1517–1521.

104. Petajan J. Sural nerve stimulation and motor control of tibialis anterior muscle in spastic paresis. Neurology 1987;37:47–52.

105. Petersen T, Klemar B. Electrical stimulation as a treatment of lower limb spasticity. Journal of Neurologic Rehabilitation 1988;2:103–108.

106. Petro D, Ellenberger C. Treatment of human spasticity with delta-9-tetrahydrocannabinol. J Clin Pharmacol 1981;21:413S–416S.

107. Pierrot-Deseilligny E. Electrophysiological assessment of the spinal mechanisms underlying spasticity. In: Rossini P, Mauguiere F, eds: New Trends and Advanced Techniques in Clinical Neurophysiology (EEG Suppl 41). Amsterdam: Elsevier, 1990:264–273.

108. Pierson S, Katz D, Tarsy D. Botulinum toxin A in the treatment of spasticity. Neurology 1994; 44(Suppl 2):A184.

109. Powers R, Campbell D, Rymer W. Stretch reflex dynamics in spastic elbow flexor muscles. Ann Neurol 1989;25:32–42.

110. Price R. Mechanical spasticity evaluation techniques. Crit Rev Phys Med Rehabil 1990;2:65–73.

111. Price R, Lehmann J, Boswell-Bessette S, et al. Influence of cryotherapy on spasticity at the human ankle. Arch Phys Med Rehabil 1993;74:300–304.

112. Putty T, Shapiro S. Efficacy of dorsal longitudinal myelotomy in treating spinal spasticity: A review of 20 cases. J Neurosurg 1991;75:397–401.

113. Reddy N, Thomas R, Canilang E, et al. Toward classification of dysphagic patients using biomechanical measurements. J Rehabil Res Dev 1994;31:335–344.

114. Robinson C, Kett N, Bolam J. Spasticity in spinal cord injured patients: 2. Initial measures and long-term effects of surface electrical stimulation. Arch Phys Med Rehabil 1988;69:862–868.

115. Rogers de Saca L, Catlin P, Segal R. Immediate effects of the toe spreader on the tonic toe flexion reflex. Phys Ther 1994;74:561–570.

116. Rosenbaum P, Russell D, Cadman D, et al. Issues in measuring change in motor function in children with cerebral palsy: A special communication. Phys Ther 1990;70:125–131.

117. Rosenbek J, Robbins J, Fishback B, et al. Effects of thermal application on dysphagia after stroke. J Speech Hearing Res 1991;34:1157–1168.

118. Rudick R, Breton D, Krall R. The GABA-agonist progabide for spasticity in multiple sclerosis. Arch Neurol 1987;44:1033–1036.

119. Seib T, Price R, Reyes M, et al. The quantitative measurement of spasticity: Effect of cutaneous electrical stimulation. Arch Phys Med Rehabil 1994;75:746–750.

120. Shader R, Greenblatt D. Drug therapy: Use of benzodiazepines in anxiety disorders. N Engl J Med 1993;328:1398–1405.

121. Shanahan T, Logemann J, Rademaker A, et al. Chin-down posture effect on aspiration in dysphagic patients. Arch Phys Med Rehabil 1993; 74:736–739.

122. Shefner J, Berman S, Sarkarati M, et al. Recurrent inhibition is increased in patients with spinal cord injury. Neurology 1992;42:2162–2168.

123. Sindou M, Jeanmonod D. Microsurgical DREZotomy for the treatment of spasticity and pain in the lower limbs. Neurosurgery 1989;24:655–670.

124. Skeil D, Barnes M. The local treatment of spasticity. Clin Rehabil 1994;8:240–246.

125. Smith C, Birnbaum G, Carter J, et al. Tizanidine treatment of spasticity caused by multiple sclerosis. Neurology 1994;44(Suppl 9):S34–S43.

126. Smith J, Greer J, Liu G, et al. Neural mechanisms generating respiratory pattern in mammalian brainstem–spinal cord in vitro. J Neurophysiol 1990;64:1149–1169.

127. Snow B, Tsui J, Bhatt M, et al. Treatment of spasticity with botulinum toxin: A double-blind study. Ann Neurol 1990;28:512–515.

128. Staas W, Cioschi H. Pressure sores: A multifaceted approach to prevention and treatment. West J Med 1991;154:539–544.

129. Staas W, Cioschi H. Neurogenic bowel dysfunction. Crit Rev Phys Rehabil Med 1989;1:11–21.

130. Stefanovska A, Rebersek S, Bajd T, et al. Effects of electrical stimulation on spasticity. Crit Rev Phys Rehabil Med 1991;3:59–99.

131. Steinbok P, Keyes R, Langill L, et al. The validity of electrophysiological criteria used in selective functional dorsal rhizotomy for treatment of spastic cerebral palsy. J Neurosurg 1994;81:354–361.

132. Stern P, Bokonjic R. Glycine therapy in 7 cases of spasticity. Pharmacology 1974;12:117–119.

133. Stover S, Lloyd L. Neurogenic bladder. Physical Medicine and Rehabilitation Clinics of North America 1993;4:211–415.

134. Thilmann A, Fellows S, Garms E. The mechanism of spastic muscle hypertonus. Brain 1991;114:233–244.

135. Tolosa E, Soll R, Loewenson R. Treatment of spasticity in multiple sclerosis with dantrolene. JAMA 1975;233:1046–1047.

136. Vaughan C, Berman B, Peacock W. Cerebral palsy and rhizotomy: A 3 year follow-up with gait analysis. J Neurosurg 1991;74:178–184.

137. Wainberg M, Barbeau H, Gauthier S. Quantitative assessment of the effect of cyproheptadine on spastic paretic gait: A preliminary study. J Neurol 1986; 233:311–314.

138. Wheeler J, Walter J, Cai W. Electrical stimulation for urinary incontinence. Crit Rev Phys Rehabil Med 1993;5:31–55.

139. Winstein C, Garfinkel A. Qualitative dynamics of disordered human locomotion: A preliminary study. J Mot Behav 1989;21:373–391.

140. Yang J, Fung J, Edamura M, et al. H-reflex modulation during walking in spastic paretic subjects. Can J Neurol Sci 1991;18:443–452.

141. Yarkony G. Pressure sores: A review. Arch Phys Med Rehabil 1994;75:908–917.

142. Yarkony G, Bass L, Keenan V, et al. Contractures complicating spinal cord injury. Paraplegia 1985; 23:265–269.

143. Yarkony G, Sahgal V. Contractures: A major complication of craniocerebral trauma. Clin Orthop 1987;219:93–98.

144. Young R. Spasticity. Neurology 1994;44(Suppl 9):S12–S20.

145. Young R, Delwaide P. Drug therapy: Spasticity. N Engl J Med 1981;304:28–33;96–99.

PART 3

Rehabilitation of Specific Neurologic Disorders

CHAPTER 7

STROKE

Rehabilitation of the 500,000 patients in the United States who suffer a stroke each year begins as soon as physicians make the diagnosis. The short-term medical treatments, interventional radiologic techniques, and surgical therapies that may limit or reverse ischemic neuronal damage are still mostly in clinical trials.[1] The errors of omission and commission during acute hospitalization that interfere with the recovery of mobility, self-care, cognition, and quality of life are often preventable. About two-thirds of survivors of stroke who are hospitalized on a short-term basis can benefit from the evaluations and recommendations of rehabilitation physicians and therapists. An increasing repertoire of compensatory and restorative approaches is becoming available to manage physical and cognitive impairments and disabilities during inpatient and outpatient care.

FISCAL IMPACT

Estimates of the total costs of stroke in the United States vary widely.[76] The approximations in Table 7–1 are drawn from several sources.[2,287] Medicare data show that people over the age of 64 years account for 87 percent of all deaths and 74 percent of all hospitalizations for cerebrovascular disease.[50]

157

Table 7–1. ESTIMATED ECONOMIC COSTS OF ALL STROKE PATIENT CARE IN 1991 ($18 BILLION)

Direct Costs (%)	
Acute hospital care	19
Nursing homes	10
Medical and social services	9
Inpatient rehabilitation	5
Physician services	<2
Chronic hospital care	2
Assistive devices	0.4
Indirect Costs (%) (lost income)	
Disability	6
Premature death	48

Estimates on these federally sponsored patients, developed by the Patient Outcomes Research Team (PORT) Study for the Agency for Health Care Policy and Research, suggested that the direct cost of stroke in 1993 was $13 billion, and the indirect cost, taking into account caregiver burden, was another $17 billion.[213] Medicare actually paid an average of $15,000 per patient, or

Table 7–2. STROKE OUTCOMES BEFORE AND AFTER DIAGNOSTIC-RELATED GROUPS (DRG)–BASED PROSPECTIVE PAYMENT SYSTEM (PPS) (1982 VERSUS 1986)

	Pre-PPS	Post-PPS
Mean length of stay (days)	16.2	11.1*
In-hospital deaths (%)	22.4	17.8*
30-day deaths	21.3	19.9
180-day deaths	35.3	34.3
Readmissions		
by 1 yr (%)	57	57
mean days	14	13

*$P = 0.01$

Source: Kahn K, Keeler E, Sherwood M, et al. Comparing outcomes of care before and after implementation of the DRG-based Prospective Payment System. JAMA 1990; 264:1984–1988.

Table 7–3 DIAGNOSTIC-RELATED GROUPS (DRG) 14: CEREBROVASCULAR DISORDER OTHER THAN TRANSIENT ISCHEMIC ATTACK (HOSPITAL COST AND UTILIZATION PROJECT, 1986)*

Number of Discharge Records	30,702
Age (y)	
Quartiles:	
25%	66
50% (median)	74
75%	81
Length of Stay (days)	
Quartiles:	
25%	4
50%	8
75%	13
Gender (%)	
Female	56.0
Male	44.0
Ethnic Origin (%)	
White	85.2
Black	11.8
Hispanic	1.6
Native American	0.1
Asian	0.6
Other	0.6
Pay Source (%)	
Medicare	77.6
Medicaid	2.7
Private insurance	14.3
Other government	0.6
Other private	4.8
Discharge Status (%)	
Routine	43.7
Long-term care	34.6
Short-term hospital care	6.0
Against advice	0.2
Died	15.5

*Agency for Health Care Policy and Research, Hospital Studies Program.

Source: Lemrow N, Adams D, Coffey R, et al. The 50 Most Frequent Diagnosis-Related Groups (DRGs), Diagnoses, and Procedures: Statistics by Hospital Size and Location. Rockville, MD. DHHS Publication No. (PHS) 90–3465, 1990:15.

over $6 billion for the first 90 days of care. Of this amount, initial hospital care accounted for 43 percent, rehospitalizations for 14 percent, and rehabilitation for 16 percent.

The rate of increase of medical costs may decline for Medicare patients, in keeping with the increasingly shorter hospital stays promoted by the Diagnostic Related Groups (DRG)–based Prospective Payment System (PPS) (Table 7–2). The DRG 14 population with acute stroke in 1986 is characterized in Table 7–3. PPS cost-containment measures, at least through 1986, have not appeared to negatively affect outcomes or to lead to more complications that could add to the cost of hospital care (see Table 7–2).[173] In countries where cost-containment measures are less imposing, social factors such as placement problems, more than the need for additional diagnostic and medical care, can account for longer lengths of hospital stay and greater costs.[305]

Shorter inpatient rehabilitation stays are also a product of Medicare reimbursement and capitated care. The mean cost across regions of the United States for inpatient rehabilitation is about twice the cost of an acute hospital stay, but only a minority of survivors of stroke receive this level of care. About 12 percent of Medicare patients are transferred for stroke rehabilitation from an acute hospitalization, although this number varies by about 5 percent across regions of the country.[76] Patients whose inpatient and outpatient rehabilitation costs are well above average have often been those who failed to become independent.[247] The greater availability of nursing homes and a decline in age-adjusted death rates,[298] which might leave more patients disabled, could raise some costs, whereas more widespread management of risk factors might decrease stroke rates and the severity of disability.

MEDICAL INTERVENTIONS DURING REHABILITATION

Most of the short-term medical and surgical therapies that might limit or reverse ischemic neuronal damage are still more

Table 7–4. POTENTIAL ACUTE STROKE INTERVENTIONS

Augment Cerebral Blood Flow
   Optimize cardiac output
   Alter rheology: hemodilution with colloid, saline, venisection, perfluorochemicals
   Lyse thrombus: tissue plasminogen activator, streptokinase, urokinase, ancrod
   Restore arterial lumen: endarterectomy, angioplasty
   Add collaterals: arterial bypass
   Treat cerebral edema
   Manage vasospasm

Limit Thrombosis
   Anticoagulation: heparin, heparinoids, warfarin, ancrod, leech proteins
   Antiplatelet agents: aspirin, ticlopidine

Protect Ischemic Neurons
   Lower energy demands: hypothermia, barbiturates
   Impede Cascade to Cell Death
      Limit lactic acidosis: normoglycemia
      Membrane sodium-potassium ionic blockade
      Block various calcium channels
      Block excitatory amino acid channels: N-methyl-D-aspartate receptor antagonists, magnesium
      Scavenge free radicals: 21-aminosteroids, vitamins C and E, mannitol, superoxide dismutase
      Protect cell membranes: GM_1 ganglioside
      Alter genes that affect cell viability: induce stress genes, e.g., heat shock proteins
      Block inflammatory components of ischemia: inhibit cytokines, cell adhesion molecules

speculative than proved (Table 7–4). Some studies raise the possibility that certain drugs including haloperidol, diazepam, phenytoin, and alpha-2–adrenergic receptor agonists and alpha-1–adrenergic receptor antagonists that are frequently used in patients admitted to hospitals because of cerebrovascular disease may negatively affect behavior and neuronal function.[118] So far, rehabilitation specialists have no means of determining whether these and other centrally acting drugs have negative effects on early neuroprotection or on subsequent mechanisms of neuroplasticity and restoration. More traditional preventive medical measures initiated in the first few days after a stroke should continue through the early course of rehabilitation, whether the patient is still in a hospital or has transferred to inpatient rehabilitation.[79,80]

An autopsy-based study (Table 7–5) revealed the most frequent causes of death related to acute stroke. Preventive measures and experienced nursing care may reduce this mortality during the acute hospital stay and the inpatient rehabilitation period.

With shorter acute hospital stays encouraged by the DRG scheme of Medicare reimbursement and by managed care organizations, physicians may have less time to monitor and to adjust their short-term therapies. In 1994, the length of stay covered for stroke without serious complications (DRG 14) was about 7.5 days. Before 1983, stroke rehabilitation programs in the United States that published the functional outcomes of their patients reported the average time from onset of stroke to transfer to their unit as ranging from 14 to 48 days.[168] For 1992, the Uniform Data Service for Medical Rehabilitation (UDS) reported a mean stroke onset to rehabilitation transfer of 20 days, but this report included non-Medicare patients, patients who developed lengthy medical complications, and, of course, patients so disabled by the stroke that they needed rehabilitation. This delay from onset to transfer has been declining as well.

In a study of patients transferred to a rehabilitation center within a mean of 10 days after a stroke, the incidence of serious medical complications found upon admission rose from 22 percent before institution of DRGs to 48 percent the year after institution.[72] Many of these complications derived from altering or starting medications during the acute hospitalization, especially antihypertensives, antiarrhythmics, platelet antiaggregants, anticoagulants, steroids, hypoglycemics, antibiotics, anticonvulsants, analgesics, and sedatives. Azotemia, hypoglycemia, hyponatremia, orthostatic hypotension, and a drug-induced encephalopathy were among the most common problems encountered. These problems delayed the

Table 7–5. **LEADING CAUSES OF DEATH WITHIN 3 MONTHS OF STROKE**

Cause of Death	Percentage (%)
Cardiac disorder	35
Acute and recurrent stroke	25
Pneumonia	15
Pulmonary embolism	10

Table 7–6. **GENERAL FREQUENCY OF INPATIENT REHABILITATION NEUROMEDICAL COMPLICATIONS**

Complications	Percentage (%) of Patients
Urinary tract infection	40
Musculoskeletal pain	30
Depression	30
Urine retention	25
Falls	25
Fungal rash	20
Hypotension	20
Hypertension	15
Hypoglycemia or hyperglycemia	15
Toxic or metabolic encephalopathy	10
Pneumonia	10
Cardiac arrhythmia	10
Malnutrition	10
Congestive heart failure	5
Angina pectoris	5
Thrombophlebitis	5
Pulmonary embolus	<5
Myocardial infarction	
Decubitus ulcer	
Recurrent stroke	
Seizure	
Azotemia	
Allergic reaction	
Gastrointestinal bleeding	

Source: Data from references 72 and 86.

start of rehabilitative therapies and contributed to additional medical morbidity.

Neuromedical complications are commonly encountered during inpatient rehabilitation (Table 7–6). A randomized trial that compared stroke management on general medical wards with that on a rehabilitation unit found that 60 percent of patients developed medical complications in each setting.[176a] In one freestanding facility in 1990, patients with an average delay of 37 days from stroke onset to rehabilitation transfer with an average 52-day stay had a mean of 3.6 medical and 0.6 neurologic complications.[86] These complications were more frequent in patients with sensorimotor and hemianopic visual loss than in those with only motor or sensorimotor impairments. The incidence of these complications was also higher in patients with the lowest Barthel Index scores on hospital admission and in those with the longest rehabilitation hospital stays. Nearly all patients required physicians' interventions for conditions that could limit rehabilitative therapies. From 5 to 15 percent of patients in rehabilitation centers require transfer back to an acute hospital setting. UDS reported an incidence of 7 percent for 26,000 patients in 1990 to 1991.[125]

Some potential medical problems must be sought proactively. When specifically monitored during physical therapy, up to one-half of patients have cardiac arrhythmias and wide variations in blood pressure, especially during stair climbing, walking, stationary bicycling, and tall kneeling.[281] Although many patients with stroke have some heart disease, the symptoms of congestive heart failure, exertional angina, and orthostatic hypotension limit therapy the most.

Cerebral Hypoperfusion

A few measures may reduce the risk of additional ischemic injury during initial attempts at mobilizing the patient with acute stroke and during early posttransfer for inpatient rehabilitation. Dysautoregulation of cerebral blood flow and systemic hypotension, superimposed upon impaired collateral blood flow, can cause focal hypoper-

fusion.[74] Thus, postural blood pressure changes, Valsalva's maneuver, and dehydration may lower cerebral blood flow and should be avoided. The most frequent errors of commission that lead to orthostatic hypotension are fluid restriction, initially from concern about cerebral edema and later from inadequate oral or intravenous intake and the treatment of hypertension.

In the elderly patient with stroke, both during and after inpatient rehabilitation, the common and sometimes subtle effects of standing hypotension cannot be emphasized enough. Postural hypotension increases with aging.[210] In an epidemiologic study of 5210 men and women aged 65 years and older, the prevalence of asymptomatic orthostatic hypotension, defined as at least a 20-mm Hg fall in the systolic pressure or a 10-mm Hg drop in diastolic pressure, was 18 percent.[289] The prevalence increased with age. Postural hypotension was significantly associated with difficulty in walking, frequent falls, transient ischemic attack, isolated systolic hypertension, and carotid artery stenosis. Exercise intolerance, fatigue, dizziness, confusion, syncope, and a decline in mental functioning[255] are potential symptoms at any age. Deconditioning, medications that induce volume depletion and dysautonomia, and diabetic neuropathies, all of which can accompany stroke and early rehabilitation, are among the medical complications that can increase the potential for postural hypotension. Finally, some of these patients probably have undertreated supine hypertension. Their blood pressure, checked when they are seated, is normal, but they have supine hypertension, which increases their risk for repeated stroke and for cardiovascular disease.

Dysphagia

Swallowing disorders affect 10 percent of elderly patients who are acutely hospitalized and 30 percent of nursing home dwellers.[89] Aspiration pneumonia and inadequate caloric intake become even more likely during an acute stroke. A prospective British study diagnosed dysphagia in 30 percent of 357 conscious patients within 48 hours of a unilateral hemispheric stroke.[17] These patients were rated as impaired if swallowing was delayed or if they coughed while swallowing 10 mL of water. Lethargy, gaze paresis, and sensory inattention were present more often than in those who swallowed normally. By 1 week, 16 percent had dysphagia. At 1 month, only 2 percent of survivors were still impaired, and, at 6 months, only 0.4 percent of survivors were impaired.

In a regional study, signs of malnutrition were found in 16 percent of patients with stroke upon hospital admission, with the greatest risk in women over the age of 74 years.[15] By hospital discharge, 23 percent were malnourished. Elderly men and patients who had infections or who received new cardiovascular drugs had the greatest risk. Clearly, clinicians must attend to the caloric intake of the disabled patient.

If oral intake is unsafe based upon a formal swallowing evaluation or if it provides fewer than 800 calories per day by 3 days after hospital admission, intravenous therapy or feeding through a small-bore nasogastric tube (NGT) is indicated. No randomized trials have been conducted to determine which method better prevents complications. NGT feedings are not benign. They can cause gastric reflux, decrease pharyngeal sensation, and become misplaced into the trachea or a bronchus. They can also lead to other pulmonary complications, epistaxis, perforation of the esophagus, and the use of physical restraints that keep patients from pulling the tube. A hint of the potential problems of tube feeding comes from a quality-of-care population study of 2824 Medicare patients who were hospitalized for first strokes in 1986.[173,286] In this population, 44 percent were unable to eat normally. About 20 percent had feeding tubes placed within the first 3 days or the last 2 days after admission. This group included 42 percent of comatose and 23 percent of noncomatose patients. The feeding tubes did not protect against the development of pulmonary infiltrates, which occurred in 10 percent of patients with dysphagia who received or did not receive an NGT, compared with 4 percent of patients who had no difficulty in swallowing. Most feeding tubes in patients remained in place at hospital discharge, and 75 percent of these patients were sent to nursing homes. Use of a feeding tube for comatose and alert patients was associated with higher mortality rates than reported in patients who did not have a feeding tube, even if they were alert and had difficulty in swallowing.

Patients with aphagia with unilateral hemispheric lesions who are going to be sent to an inpatient rehabilitation program should not undergo a gastrostomy for feedings. Most patients recover spontaneously and with therapy. Patients with bihemispheric strokes and a pseudobulbar palsy, pontomedullary lesions, and unilateral lesions of the sylvian fissure are most likely to be affected beyond the acute hospital stay. These patients are a challenge for the rehabilitation team.

TESTS

In alert, at-risk inpatients undergoing stroke rehabilitation, coughing or a wet-hoarse quality of the voice within 1 minute of continuously swallowing 90 mL of water from a cup had a sensitivity of 80 percent and a specificity of 54 percent for aspiration, demonstrated by a modified barium swallow (MBS). The bedside test had a sensitivity of 88 percent and a specificity of 44 percent for large amounts of aspiration that may be more clinically significant.[65] False-negative test results usually involved less than 10 percent aspiration of barium. Thus, this quick screen reveals most patients who aspirate on the MBS and, in the study, all who developed pneumonia, but it also includes many false-positive results. When the 3-oz water swallow test was included in a seven-part screening test for dysphagia, it was the strongest predictor of pneumonia, recurrent airway obstruction, and death.[66] These complications were 7.6 times more likely in the inpatients with stroke who failed the screen than in those who passed. In the same population, the investigators also found that pneumonia was significantly more likely to develop during 1-year follow-up of patients who aspirated a small amount, silently, or more than 10 percent on MBS, compared with those who did not, although about 3 to 6 times as many patients showed aspiration and did not develop pneumonia.[151]

The MBS is the gold standard screening test and has offered other insights into the risks related to dysphagia. In a 1-year follow-up study of 60 patients with dysphagia after stroke, aspiration pneumonia occurred in those whose videofluoroscopic studies revealed a total kinematic pharyngeal transit time of greater than 2 seconds, with the highest risk if greater than 5 seconds.[165] The presence or absence of vallecular or piriform pooling or penetration of the bolus through the true vocal cords did not correlate with subsequent clinically apparent aspiration.

A prospective study of 40 patients with strokes of middle cerebral artery distribution at a mean of 21 days (range of 15 to 60 days) after onset found differences in the pattern of swallowing based on lesion location.[270] Few of the patients showed clinical signs or symptoms of dysphagia. Compared with controls, for example, patients with lesions of the left hemisphere had a longer transit time for a bolus to pass through the pharynx. Patients with right-sided lesions had a longer total swallowing duration and a higher incidence of laryngeal penetration and aspiration of liquid. Patients with anterior lesions showed longer swallowing durations on most variables than healthy persons and those with posterior lesions. Patients with left-sided infarctions who demonstrated labial, lingual, and mandibular incoordination and some apraxia of swallowing ate safely, despite their abnormal MBS. Although clinicopathologic correlations are conjectural, the study does suggest that patients should be examined for silent aspiration of liquids within 1 month of an infarction of the right hemisphere.

MANAGEMENT

Most often after a hemispheric stroke, the swallowing reflex is delayed, the bolus slides over the base of the tongue and collects in the valleculae and hypopharynx, and sometimes the pharyngeal constrictor malfunctions. Chapter 6 describes management techniques (see Table 6–11).

A trial of three graded levels of dysphagia therapy during inpatient stroke rehabilitation randomized 115 subjects to one of the following categories:

1. One formal therapy that explained the results of an MBS and gave recommendations about food consistency and compensatory techniques; patient and family then made their own decisions.
2. The same therapy as No. 1, but a therapist reassessed the diet every other week.
3. The therapist prescribed the diet and gave instructions about compensatory techniques and recommendations daily at mealtime.[67]

Patients who aspirated more than 50 percent of all food consistencies and who continued to aspirate after attempting compensatory techniques were excluded from the trial. At discharge and at 1-year follow-up, no differences were apparent among the groups in end points of pneumonia, dehydration, calorie-nitrogen deficit, upper airway obstruction, and death. Fifteen percent reached an end point during the inpatient stay. MBS evidence of aspiration of thick liquids and solids was associated with a greater risk and early onset of pneumonia. No differences were found when patients were grouped by Barthel Index score, by stroke impairment, or by cognition. Thus, limited instruction to patients and their families can be as effective as daily, formal dysphagia therapy for most inpatients.

NGT feedings can supplement oral calories and fluid. These feedings should be given after each meal so they do not blunt the patient's appetite. If profound dysphagia persists toward the time of discharge from inpatient rehabilitation, a gastrostomy tube is a comfortable portal for nutrition, although the technique is probably no safer in preventing reflux aspiration than an NGT. Even in patients with medullary strokes that cause unilateral paresis of the pharyngeal muscle and the adductor of the larynx, along with cricopharyngeal dysfunction, however, swallowing can gradually be retrained in motivated patients.[204]

Deep Vein Thrombosis

From the first day after stroke until a patient is ambulatory in the rehabilitation ward, clinicians and staff must take a forward approach to the prevention and management of venous thromboembolism.[34] The clinical signs and symptoms of deep vein thrombosis (DVT) and pulmonary embolism (PE) are not sensitive or specific, so they cannot be considered reliable. By impedance plethysmography and, for the calf, by radioisotope scanning with fibrinogen iodine 125, venous thrombi can be found in the paretic leg within 1 week of an acute stroke in more than 50 percent of patients, although symptoms and signs are far less frequent.[301,351] Duplex ultrasonography and venography are among the best diagnostic tests. When a PE is suspected, ventilation-perfusion scanning or pulmonary angiography must be performed.

In controlled trials of prophylaxis, DVT has been found in 20 to 75 percent of untreated patients within 2 weeks of stroke.[111,215,217,332,334] From 5 to 20 percent suffered a PE, which was fatal in about 10 percent. Intermittent calf compression for the paretic leg, intermittent low-dose heparin at 5000 U q8h or q12h, and low-molecular-weight heparinoid were more effective than no intervention or the use of antiembolism hose. These interventions reduced DVT by a factor of 2 to 7, and they reduced PE by about 2 to 4. Low-dose heparin prophylaxis has been recommended by a consensus conference for all patients with nonhemorrhagic stroke, and external pneumatic calf compression has been recommended for the rest.[244] Heparinoids may be more effective than heparin.[333]

Patients with stroke who are inpatients in a rehabilitation service vary in the incidence of occult and symptomatic DVT and PE. Higher rates are reported in screening studies that use ultrasonography and impedance plethysmography for occult DVT. Higher incidences have also been associated with greater severity of leg paresis, inability to ambulate,[36,242] and hypercoagulability suggested by a shortened partial thromboplastin time.[190]

Once DVT is diagnosed, immediate heparinization to an activated partial thromboplastin time of about two times control generally allows the patient to restart activities out of bed by day 2.[155] Thus, rehabilitation efforts can usually continue without transfer to an acute setting. Warfarin is also started upon diagnosis to achieve an international normalized ratio (INR) of 2 to 3 for 6 months for the first episode of DVT.[299a,355]

Bowel and Bladder Dysfunction

Urinary incontinence and retention and bowel incontinence and obstipation are common early after a stroke. These conditions come under control with simple measures in most cases. They should be managed proactively to prevent infection and pressure sores, as well as to preserve the patient's dignity and quality of life.

Many elderly patients have a premorbid history of bladder dysfunction. Urinary dribbling and involuntary emptying affects 30 percent of the healthy, noninstitutionalized population over the age of 65 years.[324] After a stroke, many of these patients decompensate further, and previously asymptomatic patients with hemiparesis become affected. In a prospective follow-up study of 150 patients with all degrees of impairment after stroke, 60 percent were incontinent in the first week, 40 percent were incontinent at 4 weeks, and 30 percent were incontinent at 12 weeks.[31] Of patients who had no bladder control by 6 weeks, only 18 percent were continent at 1 year. Another study followed patients with a mean age of 68 years who were admitted to an inpatient rehabilitation service. By 1 month following an acute stroke, 10 percent of patients with a pure motor impairment and 70 percent of patients with the more severe combination of motor, proprioceptive, and visual hemianopic deficits had urinary incontinence.[265] At 6 months, 30 percent of the second group of patients, who presumably had suffered a full middle cerebral artery territory infarction, were still incontinent. During outpatient therapy, some patients may be too embarrassed to offer that they are incontinent. The clinician must ask specific questions.

Urodynamic studies are indicated when the cause of urinary retention or incontinence is unclear (see Chapter 6). Elevated postvoid residual volumes, over 50 mL, have been detected in 35 to 50 percent of patients with a first stroke who are admitted for rehabilitation.[110] About one-third of these patients with urine retention have bladder outlet obstruction, one-third have bladder hyporeflexia, and others have a combination of both. Cognitive dysfunction contributes to this disorder in some instances. No relationship has been found between residual volume and position during voiding, whether in bed or on a commode, for men and women. Among incontinent patients admitted to one rehabilitation unit, 37 percent had normal cystometrographic studies, another 37 percent had detrusor hyperreflexia, 21 percent had detrusor hyporeflexia, and 5 percent had detrusor-sphincter dyssynergia.[109] An unstable detrusor is the most common study abnormality associated with persistent urinary incontinence.

MANAGEMENT

Principles of management are described in Chapter 6, and commonly used medications are listed in Table 6–7. A few points are especially important. Urinary tract infections must be identified and treated. Prostatic enlargement can produce overflow incontinence in patients who can void, and it can produce obstruction with high residual urines in patients who cannot void. Timed voiding, administration of anticholinergic agents, and an external catheter are of value for the patient who is incontinent but has less than 100 mL residuals. In patients with residuals over 100 mL, drug side effects should be considered as a cause. Intermittent catheterization is best for patients who cannot void. Prostatic obstruction of the urethra that is not relieved within 2 weeks by an alpha-blocking agent such as terazosin may have to be corrected before the patient is discharged from the facility. Attempts to decrease prostate volume by blocking the conversion of testosterone to dihydrotestosterone with a drug such as finasteride may take 6 months or more to become effective.

Bowel incontinence develops in about 30 percent of patients, but it usually resolves spontaneously by 2 weeks after stroke, or it is corrected by treating the underlying medical cause.

Seizures

Seizures occur in 5 to 8 percent of patients within 24 hours to 2 weeks of an ischemic stroke.[25,184] These seizures are often focal motor, complex partial, or secondary generalized. Periodic lateralized discharges predict subsequent seizures. Seizures associated with an acute infarction usually include the cortex. Cardioembolic and thrombotic types of stroke have equal predilection for a seizure. About 12 percent of patients with a lobar or basal ganglionic intracerebral hemorrhage suffer a seizure near onset.[98] By 2 years after an infarction, 20 to 30 percent of patients with an early seizure have epilepsy, compared with 10 percent of patients without an early seizure.[132,184] For patients with parenchymatous hemorrhages, 13 percent of patients who have survived for 30 days to 2 years and 7 percent of patients who have survived for 2 to 5 years develop epilepsy.[98] Monotherapy with an anticonvulsant agent is usually effective. Recurrences often follow subtherapeutic drug levels or systemic toxic and metabolic illnesses.

Sleep Disorders

Age-related changes in sleep include nighttime wakefulness and daytime fatigue and napping.[261] During inpatient and outpatient therapy, insomnia and excessive daytime sleepiness can interfere with attention and carryover. Stimulants, alcohol, medications, discomfort, anxiety, depression, and chronically poor sleep habits can contribute. Central and obstructive sleep apnea or a mix of both can develop from brainstem and cortical lesions, especially in patients with bulbar dysfunction or in relation to a toxic or a metabolic encephalopathy. These disorders may precede the stroke, because they have been associated with a higher risk of stroke.[252] Pharyngeal muscle weakness and impaired neural control of nasopharyngeal and pharyngolaryngeal muscles during sleep because of a stroke contribute to the risk of obstructive apnea. Up to one-third of inpatients with stroke may have a sleep disorder.

A polysomnogram is indicated when the rehabilitation team observes a hypersomnolent, confused, and snoring or apneic patient. More than 5 apnea episodes per hour or 30 episodes per night is abnormal. One study found an average of 52 sleep-disordered breathing events per hour in selected subjects within 1 year of stroke.[222] The number of oxygen desaturation events and the oximetry measures during sleep-disordered breathing have correlated with Barthel Index scores at 1 and 12 months after stroke.[120]

Continuous positive airway pressure devices can help in both apneic conditions. Drugs such as protriptyline can increase upper airway muscle activity. Surgical interventions that include uvulopalatopharyngoplasty can lessen oropharynx obstruction, although this procedure may cause problems in the patient with bulbar muscle weakness.

Repeated Stroke and Death

Following a stroke, education about the natural history of cerebrovascular disease can help patients and their families to put the risk of another stroke in perspective. They must be encouraged to take the steps needed to manage risk factors and to make changes in lifestyle.

RISK FACTORS

Table 7–7 provides an estimate of the unadjusted risks of some of the predisposing vascular and cardiac disorders that internists and neurologists often address.[19] This information reminds us that the greatest risk factor for stroke is a preceding stroke. Five-year recurrence rates were 40 percent for men and 25 percent for women in the Framingham Study, in which no special effort was made to manage risk factors.[291] In the 675 patients registered with a first stroke in the Oxfordshire Community Stroke Project, the actuarial risk of suffering a recurrence was 30 percent by 5 years, 9 times the risk of the general community.[39] The risk was 13 percent in the first year, then 4 percent per year, without a clear relationship to age or stroke type. These recurrent strokes caused significant functional disability in 60 percent of cases. The second stroke is most often of the same type—atherothrombotic, cardioembolic, lacunar, subarachnoid, or parenchymatous hemorrhage—as the first stroke, so knowledge gained about the initial cause may be used as a basis for subsequent risk factor management. A search for cardioem-

Table 7–7. STROKE RATES FROM PROSPECTIVE STUDIES

AFTER AN ATHEROTHROMBOTIC STROKE:

Framingham Study:
8%/yr in males; 5%/yr females

Canadian American Ticlopidine Study:
Stroke/myocardial infarction/vascular death: 15%/yr on placebo versus 11%/yr on ticlopidine

AFTER AN ATHEROTHROMBOTIC TIA
(50% MINOR STROKES):

Canadian Acetylsalicylic Acid (ASA) Study:
Male stroke/death: 9%/yr on placebo versus 5%/yr on ASA

Ticlopidine Aspirin Stroke Study:
First yr: 6% on ASA; 3% on ticlopidine
3 yr: 15% on ASA; 10% on ticlopidine

External Carotid/Internal Carotid Bypass Study for Symptomatic Occlusive Disease:
4%/yr for inaccessible carotid/middle cerebral disease
Maximum rate 7.5%/yr with symptomatic internal carotid artery occlusion

North American Symptomatic Carotid Endarterectomy Trial
(>70% internal carotid artery stenosis; rates over 18-mo follow-up):
Ipsilateral stroke in 24.4% medical versus 7.2% surgical
Major/fatal stroke, vascular death in 12.7% medical versus 5.2% surgical

ASYMPTOMATIC OCCLUSIVE INTERNAL CAROTID ARTERY DISEASE:

Veterans Administration Medical Centers Study:
Ipsilateral stroke in 9% medical versus 4.7% surgical over 4 yr
Transient ischemic attack and stroke in 24% versus 13% (32% died)

Asymptomatic Carotid Artery Stenosis Study:
(>60% internal carotid artery stenosis; rates over 5-yr follow-up)
Stroke and death: 10.6% medical versus 4.8% surgical

ASYMPTOMATIC ATRIAL FIBRILLATION:

Stroke Prevention in Atrial Fibrillation I:
Stroke/systemic embolus: 8.3%/yr on placebo versus 1.6% on warfarin

bolic causes can be revealing when the cause is unclear; however, up to 25 percent of strokes have an uncertain (thrombotic versus embolic) cause.

Teaching during rehabilitation should include information about modifying the risk factors associated with stroke and cardiac disease. Factors include hypertension, cigarette smoking, atrial fibrillation, symptomatic or asymptomatic internal carotid artery stenosis greater than 70 percent, heavy alcohol consumption, hyperlipidemia, diabetes mellitus, and the impact of obesity and inactivity on these factors.[290] The number of cigarettes smoked increases the risk for a stroke, with rates doubling for over 40 per day, as compared with 10 per day.[363] Age-adjusted probabilities for a first stroke, based on the accumulation of risk factors, have been provided by the Framingham Heart Study and can be used to help patients understand their chronic disease.[56]

Unusual risk factors should be sought when the cause of stroke is not readily explained. A circulating antiphospholipid antibody can cause a procoagulant state. Although antiplatelet agents may suffice to reduce the risk of stroke in asymptomatic people and after a transient ischemic attack (TIA), warfarin anticoagulation may be more protective after an ischemic stroke.[278] Clinical trials are in progress. Hyperhomocystinemia in young and older people has been associated with coronary and cerebrovascular disease, as well as with stenosis of the extracranial carotid artery.[46,295] A high homocysteine level can be reduced with folate, pyridoxine, cyanocobalamin, and betaine.

MANAGEMENT

Vigorous therapy of hypertension and cessation of cigarette smoking dramatically reduce the risk of first stroke, of recurrent stroke, and of coronary artery disease. Recurrence rates for stroke decreased in one epidemiologic study as diastolic blood pressure control increased in patients with hypertension at the time of the initial stroke.[6] Remarkably, this population-based study found that 44 percent of patients with no history of hypertension had an elevated blood pressure 4 months after the first stroke, and 65 percent with a history of hypertension still had uncontrolled hypertension.[306] Even the elderly with borderline hypertension should be treated.[157] The excessive risk of stroke among female former smokers largely disappears by 4 years after cessation of smoking,[179] and the rate of progression of carotid atherosclerosis slows in people who quit, compared with those who continue.[326] One estimate suggested that optimal treatment of hypertension could prevent up to 246,000 strokes, and the elimination of cigarettes would eliminate another 62,000 strokes a year, thereby saving $20 billion in the nation's health care costs.[123]

Clinical trials suggest that ticlopidine[112] and aspirin[11] reduce the risk of repeated atherothrombotic stroke. Ticlopidine has a modest advantage over aspirin, reducing stroke rates[112,140] after TIA and first stroke by about 30 percent over several years. Warfarin reduces the risk of repeated cardioembolism. Other medical treatments, such as clopidogrel and warfarin for secondary thrombotic stroke prevention, are in clinical trials. Because cardiac mortality is even higher than the 30 to 50 percent death rate over 5 years from a second stroke, clinicians should consider evaluating selected patients with a good recovery after stroke for a noninvasive heart study, such as a treadmill test.

MORTALITY

The likelihood of long-term survival after a first stroke could affect the allocation of rehabilitation resources. Mortality has been addressed by several community-based studies in Framingham and Oxfordshire.[64,291] Overall, the risk of death from infarction is about 20 percent in the first 30 days and 30 percent for the first year. The annual average risk up to 5 years is 9 percent. The long-term survival for patients with subarachnoid and primary intracerebral hemorrhages seems much better, with most deaths occurring early. The risk of dying varies with age. In the Oxfordshire study, patients under 64 years of age had the highest risk. The relative risk of death after infarction for patients of all ages, compared with controls, was 4.8 in the first year and 2.1 for the next 5 years. The cause of death in patients who survived more than 30 days after a first stroke was a recurrent stroke in one-third and cardiovascular disease in another one-third. In the Framingham Study, however, those who survived the first year and did not have hypertension or cardiac disease had no subsequent excess mortality. Vigorous attempts at secondary prevention of vascular disease over the long run must be part of any rehabilitation effort.

RECOVERY FROM IMPAIRMENTS

Many studies in North America, Europe, and Asia have attempted to define predictors of the course of recovery after a stroke. Patient populations vary considerably. Some studies have assessed all patients seen within 48 hours to a week after an acute stroke at one hospital, others looked at one community or at a collaborating group of facilities, and others reflected only patients admitted to a rehabilitation ward within days to weeks of the stroke. Measures of impairment and disability, the completeness of the data set in retrospective studies, and biases inherent in the selected population vary as well. The natural history of recovery that can be gleaned, especially for motor impairments, provides useful insights, however. Table 7–8 shows the frequency of common impairments and disabilities present at the time clinicians would be considering the transfer of their patients for rehabilitation.

Natural History

Several epidemiologic studies have come to similar conclusions about aspects of the natural course of motor recovery. In the Framingham Study, 50 percent of patients surviving ischemic stroke had no motor deficit at 6 months after onset. A community-based, prospective study in Auckland, New Zealand, assessed 680 patients at the onset of an acute stroke. The investigators found hemiparesis in 88 percent of patients, with equal numbers graded mild (functionally insignificant), moderate, and severe (little or no movement).[30] At 1 month, 26 percent had no impairment and 39 percent were graded

Table 7–8. ESTIMATES OF THE FREQUENCY OF IMPAIRMENTS AND DISABILITY WITHIN 2 WEEKS OF STROKE

	Frequency (%)
Hemiparesis	70–85
Ambulation	70–80
Visuoperception	60–75
Activities of daily living	
Complete dependence	40–65
Assistance required	20–60
Dysarthria	55
Sitting balance	45
Depression	40
Proprioception	40
Hemianopia	20
Aphasia	20–35
Dysphagia	15–35
Hemineglect	10–35
Recent memory loss	10–20

Source: Data from references 75 and 82.

as mild. Motor impairment on this broad scale at 6 months was rated as none for 39 percent of survivors, mild for 36 percent, moderate for 10 percent, and severe for 14 percent. The likelihood of dying by 6 months was 4 times greater for patients with hemiplegia at 1 week than in patients graded as having mild weakness. Initially mild, compared with severe, motor impairment made it 10 times more likely that full recovery would follow.

A prospective study in Bristol, England's, Frenchay Health District followed 976 patients with an acute stroke and re-examined survivors at 3 weeks and 6 months.[339] The study included the 26 percent of patients who were not hospitalized. Thus, this study is a real-world look at stroke outcomes. Of the 453 patients assessed within 7 days of the stroke, 17 percent had no paralysis and 31 percent had a severe paralysis of arm and leg based on the Motricity Index score (see Chapter 5). Many with severe hemiplegia were unconscious, and 62 percent of these patients had died by 6 months. At 6 months, 47 percent of survivors had no measurable weakness in the arm or leg, much like the results of the Framingham Study. Only 9 percent had profound weakness. No patients with paralysis of the arm or leg at 3 weeks after onset achieved normal strength at 6 months. This result has an impact on planned efforts at rehabilitation. The Motricity Index scores significantly correlate with the Barthel Index.

Although clinicians may perceive that the lower extremity improves more than the upper, muscle testing suggests no difference. Based on the motor portion of the Fugl-Meyer Assessment, a study showed that the percentage of improvement in motor recovery of the arm and leg was the same in patients with anterior circulation infarcts. The fastest gains happened in the first 30 days of a 180-day follow-up.[88]

The stroke type is another factor in the natural history of improvement. In a study of 410 patients from the Stroke Data Bank of the National Institute of Neurological Diseases and Stroke (NINDS), 23 percent of patients with a pure motor stroke had improved by 10 days, whereas 5 percent with other stroke syndromes have deteriorated compared with examination on admission.[197] The mean relative improvement in those in each group with improved strength at the shoulder, wrist, hip, and ankle was also greater in the patients with pure motor stroke by 52 percent versus 40 percent. Most of these patients had lacunar infarcts. In a trial of acute heparinization versus placebo to prevent progressing stroke, in which most patients appeared to have suffered lacunar infarcts, about 1 in 4 patients had improved in the first week in neurologic scores that emphasized strength.[87]

In a longitudinal study of 41 patients starting within 1 week of a right cerebral infarction, behavioral and motor abnormalities were followed at 2-week to 4-week intervals by repeated measures with specific tests, until the patients recovered or plateaued.[150] Most patients received an unspecified amount of physical and occupational therapy. With a life-table analysis method, recovery curves showed the following: Arm and leg weakness recovered in about 40 percent by week 16; sensory extinction recovered in 80 percent by week 46; hemianopia recovered in 65 percent by week 33; unilateral spa-tial neglect on drawing recovered in 70 percent by week 13; anosognosia and neglect recovered in nearly all patients by week 20, with half of those affected recovering by week 10; motor impersistence recovered in all patients by week 55, with 45 percent recovering by week 8; and prosopagnosia and constructional apraxia on the Block Design and Rey figure (see Table 5–3) recovered in 80 percent by week 20. Patients with smaller lesions (less than 6 percent of right hemispheric volume) or hemorrhages, or younger patients, tended to recover faster from some of these impairments. The amount of recovery for many of these behaviors, compared with motor function, is consistent with the notion that recovery is better for impairments that have the most diffuse neural substrate for reorganization (see Chapter 1).

Predictive Value of Technologies

EVOKED POTENTIALS

Somatosensory-evoked potentials (SEP) and motor-evoked potentials (MEP) have been used to predict the recovery of upper extremity function.[357] The SEP stimulated by the median nerve can recover or increase its amplitude or conduction time to become more symmetric with the SEP of the unaffected hemisphere over the first 6 to 8 weeks after a stroke.[209] The presence of an SEP has correlated with a higher Barthel Index score at discharge,[45] with recovery of hand function, and, in 70 percent of cases, with independent gait.[254] These studies do not reveal a clear prognostic advantage of the SEP over the clinical examination that assesses for impaired sensation and strength, however.[124] A poor prognosis for motor recovery of the hand 4 weeks after a stroke is better predicted by the persistent absence of movement than by an absent SEP. As an assessment tool, the SEP can be helpful in its quantitative approach to somatic sensation and when, for example, a patient with aphasia or obtundation cannot report on sensory appreciation.

The MEP has been elicited by electric and magnetic cortical stimulation (see Chapter 1). It provides the equivalent of a central motor nerve conduction study. When adequately stimulated, cortical pyramidal neurons transmit a signal to anterior horn motoneurons. If the motor cortex is too severely damaged, no response is obtained. A subcortical infarct along the corticospinal tract can delay, prolong, or abolish the MEP.[208] No recovery of upper extremity function is usually predicted by an absent response, whereas a normal or delayed MEP enables one to identify the patient who is most likely to improve.[84] A study of 118 patients who had a first stroke found that a normal or delayed central motor conduction time in the first 12 to 72 hours identified the group with a high probability of survival and functional recovery at 1 year by the Barthel Index and Rankin Scale.[141] Absence of a cortical response or a very high threshold for stimulation was associated with poor function and greater probability of stroke-related death. The MEP can also reveal cortical neuron representational plasticity and reorganization after a cortical or subcortical stroke (see Chapter 1).

FUNCTIONAL IMAGING

Neurologic outcome at 2 months, based on the Mathew Scale of impairments, has been correlated with cerebral blood flow and oxygen consumption by positron emission tomography (PET) performed at 5 to 18 hours after the onset of a middle cerebral artery distribution infarction.[211] The pattern of a large cortical-subcortical area of greatly reduced perfusion and oxygen consumption carries a poor prognosis. A pattern of increased perfusion, equivalent to hyperemia, with only a small area of focally reduced oxygen consumption suggests a good recovery. Neurologic recovery has correlated better with the volume of acute hypoperfusion than with subsequent blood flow to the area of chronic infarction by single-photon emission computed tomography (SPECT).[63] A few PET studies have suggested a potential correlation between the recovery of impairments and resolution of diaschisis, the functional deactivation of tissue remote from the responsible structural lesion (see Chapter 1). A study of 50 patients with stroke obtained acute and 3-month follow-up SPECT scans that identified 168 ipsilateral sites of

diaschisis.[32a] The investigators, however, related only an increase in thalamic activity over time with an improved neurologic examination. More studies are needed to determine whether remote deafferentation may relate to mechanisms of impairment and recovery.

Impairment-Related Functional Outcomes

POPULATION STUDIES

Mathematic models that look at prognostic indicators near the onset of stroke could be useful for research into rehabilitative interventions. The goal of these models is to take multiple variables that are usually related to impairments and to anticipate functional outcomes. These models may, for example, help one to determine the nature of the target population and to allow a power calculation of the needed sample size. Modeling has run into many barriers, however, including wide biologic variability among patients over time. Early inpatient and outpatient rehabilitative efforts correspond to the rapid pace of improvement in impairments in the first 30 to 90 days after stroke. Although some impairments can improve for up to a year, continued gains in functional skills in the presence of stable impairments often evolve between 3 and 12 months after a stroke. A variety of behavioral adaptations may account for some of those late performance changes. Such adaptations are among the confounding features that make quantitative clinical models less than ideal.

Certain multivariate models have been developed for prognostication in patients with acute stroke.[114] For example, in one study, death or dependence (Glasgow Outcome Score 3 to 5) 3 months after a stroke depended upon the severity of the clinical impairment in the first 24 hours, history of previous stroke, and increasing age.[147] A prospective British district hospital study evaluated 205 consecutive patients with acute stroke seen within 48 hours of onset. Mortality and functional recovery at 6 months were related to six factors by a multivariate statistical analysis.[106] Leg and arm power and function, a weighted mental status score similar to the Mini-Mental State Examination, level of consciousness, score on a line-cancellation test for perceptual neglect, and electrocardiographic abnormalities predicted functional outcome with 67 percent accuracy and death with 83 percent accuracy. These items appear in most models that have achieved similar levels of precision for anticipating the general level of independence in functional skills.

REHABILITATION STUDIES

Although most survivors of an acute stroke do improve, studies of early impairments do not provide clear-cut information about the selection of individual patients for inpatient and outpatient rehabilitation efforts. Even carefully constructed equations that seek to help predict outcome at 6 months have not been powerful enough to anticipate the outcome for a particular patient.[18] Rehabilitation specialists should consider prognosticators of poor recovery when designing an individual's program, however.

A review of 33 studies found certain prognosticators to be potentially unfavorable for recovery if they are present at the time of transfer to a rehabilitation unit. These factors include advanced age and the neurologic impairments of profound paresis, loss of proprioception, visuospatial hemineglect, and bowel and bladder incontinence.[168] Persistently poor attention span, judgment, memory, and carryover skills negatively influence outcome as well. Motor impersistence and impaired half-hour recall have predictive value for poorer functional outcome.[238] In a study of inpatients in rehabilitation facilities, impairments in comprehension, judgment, short-term memory, and abstract thinking by testing with the Neurobehavioral Cognitive Status Examination led to longer stays, lessened ability to perform activities of daily living (ADLs) when discharged, and more outpatient therapy and home services, compared with a control group of patients in orthopedic rehabilitation.[107] Even with any combination of these prognosticators, however, many individuals still improve enough to reach a functional level that allows them to live at home.

In patients over the age of 75 years, the Orpington Prognostic Score of impair-

Table 7–9. **ORPINGTON PROGNOSTIC SCORE**

Clinical Impairment	Score
Arm Strength (Medical Research Council grade)	
5	0.0
4	0.4
3	0.8
1–2	1.2
0	1.6
Proprioception (eyes closed): Locates Affected Thumb	
Accurately	0.0
With slight difficulty	0.4
By means of the ipsilateral arm	0.8
Not at all	1.2
Balance	
Walks 10 ft without help	0.0
Maintains stance	0.4
Maintains sitting position	0.8
Has no sitting balance	1.2
Cognition (Mental test score)	
10	0.0
8–9	0.4
5–7	0.8
0–4	1.2

Source: Data from reference 175.

ments, measured 2 weeks after a stroke, had a strong correlation with functional outcome.[175] Patients who scored less than 3.2 were discharged within 3 weeks, whereas those with scores higher than 5.2 required long-term care (Table 7–9). The total score is the sum of 1.6 plus the motor, proprioception, balance, and cognition subscores. Such tools can be used to stratify patients who participate in clinical trials.

RECOVERY FROM DISABILITY

Epidemiologic Studies

Studies of community-based populations of survivors of acute stroke provide a sense of the natural history of functional recovery. The prospective Framingham Study examined the 148 people in their cohort who survived for 6 months after an acute nonhemorrhagic stroke.[130] These data need to be viewed within the context of possible differences in the types of stroke and in their morbidity and mortality over the 2 decades before 1978. It is one of the few studies, however, that compared functional disabilities in survivors of stroke with a control group matched for age and sex. As mentioned earlier, 52 percent of survivors of stroke had no motor impairment. Some of the persisting disability was related to comorbid problems and not directly to the stroke. Gresham and Granger analyzed the study's stroke-related disability with and without these comorbid conditions.[129] For patients limited in household tasks, the number disabled by the stroke alone fell from 56 to 28 percent upon "removal" of comorbidities; in patients dependent in self-care, those disabled by the stroke alone fell from 32 to 14 percent; in those dependent in mobility, from 22 to 9 percent; in those socializing less, from 59 to 32 percent; and in those living in an institution, from 15 to 4 percent.

Geriatric victims of an acute stroke often present with premorbid impairments and disabilities that may confound assessment, treatment, and expected outcomes. People over the age of 65 years have twice the disability and four times the limitation in their activities as patients who are 45 to 64 years old. Because of chronic diseases, the percentage of adults who need assistance in walking, bathing, and dressing rises from 5 percent between the ages of 65 and 74 years to 11 percent between 75 and 84 years, then to 35 percent over age 85 years. For these three age groups, assistance in shopping, chores, preparing meals, and handling money rises from 6 to 14 to 40 percent, respectively.[282]

Investigators evaluated a subgroup of 46 long-term survivors of stroke in the Framingham Study whose mean age was 77 years. The patients were given a neurologic examination, the Mini-Mental State Examination, and the Barthel Index (BI) at the onset of stroke and at 3, 6, and 12 months later.[181] Statistically significant recovery occurred in the first 3 months in the total BI score and in self-care, mobility, and language. Lesser gains were made in continence and toileting, cognition, and strength. Only language

function continued to improve beyond 6 months. The 12 patients who underwent rehabilitation were more disabled at onset (BI scores were 36 versus 68) and improved an average of 30 points in the BI in the first 3 months, compared with an increase of 16 points for patients not sent to inpatient rehabilitation. The best predictor of institutionalization after stroke for men was single status; for women, it was age and severity of disability.

The prospective Frenchay Health District Study found that 47 percent of survivors were functionally independent and 21 percent showed moderate to severe dependence at 6 months after their stroke. The ADLs recovered in a consistent order at 3 weeks and 6 months. The evolution of gains went from walking to dressing, stair climbing, and then bathing.[340]

In a retrospective study drawing on the record linkage system of the Mayo Clinic, Rankin Scores (see Table 5–14) were determined for the 251 patients who survived more than 1 week after a first stroke.[83] Their mean age was 70 years. The mean Rankin Score increased from 1.7 before the stroke to 2.8 (moderate disability) in survivors at discharge from the acute hospital stay. Before their stroke, 20 percent were rated at 3 to 5 (moderate to severe disability). This percentage increased to 75 percent at onset, then decreased to 57 percent at discharge from the acute hospital stay. This level of disability fell to 40 percent at 6 months and to about 35 percent at 1 to 3 years, although half the cohort had been lost to follow-up by then. Age over 75 years was highly associated with a Rankin Score at 1 year after stroke of 3 or more, even in the elderly with no comorbid conditions.

The ability to walk is an especially important functional outcome. A prospective study compared 64 age-matched controls with 60 patients with acute stroke who survived 13 weeks.[347] In the first week and final assessment, 25 percent of the patients with stroke could not ambulate and 23 percent were independent. Although 60 percent of the whole group became independent in ambulation and 40 percent regained normal walking speed, only 22 percent of patients initially dependent in gait recovered a normal walking speed. Speed is a good reflection of overall gait pattern.

A community-based population study that prospectively followed 800 survivors of acute stroke initially found that 51 percent were unable to walk, 12 percent walked with assistance, and 37 percent were independent.[170] Within the same facility, all who needed rehabilitation received services for an average total stay of 35 days (S.D. 41). At discharge, 22 percent could not walk, 14 percent walked with assistance, and 64 percent of survivors walked independently. About 80 percent of patients who were initially nonwalkers reached their best walking function within 6 weeks, and 95 percent reached it within 11 weeks. In patients who walked with assistance, 80 percent reached best function within 3 weeks, and 95 percent reached it within 5 weeks. Independent walking was achieved by 34 percent of the survivors who had been dependent and by 60 percent of those who initially required assistance. Recovery of ambulation correlated directly with leg strength.

Predictors of Functional Recovery

One of the more telling predictors is that the higher the admission score on the BI (Table 5–12), a valid and reliable measure of burden of care, the higher the discharge score and the greater the likelihood that the patient will return to living at home. A BI score over 61 by time of discharge is associated with living in the community 6 months later. No single score serves as a complete predictor, however.[128] The best predictor of greater disability on the BI in a population-based English study was incontinence within 72 hours of stroke.[322] This finding had a sensitivity of 60 percent and a specificity of 78 percent at 3-month follow-up, when 9 percent of patients were severely disabled, and 15 percent were moderately disabled. At 12 months, 11 percent had moderate to severe disability, for which initial incontinence was still the best predictor.

Urinary incontinence is about as good a predictor of a poorer outcome as any group of impairments.[348] Indeed, one approach to predicting outcome for inpatient rehabilitation found that the level of independence in toilet and bladder management and toilet transfers, along with adequacy of financial resources, best predicted discharge of the patient to the community, survival for more than 3 months after discharge, and no more than minimal physical assistance for ADLs.[97]

The admission score on the Functional Independence Measure (FIM) (see Table 5–9) can anticipate discharge placement. At one Canadian center, where the median time to rehabilitation admission was 52 days, followed by an average stay of 64 days, patients who scored 36 or less never returned home, and those who scored 97 or more always did.[241] From 50 to 90 percent of patients with intermediate scores returned home. Poor postural control and bladder or bowel incontinence on admission also predicted discharge to a nursing home. The lowest FIM scores were found in patients with impairments such as hemianopia, sensory loss, neglect, aphasia, and cognitive dysfunction. The absolute change in FIM scores was not predictive, except for patients with admission scores between 36 and 96 and with large gains. Other studies have also suggested that the efficiency or rate of improvement of inpatient gains in ADLs may be independent of initial disability.[144]

A retrospective study in the United States of 464 patients with nonhemorrhagic stroke who were admitted in 1991 after a mean acute hospitalization of 18 days to an inpatient rehabilitation unit drew conclusions similar to those of the Canadian study.[4] Patients spent an average of 34 days at the facility. Admission FIM scores and age were analyzed in relation to discharge FIM and placement. Admission FIM positively correlated with discharge FIM, and admission FIM negatively correlated with length of stay. Less FIM gain was found after a right, compared with a left, cerebral infarct in patients with the lowest admission FIM scores of less than 40. The greatest FIM change over time occurred in patients with admission FIM scores of 4 to 80. Those with admission scores over 80 and age less than 55 years returned home. A score of less than 40 and age over 65 years indicated discharge to a nursing home for 62 percent. For the rest of the FIM-age subgroups, only 13 percent went to nursing facilities. The admission FIM score, then, represents the burden of care on the care provider, and it may be used to group patients with stroke on admission according to their likely needs.

No reliable relationship has been found between sex or hemisphere infarcted and functional outcome. Although a long onset to rehabilitation admission, beyond 30 days, has been said to be a poor prognostic indicator,[100] other factors in a multiple regression analysis encompass this notion. The delay from onset of stroke to the start of rehabilitation seems to have a weak effect on long-term outcomes.[166]

PET studies may reveal information relevant to functional recovery. For example, a higher ipsilateral,[189] as well as global and contralateral,[145] cerebral metabolic rate for glucose within 1 to 2 weeks of an acute stroke correlated with a better functional outcome in survivors of stroke at a mean of 3 and 50 months. Low glucose consumption within the unaffected hemisphere in hypertensive patients led to poorer performance of ADLs, perhaps because of a subclinical hypertensive arteriopathy producing tissue damage that limited compensation.[145]

The Copenhagen Stroke Study related the severity of neurologic deficits using the Scandinavian Stroke Scale and functional disability by the BI to outcome and the time to best recovery.[171,172] In this community-based study, nearly all 1200 patients were evaluated by 1 week after a stroke, and all received inpatient rehabilitation evaluations and treatments in a specialized unit. The subjects were examined weekly during the hospital stay and at 6 months. After a mean hospital stay of 37 (S.D. 41) days, 11 percent of survivors had severe impairments, and 78 percent had mild or no deficits. Severe disability was found in 20 percent, moderate disability in 8 percent, mild disability in 26 percent, and no disability in 46 percent. Functional recovery was completed by 13 weeks after onset in 95 percent. Best ADLs were reached within 9 weeks by those with mild impairments, within 13 weeks by those with moderate impairments, and within 20 weeks by those with severe deficits; however, 80 percent reached their best BI score by 12 weeks. The study offers some insights into outcomes across the spectrum of unselected patients with acute stroke when a multidisciplinary team provides a Bobath approach and keeps patients in the hospital until further rehabilitation progress appears unlikely.

Functional Outcomes

In general, studies across rehabilitation units report that 70 to 80 percent of discharged patients are independent in walking with or without assistive devices, and two of three are independent in ADLs.

A prospective study from 17 stroke rehabilitation units entered 539 patients between 1980 and 1982.[127] The mean age of these patients was 69 years, the interval from onset of stroke to rehabilitation admission was 19 days, the BI admission score was 37, and the length of stay was 37 days. The mean gain in BI scores was 29 points, pushing the total mean score over 61, a number associated with a home discharge. Indeed, 70 percent of the patients returned home, whereas 17 percent were discharged to nursing facilities, 8 percent to acute care, 4 percent to another rehabilitation unit, and 6 percent died. At 6-month follow-up, the mean score was 77, 80 percent lived in the community, and 58 percent reported satisfaction with their lives. Only 21 percent were unlimited in work or homemaking, and 14 percent had died.

In the United States, more recent information from UDS describes outcomes in terms of the FIM (see Table 5–9) across 256 facilities in 44 states (Table 7–10).[126] The scores are identical to the results from 1990 and from over 15,000 cases in 1991; however, the time from onset of stroke to rehabilitation transfer fell from 22 to 20 days, and the mean length of stay declined from 32 to 28 days over this 2-year period. On follow-up, 3 months after rehabilitation discharge, the total FIM score increased to 97 units or an average of 5.4 units for all FIM items.[136] The motor domain increased 8 percent, and the cognitive domain increased 14 percent. One of the most important outcomes of successful inpatient rehabilitation is discharge placement to home. Table 7–11 shows that higher FIM scores at discharge are associated with return to the community.[335]

Table 7–10. **UNIFORM DATA SERVICE FIRST ADMISSIONS FOR STROKE REHABILITATION IN 1992 (26,634 PATIENTS)**

Mean Subscore	Admission	Discharge
Self-care	3.4	4.9
Sphincter control	3.9	5.2
Mobility	2.9	4.5
Locomotion	2.0	3.8
Communication	4.5	5.2
Social cognition	4.0	4.8
Mean FIM total	62(S.D. 22)	86(S.D. 26)
Median FIM	63	91
Mean onset (days)	20	
Length of stay	28(S.D. 18)	
FIM gain/wk	6	
Discharge (%)		
Community	76	
Long-term care	15	
Acute care	7	
Mean age (yr)	71(S.D. 12)	

FIM = Functional Independence Measure.

Table 7–11. **PERCENTAGE OF STROKE PATIENTS DISCHARGED TO THE COMMUNITY IN EACH FUNCTIONAL INDEPENDENCE MEASURE SCORE RANGE**

Score	Percentage (%)
18–29	25
30–39	30
40–49	37
50–59	45
60–64	55
65–69	58
70–74	59
75–79	67
80–84	77
85–89	80
90–99	87
100–109	92
110–119	97
>120	98

Source: Uniform Data Service newsletter, 1993.

Reding and Potes provided more detailed information about functional outcomes in a prospective study of 95 consecutive inpatients admitted to a rehabilitation center after a hemispheric stroke.[264] These investigators examined the relationship between impairment and level of independence over time. The patients were divided into three categories of impairment and examined at 2-week intervals until they reached a plateau in recovery. The investigators constructed life-table analyses of the probability of recovering mobility and overall Barthel Index functions. Over 90 percent of patients with a pure motor (M) deficit became independent in walking 150 feet by week 14, but only 35 percent of those with motor and proprioceptive (SM) loss by week 24, and 3 percent of those with motor, sensory, and hemianopic deficits (SMH) were independent by week 30. The probability of walking over 150 feet with assistance increased to 100 percent with M impairment by week 14 (80 percent by week 8), to over 90 percent in those with

SM loss by week 26, and with SMH deficits by 28 weeks after the stroke. About 65 percent achieved a BI score over 95 by 15 weeks if they had only M deficits and by 26 weeks with SM loss. Only 10 percent scored that high with SMH deficits after 18 to 30 weeks. However, 100 percent achieved a score of more than 60 by 14 weeks with M loss only, 75 percent by 23 weeks with SM deficits, and 60 percent by 29 weeks with SMH loss. Both the life-table analysis and this clinical grouping of patients make good sense for some experimental designs of stroke rehabilitation interventions.

CLINICAL TRIALS OF STROKE REHABILITATION

Clinical trials of the effectiveness of stroke rehabilitation in enhancing functional performance include comparisons of methods of service provision and strategies of therapy. Most often, one of the four following questions is asked[4,81]: Is the rehabilitation of disabilities effective? Is a particular therapeutic approach better than another? Is rehabilitation delivered in a specialized unit more effective than care in a general medical ward? What is the most efficient setting that provides a particular level of care for a patient with a given level of disability?

After reviewing 124 investigations drawn from a literature search of studies done from 1960 to 1990, Ottenbacher and Jannell carried out a meta-analysis on 36; these trials met the criteria of including patients with hemiparesis from stroke who were given a rehabilitation service in a design that compared at least two groups or conditions for change in a quantifiable functional measure.[248] Outcomes included gait, hand function, ADLs, response times, and visuoperception. From 173 statistical evaluations recorded on the 3717 patients with acute and chronic stroke in the 36 trials, the analysis showed that the average patient who received a program of focused stroke rehabilitation or a particular procedure performed better than about 65 percent of the patients in the comparison group. Greater treatment effects were associated with an earlier intervention and younger patients. No association was found with the duration of a program. The authors point out that this synthesis of data is imperfect. The review could not assess the intensity of the interventions and how well they were carried out to be able to judge the integrity of each program. They could not detect systematic biases or account for missing data.

In addition, the real impact of the changes in the variety of outcome measures used to assess an even wider variety of stroke-related functional problems is unknown. Statistical significance in this meta-analysis does not imply that a change has clinical or functional importance and does not reveal how long a benefit has lasted, nor does this approach tell rehabilitation specialists the best possible intervention for any particular problem. How improvement came about has not been made clear. Could the outcome have been facilitated by any physical or behavioral art, perhaps spurred on by spontaneous recovery? If improvement depends on specific training methods, do gains in one neurologic impairment, say visuoperceptual skills, generalize to decrease disability, for example, in dressing or ambulation? Despite

these concerns about the quality of the data used, the review does help to refine the controversy about whether studies indicate that focused programs do[262] or do not improve outcome.[73] Future clinical trials can draw upon the limitations of prior designs.

Trials of Locus of Treatment

Many trials have compared more intensive or specialized rehabilitation units to a community's standard medical ward care. Table 7–12 lists some of the better-designed randomized trials. These patients were not too slightly or too severely disabled for inpatient rehabilitation as practiced in the United States today. The mean age for patients in each trial was 65 to 75 years, and patients were randomized within a few days to 2 weeks after the stroke. None of the various outcome measures was done blinded to allocation. These trials suggest that the milieu and the usually greater frequency of rehabilitation therapies in a dedicated unit lead to better outcomes in moderately impaired patients, at least for the first 3 to 6 months after the stroke.

Several trials have gone further in examining the reasons for better outcomes in a dedicated stroke unit compared with a general medical ward. Mortality rates can be significantly lower in a dedicated unit.[191] Even with the same type and intensity of physical and occupational therapy services provided by staff members with the same level of experience, functional recovery on Barthel Index tasks was greater and faster in the dedicated unit that directed therapy toward adapting patients' residual abilities to future needs in their homes.[176] Indeed, patients in one British trial who reached the median Barthel Index score associated with discharge had significantly shorter lengths of stay after reaching that level of function when they were managed in the stroke unit compared with patients who were just as functional in a medical unit.[174] This finding suggests a better organization of assessment and goal-oriented services in a dedicated unit; however, some community studies of all survivors of stroke raise the issue that patients who receive therapy in the hospital or with an organized outpatient approach per-

Table 7–12. **RANDOMIZED TRIALS OF EARLY STROKE REHABILITATION SERVICES**

Trial	Comparison	No. Subjects	Duration (mean days)	Outcomes
Garraway et al[108]	Stroke unit versus Medical ward	155 152	55 75	50% independent at 60 days, 55% at 1 yr 32% independent at 60 days, 52% at 1 yr
Wood-Dauphinee et al[366]	Interdisciplinary team care versus Traditional care	65 65	60 60	Survival same for all patients *Males*: Motor performance and ADLs better *Females*: Motor performance poorer; ADLs same *Males*: Motor performance and ADLs poorer *Females*: Motor performance better; ADLs same
Strand et al[314]	Stroke unit versus Medical ward	110 183	21 31	Fewer patients still hospitalized at 3 mo; more independent in ADLs More patients still hospitalized at 3 mo; fewer independent in ADLs
Indredavik et al[156]	Stroke unit versus Medical ward	110 110	Up to 42 days Up to 42 days	56% discharged home; 36% in institutions; BI = 80 33% discharged home; 52% in institutions; BI = 66 (Differences still significant at 1 yr)
Kalra et al[176]	Stroke unit versus Medical ward	Mild: 31 Moderate: 75 Severe: 18 Mild: 32 Moderate: 71 Severe: 18	Mild: 13 Moderate: 48 Severe: 52 Mild: 14 Moderate: 104 Severe: 123	Moderately impaired group 75% at home 22% in institutions 81% independent by BI Moderately impaired group 52% at home 44% in institutions 60% independent by BI Mild and severe groups No significant differences

ADLs = activities of daily living; BI = Barthel Index.

form, overall, as well as patients who receive little or no remedial treatment.[62,344]

Trials of Schools of Therapy

Another group of studies has compared one school of physical therapy with another to determine whether a particular technique improves functional performance. Small randomized trials during inpatient or outpatient therapy have shown no significant differences between conventional therapy and proprioceptive neuromuscular facilitation (PNF),[311] conventional exercise and Bobath technique,[206] conventional exercise versus Bobath and Rood,[205] conventional exercise versus PNF versus Bobath,[71] electromyographic biofeedback (EMG BFB) versus Bobath technique,[21] sensorimotor integrative versus functional treatment in occupational therapy,[169] and, in an alternating treatment design, Bobath compared with the Brunnstrom method.[349] One trial gave all 75 patients functional training and stretching and randomized three groups to functional training and stretching alone, to additional active exercises, and to additional resistive exercises.[159] The third group was more independent at 1 month, but no difference was apparent by 2 months. Strength was increased in the resistive-exercise group. Although selective muscle strengthening has not been a focus of most schools of therapy, this trial alone warrants further exploration of possible links between the rate of early recovery and methods to enhance strength.

All of these trials have methodologic flaws.[13,92] For example, they likely included too few patients, given the spectrum of impairments and disabilities of patients with stroke, to detect real differences if such differences exist. Thus, they are at risk for a type II statistical error. They did not clearly address principles of training motor skills. The trials did not include outcomes related to the effect of therapists' efforts on behavioral compensation for, say, the hemiplegia, compared with changes in the performance of the affected limbs. Indeed, indices of ADL independence, the primary outcome measure in these trials, may poorly reflect the primary intention of the schools of physical therapy, which is to improve patterns of movement (see Chapter 3).

Biofeedback

BFB, particularly EMG BFB, has been used during inpatient therapy to increase or decrease selective muscle activity, but its greatest use is during outpatient care (see Chapter 3). A meta-analysis of EMG BFB for neuromuscular re-education of the arm or leg included eight randomized or matched control group studies with 190 patients. It found a significant range of gains in a variety of outcome measures.[294] This type of analysis, the quality of the studies included, and the clinical significance of the outcome measures leave the efficacy and cost of BFB still in doubt, however. Examples of the use of BFB in hemiplegia follow later in this chapter.

Acupuncture

Acupuncture has been used for centuries in China for managing acute stroke and for rehabilitation, but modern reports from Asia are, at best, descriptive of poorly measured changes in uncontrolled trials.[44] A randomized trial in Sweden showed that patients who received acupuncture plus daily physical and occupational therapies made significant improvements in balance, mobility, ADLs, quality of life, and time at home compared with patients given the same interventions without the acupuncture.[163] In this trial, treatments began a mean of 7 days after onset of hemiplegia. Bilateral manual acupuncture combined with electrical needle stimulation to the paretic side continued twice a week for 10 weeks. The differences were apparent at 1 and 3 months and persisted at 1 year after stroke onset. For example, BI scores were 45 for each group at onset, 69 for the acupuncture group versus 61 in the control group at 1 month, and 92 versus 71 at 1 year. Motor function of the hemiplegic side did not differ, however. Possible mechanisms for functional efficacy may include the special attention given to the acupuncture patients, the effects of the release of systemic or central nervous system peptides and neurotransmitters on neuronal networks, and the greater sensory stimulation that could, for example, modulate the size of neuronal representational sensorimotor maps. More research is needed, particularly that designed to assess the potential effects of stimulation of the affected arm or leg versus general sensory stimulation, as well as stimulation during goal-oriented tasks.

Pharmacotherapy

Pharmacotherapy may enhance functional gains by many potential mechanisms (see Chapters 1 and 2). A single dose of 10 mg of amphetamine, followed by physical therapy, improved the Fugl-Meyer score of motor function in a blinded, randomized trial of 8 patients who were treated within 10 days of the onset of stroke.[54] Only 2 of the 4 responders had remarkable improvements. Over 100 patients were screened for participation until the 8 chosen patients met entry and exclusion criteria.

In a double-blind, placebo-controlled trial of *d*-amphetamine, 9 patients received 10 mg of drug every morning for 14 days and then 5 mg daily for 3 days.[266] Patients were on average 35 days post stroke and were undergoing inpatient rehabilitation. Drug-treated patients were 11 years older than the 12 patients who received placebo, but they had a similar distribution of hemisphere and subcortical infarctions. At 4 weeks, motor scores on the Fugl-Meyer scale, BI scores, and Zung Depression scores were not significantly different. No drug side effects were found. The investigators needed 2 years to find suitable patients in a busy inpatient service, however.

These and other unpublished small trials raise the possibility that amphetamine may be of value when it is given at some ideal interval after stroke in a dose frequency that may not be daily and by timing the dose with specific therapy. None of these criteria have been determined, however. The use of any drug intervention faces similar difficulties.

In two small Japanese studies, thyroid-releasing hormone facilitated early functional gains and shortened the hospital stay after acute stroke and, after a single dose in a few patients with chronic stroke who were ambulatory, it increased walking speed.[234] Future studies of drugs that may modulate motor recovery should define specific, functionally important outcomes and should consider training patients in task-oriented therapies related to those outcomes.

In addition, investigators in clinical trials of drug or other interventions must be aware of the potentially detrimental effects of routinely prescribed drugs. For example, a regression analysis of a study of the effects of GM_1 ganglioside in acute stroke suggests that patients who receive benzodiazepines, dopamine, and alpha-1–adrenergic receptor antagonists, or alpha-2–adrenergic agonists, have more motor impairment in the upper extremity and greater dependence in ADLs at 84 days after the onset of stroke.[119] As noted earlier, just as amphetamine may stimulate long-term potentiation for learning and may decrease diaschisis after stroke, other drugs may block endogenous mechanisms of neuroplasticity.

Conclusions

In conclusion, the few randomized, if unblinded, clinical trials of types of physical therapy and program structure leave us with the possibility that the effect of the overall milieu of the therapy setting is more influential than are specific programs. The school of physical therapy, for example, may not matter as much as the provision of a thoughtful, broad-based approach that aims to enhance mobility and self-care skills while it provides individual and family psychosocial support. On an inpatient service, remarkably little formal therapy time is reportedly spent with each patient in some institutions in the course of a day. Although the definition of therapy time is debatable, reports range from 13 to 30 percent of the working day.[180,328] Often, the most time goes to patients who have the least function and will make the fewest gains.[345] Almost any type of clinical trial can include a comparison of differing intensities of a specific therapy.

Early active intervention seems to have a benefit on mobility and functional independence, but clinicians should define and test specific interventions. Over the short and long term, psychologic and social influences must also be taken into account. Interesting trials are described later in this chapter for particular rehabilitation problems.

INPATIENT REHABILITATION

Eligibility for Rehabilitation

A minority of survivors of stroke are referred for inpatient rehabilitation (Table 7–13). For example, when medical centers in the United States reported the discharge sites of their patients who survived a stroke between 1971 and 1982,[113] 54 to 63 percent went home, 29 to 36 percent were sent to a long-term care facility, and 3 to 17 percent went to a rehabilitation inpatient program. At the Rochester, Minnesota, center that followed 251 1-week survivors of a first stroke between 1975 and 1979, about 50 percent received evaluations by rehabilitation physicians and physical therapists; 26 percent of these patients subsequently were referred to an inpatient rehabilitation program, 40 percent were seen by occupational therapists, and 13 percent were seen by speech therapists.[83] The 14 percent of the entire group who were transferred to a rehabilitation unit after a median acute hospitalization of 17 days had a median 32-day length of stay in the unit. When a rehabilitation medical evaluation was not required before requesting a physical and occupational therapy evaluation, one facility found that acute hospitalization time was reduced from 11 to 7 days.[243] Of 1094 patients with acute stroke who were admitted to a British district hospital from 1972 to 1978, 33 percent died in the hospital, 20 percent had fully recovered by discharge, and 30 percent were too frail or ill to be offered participation in an outpatient rehabilitation trial of 4 whole days a week, leaving 11 percent able to participate.[304]

Criteria for referral to inpatient rehabilitation upon discharge from acute care generally include that a patient be medically stable enough to tolerate at least 3 hours of therapies a day, need more than minimal assistance for ambulation and self-care, be motivated and have adequate cognition and language function to participate in treatments, and have adequate social supports to anticipate a return home or to a place other than a hospital or nursing facility upon discharge. Patients in the United States who already function too independently to qualify for inpatient rehabilitation are eligible for home therapies, if these patients are physically unable to leave their homes. Other patients attend outpatient physical, occupational, and speech therapy sessions until their functional progress plateaus, based on the observations of physician and therapist, but subject to retroactive review by Medicare and most health care payers. Geriatric patients who are at too low a level to participate in an inpatient unit may still be eligible for less intensive therapies at a skilled nursing facility, and they may later qualify for transfer to an inpatient unit. The US Public Health Service offers guidelines that are similar to these criteria for clinicians to use for rehabilitation referrals.[130a]

Some general strategies for determining admission to an inpatient rehabilitation facility can be tested based on several of the studies of the natural history of stroke and rehabilitation discussed previously.[4,12,241] In patients with FIM scores over 80, a well-designed outpatient rehabilitation program can be more appropriate than inpatient care, except when the partially disabled patient has inadequate supervision at home. A clinical trial of patients with high FIM scores on admission who are randomized to the same intensity of therapy as inpatients versus outpatients would be of great interest. Patients over the age of 75 years who have rehabilitation admission FIM scores of less

Table 7–13. PLACEMENT AFTER HOSPITALIZATION FOR ACUTE ISCHEMIC STROKE

	Percentage (%)
Deceased	18–25
Nursing home care	15–30
Rehabilitation unit	5–20
Home	35–60

than 60 are at highest risk for eventual placement in a nursing facility, especially if they have suffered a stroke in the distribution of the full right middle cerebral artery. Except for patients who have the resources to provide costly care in the home upon rehabilitation discharge or who have a reversible medical problem that has made their FIM score much lower than it will be after a medical intervention, clinicians may consider nursing facility placement with less intensive attempts at therapy. This group should be reassessed for inpatient care every 2 weeks for up to several months.

Patients with admission FIM scores of 40 to 80 are most likely to improve and to return home. These patients should be admitted to a specialized rehabilitation unit. This group may also be most appropriate for clinical trials of a particular therapeutic approach to one or more disabilities. Patients with this level of function can also be used to compare hospital-based rehabilitation with what many health care payers may seek—treatment in a less expensive, skilled nursing facility.

Discharge

Discharge should occur when the patient becomes independent enough to be managed at home. When feasible, this level of functioning includes controlled bowel and bladder function and minimally assisted, or better, transfers and ambulation. Long inpatient rehabilitation stays have been associated with lower admission ADL scores, along with private funding for hospitalization and admission from places other than the home.[144] Patients under the age of 55 years who have low admission FIM scores, usually under 50, have the longest stays.[4]

One argument for the use of focused rehabilitation programs, as opposed to care in a medical ward, is that patients are perhaps more likely to be discharged from the less organized setting without adequate warning and family preparation, without durable medical equipment, and without immediate follow-up medical care or disability-oriented community care.[230] The discharge plan should include these important features.

OUTPATIENT REHABILITATION

Although functional performance improves significantly during inpatient rehabilitation, patients generally continue to improve for at least another 3 to 6 months, especially in mobility and compensatory techniques for ADLs. Follow-up studies of patients discharged to outpatient care or to no formal therapy vary greatly. For example, these studies differ in the time from onset of stroke to discharge from a facility, in the residual impairments and disabilities of the patients, and in the level of available psychosocial support. These variables make it difficult to determine the natural history of postacute rehabilitation recovery and the optimal amount and type of therapy that may help these patients.

Postacute Therapy

In the 3 months after discharge from a rehabilitation unit, UDS data, noted previously, shows about 10 percent gains in FIM scores. At 6 months to years later, most patients discharged to home have reported maintained or modestly improved gains.[8,101,194] In one 6-month, postrehabilitation follow-up study of patients with first stroke and no cognitive impairment, patients with more severe neurologic impairments at discharge showed significant, if modest, gains in their Fugl-Meyer scores and BI.[101] No formal therapy was provided in that interval. The combined mean acute and rehabilitation inpatient stay was 143 days. A subgroup over the age of 65 years appeared to improve more by functional compensation than by lessening of impairments. When self-care skills decline after discharge, the cause, in the absence of new neuromedical problems, is most often due to the caregiver's ability to provide more efficient and more convenient assistance for an ADL than the patient can accomplish independently.

CLINICAL TRIALS

In England, the Bradford Community Stroke Trial randomized 124 new stroke patients to rehabilitation therapy in a day hospital twice a week or to home therapy for up to 20 hours over 8 weeks.[368] The study also stratified patients using two levels of functional severity. Subjects were over the age of 60 years and had new, residual disability at the time of hospital discharge. The interval between stroke and acute hospital discharge was less than 4 weeks for 16 percent, 4 to 7 weeks for 31 percent, 8 to 11 weeks for 23 percent, and over 12 weeks for 30 percent. Thus, over half these patients were more than 2 months post stroke at entry. At 8 weeks, both groups showed small, significant gains. The home-treated group, which received less therapy, did better on stairs. Over one-third of patients in both groups were depressed. A general health questionnaire showed that 1 in 4 caregivers felt stressed. At 6 months, both groups had improved compared with function at discharge, but gains on the BI and Motor Club Assessment were greater for the home-treated group. Depression and emotional stress remained the same. For the modest resources expended, home physical therapy was more beneficial, but neither approach addressed psychosocial functions well.

A Nottingham study randomly allocated three groups of inpatients who had been discharged from acute and rehabilitation hospitals to either a domiciliary team or hospital-based outpatient care.[115] No differences in ADLs and scores on a quality of life profile were apparent at 6 months with these different levels of organization for therapy and support.

An older study randomized 133 patients upon discharge from acute hospitalization to 4 days of outpatient rehabilitation therapies per week, versus 3 half-days, versus regular home visits that encouraged patients to carry out what had been taught in the hospital.[304] By 6 months after the stroke, the greatest improvement in ADLs occurred in the patients who received intensive care; intermediate gains were made by the conventionally treated group, and deterioration occurred in the untreated patients. The maximum benefit was achieved by 3 months.

As a clinical generalization, formal therapy provided at least three times a week, accompanied by home practice for specific disabilities, seems more likely to enable pa-

tients to achieve their highest plateau of function in less time than informal instruction and services that limit the specificity and intensity of training.

Long-Term Therapy

If the debilitating effects of an intercurrent illness are excluded, most patients maintain their level of function following inpatient and outpatient rehabilitation for at least 2 years after a stroke, regardless of age.[32] Conditioning exercises are one of the most important recommendations to patients over the long run. Muscle strengthening and aerobic training counteract many of the potentially debilitating physiologic changes associated with aging and with a sedentary lifestyle.[354] At every follow-up visit, patients should be encouraged to walk or pedal on a stationary bicycle for at least 20 minutes a day. Along with their routine stretches and home therapy program, patients can improve balance and leg muscle strength simply by repeatedly rising from a chair. In addition, therapy that restarts a year or more after a stroke can benefit patients, at least transiently.

CLINICAL TRIALS

In a randomized, crossover trial with repeated measures of walking speed and functional activities related to ambulation, patients who were 2 to 7 years poststroke and who still walked slowly (more than 10 seconds to go 10 m if under age 60 years, more than 12.5 seconds if 60 to 69 years old, more than 16.5 seconds if over 70 years old) spent one to six sessions with a physical therapist.[338] The interventions, mostly problem solving, included re-education for gait deviations, practice on uneven surfaces and going from sit to stand, adjustments and provision of aids, and exercise to increase fitness. This modest approach led to a significant increase in speed after 3 months for the treated group, whereas the other half of the cohort declined. When the second group was treated, they improved over the subsequent 3 months, whereas the first group declined. Speed increased 9 percent and declined about 12 percent. Functional measures related to mobility did not change.

In a quasi-experimental design in which patients, on average 3 years after a stroke, were their own controls, significant improvements were demonstrated in weight shifting, balance, and ADL scores after 8 hours of physical and occupational therapy a week for 1 month.[318] The treatment emphasized skills required by the outcome measures in these motivated, ambulatory patients. Far more intensive therapy was given to 51 selected patients who could not walk and who had BI scores below 60 3 months after a stroke.[57] Subjects received from 20 to 30 hours a week of physical and occupational therapy for 1-month to 3-month intervals, repeated for up to 2 years. At 6 months after their strokes, 25 percent of these patients achieved BI scores over 70, and 18 percent reached independent ambulation. At 1 year, 68 and 64 percent did so, and at 2 years, 79 and 74 percent achieved these levels of function. Changes for the group were statistically significant at 1 year but not at 2 years.

Thus, patients maintain functional gains and can make some additional improvements in ambulation and ADLs with a directed refresher program. Brief "pulse" rehabilitation therapy aimed at a specific functional need should be considered even years after a stroke. The goal and the intervention must be well defined, and success should aim to improve the patient's quality of life.

REHABILITATIVE APPROACHES AND OUTCOMES FOR COMMON PROBLEMS

Mobility

One of the foremost goals of the patient with hemiplegia is to achieve independent ambulation. Patients who require more than minimal assistance to walk a short distance, say 10 to 15 feet, by the end of their acute hospitalization have the most common disability that leads to transfer to an inpatient rehabilitation program. The physical therapist develops strategies to improve the patient's ambulation, but the entire rehabili-

tation team reinforces techniques for head and trunk control, for sitting and standing balance, for transfers, and for a safe and energy-efficient reciprocal pattern for gait. The assessment and management of hemiparetic gait deviations are covered in Chapter 4. The most appropriate targets for gait interventions are still uncertain. Most work has centered upon balance, weight bearing, leg symmetry in swing and stance times, normalization of strength, and improvement of motor control.[27]

Some generalizations about recovery of ambulation can be made. Advanced age, prior stroke, and low initial BI scores lessen the likelihood of recovery of independent ambulation. Poor trunk control at 6 weeks after an ischemic stroke makes it unlikely that the patient will develop independent ambulation outside the home. Recovery of hip extension helps the patient to stabilize the hip and the knee during stance. Recovery of hip flexion during swing and recovery of weight-supporting knee extension during stance increase the likelihood of independent ambulation with or without an assistive device. The ability to fully straighten the affected knee from 30 degrees of flexion during single-limb stance in patients with normal leg proprioception who were more than 3 months poststroke differentiated household from community ambulators in most cases in one study.[254a] In patients with hemiparesis who could stand unsupported on a force plate during inpatient rehabilitation, measures of body sway and symmetry of weight bearing on the affected and unaffected legs showed some correlation with the ability to ambulate.[269] Coordination of movement, as well as good leg strength, however, is important. For example, one prospective study found that 11 percent of patients with normal leg power had difficulty in walking, and 15 percent of those with moderate weakness walked alone 3 weeks after a stroke.[339] The patient with hemiplegia who most predictably becomes an independent ambulator, with or without an assistive device, is the otherwise generally fit patient who has had a first pure motor stroke. As noted earlier, most patients with a large hemispheric infarction who participate in rehabilitation recover assisted ambulation for 150 feet by 7 months after the stroke.

Once inpatient therapy for gait progresses away from the hemibar or parallel bars to increasing distances walked with a quad-cane, a cane, or an ankle-foot orthosis, then stair climbing and outdoor ambulation on uneven surfaces can proceed. By then, therapy can continue in the outpatient setting, where therapists stress mobility in the home and the community. For some patients with hemiplegia, work on ambulation can go on indefinitely in an effort to improve speed and endurance.

Additional therapy has been studied in already mobile patients from the community.[149] At entry into the study, 148 patients with recent stroke walked at least 20 m independently without an assistive device. Their minimum BI was 75, and cognition and language were unimpaired. After 5 hours a week of Bobath-based physical therapy for 4 weeks, in addition to occupational therapy, these patients showed statistically significant gains in stance duration and in the symmetry of swing and push-off of both legs. The symmetry of ground reaction forces did not change. Speed over a 10-m distance and maximum distance walked changed only slightly. Thus, functional mobility did not change much with a modest intervention that emphasized balance and symmetry of movement, but not walking speed, in well-functioning patients.

The significance of stroke-induced locomotor disability cannot be underestimated. As noted earlier, the community-based Framingham Study found that 22 percent of survivors of stroke were dependent in ambulating 150 feet when examined 6 months post stroke.[130] In other studies, this figure runs as high as 35 percent. In a British population-based study of acute stroke, about 60 percent of patients who were initially dependent have become independent.[340] Only 22 percent of patients initially dependent in gait have recovered a normal walking speed over 10 m, as compared with age-matched controls, however.[347] Thus, many patients who recover the ability to ambulate without physical assistance are still disabled by their slow walking speed and can walk only short distances. This drawback may account for the reduction in their community activities.[130] Indeed, across studies of recovery of gait in patients with stroke who received rehabilitation therapy, self-selected walking speeds tend to peak in 3 to 6 months at one-third to one-half of normal for age.[33,245,268,347] Speed is a good reflection of the overall gait pattern. Usual casual walking speed for older adults is about 90 cm per second (2.95 feet per second or 2 mph).[303] Healthy geriatric patients can increase their speed to walk 50 feet in 12 seconds (130 cm per second or 2.9 mph).[267] Mean ranges for gait speed in several studies of recovery from hemiplegic stroke were 25 to 50 cm per second.[268] In a large group of patients who received conventional inpatient rehabilitation, mean speed increased from 36 (S.D. 10) feet per minute or 18 cm per second at 30 days post stroke to 75 (S.D. 11) feet per minute or 38 cm per second at 140 days.[293] More than 3 months after disabling stroke, unlimited household ambulators walk at 25 ± 10 cm per second, and unrestricted community ambulators have achieved speeds of 80 ± 15 cm per second and have better strength in the affected leg.[254a] Thus, gait speed and endurance for walking longer distances than the standard BI and FIM test of 150 feet should become the focus for mobility interventions.

SPASTICITY

On occasion, hypertonicity impedes residual voluntary movement and causes gait deviations that affect the efficiency or safety of ambulation. However, hypertonicity constricts the functional recovery of hemiplegic gait far less than other abnormalities of motor output, such as dyssynergic patterns of muscle activation, paresis, and fatigability. Any source of pain, especially from viscera or joints, can enhance spasticity and must be eliminated. Antispasticity medications, as discussed in Chapter 6, can reduce hypertonicity and, on occasion, can improve the locomotor pattern. A clear positive effect should be evident, and attempts should be made after further physical therapy to eliminate the need for these drugs, which have considerable side effects. Direct peroneal nerve stimulation timed to the step cycle to help clear the foot also can decrease plantarflexor tone. Nerve blocks and surgical management with tendon lengthening and transplants are infrequently used in geriatric patients.

ADDITIONAL APPROACHES

In addition to the approaches described in Chapter 3 for mobility and gait training, therapists have begun to explore other methods, such as bicycling,[37] isokinetic Kinetron activities (Cybex Co., Division of Lumex, Ronkonkoma, New York),[116] and strength and balance training after stroke. The amount of practice in transferring weight onto the paretic leg during stance, done to improve extensor strength, correlated with improved functional ambulation in a pilot study.[234] Balance training on a force plate to improve the symmetry of weight bearing on each leg did not generalize to improve gait in another study, however.[360]

Treadmill Training. Treadmill training by a variety of techniques has been the subject of small studies.[337] In part, this training has been tried in response to the hypothesis that task-specific training is most conducive to motor learning.[203] A 5-week, randomized trial of patients with acute hemispheric stroke compared two traditional approaches and intensities of treatment with a more intensive and focused set of interventions that included treadmill gait training.[268] At 6 weeks after stroke, the second group had a 40 percent greater gait speed than the conventional groups. At 3 months, the investigators found no differences, although all three groups had continued to improve. One conclusion was that a trial for gait training should proceed for 3 months following a stroke.

Several investigators have reported improvement in biomechanical and kinesiologic measures of locomotion using a combination of body weight support by an overhead harness and the rhythmic oscillation of the lower extremities made possible by simultaneous treadmill training.[77,103,148] Pilot studies have been limited to patients who are 2 to 12 months post stroke and who walk poorly or not at all overground.

Figure 7–1 shows the relationship between treadmill speed and speed of overground ambulation over time during body weight–supported treadmill training (BWSTT) of patients with stroke 1 year after the onset of stroke.[77] These are exemplar data from three patients with different severities of impairment. Along with seven other patients, they trained as outpatients 3 or 4 times a week. In the month before starting BWSTT, these patients received 12 sessions of conventional treatment for gait. This training did not produce a significant increase in overground walking speed. At the start of BWSTT, these patients walked with moderate assistance overground at 10 to 35 cm per second (0.2 to 0.8 mph). Body weight support was used for 6 to 8 weeks, at which point the patients were able to proceed using the harness only as a safety precaution during full weight bearing, despite subsequent increases in treadmill speed. For the overall group, speeds significantly increased. In this ongoing treatment protocol of patients with acute or chronic stroke at the University of California Los Angeles, training that includes practice at a treadmill speed that exceeds overground speed capability appears to lead to more functional overground speeds. At slow speeds, usually below 0.8 mph, many patients describe a highly cognitive approach to their stepping in which they have to pay attention to more details during each step than when they are pushed to walk at higher speeds. One mechanism that affects automaticity of stepping during BWSTT appears to be related to the angular velocity of hip extension induced by the treadmill. This mechanism is consistent with the load and hip extension studies described for cats that have undergone spinal transection and for patients with spinal cord injury (see Chapters 1 and 8).

Hesse and colleagues added 25 sessions of BWSTT to ongoing physical therapy in eight patients with stroke who could not ambulate independently 2 to 4 months after the onset of stroke and, in one case, after 14 months.[148] Initial treadmill training speeds were 7 to 11 cm per second (0.2 mph) and reached the maximum of 12 to 23 cm per second (0.5 mph) by day 8. Higher speeds were not attempted. In addition, their patients required no body weight support on average at day 6 (range of 4 to 20 days).

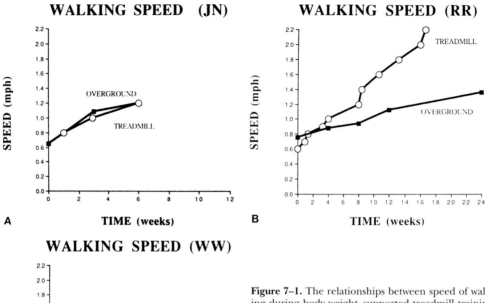

Figure 7–1. The relationships between speed of walking during body weight–supported treadmill training (BWSTT) and speed overground with asssistive devices are shown for patients who had (*A*) a severe motor impairment, (*B*) a severe sensorimotor impairment, and (*C*) a severe sensorimotor with visual field impairment. For patients A and B, increasing treadmill speeds were associated with increasing speed of overground walking. While overground walking speed did not increase with the increase in treadmill walking speed in patient C, by a kinematic assessment the quality and safety of ambulation did improve. Patient C, who had a right hemispheric infarction and visuoperceptual impairments, described a sense of fear in trying to walk faster overground.

Swing and stance times of each leg became more symmetric and gait became more independent. Mean overground velocities increased significantly from 12 (S.D. 8) cm per second to 42 (S.D. 23) cm per second, or to a mean of less than 1 mph.

In a 6-week inpatient, randomized trial at the Jewish Rehabilitation Hospital and McGill University in Montreal,[336a] BWSTT was compared with treadmill training alone. One hundred patients were entered, 50 assigned to each intervention. Entry criteria included the ability to flex the hip and to take a step with assistance if needed. The average time from the onset of stroke to entry into the trial was 77.0 days. Even after that long delay, patients had an average inpatient stay of 70 days, mostly because no outpatient therapy was available to them. The study had

a 30 percent dropout rate for the treadmill training alone group, mostly in subjects whose initial walking speed overground was below 20 cm per second. These patients could not tolerate step training even at slow treadmill speeds. Initial mean overground speed for each group was 18 cm per second. In the BWSTT group, approximately 60 percent were fully weight bearing by 10 sessions. The protocol increased the treadmill speed modestly or eliminated use of the side bars for lateral support at that point. By the end of BWSTT at 6 weeks, 82 percent were able to walk without body weight support; however, only 12 percent were able to walk on the treadmill without body weight support at 1.5 mph or more at the end of training. At 6 weeks, the average comfortable treadmill speed without body weight support for subjects assigned to both interventions was 0.9 mph, with a range of 0.1 to 2.0 mph. For the 79 subjects who completed 24 sessions of BWSTT or treadmill training alone, significant gains were found in the BWSTT group in balance, motor function, overground walking speed, and distance walked.

These studies point to the need for additional trials that compare BWSTT with conventional methods. Too many dropouts occur when no body weight support is provided during early treadmill training. The time from onset of stroke to start of the intervention, as in the Hesse studies,[148,148a] was longer than is typical for rehabilitation inpatient services in the United States. Thus, treadmill training without body weight support may be even more difficult for patients with more acute stroke. Moreover, entry criteria in the Canadian trial eliminated many of the patients—those who could not yet flex at the affected hip while standing—who most often reached a rehabilitation unit in the United States by 14 days after the onset of stroke. As in the Hesse trial, treadmill speeds during training were kept slow, a factor that may diminish the potential effects of BWSTT to enhance automatic stepping and increase overground speed.

BWSTT can reduce the gait deviations brought on by attempts at full weight loading of the paretic limb. It may allow the neural networks of the brainstem and spinal cord to receive more normal step-related sensory feedback, which could enhance automatic stepping for locomotion (see Fig. 1–6). The motor learning concept that recommends task-specific therapy has also been invoked as a rationale for treadmill training. The technique permits gait training in patients with acute stroke who have fair truncal balance but who cannot bear weight. Early use may limit muscle atrophy and reduce the risk of DVT. Randomized trials for patients with acute stroke are necessary before the technique takes hold as an adjunct intervention.

Biofeedback. As discussed in Chapter 3, feedback plays an important role in learning motor skills. It improves error detection and correction, helps guide the patient toward the desired movement, and motivates the pa-

tient. BFB probably works best for motor learning in a task-specific paradigm. EMG BFB has been used to recruit or to inhibit most muscle groups of the lower extremities during exercise and during ambulation.[20,185] Quasi-experimental and N-of-1 trials are often reported for feedback techniques to improve stride length, stance time on the paretic leg, and the symmetry of weight bearing during stance and balance tasks. The results may grab our attention, but individual studies leave one puzzled about whether any form of BFB has improved important functions more than another intervention, however. A few examples point to the potential of a range of BFB paradigms.

One 6-week randomized trial for gait dysfunction compared a control group with groups receiving three interventions: EMG BFB, functional electrical stimulation (FES), and FES plus BFB.[53] With only eight subjects in each group, the investigators found a significantly better outcome on two measures in the FES-plus-BFB group compared with the control group, but no differences between the control and the other groups. Even this one positive finding may have been related to chance alone, given the multiple measures and the sample size. On the other hand, the sample size may not have been large enough to detect differences, had they existed.

Another study of EMG BFB for ambulation in patients with chronic hemiparesis used a crossover design that revealed no clear differences between physical therapy and BFB,[164] although the outcomes analysis was probably inadequate.

Another approach converted the EMG signal for a healthy person's muscle activation pattern during gait to a changing sound pitch and asked the patients with hemiparesis to match the timing of the sounds.[361] Although this approach led to a reduction of the flexor synergy through relaxation of the tibialis anterior muscle at the onset of the swing phase, the changes are difficult to interpret without a control group. Audio-monitoring of the EMG signal did decrease footdrop during the swing phase after 15 training sessions in a small experimental group, compared with a group of patients with chronic stroke who were treated with the Bobath method alone, although step length and velocity did not changed.[158]

Feedback from changes in the joint angles of the leg has also shown promise in improving hemiplegic gait. In a randomized study of 26 patients with recent stroke who could ambulate with standby help, electrogoniometric BFB was used during training for stance and gait to correct genu recurvatum.[226] An auditory signal was activated at the moment of hyperextension and increased in pitch proportional to the degree of recurvatum. Patients who received this intervention as an adjunct to physical therapy began to improve during 4 weeks of daily treatment. These patients showed a statistically significant reduction in knee hyperextension over the subsequent 4 weeks of physical therapy alone, compared with the group that had only physical therapy during the 8 weeks. However, gait velocity and single-limb stance times did not significantly change. Although the experimental group had more subjects who could walk 5 m unaided compared with the control group, the degree of recovery did not reach statistical significance.

A small crossover study assessed the effects of ankle joint angle and soleus EMG BFB on ambulatory patients. The affected soleus muscles showed a high activation pattern during early and midstance, which restrained passive dorsiflexion, and again in late stance, which interfered with push-off.[47] Significant gains were found for gait velocity, stride length, symmetry, and push-off impulse, compared with physical therapy with a neurodevelopmental and motor learning approach. The improvement was consistent with data showing that the plantarflexors perform 80 percent of the positive work of gait, but excess plantarflexion in early stance prevents the ankle from dorsiflexing into a position at which the plantarflexors can contribute to forward impulse by an active push-off.

Thus, BFB for specific motor problems in hemiplegia can complement the training of discrete motor control for gait. Larger controlled clinical trials with well-defined paradigms and outcome measures that establish whether gains carry over to real-world settings when BFB is discontinued will determine whether the approach plays a more important role in stroke rehabilitation.

ORTHOTICS

Patients with hemiparesis who recover little ankle movement, whose foot tends to turn over during gait, or who lack enough knee control to prevent it from snapping back usually can be managed with a polypropylene ankle-foot orthosis (AFO) fitted to the patient's needs (see Chapter 3). In patients with profound sensorimotor impairment, a double upright metal brace may be indicated, but a well-constructed AFO usually suffices. Randomized trials of the utility of common assistive devices or comparisons among devices have not been performed in patients with stroke, but some studies have confirmed the clinical impression that energy demands,[352] gait speed, and the gait pattern can be improved with an AFO.[193]

FALLS

Falls and the fear of falling pose a potential problem, especially during outpatient maintenance therapy. The yearly incidence of falls increases from 25 percent among 70-year-old patients living in the community to 35 percent after the age of 75 years, and half of these elderly patients fall repeatedly.[327] Five percent of falls cause a fracture, and another 10 percent result in serious injury. After stroke, 80 percent of femoral neck fractures have been reported on the hemiplegic side, associated with muscle weakness and disuse that produces demineralization.[135] Osteoporosis may be greater in the plegic arm than in the plegic leg if the leg experiences some weight bearing. Hemiparesis, ataxia, sensory loss, hemianopia, and visuospatial and cognitive deficits, especially in patients with a right hemispheric stroke, make it yet more likely that the geriatric patient with stroke will suffer a serious injury from a fall or will limit activities for fear of falling. Patients may gain confidence by wearing a gait belt. The caregiver slips several fingers behind the back of the belt as the patient walks. Moreover, architectural barriers and obstacles such as loose rugs and raised floor thresholds should be removed from the home (see Chapter 10).

PAIN

Thoracolumbar and lower extremity pain can limit transfer training and ambulation. Treatable sources include soft tissue strain or myofascial pain, the biomechanically stressed and osteoarthritic weight-bearing joints of the lumbosacral spine and hemiplegic leg, the hyperextended knee of a genu recurvatum, the plantarflexor contracture of the heel cord, flexor spasms of the toes, postphlebitic venous obstruction, unrecognized fractures, radiculopathies, and diabetic neuropathies.

Upper Extremity Function

Loss of the use of an arm and hand, especially of the dominant upper extremity, impedes everyday activities. For some survivors of stroke, the "dead arm" acts as an immutable reminder of disability and of vulnerability to stroke. These patients constantly fidget with the paretic hand, pulling on the wrist and straightening the fingers with their "good hand." Even patients who improve to regain selective movements over mass flexion of the fingers with slow, if any, finger extension often do not recover their ability to finely coordinate and efficiently manipulate objects. Compensation, through use of the unaffected hand and assistive devices, is still the mainstay of rehabilitative interventions. Experimentally determined, more physiologically based techniques hold the promise of better outcomes.

The nonparetic arm of the patient with hemiplegia, which often serves as a control in clinical studies, also appears to be affected in subtle ways after an ipsilateral stroke. Studies of the "normal" arm have shown slower EMG recruitment patterns,[137] reduced speed and strength of hand actions,[162] paretic proximal and distal muscles,[48] and impaired sensory discrimination in the hand.[93] Test results that require continuous sensory feedback, such as reaction times and tracking, seem especially impaired, even 12 months after a stroke.[167] Pos-

sible mechanisms, discussed in Chapter 1 in the context of the hierarchic and distributed organization of the brain, include loss of commissural fiber inputs from the involved to the uninvolved hemisphere, contributions of uncrossed pathways to bilateral upper limb functions, and alterations in the modulation of subcortical, brainstem, and spinal sensorimotor regions that receive bilateral inputs. These findings help to explain why upper and lower extremity functions that are initially impaired by a contralateral stroke sometimes worsen after a subsequent ipsilateral stroke, with or without an accompanying pseudobulbar palsy. Rehabilitation specialists must identify any ipsilateral impairments that may cause disabilities and interfere with compensatory training of the "unaffected" arm.

CHRONOLOGY OF FUNCTIONAL IMPROVEMENT

In studies of selected survivors of stroke, about 10 percent recover normal function of the upper extremity, about one-third recover useful function, about one-fourth have no recovery, and one-third have some movement and limited function.[227,297] Follow-up studies vary in the timing of examinations and in the tests used to measure strength and function.

In one series, 20 percent of patients with an upper extremity that remained flaccid 2 weeks after a stroke regained functional use of the hand. None of these patients regained use of the hand if isolated motion of the fingers and some grip strength had not returned by 1 month.[342] Increases in grip strength beyond 1 month, even when accompanied by increased flexor tone, correlated with improved hand function, but not with dexterity.[315]

Only 10 percent of patients in another series who, at the time of admission to rehabilitation, had no better than movement of the arm and hand with gravity eliminated recovered independent feeding and dressing with the affected arm by the time of discharge from the facility.[246] Half of those patients with movement against gravity became independent. The rest required minimal assistance. In another study of selected patients who started inpatient or outpatient rehabilitation at a median of 12 days (range 2 to 86 days) after stroke, the affected arm significantly improved between 3 weeks and 3 months after the onset of stroke. Some patients noted improvements in more difficult upper extremity tasks between 6 months and 1 year.[302] Tests of hand function ranged from the least difficult, using both hands to open a jar, to the more difficult, using the affected hand to grasp and release a cylinder, to the most difficult, using the affected hand to comb hair and to open and close a clothespin.

A Danish community study that assessed upper extremity strength and function with BI subscores for grooming and feeding found that the best function was achieved by 95 percent within 9 weeks.[235] Patients with mild paresis improved by 6 weeks. With severe paresis, they reached best function by 11 weeks. Full function was achieved by 79 percent of those with mild paresis, but only 18 percent with severe paresis reached full function. These and other studies[9] suggest that arm and hand function for most patients tends to improve for up to 12 weeks. Patients who have fair function by 3 months note improvements for up to a year in some specific tasks. Patients who reach full recovery usually do so by 8 weeks.

Although the best predictor for the degree of recovery of the upper extremity is the amount of movement found on admission for rehabilitation, other factors include anesthesia, joint pain, contractures, apraxia, and perceptual impairments. These factors can limit gains in a particular level of motor function.

CLINICAL TRIALS

Therapeutic trials specific to the hemiparetic upper extremity have included enhanced physical interventions, avoidance of learned disuse, sensory relearning, BFB, and home-based exercise.

Enhanced Interventions. A trial compared traditional Bobath, Johnstone, and related techniques to a series of more intensive treatments. These treatments included behavioral methods to increase family and patient participation in therapy and to prevent learned nonuse of the arm. The therapists also facilitated the learning of new motor skills with tasks of graded difficulty and provided feedback on performance, used EMG BFB, and trained patients with microcomputer games.[316] Patients were evaluated by a variety of tests at a median of 10 days after the stroke, with retests at 1, 3, and 6 months. Subgroups of 64 severely and 57 mildly affected patients were also compared. The primary effect of the enhanced intervention, which included about twice the amount of therapy time, was improved arm function at 1 month. At 6 months, the mildly affected patients who received enhanced therapy, but not the severely impaired subgroup, showed significant improvements in the Nine Hole Peg Test and a motor score. Thus, a moderate addition to usual interventions benefited patients who had arm movement at entry into the trial. A better-defined set of enhanced interventions and measures with less serious floor and ceiling effects may reveal more about efficacy. This study is remarkable, however, in what it tells us about a well-designed clinical trial in one setting. It took 3 years to enroll subjects and 5 years to complete the trial.

Overcoming Nonuse. One of the mainstay interventions for improving self-care and functional skills is to compensate for the paretic limb with the unaffected limb. Several animal and clinical studies raise the possibility that those who constantly prefer to use the unaffected limb seem to learn nonuse of the paretic limb (see Chapter 1). Patients who have had at least modest recovery of the wrist and hand extensors and who are forced to use the paretic hand appear to improve its function. One study of 25 patients with chronic hemiplegic stroke and head injury who overcame a flexor synergy used a multiple-baselines design to look for an effect of enclosing the unaffected hand in a sling for 2 weeks.[365] For a series of simple functional tasks, repeated measures showed significant increases in speed and greater applied force, including grip. The quality of the shoulder, elbow, and hand movements did not appear to improve, based on observer ratings. At 1-year follow-up, these gains persisted or increased. In another study, 9 patients with chronic stroke who could extend their affected fingers and wrist were assigned either to restraint of the unaffected arm for 14 days along with 6 hours of daily practice using the affected hand or to encouragement to use the affected hand with passive ranging.[321] The restrained group showed a significant 30 percent decrease in the timed performance of a series of upper extremity functional tasks and a significant increase in the amount of use of the affected hand during daily activities. Half of the improvement in daily use was evident after 1 day of restraint plus therapy, a finding suggesting that a latent capability had succumbed to learned nonuse. Gains were maintained in a 2-year follow-up.

These trials do not provide information about upper extremity functions that had improved and then were lost between the onset of stroke and entry into the forced-use study. They do confirm that strong motivation, good cognition, and some selective hand movement are needed if gains are to be made. Training interventions must be further developed to determine whether more specific learning paradigms and activities can unmask latent function, train compensatory motor actions, and take advantage of the potential for neuronal representational plasticity. For example, patients with hemiplegia who reach with the arm, even if slowly and mostly in a synergistic pattern, may be trained to develop a fair key grip action with the nearly plegic thumb pressing against the fist. These patients may also better learn to grasp with their flexing fingers or their key grip when the palm is up, rather than facing down. Training takes repetitive, problem-solving trials and seems to work best by grasping an object that can be useful, such as a tissue or playing cards. These latent abilities should be tested for during each outpatient visit.

Sensory Re-education. Studies of cortical and thalamic representational plasticity have provided a theoretic basis for techniques of sensory re-education after stroke. If some afferent pathways and somatosensory cortical areas are intact, then receptive fields not excited by sensory inputs before an injury to neighboring neurons may be trained to appreciate inputs from the arm and hand. Rehabilitation goals are as follows:

1. To improve the appreciation of spatial and temporal patterns of skin contact as the fingers move over the edges, surfaces, and textures of objects
2. To identify and manipulate objects
3. To improve precision movements
4. To adjust grip forces
5. To prevent nonuse of the partially deafferented hand
6. To enhance daily manual activities

Successful sensory retraining was demonstrated in the 1930s when monkeys were trained to discriminate manipulated objects by shape, texture, and weight and then relearned these distinctions after a parietal lobe ablation.[288] Few studies have provided more than anecdotal or single-case examples of this recovery in human patients after stroke. Several reports suggest the potential for sensory retraining techniques.

One exploratory study showed gains in the ability of a patient with chronic stroke to use utensils after a series of interventions over the course of a year.[59] A 100-Hz current was applied to finger surfaces at intensities that evoked appreciation of the stimulus and aimed to allow the patient to identify which finger was stimulated. Velcro strips attached to a variety of objects and utensils and in geometric patterns on cardboard were used to stimulate moving touch-pressure inputs. The patients were highly motivated to accomplish their defined functional goals. A series of four single-case study designs with multiple baselines showed significant improvements in wrist proprioception and tactile discrimination of the fingers.[41] For discrimination, the investigators used finely graded ridges and grooves explored by one finger with graded progression of stimuli and no visual input. The trainers used a learning paradigm with quantitative feedback on performance and summary feedback on judgments and on the method of exploration. The training effects were specific to the individual tasks, as predicted by the motor learning literature (see Chapter 3) and by studies of sensorimotor representational maps in monkeys.[219]

In another protocol, investigators trained patients with chronic stroke to relearn sensory information and compared this group with an untreated, matched control group.

Patients correlated tactile input with what they saw in their affected hand and attempted to make purposeful exploratory movements with the hypesthetic fingers.[367] By training patients three times a week for 6 weeks in a variety of problem-solving tasks, scores for identifying the location of a touch to the fingers, the position of the elbow, two-point discrimination, and stereognosis improved significantly, especially in patients who retained some sensation after a left cerebral injury.

Although these trials have flaws in their designs, they do suggest that rehabilitation specialists should further explore and select from the infinite number of paradigms that can combine learning principles with tasks that use repetitive, meaningful multisensory inputs. More work must be undertaken to examine strategies to enhance hand function in the presence of, for example, perceptual or memory impairments. Moreover, an injury to particular cerebral structures may alter learning. This phenomenon has been demonstrated in primates when somatosensory cortical ablations impaired the learning of new motor skills, but not the execution of existing skills.[253]

Biofeedback. Surface and intramuscular EMG analysis of upper extremity movements provides some insight into alterations of voluntary movement in the patient with hemiparesis. The technique has been used to suggest and to monitor interventions. For example, volitional movement at the wrist in a group of patients with hemiparesis recruited the flexor carpi radialis (FCR) and the extensor carpi radialis (ECR) more slowly than normal. The forearm extensors showed greater recruitment slowing, more gaps in the pattern of motor unit firing, and early termination of activity when patients tried to maintain a contraction.[187] The longer the attempted contraction, the greater the co-contraction of the FCR and ECR muscles. EMG BFB was recommended but not undertaken by the investigators to try to reduce the gaps in the motor units and decrease any detrimental co-contraction of agonist and antagonist muscle groups. The relationship between EMG activity and movement is not simple, however.

When therapists found three exercises to evoke a maximal recruitment pattern of mo-

tor units in the extensor digitorum muscle of patients with hemiparesis, the exercises were tried as a way to increase wrist and finger extension.[331] Patients able to grasp a cylinder 4 to 6 weeks after a stroke were trained to repeatedly squeeze a dynamometer, to resist finger extension against a rubber band, and to throw a Ping-Pong ball for ballistic extension. No one exercise significantly improved range of motion, the speed of finger tapping, or the grasp and release of various-sized cylinders when compared with one of the other exercises or the control group. Spontaneous improvement, a small and less than optimally balanced sample population, and outcome measures that perhaps did not reflect the possible effects of the intervention probably contributed to this unsuccessful trial. More studies are needed to determine whether increasing the number of motor units that fire has any impact on upper extremity function. This goal has been pursued with the use of EMG BFB.

EMG BFB has been applied to many muscle groups of the hemiplegic upper extremity.[185] The intention is to enhance movement, to decrease the resistance of spastic antagonists, and to help regain stabilizing functions, such as its application over the trapezius and anterior deltoid to reduce shoulder subluxation.[20] In general, however, the strategy seems comparable to physical therapies, or the evidence for its efficacy is insufficient to strongly recommend the intervention.[70,200] A meta-analysis of six well-designed studies did not find support for the use of this technique in altering impairment or function.[225] A few studies are of note because of their intent and design. The relationship between EMG activity and functional activities is moot, so the mechanisms for efficacy of EMG BFB are uncertain.

One 5-week randomized trial compared a behavioral approach with EMG BFB with the Bobath neurofacilitatory technique in 29 patients with mild paresis of at least 4 months or severe motor involvement for less than 4 months.[21] On the Upper Extremity Function Test[42] and a finger tapping test, both groups improved and attained the same level of function at 9 months.

In another study of 12 patients with chronic hemiparesis, EMG BFB that aimed to reduce activity in a co-contracting muscle

ence an unpleasant coldness of the hand or arm. The skin temperature can be lower, associated with reduced blood flow.[350] Local warming, exercise, and vasoactive drugs sometimes help.

ALIEN HAND SYNDROME

The alien hand syndrome is characterized by involuntary reaching with a clumsy, paretic arm and grasping with a hand that features a powerful tonic grasp reflex. The hand tends to grab whatever touches it or what the patient sees nearby, although it usually stays within its own hemispace. The dismayed patient often clenches the hands together to control the "estranged" hand and tries to command it to behave, especially when it perseverates in clutching a nurse or therapist. Lesions of the medial frontal lobe in the anterior cerebral artery distribution that usually extend to the corpus callosum are most often associated with this dissociation between intention and action. Lateral parietal and medial occipital infarctions can produce a similar syndrome.[16] The behavior may result from uninhibited activity of a lateral cortical premotor system after damage to the medial premotor cortex that ordinarily interacts with it.[117] The alien hand comes under volitional control in most cases within 6 to 12 months, perhaps through extension of control by ipsilateral medial cortical or subcortical mechanisms.[117]

Communication Disorders

Across a range of studies, 20 to 35 percent of patients with acute stroke have impaired language at onset, and 10 to 20 percent of long-term survivors of stroke remain aphasic. The natural history of recovery interacts with rehabilitation interventions.

In a British health district of 250,000 people, 202 cases of aphasia per year were detected. By 1 month post stroke, the 165 patients who survived but had not recovered were candidates for speech therapy.[60] Another British district study of over 900 consecutive patients with acute stroke used a simple screening battery to test comprehension, expression, reading, and writing. It found that at least 24 percent of testable pa-

tients were aphasic in the first week and 20 percent at 3 weeks; only 12 percent of survivors remained aphasic at 6 months. Thus, about 40 percent of patients who tested as aphasic at 3 weeks after onset recovered by 6 months; 44 percent of patients and 57 percent of caregivers believed that speech remained abnormal, however.[341]

Over the range of aphasia severities found by testing with the Porch Index of Communicative Abilities (PICA), patients in a typical series improved in their total scores throughout the first year after a stroke and then leveled off during the second year.[236] Most gains in overall function are made in the first 3 months, except for patients with global aphasia, who tend to improve in more subtle ways over a longer time.[196] In the first 3 months, patients with aphasia tend to improve by a fixed amount rather than in proportion to the initial severity of aphasia.[91]

PREDICTORS OF RECOVERY

Age, gender, and handedness have not been as important to outcome as the extent and location of the injury, the severity of language impairments at onset, and the degree of recovery by 1 month after the onset of stroke.[152] The eventual level of language function measured by test scores tends to correlate best with the severity of the initial impairments. For example, the inability to recognize environmental sounds, agnosia, can be a poor prognostic sign for gains in comprehension.

A few studies have offered insights into gains over time. Investigators tested 17 patients with severe global aphasia and 5 patients with severe Wernicke's aphasia starting 1 to 2 months after onset with the Boston Assessment of Severe Aphasia (BASA) and at 6-month intervals for 2 years. Higher subscores for praxis (the ability to carry out buccofacial and limb commands) and for oral and gestural expression at 6 months best predicted overall BASA performance at 24 months.[236] Praxis improved significantly in the first 6 months, whereas reading and auditory comprehension increased between 6 and 12 months. Some patients with global aphasia develop less severe forms of nonfluent aphasia, but most remain within the same classification.[183] These traditional aphasic syndromes are outlined in Table 3–5. Most long-term studies of aphasia recovery suggest that auditory comprehension tends to improve more than speech output across all forms of aphasia.[299]

Neuroimaging can provide insights about recovery. Single-word and sentence-level comprehension appear especially likely to improve by 1 to 2 years in the patient with global aphasia whose frontoparietal infarct extends only to the isthmus of the subcortical temporal lobe, compared with having a lesion that includes at least half of Wernicke's area.[232] On an axial CT scan, this sparing corresponds to the temporal lobe seen from the level of the maximum width of the third ventricle to its roof, often visualized with the pineal gland. Patients with Wernicke's aphasia also tend to have better recovery of auditory comprehension by 6 to 12 months if less than half of Wernicke's cortical area is infarcted.[233] These patients can develop a milder fluent aphasia, such as a conduction or anomic type.

Patients with Broca's area aphasia also recover in ways that may be partly predicted by analyzing the location of the injury and its language sequelae. For example, many of the variations in the speech and language of patients with nonfluent aphasia arise from differential lesions of the frontal operculum, the lower motor cortex, and the subjacent subcortical and periventricular white matter.[5] Damage to the frontal operculum initially affects its function as an integrator for the limbic activational aspects of speech, the posterior temporal and inferior parietal semantic inputs for language, and the frontal motor areas for planning. The resultant language impairment is usually not permanent, however. Sparse and effortful speech and dysnomia and semantic paraphasias indicate more extensive damage to adjacent cortex and white matter projecting from limbic and posterior language-associated regions.

Metabolic imaging studies may also help to predict recovery. These studies can reveal the functional reorganization of speech and language that follows a focal injury (see Chapter 1). For example, in patients with aphasia of all types who could speak spontaneously, a higher left hemisphere regional metabolic rate for glucose by PET during speech activation at 2 weeks after the onset of stroke strongly predicted a better recovery at 4 months.[146] In patients with moderate to severe impairments within 3 weeks of a stroke, receptive language dysfunction that persisted for 2 years on the Token Test correlated with low metabolic rates for glucose in the superior temporal cortex.[177] Poor word fluency correlated with low rates in the left prefrontal cortex. Patients who recovered from Wernicke's aphasia had increased left frontal and right perisylvian activity in the face of infarction of Wernicke's area.[354a] These findings are consistent with the contribution of the preexisting parallel, distributed processing and bilateral neurocognitive networks for comprehension and speech production.

INTERVENTIONS

Studies of the efficacy of aphasia therapy after a stroke have usually set out to learn whether nonspecific approaches improve language functions. Most studies suffer from the methodologic shortcomings found in clinical trials of stroke rehabilitation interventions for mobility and self-care. Design problems include lack of randomized controls, failure to stratify subjects by particular aphasia syndromes, inadequate assessment of the extent of the cortical and subcortical lesion or of the presence of a contralateral lesion that may affect compensation, assessment and outcome tools of uncertain precision and reliability, and wide variations among patients in the time since onset of stroke, in age and education, and in comorbidities that may affect cognition and learning. Little may be specified about the type, intensity, and duration of language therapy. Moreover, aphasia assessment tests vary in the degree to which they reflect changes in functional communication. An overall score may not reveal clinically important gains in language and nonlanguage subskills.

Table 7–14 summarizes some of the better designed, large clinical trials of aphasia therapy for stroke. These conventional therapeutic approaches are described in Chapter 3. Treatments averaged 45 to 60 minutes. Dropouts were due to illness, death, disenchantment with the program, and satisfaction with the level of recovery. In these studies, patients showed average gains of 20 percent in scores on the Functional Communication Profile (FCP) and a 10 to 20 percentile change on the PICA. Patients with aphasia improved on test scores spontaneously and with nonspecific, traditional interventions. General gains continued for 6 months. The modest, sometimes equivocal effects of conventional therapy suggest the need to find techniques to assess and treat better-defined types of communication disorders. Single-case and small-group studies have shown that interventions developed for specific impairments can improve outcome beyond the time of spontaneous improvements. More work is needed to test such approaches and to determine whether they allow for practical gains in social communication.

Energy must also go into helping the patient and family cope with this disability. Although speech therapy may also seem to offer a psychotherapeutic benefit, the randomized trial of Lincoln and colleagues in Table 7–14 revealed no differences in measures of the mood of treated and of untreated patients and their families.[198] Only 10 percent of patients were rated as depressed, but nearly half their spouses had depressive symptoms at 22 weeks after the onset of the stroke. These investigators found no relationship between the PICA and FCP scores and mood.

Behavioral and Cognitive Disorders

Cerebrovascular disease produces as many neuropsychologic sequelae as a clinician can differentiate from among the components of cognition. From anosognosia to dementia, from not shaving one side of the face to mistaking a wife for a hat, rehabilitation specialists often confront subtle and profound cognitive disorders that increase disability and limit gains in mobility, ADLs, and social reintegration. After discharge from inpatient rehabilitation, patients and their families often become aware of modest cognitive limitations, but they cannot always articulate what is wrong. The paucity of brief, uniform, standardized tests with alternate forms that can be given serially to a predominantly elderly population makes the formal investigation of cognitive dysfunction difficult.

A prospective study of 227 patients with ischemic stroke revealed cognitive impairments 3 months after onset in 35 percent of patients and in 4 percent of controls.[320] Memory, orientation, language, and attention were most often affected. Large dominant and nondominant hemisphere infarcts were most frequent. As in other studies, greater intellectual impairment correlated with dependent living after hospitalization, even after adjusting for age and physical impairment.

Before a clinically evident stroke, some patients have had silent infarcts, appreciated by imaging studies. Premorbid lesions that partially disconnect neurocognitive networks can lessen the patient's ability to compensate for the new stroke or produce greater dysfunction than may have been expected from the location of the new injury. Indeed, a community study of patients with a mean age of 70 years and no evidence of stroke showed that risk factors for cerebrovascular disease independently correlated with impaired abstract reasoning, memory, and visuospatial function.[68] The following discussion looks at a few of the more common disorders that follow stroke for which specific interventions have been tried. Cognitive remediation is covered in Chapter 9.

HEMIATTENTIONAL DISORDERS

Disturbances in directed attention arise from within distributed serial and parallel neural networks. Destruction or disconnection of components produces both overlapping and clinically distinct symptoms and signs.[143,220,221,259] These signs and symptoms include hemispatial neglect, hemibody neglect, hemiakinesia, extinction of simultaneous stimuli, and anosognosia. In patients with right cerebral lesions, hemispatial neglect can be accompanied by impairments in facial recognition and in producing or appreciating emotionally toned speech. The presence of aphasia can limit testing for any of these disturbances. Severe left visual neglect in peripersonal space can coexist with minimal inattention to items in extrapersonal space.[133] Hemisensory and visual field impairments often accompany neglect and anosognosia, but these impairments are not essential.[90] Some patients with neglect sit

Table 7–14. **CLINICAL TRIALS OF GENERAL APHASIA THERAPY FOR STROKE**

Trial	Comparison (No. Subjects)	Time After Onset	Duration of Therapy	Outcomes	Comments
Basso et al[22]	Traditional therapy, emphasis on verbal responses (162) versus no therapy (119)	<2 mo: 137 2–6 mo: 86 >6 mo: 58	≥3 therapies/wk × 6 mo	On standard tests: gains in expression and comprehension in therapy groups	Not randomized; 85% had a stroke
David et al[61]	Traditional therapy (71) versus untrained volunteer support (84)	Median 4 wk; range >50 wk	2 therapies/wk × 15–20 wk	On FCP: no difference in gains	Randomized; 30% dropout; poorly defined cases
Shewan and Kertesz[299]	Linguistic (25) versus facilitation by therapist (25) versus stimulation by trained nurse (25) versus no treatment (25)	2–4 wk	Therapy to maximum gain or 1 yr (mean = 68 therapies)	On WAB: therapy groups' gains no greater than for no therapy	Subgroups too small to see group differences; auditory comprehension changed least

Lincoln et al[199]	Traditional therapy (104) versus no therapy (87)	10 wk	2 therapies/wk × 24 wk	On PICA and FCP, no difference	15% dropout; many received less than planned therapies; in 47 matched pairs who completed >50% of therapies, no difference
Wertz et al[359]	Traditional therapy (29) versus therapy with trained family (36) versus deferred 12 wk, then traditional therapy (29)	7 ± 6 wk	8–10 hr/wk × 12 wk	On PICA: traditional therapy better than no therapy at 12 wk; no difference in gains between groups at 24 wk	23% dropout; no harm apparent for delayed therapy
Hartman and Landau[139]	Traditional therapy (30) versus supportive conversation (30)	1 mo	2 therapies/wk × 6 mo	On PICA: no difference in gains at 7 and 10 mo	Equal gains in fluent and nonfluent cases

FCP = Functional Communication Profile; WAB = Western Aphasia Battery; PICA = Porch Index of Communicative Abilities.

with their trunks leaning toward their affected side, although their strength is no worse than patients who sit in the midline and do not have a neglect syndrome.[323]

Unilateral neglect arises from injuries of the posterior parietal cortex, the prefrontal cortex that encompasses the frontal eye fields, and the cingulate gyrus. These regions include representations for sensation, for motor activities such as visual scanning and limb exploration, and for motivational relevance, respectively. Lesions of the right inferior parietal lobule (Brodmann's areas 39 and 40) are particularly closely associated with neglect. This region appears necessary for awareness of external stimuli and serves as a critical node in the modular cortical-limbic-reticular network that directs attention.[353] Incoming and outgoing neural activity in this region probably helps to integrate the localization and identification of a stimulus, as well its importance to the person. Subcortical areas such as the thalamus, the striatum, and the superior colliculus interact with these networked cortical regions, perhaps coordinating the distribution of attention, so lesions in these areas can also cause impairment. Atrophy of frontal white matter and of the diencephalon contributes to persistent anosognosia.[308] The anterior and posterior extent of a lesion may also produce impairments in attentional and intentional processes that contribute to neglect.[69]

Natural History. In a community-based study of 281 3-week survivors of a first acute stroke who had only unilateral signs, visual neglect was detected in about 10 percent.[317] Subjects were tested on their ability to copy the Greek cross and to use visual reasoning to complete the Raven's Colored Progressive Matrices. Only about one-half of these patients had hemianopia or visual extinction. The neglect was modestly associated with poorer ADL scores and slower recovery, although severe neglect was rare beyond 6 months. The NINDS Stroke Data Bank also looked at the effect of hemineglect on ADL scores at 7 to 10 days and 1 year after the onset of a first stroke.[212] Patients with anosognosia, visual neglect, tactile extinction, motor impersistence, or auditory neglect had the lowest BI scores at 1 year, along with patients who were aphasic or who had greater than mild weakness, even after adjusting the data for initial ADL scores and for poststroke rehabilitation.

The detection and grading of a hemi-inattention syndrome depend on the tests used. In a serial follow-up study of patients with right hemispheric stroke, recovery occurred in unilateral spatial neglect tested by drawing in 70 percent by week 13 and in anosognosia and neglect in nearly all by week 20. The mean time to recovery of hemineglect was 11 weeks.[150] These gains may not have carried over to all functional tasks, however. Visual neglect, documented on a battery of seven tests by 3 days after a stroke, was greater in patients with right hemisphere lesions than in left hemisphere lesions.[313] In this report and others, right-sided inattention on testing has been detected in 15 to 40 percent of patients without aphasia and with acute left cerebral infarcts, although this feature is clinically most prominent after right brain injury. Recovery was fastest within 10 days, regardless of side of stroke, and it plateaued at 3 months, when most patients had little visual neglect. Severe visual neglect and anosognosia at 3 days was a predictor of persistent impairment at 6 months. Only 14 of 84 patients with initial neglect showed moderate or severe dependence in ADLs on the BI in follow-up.[312] Interventional studies may consider matching subjects by scores on this test battery and by the time from the onset of the stroke to the time of testing.

Unilateral neglect, then, has multiple components. When the most clinically obvious components resolve, the patient may seem cured, but many patients have lingering impairments. For example, early after a right hemisphere stroke, patients show a strong and consistent rightward attentional bias in addition to an inability to reorient their attention leftward.[214] Twelve months later, the attentional bias continues, but they can fully reorient to left hemispace when they perform line bisection and cancellation tasks.

Interventions. The choice of interventions can be based upon the theory of unilateral spatial neglect to which the rehabilitation team ascribes.[134] For example, a therapist can manage the patient as if the underaroused right hemisphere has difficulty in processing sensory inputs. A powerful bias of the left hemisphere for attention to contralateral space can lead to an imbalance after right brain injury, requiring other strategies of therapy. Selective inability to disengage from inputs from ipsilateral space may need to be addressed. Other strategies may need to be developed if the mental representation of contralesional space has been degraded or if a unilateral impairment in the activation of motor programs delays or prevents the intention to move to the contralesional side. Multiple neurocognitive mechanisms probably interact to cause neglect. Approaches to treatment can try to distinguish among and to combine several putative mechanisms, then move to another mechanism if the initial theory-based intervention is not successful.

Certain strategies have been studied that aim to remediate hemi-inattentional phenomena during stroke rehabilitation (Table 7–15). One of the traditional inpatient approaches has been to orient the bed so that the patient's neglected hemispace is toward the entrance to the room or a visitor's seat. This orientation may draw the patient's visual search into that field. A study that compared bed orientation toward and away from the field showed no difference in functional outcome.[207] No single, isolated strategy is likely to improve visual tracking toward neglected hemispace, however.

Gordon, Diller, and their colleagues designed a program at New York University to treat visuoperceptual disorders after a right brain injury.[121] Therapists trained patients

visually to scan from left to right by providing an anchoring target on the left. A red ribbon to the left of the meal tray or margin of a magazine served as the cue that the patient sought. Other techniques included gradually decreasing the density of the stimuli used to draw attention to left hemispace and pacing the tracking of visual patterns. In addition, patients were treated for deficits in sensory awareness and spatial organization by receiving feedback on the position of tactile stimuli to their backs and by visually estimating the size of rods. More complex visuoperceptual impairments were managed by engaging patients in tasks that required them to organize and sequentially analyze spatial information, partly by verbalizing what they saw as they scanned from left to right. Although patients improved in the tests for left inattention during inpatient care, a control group reached a similar level of gains on the training tasks 4 months after discharge. In addition, the gains did not generalize to real-world tasks.

In a study of 32 patients randomly allocated to conventional occupational therapy or to a program of perceptual training such as the New York University protocol, no functional differences were found.[201] Patients tended to improve with both techniques. Variations on this remediation approach have revealed gains in spontaneous exploration of the environs in some studies of chronic hemineglect.[256]

In a single-case design carried out with tasks related to ADLs instead of only paper-and-pencil and reading activities, gains in visuospatial attention, visuoconstruction, and ADLs, but not in visual memory, were achieved with a therapy program that began 8 months after a stroke.[138] The patient had suffered a posterior cerebral artery occlusion and thalamo-occipital infarction seen on an MRI scan (Fig. 7–2A). Therapists established effective external visual and verbal cues, and the patient verbalized strategies appropriate to a variety of settings. Then the cues were gradually withdrawn. Improvement occurred despite right hemisphere hypometabolism on a 2-deoxyglucose PET scan (Fig. 7–2B). Some of the effectiveness may also have been related to training that increased incorporation of movements of the patient's anesthetic but only moderately pa-

Table 7–15. **INTERVENTIONS FOR HEMINEGLECT**

Multisensory cues, then fading cues
Verbal elaboration of visual analysis
Environmental adaptations
Videotape and view activities of daily living
Computer training
Left limb movement in left hemispace
Hemibody sensorimotor stimulation
Head and trunk midline adjustments
Vestibular stimulation
Pharmacotherapy
Prism glasses

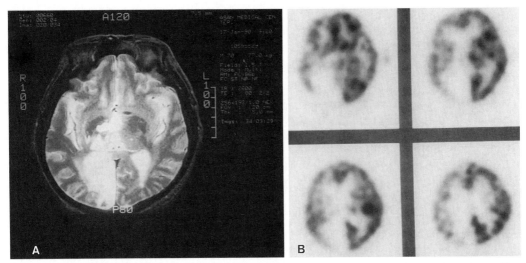

Figure 7–2. (A) T$_2$-weighted magnetic resonance imaging (MRI) scan performed 8 months after the patient suffered an occlusion of the right posterior cerebral artery, causing a persistent left hemianesthesia, hemianopia, hemineglect, and mild hemiparesis. The infarction includes the mesial occipital lobe, the thalamus, and a portion of the posterior limb of the internal capsule.

(B) A positron emission tomography (PET) scan performed at the same poststroke interval with^{18}F fluorodeoxyglucose reveals the areas of infarction (no metabolic activity) along with global transsynaptic hypometabolism of the uninjured right hemisphere.

retic left arm. In another study, left arm and hand movements seemed to activate a spatial reference system and enhance attention to peripersonal space on the left.[272] The midline of the trunk may also serve as a physical anchor for the calculation of the position of external objects in relation to the body.[178] This phenomenon can also be used in orientation strategies; however, some patients with hemineglect use an environmental rather than a body-centered frame of reference.[218] Perceptual remediation approaches may need modification to include greater functional task specificity and perhaps increased interaction with the affected hemibody if they are to lead to associated functional gains.

Many training devices, particularly computers, have been used to try to decrease visual neglect. A randomized trial of microcomputer-based scanning and attentional tasks showed no benefit.[271] One study attempted to retrain visual searching to the left hemienvironment by providing audio-feedback from eye movement–recording glasses whenever patients failed to look to the left for 15 seconds.[200] Although some patients increased their spontaneous scanning, other tests showed no change in left hemi-inattention. An electronic apparatus that flashed a fixation point and a stimulus point at another position on a screen was designed to train saccadic and exploratory eye movements.[258] It did improve visual exploration during the test but did not reduce the size of the hemianopic field as the investigators had hoped.

Therapeutic strategies for visual field impairments are often attached to strategies for visual hemi-inattention. Some proposed interventions reduce hemianopic defects that arise without visual neglect. This approach has been driven, in part, by the finding that spontaneous recovery of visual field defects has been reported in fewer than 20 percent of patients within 3 months of stroke.[369] One compensatory procedure has systematically trained ocular saccadic scanning within the scotoma on a computer screen and in daily activities.[182] This procedure has led to an increase in the field of search by a mean of 30 degrees, has reduced the size of the scotoma in some patients, and has led to a transfer of the gains to some relevant ADL functions.

Related strategies have been proposed to identify and to enhance aspects of visual perception, both conscious and unconscious, in the affected hemianopic field, based on studies of the phenomenon of blindsight.[52] Some instances of blindsight probably involve sparing of a portion of the visual cortices (see Chapter 1).

Another approach needs more study and perhaps may benefit from better materials. A randomized trial with 15-diopter Fresnel prisms applied over the affected hemifield to shift a peripheral image toward the central retinal meridian improved scores on standard tests of visuoperception, but results did not generalize to improvement in ADLs and mobility over 4 weeks of inpatient use.[280] The prisms may have drawn attention to the neglected visual field by bringing images to the fore. Tabletop activities, such as finding food on a tray, may be expected to improve.

Transient, moving visual stimuli may activate the superior colliculus on a hemianopic side and draw attention to that hemispace. Data suggest that hemispatial neglect can arise from disinhibition of orienting mechanisms of the intact side of the brain[186] or from inhibition of the superior colliculus on the hemianopic side by the contralateral colliculus.[307] These concepts provided a rationale for other therapeutic strategies. The eye ipsilateral to the right cerebral infarct was patched or visual stimuli were presented in the left field during a line bisection task.[40] Both procedures improve the results of tests of left attention.

Vestibular stimulation with cold in the left ear or with warmth in the right ear to evoke a slow phase of nystagmus and pastpointing to the left produced transient improvement in tests of left neglect.[285] Similar transient improvements have been reported not only in neglect, but in other associated signs, including somatophrenia, anosognosia, and sensory and motor deficits.[277,336] Stimulation of subcortical structures that play a role in attentional pathways may be the mechanism that caused these surprising findings. Vestibular input may also change the perception of the midline of peripersonal space. The findings suggest that one mechanism of spatial neglect is related to a defect in systems that combine visual and vestibular information for spatial orientation.[218] These sensory inputs are probably integrated in the inferior parietal lobule. Vestibular studies need replication. One approach would be to incorporate a more lasting vestibular stimulus, such as electrical stimulation over the mastoid process.[224]

The dopamine agonist, bromocriptine, reduced signs of neglect during cancellation tasks in two patients with chronic stroke. The visual inattention recurred after its withdrawal. The drug has benefited some patients after traumatic injuries.[105,216] Much larger studies are needed to determine which neurotransmitters may modulate the pathways for attention.

MEMORY DISTURBANCES

Recall of recent events can become impaired after a stroke. Wade and colleagues followed a community cohort of 138 3-month survivors of stroke who were not too confused or aphasic to participate. This restriction eliminated 50 of their initial patients. Using the Wechsler Memory Scale subtests, these investigators found no difference in immediate digit span recall when patients were compared with age-matched healthy persons.[343] Abnormally low scores were found in 29 percent on the immediate recall of a story on the Logical Memory Test, however, as well as in 39 percent on drawing four shapes recently presented, a visual memory test. Delayed recall at 30 minutes correlated with immediate recall impairments. Significant improvements were made in these two tests by 6 months after the stroke. Poor visual recall or some related cognitive ability not directly assessed, such as visuoperception, has been associated with poor performance of ADLs. The Oxfordshire Stroke Project found that 14 percent of 328 long-term survivors of stroke were severely impaired on the Rivermead Behavioral Memory Test at a mean of 4 years after their stroke.[64] None of the control group scored as poorly.

Specific disorders in memory have been related to the location of the infarction. For example, left cerebral lesions tend to affect verbal recall, whereas right-sided lesions can diminish visual memory.[330] The number and location of subcortical ischemic lesions found on computed tomography (CT) scan have been associated with poorer scores on neuropsychologic tests.[51] Impairments of visuospatial function and concentration were significantly related to the number of small lesions (an average of three). Periventricular lucencies and ventricular enlargement were related to impaired performance on tests that depended on memory and language. Bilateral posterior cerebral artery infarctions that damage the hippocampus or its immediate connections can produce anterograde amnesia. Anterograde and sometimes lesser retrograde amnesia with confabulation can follow the rupture of an anterior communicating artery aneurysm, along with a wide range of other cognitive impairments.[58] Irle and colleagues found severe mnemonic impairments when inferior and medial frontal lesions included more than 1 cm of the head of the caudate nucleus, extended into the anterior limb of the internal capsule, and damaged the cholinergic cells of the diagonal band of Broca, the substantia innominata, and the ventral striatum.[161]

Bromocriptine improved learning by enhancing the ability to make verbal associations after a confined mediobasal forebrain injury in one patient.[78] Other impairments from limited lesions that selectively interfere with a particular neurotransmitter projection may partially respond to drug interventions. Remediation is usually limited to aids such as calendars, notebooks, visual imagery, and a supportive milieu (see Chapter 9).

DEMENTIA

In a cohort followed after hospitalization for stroke, 26 percent over the age of 60 years had dementia, one-half related to stroke alone and another one-third related to stroke plus Alzheimer's disease.[319] Although clinical criteria for the diagnosis are controversial, 20 to 30 percent of cases of dementia are probably due to multiple infarcts, and another 15 percent of cases probably occur in combination with the degenerative findings of Alzheimer's disease.[38,240] Vascular disease contributed to 25 percent of cases of dementia in an autopsy series.[329] Risk factors for vascular dementia include hypertension, advanced age, and fewer years of education.[319] MRI and cerebral metabolic imaging studies can help detect the tissue

damage that contributes to impairments. Recognition of a mild dementia by the rehabilitation team should lead to the primary available interventions, which include education about the impairments, external reminders, and psychosocial support.

AFFECTIVE DISORDERS

Mood disturbances are common after a stroke.[276] Not only are they the consequence of the uncertainty and bereavement that may accompany the abrupt onset of disability, but also neuroanatomic and neurochemical alterations play a role.

Incidence. Reports suggest a prevalence of depression in 25 to 50 percent of patients from 3 weeks to 1 year after a stroke.[99,275,346] The community-based Framingham Study gave most of its 6-month survivors of stroke the Center for Epidemiologic Studies Depression Scale.[362] Depression was found in 47 percent of patients, as well as in 25 percent of age-matched and sex-matched controls, with no difference in incidence between those with left-sided and right-sided lesions. In a population-based cohort of Swedish patients with stroke whose mean age was 73 years, the prevalence of major depression was 25 percent at hospital discharge, 30 percent at 3 months post stroke, 16 percent at 1 year, 19 percent at 2 years, and 29 percent at 3 years.[14] A left anterior infarct, dysphasia, and living alone helped to predict depression upon hospital discharge. Dependence in ADLs and limited social contacts at 3 months, and few social contacts at 1 and 2 years, contributed to depression. At 3 years, when 25 percent of the cohort had died, a relationship was evident between cerebral atrophy and depression. Of patients who were depressed before 3 months, 60 percent recovered at the 1-year follow-up. Rates of recovery from early-onset major depression by 1 year after stroke run from 50 to 80 percent in patients from other countries and in other socioeconomic classes.[273,346]

Not all population-based studies have revealed a higher incidence of depression after stroke than expected, however.[154] Moreover, occasional studies have found mood disorders of anxiety and depression in, for example, 45 percent of older rehabilitation inpatients, whether they are in a stroke unit or an orthopedic service.[107]

Differences among studies of depression after stroke arise from factors that include the age of patients and the means by which the mood disorder is identified. Epidemiologic studies show that many of the affective, cognitive, and somatic symptoms of depression appear in 15 percent of community dwellers over the age of 65 years. The prevalence of major depression in late life is approximately 3 percent in the community, and the rate is 13 percent per year in nursing homes.[249] The severity and duration of untreated community-wide depression vary widely. The additive effects of psychosocial and medical problems, physiologic changes with aging, functional disabilities, and other factors that may contribute to depression in the elderly remain uncertain. Rehabilitation specialists especially want to be alert to premorbid affective disorders and frailty, alcohol abuse, inadequate psychosocial supports, and poor socioeconomic status as contributors to depression.

Another confounding problem arises in distinguishing between neurobehavioral sequelae of stroke and the side effects of hospitalization. Some patients with a right cerebral lesion minimize impairments and distress and appear indifferent. This affect can mask depression.[279] Minor and major depression has been detected in patients with anosognosia.[308] Aprosody and nonverbal, vegetative behavior can be mistaken for depressive signs in patients who are not depressed. Many of the somatic and cognitive complaints that suggest depression can, particularly during inpatient hospitalization, reflect treatable problems. For example, a noisy neighbor or shoulder pain can lead to sleep deprivation, fatigue, and poor concentration. Adverse reactions to any centrally acting medication can produce loss of energy, poor appetite, and systemic somatic complaints. Somatic complaints after stroke or after any serious illness are common. In isolation, these complaints do not imply a mood disorder.

Studies of incidence also vary in the timing of the assessment for depression and in the assessment instrument or interview technique used to make a diagnosis. Although many self-rating and examiner-rated scales are sensitive to the presence of depression, particularly in geriatric patients with stroke,[3] a formal interview is best. The diagnosis of a major depressive episode can be made with some confidence if patients meet at least five of the nine criteria in the *Diagnostic and Statistical Manual of Mental Disorders,* fourth edition (*DSM-IV,* American Psychiatric Association), for daily symptoms that last at least 2 weeks and represent a change from previous functioning (Table 7–16).[14] These symptoms must include depressed mood or loss of interest or pleasure. Clinicians may classify patients who are depressed after a stroke as meeting the criteria for *DSM-IV* 293.83, which is Mood Disorder Due to a General Medical Condition (in this instance, to stroke).

Anatomic Correlations. Major depression has been associated with left frontal lobe and basal ganglion infarction. Minor or dysthymic depression tends to accompany left and right posterior lesions.[274] PET studies have also begun to show a relationship between depression and metabolic activity in a left limbic thalamoprefrontal cortical circuit

Table 7–16. *DIAGNOSTIC AND STATISTICAL MANUAL (DSM-IV) CRITERIA FOR MAJOR DEPRESSIVE EPISODE*

Depressed mood most of the day, nearly every day, by subjective report or the observation of others

Loss of interest or pleasure in most activities almost daily

Large change in weight, appetite, or both

Insomnia or hypersomnia nearly daily

Fatigue or loss of energy

Psychomotor retardation or agitation observed by others

Feelings of worthlessness or excessive or inappropriate guilt

Impaired concentration, thinking, or decisiveness

Recurrent thoughts of death or suicide

Source: American Psychiatric Association. *Diagnostic and Statistical Manual of Mental Disorders,* 4th ed. Washington, DC: American Psychiatric Press, 1994, with permission.

that includes the amygdala.[85] The dorsolateral frontal lobe and proximity to the frontal pole have been correlated with the severity of depression. Some studies suggest, however, equal likelihood for major and minor depression in patients with left and right cerebral infarctions.[122] Lesion location may be most influential only early after a stroke. These findings, although not universally corroborated,[300] represent important clinicopathologic correlations for neuropsychiatric research.

Disruption of left frontal noradrenergic, dopaminergic, and serotonergic projections can contribute to depression.[274] Neurotransmitter alterations and compensatory mechanisms, such as upregulation and downregulation of receptors, can help to explain the curative effects of antidepressant medications and the tendency for untreated depression to diminish over time.[273]

A biochemical marker for depression[104] or for patients who may respond to medication[236] has been sought. The dexamethasone suppression test is considered positive if a nighttime dose of 1 mg fails to suppress the next day's 4 PM cortisol level below 5 μg/dL. Among reports using a variety of measures of poststroke depression, the test's sensitivity ranged from 15 to 75 percent. Its specificity varied from 15 to 90 percent.[131] For an individual patient, the test has little meaning.

Anxiety is also common in patients with cortical lesions in studies of stroke-related affective disorders. Mania has been associated with right cerebral lesions, particularly if limbic projections are involved.[310] Apathy was found in about one-quarter of patients within 10 days of a stroke. It was associated with greater cognitive impairment, poorer ADLs, and some cases of major, but not minor, depression.[309]

Treatment. Ratings of depression correlate more closely with function by 3 to 6 months after a stroke than near the onset of a stroke.[14] At 2 years after the onset of stroke, patients with early major and minor untreated depression lagged behind their nondepressed peers in ADLs and language recovery, often even when the depression had resolved earlier.[250] Moreover, patients who suffer with more severe and persistent depression are more severely disabled. For years after a stroke, depression, level of social activities, ADLs, and family stress tend to correlate.[10] These findings suggest that drug therapy, psychosocial interventions, and even electroconvulsive therapy[229] should be considered for patients with major depression. Clinicians should also approach dysthymic depressive symptoms aggressively to optimize gains whenever progress in rehabilitation falls short of expectations.

Drugs including methylphenidate, nortriptyline,[202] trazodone,[263] fluoxetine, and most other antidepressants[104] lessen depression and can improve ADL scores and cognition.[310] For example, a selective serotonin reuptake inhibitor (SSRI), citalopram, was effective within 3 to 6 weeks in 65 percent of patients who had become depressed 7 or more weeks after a stroke, compared with recovery in 15 percent who received a placebo.[7]

Emotional incontinence, with involuntary weeping, grimacing, and laughing, occurs in about 15 percent of patients within the first year after stroke.[153] This pseudobulbar affect, which disturbs most patients, can respond to antidepressants.[296] Drug dosages, especially for the elderly, should be gradually increased. Low dosages may be effective for depression or pseudobulbar emotional incontinence, such as 10 mg of methylphenidate, 10 mg of fluoxetine, or 25 mg to 50 mg of desipramine.

Close clinical monitoring for adverse reactions to the antidepressants is important during inpatient and outpatient rehabilitation. Sedation, insomnia, anticholinergic effects on bowel, bladder, and salivation, orthostatic hypotension, cardiac arrhythmias, anxiety, and extrapyramidal symptoms can be especially deleterious to the elderly patient with stroke.[260] The *serotonin syndrome* can develop within a day after initiating or increasing the dose of any of the tricyclic antidepressants except desipramine, all of the SSRIs, and in combination with medications such as bromocriptine, tryptophan, meperidine, amphetamine, and dextromethorphan.[26] Excess synaptic serotonin and modulation of serotonin's regulation of dopamine in the striatum and hippocampus probably cause the syndrome. Clonus, confusion, and agitation can result. Extrapyramidal features include rigidity, restlessness, movement disorders, and tremors. Autonomic symptoms include shivering, low-grade fever, autonomic instability, nausea, diarrhea, flushing, and sweating. Rhabdomyolysis, coma, and death have been reported as well. Clinically, this syndrome looks like the neuroleptic malignant syndrome that rarely develops about a week after starting or increasing a dopamine receptor blocker.

Sexual Function

Most men and women who have been sexually active experience sexual dysfunction after a stroke.[223] Sexual desire often persists. Subtle premorbid problems associated with diabetes, cardiovascular medications, and vascular disease can be exacerbated by poststroke neural dysfunction, decreased mobility, pain, and new medications. These problems can produce impotence, which is also an age-related disorder that increases beyond an incidence of 25 percent in men over the age of 65 years. Some patients benefit from eliminating or switching drugs, particularly cardiovascular, antispasticity, and antidepressant agents. The patient and spouse can be encouraged to explore different sexual techniques; however, clinical factors may play a lesser role than maladjustments related to psychologic and interpersonal difficulties.[29] Counseling is especially important, for example, for patients who lose self-esteem or fear rejection because the partner is now a caretaker.

Community Reintegration

SOCIAL SUPPORT

Sudden disability from stroke potentially creates havoc, especially for the family of the geriatric patient. All too often, the burden of decision making falls on an elderly spouse or on children who have not been involved in the daily lives of their parent. Social workers who have good rapport with the patient and at least one member of the family can smooth the transition of both patient and family from inpatient to outpatient care. Social workers help to build social ties for the patient and to deal with the organization of needed services, with financial issues, and with adjustment reactions. A randomized trial of 185 patients who were well matched showed that caregiver counseling with problem solving by a social worker led to better patient and family adjustment than classroom education about stroke care. Both approaches were more effective than routine medical and nursing care at 6 and 12 months after a stroke.[95]

ADJUSTMENT

Adjustment of the patient has been related to family functioning. Patients from families that have discussed their emotions and have had good problem-solving and communications skills before the stroke show better adjustment and compliance with treatment, the fewest rehospitalization days, and the greatest independence in ADLs.[94] Some studies have found a decline in the quality of life several years after a stroke, particularly in home and leisure activities. This decline did not always relate to depression or dependence in ADLs.[237]

For the 30 percent of patients with stroke who are under the age of 65 years, a return to employment represents an important aspect of community reintegration. The likelihood of returning to work at about 18 months after a stroke in a Japanese population under the age of 65 years depended on having normal strength and no apraxia.[292] Having a white-collar job tended to promote a return to work over having a blue-collar occupation. Across American and European studies of patients under the age of 60 years who had been working, 30 to 80 percent returned to employment. High BI scores, the absence of aphasia, short inpatient rehabilitation stays, and younger age at onset help to predict this outcome.[24] Most of the patients in these follow-up studies worked fewer hours or modified their activities, however.

To develop interventions that are important to patients and families, rehabilitation specialists need more information about factors that denigrate or improve the quality of life after stroke.

SUMMARY

Impairments and disabilities tend to improve for at least 3 to 6 months after stroke. Inpatient rehabilitation allows patients to have close medical and nursing supervision, heads off complications of immobility and comorbid diseases, and attempts to shift the curve of recovery over time to give more patients greater functional independence. Inpatient rehabilitation is also a time for patient and family adjustment and for education that seeks to reduce the risk factors for recurrent stroke. The goal of the rehabilitation team is to make patients independent enough in mobility, swallowing, and self-care to be able to return home. The team uses outpatient care and, even later, intermittent pulses of therapy to solve ongoing problems that limit home and community activities and quality of life. Many strategies draw upon neuroscientific mechanisms of plasticity, learning theories, and the social sciences. These strategies must take into account the special biologic and psychosocial adaptations of the elderly and the realities of financing health care. Still better strategies, some of which may include replacement of cell lines in gray matter and use of neurotrophic factors to permit the extension of axons through white matter, put to the test by well-designed clinical trials, will place rehabilitation specialists beyond the boundaries of today's "Imaginot Line."

REFERENCES

1. Adams H, Brott T, Crowell R, et al. Guidelines for the management of patients with acute ischemic stroke. Stroke 1994;25:1901–1914.
2. Adelman S. Economic impact. Stroke 1981; 12(Suppl 1):69–78.
3. Agrell B, Dehlin O. Comparison of six depression rating scales in geriatric stroke patients. Stroke 1989;20:1190–1194.
4. Alexander M. Stroke rehabilitation outcome: A potential use of predictive variables to establish levels of care. Stroke 1994;25:128–134.
5. Alexander M, Naeser M, Palumbo C. Broca's area aphasias. Neurology 1990;40:353–362.
6. Alter M, Friday G, Lai S, et al. Hypertension and risk of stroke recurrence. Stroke 1994;25:1605–1610.
7. Andersen G, Vsetergaard K, Lauritzen L. Effective treatment of poststroke depression with the selective serotonin reuptake inhibitor citalopram. Stroke 1994;25:1099–1104.
8. Anderson E, Anderson T, Kottke F. Stroke rehabilitation: Maintenance of achieved goals. Arch Phys Med Rehabil 1977;58:345–352.
9. Andrews K, Brocklehurst J, Richards B, et al. The rate of recovery from stroke and its measurement. International Rehabilitation Medicine 1981; 3:155–161.
10. Angeleri F, Angereri V, Foschi N, et al. The influence of depression, social activity, and family stress on functional outcome after stroke. Stroke 1993; 24:1478–1483.
11. Antiplatelet Trialists' Collaboration. Collaborative overview of randomised trials of antiplatelet therapy. Br Med J 1994;308:81–106.
12. Asberg K, Nydevik I. Early prognosis of stroke outcome by means of Katz index of activities of daily living. Scand J Rehabil Med 1991;23:187–191.
13. Ashburn A, Partridge C, De Souza L. Physiotherapy in the rehabilitation of stroke: A review. Clinical Rehabilitation 1993;7:337–345.
14. Astrom M, Adolfsson R, Asplund K. Major depression in stroke patients: A 3-year longitudinal study. Stroke 1993;24:976–982.
15. Axelsson K. Nutritional status in patients with acute stroke. Acta Medica Scandinavia 1988; 224:217–224.
16. Banks G, Short P, Martinez J, et al. The alien hand syndrome. Arch Neurol 1989;46:456–459.
17. Barer D. The natural history and functional consequences of dysphagia after hemispheric stroke. J Neurol Neurosurg Psychiatry 1989;52:236–241.
18. Barer D, Mitchell J. Predicting the outcome of acute stroke: Do multivariate models help? Q J Med 1989;261:27–39.
19. Barnett H, Eliasziw M, Meldrum H. Drugs and surgery in the prevention of ischemic stroke. N Engl J Med 1995;332:238–248.
20. Basmajian J. Biofeedback for neuromuscular rehabilitation. Crit Rev Phys Rehabil Med 1989;1:37–58.
21. Basmajian J, Gowland C, Finlayson A, et al. Stroke treatment comparison of integrated behavioral therapy vs. traditional physical therapy programs. Arch Phys Med Rehabil 1987;69:401–406.
22. Basso A, Capitani E, Vignolo L. Influence of rehabilitation on language skills in aphasic patients. Arch Neurol 1979;36:190–196.
23. Bate P, Matyas T. Negative transfer of training following brief practice of elbow tracking movements with electromyographic feedback from spastic antagonists. Arch Phys Med Rehabil 1992;73:1050–1058.
24. Black-Schaffer R, Osberg J. Return to work after stroke: Development of a predictive model. Arch Phys Med Rehabil 1990;71:285–290.
25. Bladin C, Johnston P, Smurawska L, et al. What causes seizures after stroke? Stroke 1994;25:245.
26. Bodner R, Lynch T, Lewis L, et al. Serotonin syndrome. Neurology 1995;45:219–223.
27. Bohannon R. Gait performance of hemiparetic

stroke patients: Selected variables. Arch Phys Med Rehabil 1987;68:777–781.

28. Bohannon R, Larkin P, Horton M. Shoulder pain in hemiplegia: Statistical relationship with five variables. Arch Phys Med Rehabil 1986;67:514–516.

29. Boldrini P, Basaglia N, Calanca M. Sexual changes in hemiparetic patients. Arch Phys Med Rehabil 1991;72:202–207.

30. Bonita R, Beaglehole R. Recovery of motor function after stroke. Stroke 1988;19:1497–1500.

31. Borrie M, Campbell A, Caradoc-Davies T, et al. Urinary incontinence after stroke: A prospective study. Age Ageing 1986;15:177–181.

32. Borucki S, Volpe B, Reding M. The effect of age on maintenance of functional gains following stroke rehabilitation. Journal of Neurologic Rehabilitation 1992;6:1–5.

32a. Bowler JV, Wade J, Jones B, et al. Contribution of diaschisis to the clinical deficit in human cerebral infarction. Stroke 1995;26:1000–1006.

33. Brandstater M, deBruin H, Gowland C, et al. Hemiplegic gait: Analysis of temporal variables. Arch Phys Med Rehabil 1983;64:583–587.

34. Brandstater M, Roth E, Siebens H. Venous thromboembolism in stroke. Arch Phys Med Rehabil 1992;73:S379–S391.

35. Braus D, Krauss J, Strobel J. The shoulder-hand syndrome after stroke: A prospective clinical trial. Ann Neurol 1994;36:728–733.

36. Bromfield E, Reding M. Relative risk of deep vein thrombosis or pulmonary embolism post stroke based on ambulatory status. J Neurol Rehab 1988; 2:51–57.

37. Brown D. Bicycle ergometer and electromyographic feedback for treatment of muscle imbalance in patients with spastic hemiparesis. Phys Ther 1987;67:1715–1719.

38. Brust J. Vascular dementia is overdiagnosed. Arch Neurol 1988;45:799–801.

39. Burn J, Dennis M, Bamford J, et al. Long-term risk of recurrent stroke after a first-ever stroke. Stroke 1994;25:333–337.

40. Butter C, Kirsch N. Combined and separate effects of eye patching and visual stimulation on unilateral neglect following stroke. Arch Phys Med Rehabil 1992;73:1133–1139.

41. Carey L, Matyas T, Oke L. Sensory loss in stroke patients: Effective training of tactile and proprioceptive discrimination. Arch Phys Med Rehabil 1993;74:602–611.

42. Carroll D. Quantitative test of upper extremity function. J Chronic Dis 1965;18:474–477.

43. Chalsen G, Fitzpatrick K, Bean S, Reding M. Prevalence of the shoulder-hand pain syndrome in an inpatient rehabilitation population. Journal of Neurologic Rehabilitation 1987;1:137–141.

44. Chen Y, Fang Y. 108 cases of hemiplegia caused by stroke. Acupunct Electrother Res 1990;15:9–17.

45. Chester C, McLaren C. Somatosensory evoked response and recovery from stroke. Arch Phys Med Rehabil 1989;70:520–525.

46. Clarke R, Daly L, Robinson K, et al. Hyperhomocystinemia: An independent risk factor for vascular disease. N Engl J Med 1991;324:1149–1155.

47. Colborne G, Olney S, Griffin M. Feedback of ankle joint angle and soleus electromyography in the re-

habilitation of hemiplegic gait. Arch Phys Med Rehabil 1993;74:1100–1106.

48. Colebatch J, Gandevia S. The distribution of muscular weakness in upper motor neuron lesions affecting the arm. Brain 1989;112:749–763.

49. Collins J, Shaver M, Disher A, et al. Compromising abnormalities of the brachial plexus as displayed by magnetic resonance imaging. Clinical Anatomy 1995;8:1–16.

50. Control CFD. Cerebrovascular disease mortality and Medicare hospitalization, 1980–1990. JAMA 1992;268:858–859.

51. Corbett A, Bennett H, Kos S. Cognitive dysfunction following subcortical infarction. Arch Neurol 1994;51:999–1007.

52. Cowey A, Stoerig P. The neurobiology of blindsight. Trends Neurosci 1991;14:140–145.

53. Cozean C, Pease W, Hubbell S. Biofeedback and functional electric stimulation in stroke rehabilitation. Arch Phys Med Rehab 1988;69:401–405.

54. Crisostomo E, Duncan P, Propst M, et al. Evidence that amphetamine with physical therapy promotes recovery of motor function in stroke patients. Ann Neurol 1988;23:94–97.

55. Crow J, Lincoln N, Nouri F, et al. The effectiveness of EMG biofeedback in the treatment of arm function after stroke. International Disability Studies 1989;11:155–162.

56. D'Agostino R, Wolf P, Belanger A, et al. Stroke risk profile: Adjustment for antihypertensive medication. Stroke 1994;25:40–43.

57. Dam M, Tonin P, Casson S, et al. The effects of long-term rehabilitation therapy on poststroke hemiplegic patients. Stroke 1993;24:1886–1891.

58. Damasio A, Graff-Radford N, Damasio H, et al. Amnesia following basal forebrain lesions. Arch Neurol 1985;42:263–271.

59. Dannenbaum R, Dykes R. Sensory loss in the hand after sensory stroke: Therapeutic rationale. Arch Phys Med Rehabil 1988;69:833–839.

60. David R, Enderby P. Speech therapy for aphasia: Operating a rationed service. Clinical Rehabilitation 1990;4:245–252.

61. David R, Enderby P, Bainton D. Treatment of acquired aphasia: Speech therapists and volunteers compared. J Neurol Neurosurg Psychiatry 1982; 45:957–961.

62. Davies P, Bamford J, Warlow C. Remedial therapy and functional recovery in a total population of first-stroke patients. Int Disabil Studies 1989; 11:40–44.

63. Davis S, Chua M, Lichtenstein M, et al. Cerebral hypoperfusion in stroke prognosis and brain recovery. Stroke 1993;24:1691–1696.

64. Dennis M, Burn J, Sandercock P, et al. Long-term survival after first-ever stroke: The Oxfordshire community stroke project. Stroke 1993;24:796–800.

65. DePippo K, Holas M, Reding M. Validation of the 3-oz water swallow test for aspiration following stroke. Arch Neurol 1992;49:1259–1261.

66. DePippo K, Holas M, Reding M. The Burke Dysphagia Screening Test: Validation of its use in patients with stroke. Arch Phys Med Rehabil 1994; 75:1284–1286.

67. DePippo K, Holas M, Reding M, et al. Dysphagia

therapy following stroke: A controlled trial. Neurology 1994;44:1655–1660.

68. Desmond D, Tatemichi T, Paik M, et al. Risk factors for cerebrovascular disease as correlates of cognitive function in a stroke-free cohort. Arch Neurol 1993;50:162–166.

69. D'Esposito M, McGlinchey-Berroth R, Alexander M, et al. Dissociable cognitive and neural mechanisms of unilateral visual neglect. Neurology 1993; 43:2636–2644.

70. De Weerdt W, Harrison M. The efficacy of electromyographic feedback for stroke patients: A critical review of the main literature. Physiotherapy 1986; 72:108–113.

71. Dickstein R, Hockerman S, Pillar T, et al. Stroke rehabilitation: Three exercise therapy approaches. Phys Ther 1986;66:1233–1238.

72. Dobkin B. Neuromedical complications in stroke patients transferred for rehabilitation before and after DRGs. Journal of Neurologic Rehabilitation 1987;1:3–8.

73. Dobkin B. Focused stroke rehabilitation programs do not improve outcome. Arch Neurol 1989; 46:701–703.

74. Dobkin B. Orthostatic hypotension as a risk factor for symptomatic cerebrovascular disease. Neurology 1989;38:30–34.

75. Dobkin B. The rehabilitation of elderly stroke patients. Clin Geriatr Med 1991;7:507–523.

76. Dobkin B. The economic impact of stroke. Neurology 1995;45(Suppl):S1–S6.

77. Dobkin B, Fowler E, Gregor R. A strategy to train locomotion in patients with chronic hemiplegic stroke. Ann Neurol 1991;30:278.

78. Dobkin B, Hanlon R. Dopamine agonist treatment of antegrade amnesia from a mediobasal forebrain injury. Ann Neurol 1992;33:313–316.

79. Dobkin B, Starkman S. The patient with stroke. In: Herr R, Cydulka R, eds: Emergency Care of the Compromised Patient. Philadelphia: JB Lippincott, 1994:67–78.

80. Dobkin B, Starkman S. Cerebral vascular emergencies. In: Grenvik A, Shoemaker W, eds: Textbook of Critical Care. Philadelphia: WB Saunders, 1995.

81. Dobkin BH. Controversies in neurology: Focused stroke rehabilitation programs do not affect outcome. Arch Neurol 1989;46:701–703.

82. Dombovy M. Stroke: Clinical course and neurophysiologic mechanisms of recovery. Crit Rev Phys Med Rehabil 1991;2:171–188.

83. Dombovy M, Basford J, Whisnant J, et al. Disability and use of rehabilitation services following stroke in Rochester, Minnesota. Stroke 1987;18:830–836.

84. Dominkus M, Griswold W, Jelinck V. Transcranial electrical motor evoked potentials as a prognostic indicator for motor recovery in stroke patients. J Neurol Neurosurg Psychiatry 1990;53:745–780.

85. Drevets W, Videen T, Price J, et al. A functional anatomical study of unipolar depression. J Neurosci 1992;12:3628–3641.

86. Dromerick A, Reding M. Medical and neurological complications during inpatient stroke rehabilitation. Stroke 1994;25:358–361.

87. Duke R, Bloch R, Turpie A, et al. Intravenous heparin for the prevention of stroke progression in acute partial stable stroke: A randomized controlled trial. Ann Intern Med 1986;105:825–828.

88. Duncan P, Goldstein L, Horner R, et al. Similar motor recovery of upper and lower extremities after stroke. Stroke 1994;25:1181–1188.

89. Elliot J. Swallowing disorders in the elderly. Geriatrics 1988;43:95–113.

90. Ellis S, Small M. Denial of illness in stroke. Stroke 1993;24:757–759.

91. Enderby P, Wood V, Wade D, et al. Aphasia after stroke: A detailed study of recovery in the first 3 months. International Rehabilitation Medicine 1987;8:162–165.

92. Ernst E. A review of stroke rehabilitation and physiotherapy. Stroke 1990;21:1081–1085.

93. Essing J, Gersten J, Yarnell P. Light touch thresholds in normal persons and cerebral vascular disease patients. Stroke 1980;11:528–533.

94. Evans R, Bishop D, Matlock A-L, et al. Prestroke family interaction as a predictor of stroke outcome. Arch Phys Med Rehabil 1987;68:508–517.

95. Evans R, Matlock A-L, Bishop D, et al. Family intervention after stroke: Does counseling or education help? Stroke 1988;19:1243–1249.

96. Faghri P, Rodgers M, Glaser R, et al. The effects of functional electrical stimulation on shoulder subluxation, arm function recovery, and shoulder pain in hemiplegic stroke patients. Arch Phys Med Rehabil 1994;75:73–79.

97. Falconer J, Naughton B, Dunlop D, et al. Predicting stroke inpatient rehabilitation outcome using a classification tree approach. Arch Phys Med Rehabil 1994;75:619–625.

98. Faught E, Peters D, Bartolucci A, et al. Seizures after primary intracerebral hemorrhage. Neurology 1989;39:1089–1093.

99. Feibel J, Springer C. Depression and failure to resume social activities after stroke. Arch Phys Med Rehabil 1982;63:276–278.

100. Feigenson J, McCarthy M, Greenberg S, et al. Factors influencing outcome and length of stay in a stroke rehabilitation unit. Stroke 1977;8:651–662.

101. Ferrucci L, Bandinelli S, Guralnik J, et al. Recovery of functional status after stroke: A postrehabilitation follow-up study. Stroke 1993;24:200–205.

102. Fields R. Electromyographically triggered electric muscle stimulation for chronic hemiplegia. Arch Phys Med Rehabil 1987;68:407–414.

103. Finch L, Barbeau H. Hemiplegic gait: New treatment strategies. Physiother Can 1986;38:36–41.

104. Finklestein S, Weintraub R, Karmouz N, et al. Antidepressant drug treatment for poststroke depression: Retrospective study. Arch Phys Med Rehabil 1987;68:772–776.

105. Fleet W, Valenstein E, Watson R, et al. Dopamine agonist therapy for neglect in humans. Neurology 1987;37:1765–1770.

106. Fullerton K, Mackenzie G, Stout R. Prognostic indices in stroke. Q J Med 1988;66:147–162.

107. Galski T, Bruno R, Zorowitz R, et al. Predicting length of stay, functional outcome, and aftercare in the rehabilitation of stroke patients. Stroke 1993;24:1794–1800.

108. Garraway W, Akktar A, Hockey L, et al. Management of acute stroke in the elderly: Follow up of a controlled trial. 1980;2:827–829.

109. Gelber D, Good D, Laven L, et al. Causes of urinary incontinence after acute hemispheric stroke. Stroke 1993;24:378–382.
110. Gelber D, Jozefczyk P, Good D, et al. Urinary retention following acute stroke. Journal of Neurologic Rehabilitation 1994;8:69–74.
111. Gelmers H. Effects of low-dose subcutaneous heparin on the occurrence of deep vein thrombosis in patients with ischemic stroke. Acta Neurol Scand 1980;61:313–318.
112. Gent M, Blakely JA, CATS Group. The Canadian-American Ticlopidine Study in thromboembolic stroke. Lancet 1989;1:1215–1220.
113. Gibson CJ. Patterns of care for stroke survivors. Stroke 1990;21(Suppl II):38–39.
114. Gladman J, Harwood D, Barer D. Predicting the outcome of acute stroke: Prospective evaluation of five multivariate models and comparison with simple methods. J Neurol Neurosurg Psychiatry 1992;55:347–351.
115. Gladman J, Lincoln N, Barer D. A randomised controlled trial of domiciliary and hospital-based rehabilitation for stroke patients after discharge from hospital. J Neurol Neurosurg Psychiatry 1993;56:960–966.
116. Glasser L. Effects of isokinetic training on the rate of movement during ambulation in hemiparetic patients. Phys Ther 1986;66:675–676.
117. Goldberg G, Bloom K. The alien hand sign. Am J Phys Med Rehabil 1990;69:228–238.
118. Goldstein L, Davis J. Physician prescribing patterns following hospital admission for ischemic cerebrovascular disease. Neurology 1988;38:1806–1809.
119. Goldstein LB, Sygen in Acute Stroke Study Investigators. Common drugs may influence motor recovery after stroke. Neurology 1995;45:865–871.
120. Good D, Henkle J, Gelber D, et al. Sleep disordered breathing predicts poor functional outcome one year after stroke. J Neuro Rehab 1994;8:86.
121. Gordon W, Diller L, Lieberman A, et al. Perceptual remediation in patients with right brain damage: A comprehensive program. Arch Phys Med Rehabil 1985;66:353–359.
122. Gordon W, Hibbard M, Ross E, et al. Issues in the diagnosis of post-stroke depression. Rehabilitation Psychology 1991;36:71–87.
123. Gorelick P. Stroke prevention. Stroke 1994;25:220–224.
124. Gott P, Karnaze D, Fisher M. Assessment of median somatosensory evoked potentials in cerebral ischemia. Stroke 1990;21:1167–1171.
125. Granger C, Hamilton B. The Uniform Data System for Medical Rehabilitation report of first admissions for 1991. Am J Phys Med Rehabil 1993;72:33–38.
126. Granger C, Hamilton B. The Uniform Data System for Medical Rehabilitation report of first admissions for 1992. Am J Phys Med Rehabil 1994;73:51–55.
127. Granger C, Hamilton B, Gresham G. The Stroke Rehabilitation Outcome Study. Part 1: General description. Arch Phys Med Rehabil 1988;69:506–509.
128. Granger C, Lewis L, Peters N, et al. Stroke rehabilitation: Analysis of repeated Barthel index measures. Arch Phys Med Rehabil 1979;60:14–17.
129. Gresham GE, Granger CV. Overview: Patient evaluation and treatment program. In: Brandstater ME, Basmajian JV, eds: Stroke Rehabilitation. Baltimore: Williams & Wilkins, 1987:399–405.
130. Gresham GE, Phillips TF, Wolf PA. Epidemiologic profile of long-term stroke disability: The Framingham Study. Arch Phys Med Rehabil 1979;61:487–491.
130a. Gresham GE, Duncan P, Stason W, et al. Post-Stroke Rehabilitation: Assessment, Referral, and Patient Management. Clinical practice guideline, No. 16. Agency for Health Care Policy and Research Pub No. 95–0663, May 1995, Rockville, MD.
131. Grober S, Gordon W, Sliwinski M, et al. Utility of the dexamethasone supression test in the diagnosis of poststroke depression. Arch Phys Med Rehabil 1991;72:1076–1079.
132. Gupta S, Naheedy M, Elias D, et al. Postinfarction seizures. Stroke 1988;19:1477–1481.
133. Halligan P, Marshall J. Left neglect for near but not far space in man. Nature 1991;350:498–500.
134. Halligan P, Marshall J. Spatial neglect: Position papers on theory and practice. Neuropsychological Rehabilitation 1994;4:103–230.
135. Hamdy R, Krishnaswamy G, Cancellaro V, et al. Changes in bone mineral content and density after stroke. Am J Phys Med Rehabil 1993;72:188–191.
136. Hamilton B, Granger, CV. Disability outcomes following inpatient rehabilitation for stroke. Phys Ther 1994;74:494–503.
137. Hammond M, Kraft G, Fitts S. Recruitment and termination of EMG activity in the hemiparetic forearm. Arch Phys Med Rehabil 1988;69:106–110.
138. Hanlon R, Dobkin B. Effects of cognitive rehabilitation following a right thalamic infarct. J Clin Exp Neuropsychol 1992;14:433–447.
139. Hartman J, Landau W. Comparison of formal language therapy with supportive counseling for aphasia due to acute vascular accident. Arch Neurol 1987;44:646–649.
140. Hass WK, Easton JD, Tass Group. A randomized trial comparing ticlopidine hydrochloride with aspirin for the prevention of stroke in high-risk patients. N Engl J Med 1989;321:501–507.
141. Heald A, Bates D, Cartlidge N, et al. Longitudinal study of central motor conduction time following stroke: 2. Central motor conduction measured within 73 h after stroke as a predictor of functional outcome at 12 months. Brain 1993;116:1371–1385.
142. Hecht J. Subscapular nerve block in the painful hemiplegic shoulder. Arch Phys Med Rehabil 1992;73:1036–1039.
143. Heilman K, Valenstein E, Watson R. The neglect syndrome. In: Vinken P, Bruyn G, eds: Handbook of Clinical Neurology. Amsterdam: North-Holland, 1985:153.
144. Heinemann A, Roth E, Cichowski K, et al. Multivariate analysis of improvement and outcome following stroke rehabilitation. Arch Neurol 1987;44:1167–1172.
145. Heiss W-D, Emunds H-G, Herbolz K. Cerebral glucose metabolism as a predictor of rehabilitation after ischemic stroke. Stroke 1993;24:1784–1788.
146. Heiss W-D, Kessler J, Karbe H, et al. Cerebral glucose metabolism as a predictor of recovery from

aphasia in ischemic stroke. Arch Neurol 1993; 50:958–964.

147. Henon H, Godefroy O, Leys D, et al. Early predictors of death and disability after acute cerebral ischemic event. Stroke 1995;26:392–398.

148. Hesse S, Bertelt C, Schaffrin A, et al. Restoration of gait in nonambulatory hemiparetic patients by treadmill training with partial body-weight support. Arch Phys Med Rehabil 1994;75:1087–1093.

148a. Hesse S, Bertelt C, Jahnke M, et al. Treadmill training with partial body weight support compared to physiotherapy in nonambulatory hemiparetic patients. Stroke 1995;26:976–981.

149. Hesse S, Jahnke M, Bertelt C, et al. Gait outcome in ambulatory hemiparetic patients after a 4-week comprehensive rehabilitation program and prognostic factors. Stroke 1994;25:1999–2004.

150. Hier D, Mondlock J, Caplan L. Recovery of behavioral abnormalities after right hemisphere stroke. Neurology 1983;33:337–350.

151. Holas M, DePippo K, Reding M. Aspiration and relative risk of medical complications following stroke. Arch Neurol 1994;51:1051–1053.

152. Holland A, Greenhouse J, Fromm D, et al. Predictors of language restitution following stroke: A multivariate analysis. J Speech Hear Res 1989; 32:232–238.

153. House A, Dennis M, Moridge L, et al. Emotionalism after stroke. Br Med J 1989;298:991–994.

154. House A, Dennis M, Moridge L, et al. Mood disorders in the year after first stroke. Br J Psychiatry 1991;158:83–92.

155. Hull R, Raskob G, Rosenbloom D, et al. Heparin for 5 days as compared with 10 days in the initial treatment of proximal venous thrombosis. N Engl J Med 1990;322:1260–1264.

156. Indredavik B, Bakke F, Solberg R, et al. Benefit of a stroke unit: A randomized controlled trial. Stroke 1991;22:1026–1031.

157. Insura J, Sacks H, Lau T, et al. Drug treatment of hypertension in the elderly: A meta-analysis. Ann Intern Med 1994;121:355–362.

158. Intiso D, Santilli V, Grasso M, et al. Rehabilitation of walking with electromyographic biofeedback in foot-drop after stroke. Stroke 1994; 25:1189–1192.

159. Inuba M, Edberg E, Montgomery J, et al. Effectiveness of functional training, active exercise and resistive exercise for patients with hemiplegia. Phys Ther 1973;53:28–35.

160. Inuba M, Piorkowski M. Ultrasound in treatment of painful shoulders in patients with hemiplegia. Phys Ther 1972;52:737–741.

161. Irle E, Wowra B, Kunert H, et al. Memory disturbances following anterior communicating artery rupture. Ann Neurol 1992;31:473–480.

162. Jebsen R, Griffith E, Long E, et al. Function of the "normal" hand in stroke patients. Arch Phys Med Rehabil 1971;52:170–174.

163. Johansson K, Lingren I, Widner H, et al. Can sensory stimulation improve the functional outcome in stroke patients? Neurology 1993;43:2189–2192.

164. John J. Failure of electrical myofeedback to augment the effects of physiotherapy in stroke. Int J Rehabil Res 1986;9:35–40.

165. Johnson E, McKenzie S, Sievers A. Aspiration pneumonia in stroke. Arch Phys Med Rehabil 1993;74:973–976.

166. Johnston M, Keister M. Early rehabilitation for stroke patients: A new look. Arch Phys Med Rehabil 1984;65:437–441.

167. Jones R, Donaldson I, Parkin P. Impairment and recovery of ipsilateral sensory-motor function following unilateral cerebral infarction. Brain 1989; 112:113–132.

168. Jongbloed L. Prediction of function after stroke: A critical review. Stroke 1986;17:765–776.

169. Jongbloed L, Stacey S, Brighton C. Stroke rehabilitation: Sensorimotor integrative treatment versus functional treatment. Am J Occup Ther 1989; 43:391–397.

170. Jorgensen H, Nakayama H, Raaschou H, et al. Recovery of walking function in stroke patients: The Copenhagen Stroke Study. Arch Phys Med Rehabil 1995;76:27–32.

171. Jorgensen H, Nakayama H, Raaschou H, et al. Outcome and time course of recovery in stroke. Part 1: Outcome. The Copenhagen Stroke Study. Arch Phys Med Rehabil 1995;76:399–405.

172. Jorgensen H, Nakayama H, Raaschou H, et al. Outcome and time course of recovery in stroke. Part II: Time course of recovery. The Copenhagen Stroke Study. Arch Phys Med Rehabil 1995; 76:406–412.

173. Kahn K, Keeler E, Sherwood M, et al. Comparing outcomes of care before and after implementation of the DRG-based Prospective Payment System. JAMA 1990;264:1984–1988.

174. Kalra L. The influence of stroke unit rehabilitation on functional recovery from stroke. Stroke 1994; 25:821–825.

175. Kalra L, Crome P. The role of prognostic scores in targeting stroke rehabilitation in elderly patients. J Am Geriatr Soc 1993;41:396–400.

176. Kalra L, Dale P, Crome P. Improving stroke rehabilitation: A controlled trial. Stroke 1993;24:1462–1467.

176a. Kalra L, Yu G, Wilson K, et al. Medical complications during stroke rehabilitation. Stroke 1995; 26:990–994.

177. Karbe H, Kessler J, Herholz K, et al. Long-term prognosis of poststroke aphasia studied with positron emission tomography. Arch Neurol 1995; 52:186–190.

178. Karnath H, Schenkel P, Fischer B. Trunk orientation as the determining factor of the contralateral deficit in the neglect syndrome and as the physical anchor of the internal representation of body orientation in space. Brain 1991;114:1997–2014.

179. Kawachi I, Colditz G, Stampler M, et al. Smoking cessation and decreased risk of stroke in women. JAMA 1993;269:232–236.

180. Keith R, Cowell K. Time use of stroke patients in three rehabilitation hospitals. Soc Sci Med 1987; 24:529–533.

181. Kelly-Hayes M, Wolf P, Kannel W, et al. Factors influencing survival and the need for institutionalization following stroke: The Framingham Study. Arch Phys Med Rehabil 1988;69:415–419.

182. Kerkhoff G, MunBinger U, Meier E. Neurovisual rehabilitation in cerebral blindness. Arch Neurol 1994;51:474–481.

183. Kertesz A, McCabe P. Recovery patterns and prognosis in aphasia. Brain 1977;100:1–18.

184. Kilpatrick C, Davis S, Hopper J, et al. Early seizures after acute stroke. Arch Neurol 1992;49:509–511.

185. King T. Electromyographic biofeedback treatment in hemiplegia. Crit Rev Phys Rehabil Med 1994; 6:259–272.

186. Kinsbourne M. Mechanisms of unilateral neglect. In: Jennerod M, ed: Neurophysiological and Neuropsychological Aspects of Unilateral Neglect. New York: Elsevier, 1985:69–86.

187. Kraft G, Fitts S, Hammond M. Techniques to improve function of the arm and hand in hemiplegia. Arch Phys Med Rehabil 1992;73:220–227.

188. Kumar R, Mehta A, Chew T. Shoulder pain in hemiplegia: The role of exercise. Am J Phys Med Rehabil 1990;69:205–208.

189. Kushner M, Reivich M, Fieschi C, et al. Metabolic and clinical correlates of acute ischemic infarction. Neurology 1987;37:1103–1110.

190. Landi G, D'Angelo A, Coccardi E, et al. Venous embolism in acute stroke: Prognostic importance of hypercoagulability. Arch Neurol 1992;49:279–283.

191. Langhorne P, Williams B, Gilchrist W, et al. Do stroke units save lives? Lancet 1993;342:395–398.

192. Leandri M, Parodi C, Rigardo S. Comparison of TENS treatments in hemiplegic shoulder pain. Scand J Rehabil Med 1990;22:69–72.

193. Lehmann J, DeLateur B, Fowler R. Stroke: Does rehabilitation affect outcome? Arch Phys Med Rehab 1975;56:375–381.

194. Lehmann J, Condon S, Price R, et al. Gait abnormalities in hemiplegia: Their correction by ankle-foot orthoses. Arch Phys Med Rehabil 1987; 68:763–771.

195. Lemrow N, Adams D, Coffey R, et al. The 50 Most Frequent Diagnosis-Related Groups (DRGs), Diagnoses, and Procedures: Statistics by Hospital Size and Location. Rockville, MD: DHHS Publication No. (PHS) 90–3465, 1990:15.

196. Lendrem W, Lincoln N. Spontaneous recovery of language in patients with aphasia between 4 and 35 weeks after stroke. J Neurol Neurosurg Psychiatry 1985;48:733–738.

197. Libman R, Sacco R, Shi M, et al. Neurologic improvement in pure motor hemiparesis. Neurology 1992;42:1713–1716.

198. Lincoln N, Jones A, Mulley G. Psychological effects of speech therapy. J Psychosom Res 1985;29:467–474.

199. Lincoln N, Mulley G, Jones A, et al. Effectiveness of speech therapy for aphasic stroke patients. Lancet 1984;1:1197–1200.

200. Lincoln N, Sackley C. Biofeedback in stroke rehabilitation. Crit Rev Phys Rehabil Med 1992;4:37–47.

201. Lincoln N, Whitting S, Cockburn J, et al. An evaluation of perceptual training. International Rehabilitation Medicine 1985;7:90–101.

202. Lipsey J, Robinson R. Nortriptyline treatment of poststroke depression. Lancet 1984;1:297–299.

203. Lister M, ed. Contemporary Management of Motor Control Problems: Proceedings of the II Step Conference. Alexandria, VA: Foundation for Physical Therapy, 1991:278.

204. Logemann J, Kahrilas P. Relearning to swallow after stroke: Application of maneuvers and indirect biofeedback. Neurology 1990;40:1136–1138.

205. Logigian M, Samuels M, Falconer J. Clinical exercise trial for stroke patients. Arch Phys Med Rehabil 1983;64:364–367.

206. Lord J, Hall K. Neuromuscular reeducation versus traditional programs for stroke rehabilitation. Arch Phys Med Rehabil 1986;67:88–91.

207. Loverro J, Reding M. Bed orientation and rehabilitation outcome for patients with stroke and hemianopsia or visual neglect. Journal of Neurologic Rehabilitation 1988;2:147–150.

208. Macdonell R, Donnan G, Bladin P. A comparison of somatosensory evoked and motor evoked potentials in stroke. Ann Neurol 1989;25:68–73.

209. Macdonell R, Donnan G, Bladin P. Serial changes in somatosensory evoked potentials following cerebral infarction. Electroencephalogr Clin Neurophysiol 1991;80:276–280.

210. Mader S. Aging and postural hypotension. J Am Geriatr Soc 1989;37:129–137.

211. Marchal G, Serrati C, Baron J, et al. PET imaging of cerebral perfusion and oxygen consumption in acute ischaemic stroke: Relation to outcome. Lancet 1993;341:925–927.

212. Marshall R, Sacco R, Lee S, et al. Hemineglect predicts functional outcome after stroke (abstract). Ann Neurol 1994;36:298.

213. Matchar D, Duncan P. Cost of stroke. Stroke Clinical Updates. National Stroke Association 1994; 5:9–12.

214. Mattingley J, Bradshaw JL, Bradshaw JA, et al. Residual rightward attentional bias after apparent recovery from right hemisphere damage: Implications for a multicomponent model of neglect. J Neurol Neurosurg Psychiatry 1994;57:597–604.

215. McCarthy S, Turner J. Low-dose subcutaneous heparin in the prevention of deep-vein thrombosis and pulmonary emboli following acute stroke. Age Ageing 1986;15:84–88.

216. McNeny R, Zasler N. Neuropharmacologic management of hemi-inattention after brain injury. NeuroRehabilitation 1991;1:72–78.

217. Mellbring G, Strand T, Eriksson S. Venous thromboembolism after cerebral infarction and the prophylactic effect of dextran 40. Acta Medica Scandinavia 1986;220:425–429.

218. Mennemeier M, Chatterjee A, Heilman K. A comparison of the influences of body and environment centred reference frames on neglect. Brain 1994; 117:1013–1021.

219. Merzenich M, Recanzone G, Jenkins W, et al. Adaptive mechanisms in cortical networks underlying cortical contributions to learning and nondeclarative memory. In: Cold Spring Harbor Symposia on Quantitative Biology. Cold Spring Harbor, NY: Cold Spring Harbor Laboratory Press, 1990:873–887.

220. Mesulam M. A cortical network for directed attention and unilateral neglect. Ann Neurol 1981; 10:309–325.

221. Mesulam M-M. Large-scale neurocognitive networks and distributed processing for attention, language, and memory. Ann Neurol 1990;28:597–613.

222. Mohsenin V, Valor R. Sleep apnea in patients with hemispheric stroke. Arch Phys Med Rehabil 1995; 76:71–76.

223. Mongra T, Lawson J, Inglis J. Sexual dysfunction in stroke patients. Arch Phys Med Rehabil 1986; 67:19–22.

224. Moore D, Hoffman L, Honrubia V, et al. Electrically evoked vestibulo-ocular reflex: Normal subjects. Otolaryngology and Head and Neck Surgery 1991;104:219–224.

225. Moreland J, Thomson M. Efficacy of electromyographic biofeedback compared with conventional physical therapy for upper-extremity function in patients following stroke: A research overview and meta-analysis. Phys Ther 1994;74:534–543.

226. Morris M, Matyas T, Bach T, et al. Electrogoniometric feedback: Its effect on genu recurvatum in stroke. Arch Phys Med Rehabil 1992;73:1147–1154.

227. Moskowitz E, Lightbody F, Freitag N. Long-term follow-up of the poststroke patient. Arch Phys Med Rehabil 1972;53:167–172.

228. Moyna C, Lantz L, Solomon B, et al. Continuous passive motion for the prevention of shoulder-hand syndrome post stroke. J Neuro Rehab 1994; 8:87–88.

229. Murray G, Shea V, Conn D. Electroconvulsive therapy for post-stroke depression. J Clin Psychiatry 1986;47:258–260.

230. Murray S, Garraway W, Akhtar A, et al. Communication between home and hospital in the management of acute stroke in the elderly: Results from a controlled trial. Health Bull 1982;40:214–218.

231. Naeser M, Alexander M, Stiassny-Elder D, et al. Acupuncture in the treatment of hand paresis in chronic and acute stroke patients. Clinical Rehabilitation 1994;8:127–141.

232. Naeser M, Gaddie A, Palumbo C, et al. Late recovery of auditory comprehension in global aphasia. Arch Neurol 1990;47:425–432.

233. Naeser M, Helm-Estabrooks N, Haas G, et al. Relationship between lesion extent in 'Wernicke's' area on computed tomographic scan and predicting recovery of comprehension in Wernicke's aphasia. Arch Neurol 1987;44:73–82.

234. Nakamura R. Recovery of gait in hemiparetic stroke patients. In: Shimamura M, Grillner S, Edgerton V, eds: Neurobiological Basis of Human Locomotion. Tokyo: Japan Scientific Societies Press, 1991:425–435.

235. Nakayama H, Jorgensen H, Raaschou H, et al. Recovery of upper extremity function in stroke patients: The Copenhagen Stroke Study. Arch Phys Med Rehabil 1994;75:394–398.

236. Nicholas M, Helm-Estabrooks N, Ward-Lonergan J, et al. Evolution of severe aphasia in the first two years post onset. Arch Phys Med Rehabil 1993; 74:830–836.

237. Niemi M-L, Laaksonen R, Kotila M, et al. Quality of life 4 years after stroke. Stroke 1988;19:1101–1107.

238. Novack T, Haban G, Graham K, et al. Prediction of stroke rehabilitation outcome from psychologic screening. Arch Phys Med Rehabil 1987;68:729–734.

239. Nugent J, Schurr K, Adams R. A dose-response relationship between amount of weight-bearing exercise and walking outcome following cerebrovascular accident. Arch Phys Med Rehabil 1994; 75:399–402.

240. O'Brien M. Vascular dementia is underdiagnosed. Arch Neurol 1988;45:797–798.

241. Oczkowski W, Barreca S. The Functional Independence Measure: Its use to identify rehabilitation needs in stroke survivors. Arch Phys Med Rehabil 1993;74:1291–1294.

242. Oczkowski W, Ginsberg J, Shin A, et al. Venous thromboembolism in patients undergoing rehabilitation for stroke. Arch Phys Med Rehabil 1992; 73:712–716.

243. Odderson I, McKenna B. A model for management of patients with stroke during the acute phase. Stroke 1993;24:1823–1827.

244. Office of Medical Applications Research, National Institutes of Health. Consensus conference: Prevention of venous thrombosis and pulmonary embolism. JAMA 1986;256:744–749.

245. Olney S, Griffin M, Monga T, et al. Work and power in gait of stroke patients. Arch Phys Med Rehabil 1991;72:309–314.

246. Olsen T. Arm and leg paresis as outcome predictors in stroke rehabilitation. Stroke 1990;21:247–251.

247. Osberg J, Haley S, McGinnis G, et al. Characteristics of cost outliers who did not benefit from stroke rehabilitation. Am J Phys Med Rehabil 1990; 69:117–125.

248. Ottenbacher K, Jannell S. The results of clinical trials in stroke rehabilitation research. Arch Neurol 1993;50:37–44.

249. Panel NCD. Diagnosis and treatment of depression in late life. JAMA 1992;268:1018–1024.

250. Parikh R, Robinson R, Lipsey J, et al. The impact of poststroke depression on recovery of activities of daily living over a 2-year follow-up. Stroke 1990; 47:785–789.

251. Parker V, Wade D, Langton-Hewer R. Loss of arm function after stroke: Measurement, frequency and recovery. International Rehabilitation Medicine 1986;8:69–74.

252. Partinen M, Palomaki H. Snoring and cerebral infarction. Lancet 1985;1:1325–1326.

253. Pavlides C, Miyashita E, Asanuma H. Projection from the sensory to the motor cortex is important in learning motor skills in the monkey. J Neurophysiol 1993;70:733–741.

254. Pavot A, Ignacia D, Kutavanish A, et al. Prognostic value of somatosensory evoked potentials in cerebrovascular accidents. Electromyogr Clin Neurophysiol 1986;26:333–340.

254a. Perry J, Garrett M, Gromley J, et al. Classification of walking handicap in the stroke population. Stroke 1995;26:982–989.

255. Pilgrim J. Low blood pressure, low mood? Br Med J 1992;304:75–78.

256. Pizzamiglio L, Antonucci G, Judica A, et al. Chronic rehabilitation of the hemineglect disorder in chronic patients with unilateral right brain damage. Journal of Clinical and Experimental Neuropsychology 1992;14:901–923.

257. Poduri K. Shoulder pain in stroke patients and its

effects on rehabilitation. Journal of Stroke and Cerebrovascular Diseases 1993;3:261–266.

258. Pommerenke K, Markowitsch H. Rehabilitation training of homonymous visual field defects in patients with postgeniculate damage of the visual system. Restorative Neurology and Neuroscience 1989;1:47–63.

259. Posner M, Peterson S. The attention system of the human brain. Annu Rev Neurosci 1990;13:25–42.

260. Potter W, Rudorfer M, Manji H. The pharmacologic treatment of depression. N Engl J Med 1991;325:633–642.

261. Prinz P, Vitiello M, Raskind M, et al. Geriatrics: Sleep disorders and aging. N Engl J Med 1985;323:520–526.

262. Reding M, McDowell F. Focused stroke rehabilitation programs improve outcome. Arch Neurol 1989;46:700–701.

263. Reding M, Orto L, Winter S, et al. Antidepressant therapy after stroke. Arch Neurol 1986;43:763–765.

264. Reding M, Potes E. Rehabilitation outcome following initial unilateral hemispheric stroke: Life table analysis approach. Stroke 1988;19:1354–1364.

265. Reding M, Winter S, Thompson M. Urinary incontinence after unilateral hemispheric stroke. Journal of Neurologic Rehabilitation 1987;1:25–30.

266. Reding MJ, Solomon B, Borucki S. The effect of dextroamphetamine on motor recovery after stroke. Neurology 1995;45(Suppl 4):A222.

267. Reuben D, Siu A. An objective measure of physical function of elderly outpatients. J Am Geriatr Soc 1990;38:1105–1112.

268. Richards C, Malouin F, Wood-Dauphinee S, et al. Task-specific physical therapy for optimization of gait recovery in acute stroke patients. Arch Phys Med Rehabil 1993;74:612–620.

269. Ring H, Mizrahi J. Biomechanical sway measurements in the evaluation of stroke patients. NeuroRehabilitation 1992;2:27–35.

270. Robbins J, Levine R, Maser A, et al. Swallowing after unilateral stroke of the cerebral cortex. Arch Phys Med Rehabil 1993;74:1295–1300.

271. Robertson I, Gray J, Pentland B, et al. Microcomputer-based rehabilitation for unilateral left visual neglect: A randomized controlled trial. Arch Phys Med Rehabil 1990;71:663–668.

272. Robertson I, North N. Spatio-motor cueing in unilateral neglect: The role of hemispace, hand and motor activation. Neuropsychologia 1992;30:553–563.

273. Robinson R, Bolduc M, Price T. Two-year longitudinal study of poststroke mood disorders. Stroke 1987;18:837–843.

274. Robinson R, Kubos K, Starr L, et al. Mood disorders in stroke patients: Importance of location of lesion. Brain 1984;187:81–93.

275. Robinson R, Price T. Post-stroke depressive disorders: A follow up study of 103 outpatients. Stroke 1982;13:635–640.

276. Robinson R, Starkstein S. Current research in affective disorders following stroke. J Neuropsychiatry Clin Neurosci 1990;2:1–14.

277. Rode G, Charles N, Perenin M-T, et al. Partial remission of hemiplegia and somatoparaphrenia through vestibular stimulation in a case of unilateral neglect. Cortex 1992;28:203–208.

278. Rosove M, Brewer P. Therapy for the antiphospholipid antibody syndrome. Ann Intern Med 1992;117:303–308.

279. Ross E, Rush A. Diagnosis and neuroanatomical correlates of depression in brain-damaged patients: Implications for a neurology of depression. Arch Gen Psychiatry 1981;38:1344–1354.

280. Rossi P, Kheyfets S, Reding M. Fresnel prisms improve visual perception in stroke patients with homonymous hemianopia or unilateral visual neglect. Neurology 1990;40:1597–1599.

281. Roth E, Mueller K, Green D. Cardiovascular response to physical therapy in stroke rehabilitation. NeuroRehabilitation 1992;2:7–15.

282. Rowe JW. Health care of the elderly. N Engl J Med 1985;312:827–835.

283. Roy C. Shoulder pain in hemiplegia: A literature review. Clinical Rehabilitation 1988;2:35–44.

284. Roy C, Sands M, Hill L. Shoulder pain in acutely admitted hemiplegia. Clin Rehabil 1994;8:334–340.

285. Rubens A. Caloric stimulation and unilateral visual neglect. Neurology 1985;35:1019–1024.

286. Rubenstein L, Brook R, Dobkin B, et al. When stroke patients can't swallow: How difficulty swallowing and feeding tubes affect outcomes. Journal of the American Geriatric Society, 19 (in press).

287. Rubin R, Gold W, Kelley D, et al. The Cost of Disorders of the Brain. National Foundation for Brain Research, 1992.

288. Ruch T, Fulton J, German W. Sensory discrimination in monkey, chimpanzee and man after lesions of the parietal lobe. Arch Neurol Psychiatry 1938;39:914–918.

289. Rutan G, Hermanson B. Orthostatic hypotension in older patients: The Cardiovascular Health Study. Hypertension 1992;19:508–519.

290. Sacco R. Risk factors and outcomes for ischemic stroke. Neurology 1995;45(Suppl 1):S10–S14.

291. Sacco R, Wolf P, Kannel W, et al. Survival and recurrence following stroke: The Framingham study. Stroke 1982;13:290–296.

292. Saeki S, Ogata H, Okubo T, et al. Return to work after stroke. Stroke 1995;26:399–401.

293. Satta N, Benson S, Reding M, et al. Walking endurance is better than speed or FIM walking subscore for documenting ambulation recovery after stroke. Stroke 1995;26:157.

294. Schleenbaker R, Mainous A. Electromyographic biofeedback for the neuromuscular reeducation of the hemiplegic stroke patient: A meta-analysis. Arch Phys Med Rehabil 1993;74:1301–1304.

295. Selhub J, Jacques P, Bostom A, et al. Association between plasma homocysteine concentrations and extracranial carotid-artery stenosis. N Engl J Med 1995;332:286–291.

296. Seliger G, Hornstein A, Flax J, et al. Fluoxetine improves emotional incontinence. Brain Inj 1991;5:1–4.

297. Shah S, Corones J. Volition following hemiplegia. Arch Phys Med Rehabil 1980;61:523–528.

298. Shahar E, McGovern P, Sprafka J, et al. Improved survival of stroke patients from 1980 to 1990: The Minnesota Heart Survey. Stroke 1994;25:245.

299. Shewan C, Kertesz A. Effects of speech and language treatment on recovery from aphasia. Brain Lang 1984;23:272–299.

299a. Schulman S, Rhedin A-S, Lindmarker P, et al. A comparison of six weeks with six months of oral anticoagulant therapy after a first episode of venous thromboembolism. N Engl J Med 1995; 332:1661–1665.

300. Sinyor D, Jacques P, Kaloupek D, et al. Poststroke depression and lesion location. Brain 1986; 109:537–546.

301. Sioson E. Deep vein thrombosis in stroke patients: An overview. J Stroke Cerebrovasc Dis 1992;2:74–78.

302. Skilbeck C, Wade D, Langton-Hewer R, et al. Recovery after stroke. J Neurol Neurosurg Psychiatry 1983;46:5–8.

303. Smidt G, ed. Gait in Rehabilitation. New York: Churchill Livingstone, 1990:329.

304. Smith D, Goldenberg E, Ashburn A. Remedial therapy after stroke: A randomized controlled trial. Br Med J 1981;282:517–520.

305. Smurawska L, Alexandrov A, Bladin C, et al. Cost of stroke. Stroke 1994;25:271.

306. Sobel E, Alter M, Davinipour Z, et al. Control of hypertension, arrhythmia, and MI 4 months after stroke in a whole population. Neurology 1990; 40(Suppl 1):421.

307. Sprague J. Interaction of cortex and superior colliculus in mediation of visually guided behavior in the cat. Science 1966;153:1544–1547.

308. Starkstein S, Fedoroff J, Price T, et al. Anosognosia in patients with cerebrovascular lesions. Stroke 1992;23:1446–1453.

309. Starkstein S, Fedoroff J, Price T, et al. Apathy following cerebrovascular lesions. Stroke 1993; 24:1625–1630.

310. Starkstein S, Robinson R. Affective disorders and cerebral vascular disease. Br J Psychiatry 1989; 154:170–182.

311. Stern P, McDowell F, Miller J, et al. Effects of facilitation exercise techniques in stroke rehabilitation. Arch Phys Med Rehabil 1970;51:526–531.

312. Stone S, Patel P, Greenwood R. Selection of acute stroke patients for treatment of visual neglect. J Neurol Neurosurg Psychiatry 1993;56:463–466.

313. Stone S, Patel P, Greenwood R, et al. Measuring visual neglect in acute stroke and predicting its recovery: The Visual Neglect Recovery Index. J Neurol Neurosurg Psychiatry 1992;55:431–436.

314. Strand T, Asplund K, Eriksson S, et al. A non-intensive stroke unit reduces functional disability and the need for long term hospitalization. Stroke 1985;17:377–381.

315. Sunderland A, Tinson D, Bradley L, et al. Arm function after stroke. J Neurol Neurosurg Psychiatry 1989;52:1267–1272.

316. Sunderland A, Tinson D, Bradley E, et al. Enhanced physical therapy improves recovery of function after stroke: A randomised controlled trial. J Neurol Neurosurg Psychiatry 1992;55:530–535.

317. Sunderland A, Wade D, Langton-Hewer R. The natural history of visual neglect after stroke. International Disability Studies 1987;9:55–59.

318. Tangeman P, Banaitis D, Williams A. Rehabilitation of chronic stroke patients: Changes in functional performance. Arch Phys Med Rehabil 1990; 71:876–880.

319. Tatemichi T, Desmond D, Mayeux R, et al. Dementia after stroke. Neurology 1992;42:1185–1193.

320. Tatemichi T, Desmond D, Stern Y, et al. Cognitive impairment after stroke: Frequency, patterns, and relationship to functional abilities. J Neurol Neurosurg Psychiatry 1994;57:202–207.

321. Taub E, Miller N, Novack T, et al. Technique to improve chronic motor deficit after stroke. Arch Phys Med Rehabil 1993;74:347–354.

322. Taub N, Wolfe C, Richardson E, et al. Predicting the disability of first-time stroke sufferers at 1 year. Stroke 1994;25:352–357.

323. Taylor D, Ashburn A, Ward C. Asymmetrical trunk posture, unilateral neglect and motor performance following stroke. Clinical Rehabilitation 1994;8:48–53.

324. Teasdale T, Taffet G, Luchi R, et al. Urinary incontinence in a community-residing elderly population. J Am Geriatr Soc 1988;36:600–606.

325. Teasell R. Pain following stroke. Crit Rev Phys Med Rehabil 1992;3:205–217.

326. Tell G, Howard G, McKinney W, et al. Cigarette smoking cessation and extracranial carotid atherosclerosis. JAMA 1989;261:1178–1180.

327. Tinetti M, Speechley M. Prevention of falls among the elderly. N Engl J Med 1989;320:1055–1059.

328. Tinson D. How stroke patients spend their days. International Disability Studies 1989;11:45–49.

329. Tomlinson B, Blessed G, Roth M. Observations on the brains of demented old people. J Neurol Sci 1970;11:205–242.

330. Trahan D, Larrabee G, Quintana J. Visual recognition memory in normal adults and patients with unilateral vascular lesions. J Clin Exp Neuropsychol 1990;12:857–872.

331. Trombly C, Thayer-Nason L, Bliss G, et al. The effectiveness of therapy in improving finger extension in stroke patients. Phys Ther 1986;40:612–617.

332. Turpie A, Gallus A, Beattie W, et al. Prevention of venous thrombosis in patients with intracranial disease by intermittent pneumatic compression of the calf. Neurology 1977;27:435–438.

333. Turpie A, Gent M, Cote R, et al. A low-molecular-weight heparinoid compared with unfractionated heparin in the prevention of deep vein thrombosis in patients with acute ischemic stroke. Ann Intern Med 1992;117:353–357.

334. Turpie A, Hirsh J, Jay R, et al. Double-blind randomised trial of ORG 10172 low-molecular-weight heparinoid in prevention of deep-vein thrombosis in thrombotic stroke. Lancet 1987;1:523–526.

335. Uniform Data Service, Data Management Service. UDS Update. Buffalo, NY: State University of New York at Buffalo, 1993.

336. Vallar G, Sterzi R, Bottini G, et al. Temporary remission of left hemianesthesia after vestibular stimulation: A sensory neglect phenomenon. Cortex 1990;26:123–131.

336a. Visantin M, Korner-Bitensky N, Barbean H, et al.

A new approach to retraining gait following stroke through body weight–supported treadmill stimulation. Presented at World Confederation for Physical Therapy Congress, Washington, DC, June 25–30, 1995.

337. Waagford J, Levangie P, Certo C. Effects of treadmill training on gait in a hemiparetic patient. Phys Ther 1990;70:549–560.

338. Wade D, Collen F, Robb G, et al. Physiotherapy intervention late after stroke and mobility. Br Med J 1992;304:609–613.

339. Wade D, Hewer R. Motor loss and swallowing difficulty after stroke: Frequency, recovery, and prognosis. Acta Neurol Scand 1987;76:50–54.

340. Wade D, Langton-Hewer R. Functional abilities after stroke: Measurement, natural history and prognosis. J Neurol Neurosurg Psychiatry 1987;50:177–182.

341. Wade D, Langton-Hewer R, David R, et al. Aphasia after stroke: Natural history and associated deficits. J Neurol Neurosurg Psychiatry 1986;49:11–16.

342. Wade D, Langton-Hewer R, Wood V. The hemiplegic arm after stroke. J Neurol Neurosurg Psychiatry 1983;46:521–524.

343. Wade D, Parker V, Langton-Hewer R. Memory disturbance after stroke: Frequency and associated losses. International Rehabilitation Medicine 1987;8:60–64.

344. Wade D, Skilbeck C, Bainton D, et al. Controlled trial of a home-care service for acute stroke patients. Lancet 1985;1:323–326.

345. Wade D, Skilbeck C, Langton-Hewer R, et al. Therapy after stroke: Amounts, determinants and effects. International Rehabilitation Medicine 1984;6:105–110.

346. Wade D, Smith J, Legh-Smith J, et al. Depressed mood after stroke: A community study of its frequency. Br J Psychiatry 1987;151:200–206.

347. Wade D, Wood V, Heller A, et al. Walking after stroke. Scand J Rehabil Med 1987;19:25–30.

348. Wade D, Wood V, Langton-Hewer R. Recovery after stroke: The first 3 months. J Neurol Neurosurg Psychiatry 1985;48:7–13.

349. Wagenaar R, Meijer O, Kuik D, et al. The functional recovery of stroke: A comparison between neuro-developmental treatment and the Brunnstrom method. Scand J Rehabil Med 1990;22:1–8.

350. Wanklyn P, Ilsley D, Greenstein, et al. The cold hemiplegic arm. Stroke 1994;25:1765–1770.

351. Warlow C, Ogston D, Douglas A. Deep venous thrombosis of the legs after stroke. Br Med J 1976;1:1178–1183.

352. Waters R, Yakura J. The energy expenditure of normal and pathological gait. Crit Rev Phys Rehabil Med 1989;1:183–209.

353. Watson R, Valenstein E, Day A, et al. Posterior neocortical systems subserving awareness and neglect. Arch Neurol 1994;51:1014–1021.

354. Wei J. Age and the cardiovascular system. N Engl J Med 1992;327:1735–1739.

354a. Weiller C, Isensee C, Rijntjes M, et al. Recovery from Wernicke's aphasia: A positron emission tomographic study. Ann Neurol 1995;37:723–732.

355. Weinmann E, Salzman E. Deep-vein thrombosis. N Engl J Med 1994;331:1630–1641.

356. Weiss L, Alfano A, Bardfeld P, et al. Prognostic value of triple phase bone scanning for Reflex Sympathetic Dystrophy in hemiplegia. Arch Phys Med Rehabil 1993;74:716–719.

357. Werner R, Goldberg G. Clinical applications of evoked potential testing. Crit Rev Phys Rehabil Med 1992;4:105–131.

358. Werner R, Priebe M, Davidoff G. Reflex sympathetic dystrophy syndrome associated with hemiplegia. NeuroRehabilitation 1992;2:16–22.

359. Wertz R, Weiss D, Aten J, et al. Comparison of clinic, home, and deferred language treatment for aphasia. Arch Neurol 1986;43:653–658.

360. Winstein C, Gardner E, McNeal D. Standing balance training: Effect on balance and locomotion in hemiparetic adults. Arch Phys Med Rehabil 1989;70:755–762.

361. Wissel J, Ebersbach G, Gutjahr L, et al. Treating chronic hemiparesis with modified biofeedback. Arch Phys Med Rehabil 1989;70:612–617.

362. Wolf P, Bachman D, Kelly-Hayes M, et al. Stroke and depression in the community: The Framingham Study. Neurology 1990;40(Suppl 1):416.

363. Wolf P, D'Agostino R, Kannel W, et al. Cigarette smoking as a risk factor for stroke. JAMA 1988;259:1025–1029.

364. Wolf S, LeCraw D, Barton L. Comparison of motor copy and targeted biofeedback training techniques for restitution of upper extremity function. Phys Ther 1989;69:719–735.

365. Wolf S, Lecraw D, Barton L, et al. Forced use of hemiplegic upper extremities to reverse the effect of learned nonuse among chronic stroke and head-injured patients. Exp Neurol 1989;104:125–132.

366. Wood-Dauphinee S, Shapiro S, Bass E, et al. A randomized trial of team care following stroke. Stroke 1984;15:864–872.

367. Yekutiel M, Guttman E. A controlled trial of the retraining of the sensory function of the hand in stroke patients. J Neurol Neurosurg Psychiatry 1993;56:241–244.

368. Young J, Forster A. The Bradford community stroke trial: Results at six months. Br Med J 1992;304:1085–1089.

369. Zihl J, von Cramon D. Visual field recovery from scotoma in patients with postgeniculate damage. Brain 1985;108:439–469.

370. Zorowitz RD, Idank D, Ikai T, et al. Shoulder subluxation after stroke: A comparison of four supports. Arch Phys Med Rehabil 1995;76:763–771.

CHAPTER 8

SPINAL CORD INJURY

Spinal cord dysfunction accounts for 6 percent of the first-time admissions for rehabilitation in the Uniform Data System (UDS) for Medical Rehabilitation. About half of these patients have myelopathies from neoplasms, spondylosis, acute disk herniations, and myelitis from many causes. Traumatic spinal cord injury (SCI) accounts for the rest. Emergency medical and surgical services have improved early survival and outcomes for patients with acute traumatic SCI. Several controlled clinical trials of acute pharmacologic interventions have shown modest but significant benefits. Methylprednisolone (30 mg/kg bolus and 5.4 mg/kg per hour for 23 hours) improved strength, if started within 8 hours of SCI, in the second National Acute Spinal Cord Injury Study (NASCIS).[11,12] GM_1 ganglioside also improved function.[60] Other drug interventions found to be useful in animal studies of hypoxic-ischemic injury will also move forward to human efficacy trials during this decade. Drug, implant, and other biologic interventions that affect mechanisms of neuroplasticity (see Chapter 2) are also likely to move toward human trials of their restorative effects.

Long-term medical, rehabilitative, and educational programs have improved longevity and quality of life for persons with SCI. Most of the gains in functional independence and community reintegration continue to be made through improved technologies for assistive devices and efforts to limit environmental handicaps. This chapter emphasizes traumatic SCI, but the discussion is applicable to the problems encountered in the care of patients with other causes of myelopathy.

EPIDEMIOLOGY

Estimates of the prevalence of traumatic SCI in the United States range from 525 to 1124 cases per million population, or about 200,000 survivors.[74] The yearly incidence of hospitalized patients with SCI is about 32 per million or 8000 to 10,000 additional victims each year. Patients with nontraumatic SCI probably equal this incidence.

The 13 facilities that comprise the Model Spinal Cord Injury Systems Program provide useful estimates of demography, complications, and outcomes.[3,140] Their database, called the National Spinal Cord Injury Statistical Center (NSCISC), has pooled data on 9647 patients with traumatic SCI. These subjects survived more than 24 hours after hospital admission or entered within 1 year of an injury sustained between 1973 and 1985. The mean age was 29 years, the most frequently occurring age was 19 years, and males outnumbered females by 4 to 1. The causes of SCI varied with age, race, and economic status. They included motor vehicle accidents (48 percent), falls (21 percent), sports accidents (14 percent), and violent acts (14 percent). For example, young white males were more apt to be injured in vehicular accidents and black males, by acts of violence. More than 90 percent of sports-related SCI resulted in complete or incomplete quadriplegia. Diving, surfing, gymnastics, and football are among the leading causes. Over the past 10 years, gunshot wounds and stabbings have increased as automobile accidents have declined as causes of SCI.

Overall mortality in model systems was 3.6 percent in the first year; it declined to 1.8 percent in the second year and then was about 1 percent per year over the next 10 years.[37] Survival varied, however, especially with age at onset and completeness of the lesion. For example, at the end of 12 years, 95 percent of patients with incomplete paraplegia dating from a mean age of 19 years were alive, but only 72 percent survived from a mean age of 59 years. Younger patients with incomplete quadriplegia had a similar survival, but only 52 percent of older patients with this impairment were still alive. In patients with complete quadriplegia, 87 percent of the younger and only 18 percent of the older group survived 12 years. Life expectancy for these older patients was 10 percent of normal. The most common causes of mortality in the Model Systems cohort were respiratory (21 percent), cardiac (18 percent), septic (9 percent), and ill-defined (8 percent) complications, pulmonary emboli (8 percent), and suicide (6 percent).

FISCAL IMPACT

In 1989 dollars, acute hospitalization and rehabilitation costs at Model Systems sites ranged from $72,000 for incomplete paraplegia to over twice that for complete quadriplegia. Lifetime direct costs were estimated at $210,000 to $275,000 for paraplegia and at $462,000 to $571,000 for incomplete to complete quadriplegia.[3] In a 1983 study of trauma centers in Maryland, the average 1-year costs for SCI care of patients aged 16 to 45 years who required inpatient rehabilitation was $105,000, similar to the costs for care of patients with severe head trauma. Half of those dollars covered initial care, 30 percent went for inpatient rehabilitation, 9 percent for subsequent hospitalizations, and 3 percent for outpatient visits.[104] A gross approximation of the national yearly costs for new SCI cases using Model Systems data for 1989 is $2.5 billion in direct expenses and $3.7 billion in indirect expenses. Indirect costs include caregiver expenses and lost wages. Using national estimates of new cases and existing cases, the yearly initial hospitalization costs in 1991 dollars are $19 billion, and total annual costs of direct care are $3 billion.[130]

Hospital costs can grow quickly. A mean length of stay of 28 days for care of pressure sores in 1994 cost $24,000. About one-third of the patients discharged from Model Systems Program were rehospitalized in the first and second postinjury years. Subsequent readmissions occurred for the next 10 years (through 1986) at 25 percent yearly, for an average stay of 25 days.[35] In recent years, duration of readmission stays has fallen, perhaps by as much as one-third. One prospective study of 87 independently living adults found an average of 1.3 yearly admissions for 17 days, 1.7 emergency room visits, and 22 outpatient telephone or in-person medical contacts.[113] Although no variables predicted hospital admission, the number of days hospitalized was related to greater age, fewer years of education, more days hospitalized in the previous year, and lower self-assessment of health.

Indirect costs related to the value of expected wages in the absence of SCI, minus the actual wages over the remaining work life of the patient, have been estimated. The analysis depends upon the year of the injury, age, race, level of independence in activities of daily living (ADLs) and mobility, education, martial status, employment status at the time of injury, inflation rates, and other variables. In 1992 dollars, Model Systems data estimated that a 25-year-old patient with a C-1 to C-4 lesion and Frankel grade A, B, or C would incur a lifetime indirect cost of $1 million.[38] A patient with a Frankel grade D lesion at any level would lose $680,000.

PATHOPHYSIOLOGY

The neuropathology of SCI offers insights into the types of neurologic deficits that follow spinal cord trauma, the potential for sparing of fiber tracts that could contribute to clinical function, and factors associated with late recovery or decline.

Serious spinal column injuries are usually classified as follows:

1. Flexion with anterior wedging of the vertebral body, especially at the T-12 or L-1 level
2. Flexion dislocation with anterior dislocation, especially at cervical levels
3. Extension with anterior disk rupture, sometimes with anterior spinal artery compromise
4. Axial compression with vertebral body fragmentation and fragment extrusion[85]

Forces that displace the vertebral column also impart compressive forces on the spinal cord and cause concussion, contusion, and sometimes laceration, with partial or complete tissue disruption. Clinically incomplete SCI occurs more often than complete SCI after a fall in patients with cervical spondylosis and after gunshot wounds at any level that do not penetrate the canal. Complete injuries are more frequent after bilateral cervical facet dislocations, flexion-rotation of the thoracolumbar spine, and gunshot wounds that penetrate the canal.[153a]

The earliest visible changes after severe SCI include petechial hemorrhages, edema, and disruption of the parenchyma. Inflammatory responses and a cascade of secondary injury mechanisms, perhaps triggered or perpetuated by calcium ion fluxes into cells, lead to additional autodestruction.[174] By 24 hours, central hemorrhagic myelomalacia is evident over at least several spinal cord segments. Bare axis cylinders are around the lesion, which involves central gray and white matter more than peripheral structures. By 5 days, glial cells replace the macrophages in the necrotic tissue and begin to form a cavity that will be crossed by gliovascular bundles.[85] By 6 months, secondary wallerian degeneration is found in the posterior columns above the lesion and in the descending tracts below it.

Magnetic resonance imaging (MRI) has begun to offer insights into likely spinal cord pathology and may aid in prognostication. In chronic SCI, a low T_1-weighted and high T_2-weighted signal intensity in gray matter points to necrosis and myelomalacia.[120] In patients with quadriplegia with acute SCI, a high-intensity T_1 signal or a low-intensity T_2-weighted image, indicating an intramedullary hemorrhage, directly related to the most severe impairments.[106] All 15 patients in this study had motor complete lesions, whereas the 9 patients without hemorrhages had incomplete lesions. Improvement in Frankel grade and in muscle strength was far more likely in patients without a hemorrhage at 1-year follow-up. MRI can also visualize spinal cord transection.

Tissue sparing or regeneration is, of

course, central to any possibility of significant recovery of function. Although nerve root atrophy at the level of central gray matter necrosis accompanies the chronic injury, regeneration of anterior and posterior roots, as in a posttraumatic neuroma, often develops. In addition, ascending and descending fiber tracts are found in the walls of the central cavity. Thus, the milieu of a contusion supports some morphologic neuroplasticity. Fetal tissue transplants have been used to fill these cavities in rats and cats and appear to permit still greater inductive processes.[127] Implants, combined with other axonal growth strategies, then, may augment spared tissue (see Chapter 2).

The extent of anatomic and physiologic sparing has been evaluated in several additional ways. Most studies of SCI pathology reveals a central spinal cord syndrome at the segmental level of injury. Diffuse axonal disruption and demyelination at cervical levels, however, particularly of the medial dorsal columns, can be more prominent.[16] Animal models of SCI suggest that axonal destruction can be selective under experimental conditions. Greater injury occurs more deeply, relatively sparing axons near the pia mater, and involves larger-diameter myelinated axons.[8] What may be especially important for some recovery is the tendency for propriospinal tracts, an alternate slower-conducting pathway, to remain intact.[2] Spared tracts may not function normally, however.

One autopsy study revealed that 28 percent of 130 patients with SCI who survived for 4 days to 14 years had no sensation or voluntary movement below the lesion but had some anatomic continuity of spinal cord parenchyma across the lesion.[85] These patients may represent clinically discomplete cases in whom more careful neurophysiologic testing may reveal the intact descending influences.[132] Experimental studies show that the conduction properties of axons that project through a lesion can be abnormal; this block prevents recovery, for example, of hindlimb function in a cat model of spinal cord contusion.[7] Of interest, 4-aminopyridine in a related model sometimes improves conduction by its effect on potassium channel blockade.[9]

Although no studies have correlated mor-phologic changes with neurophysiologic and clinical changes in patients, one can anticipate their connection to modulations in reflexes, phantom sensations, spasms, and perhaps to some signs of restitution as the plasticity of spinal circuits evolves. Late neurologic deterioration can occur from disorders related to the initial injury, such as enlarging neuroma, syringomyelia, and spinal stenosis or other degenerative changes of the vertebral column.

SPECIFIC ASSESSMENT AND OUTCOME SCALES

The American Spinal Injury Association's (ASIA) 1992 revision of *Standards for Neurological and Functional Classification of Spinal Cord Injury* has become the most widely used format for categorizing motor and sensory examinations (Fig. 8–1). The motor score does not measure the abdominal muscles, which can act as hip flexors by tilting the pelvis. The sensory scale specifies only pin and light touch. The zone of partial preservation refers to the dermatomes and myotomes caudal to a complete injury that retain partial sensorimotor function. This zone is usually confined to several segments and to the region of the gray matter injury. The ASIA Impairment Scale describes the completeness of the level of injury (Table 8–1). It modifies the commonly used Frankel classification by its emphasis on sacral dermatomal sensation. Commonly used clinical measures of spasticity in SCI studies include the Ashworth Scale, a spasm frequency score,[114] and deep tendon reflex ratings (see Chapter 5).

Studies of outcome after SCI have used a variety of functional assessments. The Modified Barthel Index (MBI), a 100-point scale, is valid, reliable, and sensitive to functional change over time in patients with SCI.[67] ASIA has recommended the Functional Independence Measure (FIM) (see Table 5–9). The MBI and an adaptation of the FIM that eliminates the cognition, communication, and social adjustment subscales correlate well, especially on the self-care subscores.[129]

The Quadriplegia Index of Function has good interobserver reliability and is more

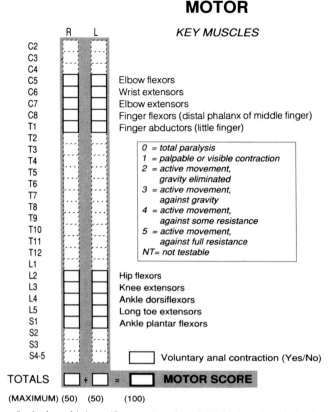

Figure 8–1. Standard neurologic classification of spinal cord injury. (**Source:** American Spinal Injury Association.)

sensitive than the Barthel Index (BI) and Kenny Self-Care Evaluation for small but important functional gains.[70] It includes 10 categories with relative weights for each component activity that add up to a normal score of 100. The Craig Handicap Assessment and Reporting Technique uses a 100-point behavioral scale for each of the dimensions of physical independence, mobility, social integration, vocation, and economic self-sufficiency, in addition to a total score that compares the person with SCI with able-bodied controls.[164]

Health-related quality-of-life (QOL) measures are just beginning to make their way into rehabilitation of SCI. These measures aim to describe how well an individual functions in daily life and to emphasize the patient's preferences for and satisfaction with the patient's own physical, mental, and social well-being and overall health. Until recently, visual analog scale ratings and mea-

sures such as the Life Satisfaction Index have been employed.[53] Chapter 5 describes other potential core measures. Studies that combine measures of impairment, disability, handicap, and QOL might contribute to our understanding of the interrelationships among preinjury variables such as employment, postrehabilitation issues such as family and economic supports, and expected outcomes for subgroups of patients with specific anatomic levels and completeness of SCI.

Impairment scores tend not to change during the rehabilitation of SCI, and impairment-based and disability-based scales do not reliably interconvert.[158] Both scales are needed, along with an assessment of QOL, to describe patients. It is not yet clear which measures are valid indicators of progress or lack of progress in rehabilitation or are measures of the effectiveness of a therapy program.

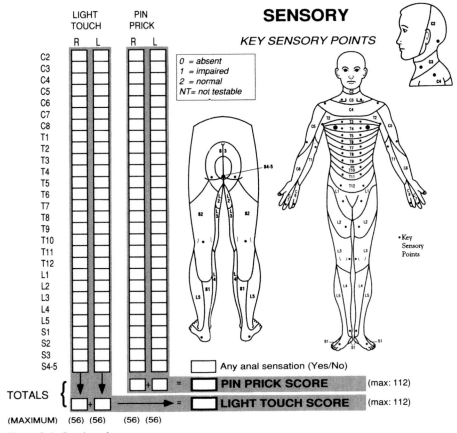

Figure 8–1. Continued.

ACUTE REHABILITATIVE INTERVENTIONS

Mortality and morbidity after SCI first began to fall and functional outcomes began to improve in 1944. This improvement accompanied the creation of specialized programs such as the British National Spinal Cord Injuries Centre at Stoke Mandeville Hospital under Sir Ludwig Guttmann. From 1973 to 1986, the American participants in the Model Systems Program found a 66 percent decrease in the risk of dying within 2 years of a traumatic SCI. These investigators also reported a significant decline in the percentage of patients who required rehospitalization and in the number of days hospitalized in the second year.[36]

Specialty Units

Data from several of the participants in the Model Systems Program in the early 1980s suggest that initial care in a specialized unit for care of acute SCI and early transfer to a spinal rehabilitation inpatient program may shorten total inpatient stays and reduce some medical complications. Patients treated in a unit for acute SCI and then transferred to the inpatient rehabilitation program at the same facility after a mean of 27 days were compared with matched patients who were transferred at a mean of 60 days from a general hospital unit.[76] Both groups were admitted at similar functional levels. The number of pressure sores, long bone fractures, surgical procedures, and internal injuries and the incidence of deep vein thrombosis were similar at the time of

Table 8–1. **AMERICAN SPINAL INJURY ASSOCIATION (ASIA) IMPAIRMENT SCALE**

A = Complete: No motor or sensory function is preserved in the sacral segments S-4–S-5

B = Incomplete: Sensory but not motor function is preserved below the neurologic level and extends through the sacral segments S-4–S-5

C = Incomplete: Motor function is preserved below the neurologic level, and the majority of key muscles below the neurologic level have a muscle grade less than 3

D = Incomplete: Motor function is preserved below the neurologic level, and the majority of key muscles below the neurologic level have a muscle grade greater than or equal to 3

E = Normal: Motor and sensory function is normal

Clinical Syndromes
Central cord
Brown-Séquard
Anterior cord
Conus medullaris
Cauda equina

Source: American Spinal Injury Association.

transfer. Despite the 33-day difference in time from onset of SCI to transfer for rehabilitation, both groups were discharged with similar overall gains. They spent the same amount of time in rehabilitation, a mean of about 70 days for paraplegia and 86 days for quadriplegia. Thus, the specialty unit appeared to offer more efficient care, but not necessarily better medical care. At one specialty center for SCI, the average acute hospitalization time in 1972 of 39 days for patients with nonmultiple trauma and 49 days for patients with multiple trauma declined to only 17 days for both by 1988.[3] Presumably, the expertise of a dedicated center contributed to more efficient care. In another retrospective study, patients with quadriplegia who were transferred to rehabilitation from a specialty trauma unit within 11 days had fewer pressure sores and respiratory complications than patients transferred later, but the complications of the patients with paraplegia did not differ.[119]

Surgical Interventions

Surgical interventions during the acute hospital stay often affect a patient's rehabilitation. The type and timing of decompressive and stabilizing spinal operations have an uncertain relation to preventing additional spinal cord dysfunction, to enhancing recovery, and to affecting length of stay and long-term complications.[48,166,167] Surgery does correct instability, especially in areas at greatest risk, such as the thoracolumbar junction and the lumbar and midcervical regions. It also corrects angulation and displacement deformities. For example, one advantage of operative treatment of a lumbar fracture is to maintain enough of a lumbar lordosis to keep the patient's center of gravity behind the flexion-extension axis of rotation of the hips.[48] This stability assists ambulation with braces.

In the 10 centers that participated in the second NASCIS study of methylprednisolone, which excluded patients with gunshot wounds and children under the age of 13 years, only 13 percent of 487 patients did not have a spinal fracture, a dislocation, or both. In the first 6 weeks after SCI, operative procedures by an anterior approach were performed in 12 percent and posteriorly in 51 percent, with a fusion in 46 percent and internal fixation in 43 percent.[11] A lateral approach for spinal cord decompression, along with a variety of hardware placements that include short and long rods for spinal stabilization, find uses that depend on anatomical and clinical needs.

Immediate care of SCI and early rehabilitation efforts often include the use of external stabilization techniques. Devices include the halo vest and orthoses such as a Philadelphia collar for cervical injuries and a thermoplastic, custom-molded body jacket that gives total thoracolumbar contact and three-point fixation to allow healing after a fracture or operative fusion. Lower extremity fractures, especially of the femur, occur in up to 5 percent of patients with acute SCI and lead to a variety of orthopedic interventions, such as the application of casts and appliances. Plastic jackets and casts that may have to be worn for up to 4 months further limit mobility and increase assistance needed by patients with SCI during their early rehabilitation.

Medical Complications

Early rehabilitation efforts should also include measures to limit acute medical complications. The second NASCIS study revealed similar morbidity rates among its three randomized treatment groups (Table 8–2). Urinary tract infections, pneumonia, and pressure sores led the list.

Patients with cervical and upper thoracic injuries and complete lesions have greater early morbidity than patients with lower spinal or incomplete lesions. Ventilatory dysfunction, aspiration, dysautonomia with upright hypotension or paroxysmal hypertension, neurogenic bowel with impactions, neurogenic bladder with retention and infections, catabolic state, and gastric atony are especially likely to complicate early management. Hypercalciuria and hypercalcemia related to immobilization may also require therapy.[110] Central and musculoskeletal pain, as well as grief reactions, require immediate attention.

Table 8–2. **MEDICAL COMPLICATIONS IN 487 PATIENTS WITHIN 6 WEEKS OF ACUTE SPINAL CORD INJURY**

Complication	Percentage (%)
Urinary tract infection	46
Pneumonia	28
Decubitus ulcer	18
Paralytic ileus	9
Cardiac arrhythmia	6
Sepsis	6
Thrombophlebitis	5
Wound infection	4
Gastrointestinal hemorrhage	3
Pulmonary embolus	3
Congestive heart failure	1

Source: Adapted from Bracken M.[12]

DEEP VEIN THROMBOSIS

The risk of deep vein thrombosis (DVT), detected by a radiolabeled fibrinogen scan, impedance plethysmography, or Doppler blood flow study, appears greatest in the first 2 weeks postinjury and reaches 25 to 100 percent over 12 weeks.[112] Paraplegia and flaccidity cause stasis, and systemic factors add a hypercoagulable state. Symptomatic thrombophlebitis and pulmonary embolism are less common.

In a randomized trial, thromboembolism was detected in 31 percent of patients with Frankel A and B lesions given 5000 units of subcutaneous heparin twice a day within 72 hours of injury. It was detected in only 7 percent of patients whose dose of heparin was adjusted every 12 hours to achieve a partial thromboplastin time of 1.5 times control values.[69] Over the average of 7 weeks of anticoagulation, bleeding complications were greater in the adjusted-dose group, especially at sites of trauma.

Mechanical and other drug interventions have also been of value for prophylaxis. Compared with intermittent heparin alone, studies suggest that the administration of low-molecular-weight heparins,[69a] the administration of a low dose of standard heparin plus electrical stimulation of the calves, or the use of external compression stockings lowered the incidence of positive tests for DVT.[112] Aspirin and external leg compression can also have benefit when heparin is contraindicated. Prophylaxis in the absence of symptoms or systemic medical complications continues for 8 to 12 weeks. The incidence of DVT in persons with chronic SCI is similar to or lower than the incidence in the nonambulatory surgical or medical patient, that is, less than 10 percent for acute and chronic DVT.[88]

RESPIRATORY COMPLICATIONS

Acute SCI carries a high risk of respiratory complications that can affect subsequent rehabilitation. Model Systems Program data found that 67 percent of patients admitted within 48 hours of a C-1 to T-12 SCI developed one or more complications.[83] The completeness of the injury had no clear impact on incidence. With levels of injury at C-1 to C-4, 84 percent were affected, most often with pneumonia (63 percent), ventilatory failure (40 percent), and atelectasis (40 percent). At C-5 to C-8, 60 percent had a complication with atelectasis (34 percent), pneumonia (28 percent), and ventilatory failure (23 percent). At T-1 to T-12, 65 percent had a complication, most often pleural effusion (38 percent), atelectasis (37 percent), and pneumothorax (32 percent). Although ventilatory failure began on average 5 days after SCI, pneumonia occurred on average at 25 days. Management includes standard respiratory prophylactic measures and vigilance, especially upon transfer of the patient for rehabilitation. Overnight oximetry measurements in patients who were extubated or who have cervicothoracic injuries may reveal significant periods of oxygen desaturation.

On occasion, a patient with a high cervical lesion who requires ventilatory support refuses treatment. Although this refusal is a moral and legal right in a competent person, the ethical procedures of informed consent and refusal always create uncertainty and dilemmas. Guidelines for discussion have been proposed.[121] These guidelines emphasize a gradual, supportive process that provides information about long-term psychosocial function after SCI, demonstrates technologic aids, and deals with misconceptions about depression, vocational possibilities, and quality of life.

EFFECT OF EARLY TRANSFER TO REHABILITATION

Figures for the interval from onset of SCI to time of transfer to rehabilitation facilities have varied widely. The UDS database for 1992 reveals certain trends. Its 1719 patients with traumatic SCI had a mean interval of 37 days until transfer, and the 2566 patients with nontraumatic SCI had a mean of 30 days, a figure that represents a fall from 1990 of 7 and 4 days, respectively. Economic pressures are likely to continue to shorten acute inpatient hospitalizations. This change may have a beneficial effect. Shorter intervals between injury and the start of a full rehabilitation program may prevent errors of omission and commission that lead to medical and psychologic complications. On the other hand, greater vigilance for lingering

medical problems will be required by rehabilitation specialists. Shorter hospital stays also mean that rehabilitation planning with patient and family should start within the first week after hospital admission. This planning includes work with insurers, visits to facilities by family or friends, discussions of short-term training activities and goals, and giving the patient the benefit of an open-ended prognosis.

SENSORIMOTOR CHANGES AFTER PARTIAL AND COMPLETE SPINAL CORD INJURY

Acute surgical and neuromedical interventions are based upon the quest to diminish or reverse sensorimotor impairments. The natural history and the causes of early and late changes in these impairments give clinicians some of the data trends that aid in their discussions with patients and the rehabilitation team.

Early Changes

The second NASCIS study provides some general information about sensorimotor changes over the first year after traumatic SCI.[11,12] The investigators used a motor scale with gradations of 0 to 5 covering 14 unilateral upper and lower extremity nerve root levels. The maximal score denoting normal strength was 70. The mean admission score was 16. Six weeks after entry, patients admitted with complete lesions who received methylprednisolone had increased their motor scores compared with the placebo group by 6.2 versus 1.3 points. At 6 months and 1 year, the difference was a statistically significant 17 versus 12 points. No correlation was attempted between this modest gain in strength and any functional recovery. The evaluation of 29 segments from C-2 to S-5 on a scale of 1 (absent) to 3 (normal) revealed that pinprick improved in 33 percent of patients receiving the drug and in 17 percent of patients receiving placebo by 6 weeks, but nonsignificant changes were found at 6 months and 1 year to pinprick (11 versus 8) and to touch (9 versus 6).

Table 8–3. **CHANGE IN COMPLETENESS OF SPINAL CORD INJURY DURING INPATIENT REHABILITATION**

Frankel Grade	Percentage at Onset (%)	Improved (%)	No Change (%)	Worsened (%)	Percentage at Discharge (%)
A	52	10	90	—	47
B	13	45	50	4	9
C	13	56	41	3	9
D	22	7	91	2	32
E	—	—	—	—	2

Source: Adapted from Stover S.[140]

Model Systems Program data on nearly 5000 patients with traumatic SCI who were admitted within 24 hours to the study show the natural history of recovery in terms of the Frankel grade at acute hospitalization and at discharge from inpatient rehabilitation, a span of about 3 to 4 months.[35] Table 8–3 shows the percentage of patients who improved at least one Frankel grade.

Table 8–4 shows the overall Model Systems Program database of neurologic levels and Frankel grades for 9647 subjects admitted for acute care or rehabilitation within 1 year of injury through 1985.[140] Patients with thoracic lesions tended to have complete sensorimotor impairments and those with lumbosacral levels usually started out with incomplete motor impairments. In this larger and more heterogeneous group, discharge Frankel grades changed from admission in 7 percent of patients with Frankel A

lesions, in 37 percent of patients with B lesions, in 54 percent of patients with C lesions, and in 6 percent of those with D lesions. About 40 percent of the small number of patients with Frankel A lesions who improved reached grade B, and about 30 percent reached grades C and D. Of the patients with Frankel B lesions who improved, about 35 percent reached a C, 50 percent a D, and 0.7 percent recovered. Of those admitted at grade C who improved, most reached a D, and 1.6 percent recovered. Lesser changes were described in a small number of patients for up to 18 months and, rarely, beyond that.

Late Changes

Gains in sensorimotor function at 1 or more years after SCI are unusual and follow several patterns. One study of 69 patients

Table 8–4. **COMPLETE NATIONAL SPINAL CORD INJURY STATISTICAL CENTER DATA FOR DISTRIBUTION OF NEUROLOGIC LEVELS AND FRANKEL GRADES***

Frankel Grade	C-1–C-4 (%)	C-5–C-8 (%)	T-1–T-6 (%)	T-7–T-12 (%)	L-1–L-5 (%)	S-1–S-5 (%)	All Levels (%)
A	45	45	80	66	17	0	51
B	8	14	6	7	7	0	10
C	13	9	4	6	11	4	8
D	34	32	9	20	64	96	30
E	0.2	0.1	0	0.1	0.1	0	1

*N = 9647.
Source: Adapted from Stover S.[140]

found an increase in the Frankel grade in about 35 percent of patients between the first year and the fifth year after injury and deterioration in 12 percent.[126] Between 1-year and 3-year examinations and 3-year and 5-year examinations, these gains were generally from an A to a B or from a D to an E. No specific therapies were used over this time. Sensation did improve in some patients, and, as may be expected, patients with good motor function can continue to improve within the limits of the Frankel scale. No patient with plegia at 1 year subsequently developed any useful motor function, however.

PARAPLEGIA

In a longitudinal investigation, 148 patients who had complete paraplegia at 1 month after SCI were examined again 1 year after injury to detect any change in strength and in sensation to pinprick and light touch.[156] Half were victims of gunshot wounds. The sensory levels in these cases tended to improve by 1 to 3 dermatomes in the first year. No one with an SCI at a neurologic level above T-9 regained any motor function, and 142 remained completely impaired. Of patients with an SCI at a level at or below T-9, 38 percent improved by a mean of about 1 grade of strength in the hip flexors and knee extensors. Of those with an SCI at an initial level at or below T-12, 20 percent regained enough strength in those hip and knee muscles to walk with conventional orthoses and crutches. Six of the patients converted to incomplete SCI more than 4 months after injury, using a sacral sparing definition. Only 2 of the entire group developed ankle or toe movement. Intact lower abdominal muscles early after SCI predicted hip flexor recovery at 1 year. Early hip flexor function anticipated strengthening of the knee extensors. In the second year, a few patients with lesions below T-11 had slight motor improvement. Consistent with studies of recovery of the upper extremities, increases in muscle strength in these patients with complete paraplegia tended to occur in the lowest muscle that had any residual strength and in muscles just below that neurologic level.

The same investigators followed patients with incomplete paraplegia with these analyses.[151] Motor recovery was independent of the level of injury, although patients with SCI at levels above T-12 had less strength at 1 month than those with SCI at levels at or below T-12. Lower extremity ASIA motor scores increased an average of 12 (S.D. 9) points between 1 month and 1 year, with a plateau in motor recovery for most patients occurring at 6 months.

QUADRIPLEGIA

The course of recovery of motor function in the upper extremities in patients with quadriplegia has received increasing attention, because anticipated changes may affect plans for assistive devices and tendon transpositions. Moreover, any new intervention aimed at improving motor activity or functional use of the upper extremities must take into account the mechanisms that underlie late spontaneous improvements.

In a study of 150 patients with acute C-4, C-5, and C-6 Frankel A and B SCI who were followed for 2 years, many patients continued to improve from a grade of less than 3 out of 5 (3/5) strength in an upper extremity group to grade 3/5 or greater, beyond the time of their inpatient rehabilitation.[42] Patients with some motor power in muscles within the zone of partial preservation in the first week after SCI recovered earlier and to a greater degree than did those with muscles graded 0/5. For example, in about 70 to 80 percent of patients with C-4 SCI with some initial biceps (C-5) power and patients with C-5 SCI with any initial wrist extension (C-6), the median grade of strength in those muscles reached 4/5 at 6 months and plateaued at 12 months. Over 90 percent achieved at least 3/5 power within a year, whereas only 45 percent with no initial power improved by 1 year, although 64 percent reached this level by 2 years.

In another group of patients with incomplete tetraplegia, mean upper and lower extremity ASIA motor scores increased between 1 month and 1 year after injury.[152] The rate of recovery rapidly declined over the first 6 months and plateaued. Upper and lower extremity motor scores increased from means of about 13 (S.D. 12) at 1 month to 25 (S.D. 12) at 1 year.

Predictions about sensorimotor recovery in patients with complete tetraplegia may be more reliable 30 days after injury, past the time of acute medical and surgical complications that can interfere with testing. Strength and sensation were examined prospectively using ASIA scales in 61 patients with traumatic SCI during rehabilitation at 1 month, monthly for 6 months, and at 1 year after injury.[150] Six of these patients had conversion to an incomplete SCI by about 2 months to, in one instance, 30 months after injury. Their functional motor recovery was no greater than that of the rest of the cohort, however. Thus, 90 percent have remained completely impaired, with no voluntary movement of a lower extremity. Gains did evolve in the arms and hands. Upper extremity muscles graded 1/5 or 2/5 at 1 month had a 97 percent chance of improving to grade 3/5 by 1 year. Muscles graded 0/5 and located one neurologic level below the most caudal level that had any motor function reached 3/5 or greater strength in 27 percent of cases by 1 year. Only 1 percent achieved this gain in muscles two levels below the lowest voluntarily active muscle, however, and only 4 percent regained any measurable strength. Motor scores increased an average of 8.6 (S.D. 4.7), with the rate of motor recovery rapidly declining by 6 months.

In these patients with quadriplegia, sensation often did not improve in dermatomes that were at the same cervical level as the muscles that improved from 0/5 to at least 3/5 strength. Another study of the recovery of sensation in patients with Frankel A lesions showed that about 80 percent of patients with C-5 to C-8 SCI improved within 3 months at one sensory level to pinprick or touch in the zone of partial preservation.[52]

Mechanisms of Sensorimotor Recovery

The rapid recovery of sensation at one to several levels can be attributed to reversal of a conduction block at the root level, perhaps in concert with overlapping dermatomes.

Rapid motor recovery at the zone of injury or in the zone of partial preservation may arise from reversal of local metabolic dysfunction or of a conduction block in spared central motor pathways and ventral roots. In one study that attempted to assess conduction block, cortical magnetic stimulation of motor-evoked potentials in the first 6 hours after SCI did not provide information about the likelihood of motor recovery in weak muscles near the injury or in paralyzed muscles just below the level of injury.[103] Impaired synchronization of descending excitatory volleys to motoneurons was found 6 weeks after injury in some of the muscles that had recovered. Thus, this technique appears to have little predictive value about recovery. Other biologic mechanisms of motor gains at the level of injury include peripheral sprouting of the motor terminals from intact or metabolically recovered motoneurons and muscle fiber hypertrophy with exercise.

Cortical representational plasticity may also play a role that can be manipulated with drug and physical interventions. For example, cortical magnetic stimulation has enhanced the excitability of motor pathways that target the muscles just rostral to the level of an SCI, which may point to an expansion of the representation to those muscles that includes cortical neurons that had activated muscles below the level. The technique has evoked paresthesias in the anesthetic legs below a thoracic lesion possibly because of a similar mechanism.[23,144] Reorganization has also been suggested in patients with dysesthetic pain below the level of injury. Patients with pain, compared with patients with SCI without pain, and compared with controls, have had better two-point discrimination above the lesion.[137] This finding suggests an increase in the size of the somatosensory cortical areas allotted to the skin, perhaps induced by the constant dysesthetic sensory input. Thus, cortical motor and sensory representations for the muscles and dermatomes around the level of the SCI can reorganize and enlarge their representational maps in a way that may lessen sensorimotor impairment. Task-oriented motor learning paradigms for training may enhance this reorganization (see Chapter 1).

Other tools may provide insights into recovery, as well as predictors for gains. As noted earlier, MRI has begun to add information about the prognosis for sensorimotor recovery beyond what the clinical examination reveals. The combination of sensory-evoked potentials and clinical assessments of pain and joint position sense had some predictive use for motor recovery after cervical SCI in one study.[97] Other investigators found little additional prognostic information from evoked potentials beyond the information offered by the early clinical examination, however.[83a,86] The presence of a sensory-evoked potential from the lower extremity shows dorsal column intactness, but its absence does not provide a measure of confidence about the potential for motor recovery.

Other neurophysiologic tests that could help to determine the completeness and the caudal spread of a lesion would have clinical value. One proposed test battery looks for a discomplete lesion.[132] It examines muscle activity in response to tendon vibration and to activation of muscles below the lesion by reinforcement maneuvers above the lesion and by attempts at voluntary suppression of plantar withdrawal reflexes. The developers of this clinical battery, however, allowed patients to increase their intra-abdominal or intrathoracic pressure during a Jendrassik's maneuver, which was performed by the upper extremities above the cord lesion. The pressure rise may have stimulated afferents below the lesion, causing reflexive EMG activity in the legs that could be misinterpreted as revealing intact pathways descending across the level of injury.

Reinforcement of an H-reflex in an arm and leg muscle by an auditory stimulus offers another approach to determining the presence of intact descending activity.[47] This audiospinal reflex facilitates reticulospinal input to cervical and lumbosacral motoneurons. Thus, testing for reflex modulation may provide information about the intactness of a white matter tract that is important for motor and, especially, locomotor activity.

Electromyography (EMG) may be misleading when one is looking for denervation to try to detect the lowest level of anterior horn neuronal dysfunction. Peripheral nerves are prone to compression, which causes neurogenic findings in associated muscles. Moreover, fibrillation potentials and positive sharp waves have been reported in lower extremity muscles on EMG examination in the first few months after complete cervical SCI.[18] By 1 year, this spontaneous activity was found in more distal muscles and tended to disappear in muscle groups with hypertonicity. This proximal-to-distal gradient was also described after stroke with hemiplegia. It may be related to the loss of a trophic influence on lower motoneurons disconnected from the upper motoneuron.

FUNCTIONAL OUTCOMES

Self-Care Skills

In prospective and retrospective reports of functional outcomes, patients with acute SCI generally improve between onset of injury and discharge from inpatient rehabilitation. They tend to maintain or improve their self-care skills and mobility at least over the subsequent several years. The lowest level of intact neurologic motor activity, along with completeness of sensorimotor impairments and age at onset, helps to predict functional capabilities (Table 8–5).

The level of independent or assisted activity achieved with training depends on many interacting factors. These factors include the patient's residual strength and sensation, the ability to substitute muscles such as the shoulder abductors to produce elbow flexion, the limitations imposed by joint immobility and musculoskeletal pain, hypertonicity and spasms, body weight, simple and high-technology assistive devices, recurrent medical complications, psychosocial and vocational supports, the importance of the activity to the individual, and the amount of time and energy it takes to accomplish a task, especially after discharge from inpatient therapy. For example, 10 subjects, ages 11 to 40 years, were tested for independence in dressing 2 to 10 months after rehabilitation for C-6 quadriplegia. All patients were able to perform this task within 1 hour, a common therapy goal.[157] All these patients routinely asked for assistance from an attendant or from the family, however, because dressing took too much time or effort. As in every

Table 8–5. **GENERAL RELATIONSHIPS BETWEEN MOTOR LEVEL AND POTENTIAL FOR FUNCTIONAL SKILLS**

Level of Injury	Feeding	Dressing	Bowel/Bladder Care	Transfers	Wheelchair Rolling	Vehicle Transport	Communication
C-3–C-4: bulbar, diaphragm, neck, and shoulder elevation action	Drinking with straw; coughing	Dependent	Dependent	Dependent; use lift or sliding board	Electric wheelchair, pneumatic or chin control; trunk support, abdominal binder	Dependent	Typing at computer with mouthstick/microswitch; adapted phone; environmental control unit
C-5: shoulder and elbow flexor action	Assisted for setup, hand cuff for utensils	Assisted for arms	Dependent	Assisted with sliding board	Electric wheelchair; manual wheelchair with wheel lugs	Dependent or hand control system	As above
C-6: wrist extension, tenodesis grasp	Independent with universal cuff	Independent for arms	Independent bowel care; assist with self-catherization	Independent with sliding board	Manual wheelchair with lugs	Driving of adapted van	Writing, typing with cuff/devices
C-7: elbow extension, wrist flexion, grasp	Independent	Independent with devices	Independent; mirror use, suppository insertion	Independent by depression lift, except from floor	Manual wheelchair	Independent with hand controls	Independent with devices
C-8: finger flexion and extension T-1: functioning as a paraplegic	Independent	Independent	Independent	Independent on all surfaces	Independent, standard wheel rims	As above	Independent

rehabilitation setting, realistic goals for functioning depend on a patient's motivation and lifestyle choices.

Strength in the upper extremities should be a good predictor of recovery of ADL. Motor scores assessed at 72 hours after injury rather than at 24 hours may be a better predictor of functional outcome.[14] In one study, the Motor Index Score correlated with the Modified Barthel Index (MBI) in patients with quadriplegia at admission and discharge.[96] In patients with paraplegia, the score correlated with the self-care subscores only at discharge.

Functional assessment tools have been used to describe gains after SCI. Using the MBI with 1382 patients, one of the Model Systems Program participants found that scores between admission and discharge improved from 42 to 80 for patients with incomplete paraplegia, from 35 to 71 for patients with complete paraplegia, from 19 to 60 for patients with incomplete quadriplegia, and from 8 to 30 for patients with complete quadriplegia.[173] At 3-year follow-up, at least 86 percent of each group maintained or improved the level of ADL independence for specific skills.[171] Excluding ambulation and stair climbing, nearly all patients with paraplegia had become independent except for bowel and bladder management, of whom about 20 percent required assistance. For patients with incomplete quadriplegia, functional skills were independent in 50 to 70 percent. For patients with complete quadriplegia, the various skills were accomplished independently in 10 to 25 percent.

Independence in ADLs was inversely related to increasing age in one study. Across all Frankel grades and neurologic levels, independence in ADLs at hospital discharge was found in 18 percent of patients younger than 15 years old, in about 37 percent at ages 16 to 45 years, in 15 percent at 46 to 60 years, and only in 8 percent over the age of 60 years.[34]

In 1988, the Model Systems Program database began to collect the FIM at the time of admission and discharge from rehabilitation. In an analysis of 750 patients, the mean score upon admission to rehabilitation was 73 for incomplete paraplegia, 68 for complete paraplegia, 59 for incomplete quadriplegia, and 47 for complete quadriplegia.[35]

The mean length of hospital stay over this period was 92 days for patients with quadriplegia and 75 days for those with paraplegia. The mean gain was about 36 points for all but those with complete quadriplegia, who improved 15 points. Table 8–6 lists the 6 subscores on the FIM for first admissions to rehabilitation taken from the 1992 UDS database of 2566 patients with nontraumatic SCI and 1719 patients with traumatic SCI.[68] These numbers provide some insight into the functional outcomes related to general rehabilitative interventions.

Ambulation

In general, ambulation for exercise becomes a possibility for patients with ASIA A lesions from T-2 to T-10. Physical assistance or guarding is necessary, along with knee-ankle-foot orthoses (KAFOs) and forearm crutches or a walker. In patients with lesions at T-11 to L-2, independent ambulation with KAFOs or ankle-foot orthoses (AFOs) and forearm crutches is possible, but it is often limited to indoor activity and some stair climbing. In patients with lesions at L-3 and below, community ambulation can be independent, with AFOs and forearm crutches or canes. For a given patient during rehabilitation, the ability to ambulate depends upon the completeness of the injury, residual strength, age, motivation, and, for some severely impaired people, the ability to incorporate less commonly used techniques such as functional electrical stimulation.

NATURAL HISTORY OF RECOVERY

Prospective studies of the recovery of ambulation that enter patients soon after acute SCI provide some working prognostic categories that help in discussions and planning with patients and their families.

A prospective study of 157 consecutive patients with SCI who had been admitted through an emergency room demonstrated that 24 percent of patients who initially had quadriplegia and 38 percent of patients with paraplegia were functional ambulators with or without an orthosis 1 year later.[30] About half had complete lesions on admission, and 20 percent of the cohort died by the time of

Table 8–6. **CHANGES IN FUNCTIONAL INDEPENDENCE MEASURE (FIM) SCORES DURING FIRST UNIFORM DATA SERVICE ADMISSION FOR SPINAL CORD INJURY IN 1992**

Mean Subscore	NONTRAUMATIC		TRAUMATIC	
	Admission	Discharge	Admission	Discharge
Self-care	4.0	5.4	3.1	4.8
Sphincter control	3.9	5.2	2.6	4.3
Transfers	2.9	4.7	2.3	4.4
Locomotion	2.0	3.9	2.0	3.7
Communication	6.3	6.5	6.4	6.6
Social cognition	5.8	6.2	5.9	6.4
Mean FIM total	74.2 (S.D. 19)	96.1 (S.D. 22)	65.3 (S.D. 21)	90.4 (S.D. 24)
Median FIM total	75	102	75	98
Mean age (yr)	64 (S.D. 17)		42 (S.D. 20)	
Mean onset, days	30		37	
Length of stay	27 (S.D. 22)		45 (S.D. 39)	
Discharge (%)				
Community	84		82	
Long-term care	8		7	
Short-term care	7		5	

Source: Adapted from Granger C, Hamilton B.[68]

follow-up. The greater their strength and sensation, the more likely it was that ambulation would recover. Using the Frankel Scale to study a series of patients with quadriplegia, 39 percent of those graded Frankel B at 72 hours after SCI and 87 percent of patients graded Frankel C and D with cervical lesions on admission (those who died or were lost to follow-up were excluded) recovered a functional gait.[111] Other studies reveal less favorable outcomes, however.

In a series of 190 patients with complete paraplegia with levels between T-1 and T-10, only 2 to 7 percent evolved partial motor recovery, and only 1 to 3 percent were ambulatory at 1 year.[50] Nine to 29 percent of patients with complete lesions at T-11 to L-1 recovered partial motor function, perhaps because the cauda equina was affected initially. Only 3 percent ambulated, however.

Patients with Frankel B lesions are an especially interesting group to follow. The Model Systems Program database included almost 1000 such patients. Forty percent improved their motor function after admission classification, and 20 percent of the entire

group eventually ambulated. In another study, when 27 patients with SCI were classified within 72 hours of onset as Frankel B, 2 of 18 with intact touch and no pinprick sensation below the lesion recovered reciprocal ambulation for at least 200 feet with or without orthoses and assistive devices; however, 8 of 9 patients with partial or complete pinprick appreciation improved to Frankel D and E and could ambulate.[29] Preserved sacral pinprick sensation in patients with incomplete quadriplegia and paraplegia in the first month after injury also significantly improved the prognosis for lower extremity motor recovery and subsequent ambulation in other studies.[152] Thus, a thorough sensorimotor examination can have predictive value.

STRENGTH AND RECOVERY

The strength of the lower extremities determines the amount of work performed by the upper extremities for support, which, in turn, determines the rate of oxygen consumption and the practicality of ambula-

Table 8–7. **RELATIONSHIP BETWEEN STRENGTH AT 1 MONTH AND PERCENTAGE OF PATIENTS IN EACH IMPAIRMENT GROUP WHO ACHIEVE COMMUNITY AMBULATION 1 YEAR AFTER SPINAL CORD INJURY**

American Spinal Injury Association (Lower Extremity Motor Score)	Complete Paraplegia (%)	Incomplete Paraplegia (%)	Incomplete Tetraplegia (%)
0	<1	33	0
1–9	45	70	21
10–19	—	100	63
20+	—	100	100
Percentage achieving ambulation (%)	5	76	46

Source: Adapted from Waters R, Adkins R, Yakura J, et al.[150]

tion.[155] In a group of patients with SCI-induced quadriplegia and paraparesis, most of whom ambulated with orthoses and assistive devices, gait velocity, oxygen cost per meter walked, and peak axial load placed on assistive devices correlated inversely with lower limb strength. Patients usually became community ambulators when strength reached 60 percent or greater of normal in their hip flexors, abductors, and extensors and in their knee flexors and extensors. These investigators used the Ambulatory Motor Index (AMI), a four-point scale in which 0 is absent movement, 1 is trace or poor, 2 is fair strength or movement against gravity, and 3 is movement against some resistance or normal. Community ambulators had pelvic control with at least a 2 in the hip flexors and a 2 at one knee extensor, so that they needed no more than one KAFO for a reciprocal gait pattern. To provide some perspective as to what effort was required to ambulate, the oxygen cost was about four times higher to walk half as fast as healthy controls, who used 0.15 mL/kg × m. As the AMI fell from a mean of 60 to 31 percent, patients went from requiring no KAFO to needing two, the load on the arms rose from a mean of 14 up to 79 percent, and the oxygen cost rose from a mean of 0.37 to 1.15.

As noted earlier, many studies show that strength is an early predictor of the likelihood of ambulation.[96] A study using the ASIA motor score found that 20 of 23 patients with incomplete tetraplegia who had an ASIA lower extremity motor score (LEMS) of 10 or more (the maximum normal score is 50) at 1 month after injury became community ambulators with crutches and orthoses by 1 year.[152] These patients subsequently achieved relatively effortless community ambulation if the LEMS improved to at least 30. In comparison, scores of 20 or less were associated with limited ambulation at slower average velocities, higher heart rates, greater energy expenditure, and greater peak axial loads on assistive devices.[153] Table 8–7 summarizes some of the contributions from Waters and colleagues on the likelihood of ambulation, based on the ASIA LEMS at 1 month after SCI.[152]

REHABILITATION OUTCOMES

Outcomes for ambulation after SCI vary with the cohort followed. In a study of 866 patients across all ages, Frankel grades, and neurologic levels, about 18 percent were independent in ambulation at the time of discharge from inpatient rehabilitation.[34] In another series of patients with SCI admitted for rehabilitation, about half of the patients with incomplete paraparesis and quadriparesis ambulated 150 feet with assistive equipment at discharge.[168] In a study of 711 patients with acute SCI followed up for 3 years after inpatient rehabilitation, only 10 percent of the patients with incomplete paraparesis and 13 percent of those with quadriparesis were independent enough to ambulate 50 m or to climb stairs, however.[171,172] No patients with complete lesions were independent.

Up to 95 percent of patients with symmetric incomplete quadriplegia from a traumatic central spinal cord syndrome recover functional ambulation between discharge and 1 year after injury, although the rate may fall to half that in patients over the age of 50 years.[124] Older patients often present with chronic cervical spinal stenosis. The initial leg strength is usually better than upper limb strength in patients with a central spinal cord syndrome. With sensory sparing of pinprick appreciation in sacral dermatomes, especially in patients with an anterior spinal cord syndrome, up to 90 percent of patients can ambulate by discharge from rehabilitation.

INTERVENTIONS AND OUTCOMES FOR COMMON FUNCTIONAL PROBLEMS

Mobility

GENERAL STRATEGIES

Inpatient rehabilitation begins with therapies to improve trunk control, endurance for sitting and exercise, autonomic reflexes, and selective strength in normal and paretic muscles. Functional training includes wheelchair mobility, activities to unload pressure points, and sliding board transfers. No randomized trials have compared therapeutic approaches for mobility. In a study of chronic SCI, patients were randomized to 8 to 16 weeks of three common rehabilition strategies: physical exercise therapy, neuromuscular electrical stimulation, and EMG biofeedback.[90] The patients made equal gains in muscle strength below the lesion, in self-care, and in mobility measures that did not include ambulation.

The patient with an incomplete lesion who has 3/5 strength or better at the hip flexors and knee extensors of at least one leg has a good chance to progress in standing

and stepping in the parallel bars with assistance and temporary orthoses. As described previously, residual supraspinal input, as measured by upper and lower extremity strength, the energy cost of locomotion, and the patient's level of conditioning and motivation tend to predict who may become rehabilitated into community ambulation using traditional orthoses and assistive devices. The patient with acute SCI who has any voluntary activity in the hip muscles is the ideal candidate for immediate selective arm and leg strengthening exercises and a conditioning program. This regimen can aid progress toward ambulation and may limit any early regression related to disuse atrophy. For most patients with incomplete quadriplegia and paraplegia, it is probably most cost-efficient to train for standing and stepping during outpatient care.

The rehabilitation team must educate the patient about the longer-term procedures and performance requirements needed to achieve any particular functional level of ambulation. Many people cling to the belief, for at least the first 6 months after a complete SCI, that they will recover and walk. As patients reintegrate into home and community, they can sensibly formulate their needs and desires. Most patients eventually come to rely on their wheelchairs, rather than upon complex orthotics that allow a slow and effortful gait that does not fit into their lifestyle.

The patient can aim for one or, depending on circumstances, a combination of the following levels of activity with assistive devices as needed.[84]

1. *Passive standing only.* Standing may reduce spasticity, prevent contractures, decrease osteoporosis, and improve circulatory reflexes and renal function. Passive standing can be accomplished with adequate truncal control by using a tilt table, a stationary or power standing frame, or a stand-up wheelchair. This type of wheelchair is handy for tasks at home or work. Bilateral KAFOs or hip-KAFOs may also be used.
2. *Short-distance ambulation for exercise only.* This type of ambulation adds the potential for cardiovascular conditioning. Patients at this level usually require help to don an orthosis, to stand up,

and to achieve balance. They may be aided by some variation of a KAFO, including temporary use of an adjustable lower extremity telescopic orthosis (LETOR). The Vannini-Rizzoli Stabilizing Limb Orthosis plantarflexes the foot to stabilize the knee and lets the patient shift weight forward and to the side of the weighted foot to pendulum-swing the unweighted foot.[102] A reciprocating-gait orthosis (RGO) allows some patients with paraplegia to use trunk extension to produce hip flexion in the swing limb for stepping with the support of a walker. A hip-guidance orthosis (HGO) is also a rigid, long leg brace interfaced to a rigid trunk and pelvic structure by low-resistance hip joints. A swivel walker then assists in stepping.

3. *Functional indoor ambulation.* At this level, patients tend to walk at home or at work and to use a wheelchair for longer distances in the community. They are independent in putting on and removing orthoses and in arising from the floor or a chair. The energy cost of walking tends to determine the practicality of activity.

Functional neuromuscular stimulation (FNS), alone or combined with an RGO, HGO, or other assistive and bracing devices, can allow stepping over modest distances.[107,135] Some FNS systems have 48 channels of fine wire electrodes to control the muscles of the trunk, hips, knees, and ankles.[108] A belt-mounted computer controls the sequence, frequency, and intensity of stimulation. Some patients with paraplegia have been able to step on even surfaces for about 1000 m at speeds of up to 1 m per second. Some patients can climb stairs.

Less complex systems place surface or implanted electrodes in the quadriceps muscle to allow the patient to stand up and flex the hip. Depending on the system's design and the patient's strength, the hamstrings, gluteals, and ankle dorsiflexors are stimulated in a sequence for stepping. For example, the custom-designed Louisiana State University's RGO allows a patient with

paraplegia to stand fully balanced for long periods. Locomotion is achieved by simultaneous electrical stimulation of one quadriceps and the contralateral hamstrings to allow the swing of one leg and simultaneous push-off of the contralateral leg.[78] A thumb switch on the walker triggers a four-channel reciprocal stimulator. A lengthy strengthening and fitness program must precede the use of these devices, however.

Devices such as the hybrid systems hold the promise of reducing the energy cost needed for standing up and stepping compared with the use of KAFOs with forearm crutches and a swing-through gait, or bracing with an RGO or HGO, or using FNS alone.[78,81,125] In patients who can stand or who can even take a few steps, simple one- to four-channel FNS systems have not reduced energy costs or increased walking speed to a functionallly useful degree.[138]

The United States Food and Drug Administration approved the Parastep 1 System in 1994. It uses a microcomputer-controlled, battery-powered stimulator that coordinates signals to the peroneal nerve and the quadriceps and gluteal or paraspinal muscles of each leg. In a multicenter trial, 129 patients with paraplegia and incomplete quadriplegia were trained.[20] More than half did not finish. To ambulate a mean of 430 feet required about 35 training sessions over 100 days. A 2-year follow-up of trainees found that 78 percent still used the device at least three times a week for household/distance ambulation. The device requires good upper body strength, finger dexterity, and stamina. Patients should be free of significant cardiopulmonary disease, osteoporosis, and epilepsy. Falls from loss of balance or a power failure could cause serious injury.

4. *Independent community ambulation.* The patient must achieve a low energy cost for walking at a reasonable speed over typical community distances. An FNS, orthotic, or hybrid system for the patient with ASIA A to C thoracic SCI has

yet to be shown to allow practical community mobility. Various systems that require extensive training are marketed to people with SCI. Anecdotal endorsements find their way into advertisements; however, no data yet support the long-term satisfaction and use of these devices or their cost-effectiveness in, for example, the workplace. The minimal goals for designers are a safe and cosmetically acceptable system that permits the patient to arise from the floor, to stand for at least an hour, to step at a velocity in the range of 50 m per minute for at least 1000 m, and to have nonfatiguing mobility on uneven surfaces, ramps, and stairs.

EXPERIMENTAL STRATEGIES FOR STEPPING

As described in Chapter 1, the hindlimbs of adult animals that have undergone thoracic spinal transection can be trained to step on a moving treadmill belt. Using a similar protocol, several groups have demonstrated the feasibility of using body weight–supported treadmill training (BWSTT) to enable some patients with chronic incomplete paraplegia to walk.[5,159]

Up to 50 percent of the body weight of these patients is suspended in a harness connected to an overhead hydraulic lift (Fig. 8–2). The weight support is adjusted so that the knees neither buckle nor hyperextend during stance. Therapists manually assist the legs when needed so patients can step with a pattern that approaches normal on a slowly moving treadmill belt. This intervention can require an assistant for each leg and another to help stabilize the hips and trunk from behind the patient. The aim is to gradually achieve full weight bearing at increasing treadmill velocities. When one or both legs have some voluntary activity, weight support and treadmill speed are adjusted to try to eliminate hip hiking, toe drag, and initial contact with the forefoot rather than a heel strike, as well as other typical spastic paretic gait deviations.

In many cases, sensory inputs enhance the motor output during BWSTT.[43,45] Thigh pinching and electrical stimulation over the dorsum of the foot sometimes increase hip

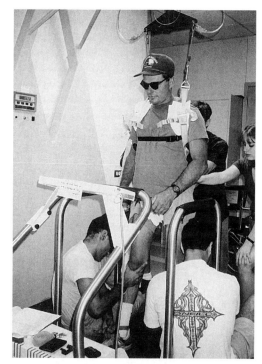

Figure 8–2. A patient with complete spinal cord injury (SCI) undergoing body weight–supported treadmill training (BWSTT) in a suspension apparatus.

flexion when timed to the swing phase. These inputs may activate a motor pattern through spinal flexor reflex afferent pathways. Limb loading, especially at the end of the stance phase when the hip goes into extension, often elicits automatic hip flexion.

Patients who have some residual descending neural input but are able to walk little or not at all can achieve independent BWSTT walking.[6,39,147,160,161] The training has allowed selected patients to walk slowly overground for the first time or to improve the distance and velocity of their walking with assistive devices. The strategy, combined with the 5-HT antagonist cyproheptadine and the alpha-2–nonadrenergic agonist clonidine, improves aspects of stepping.[59] Clinical trials with this strategy are in progress in Canada, Germany, and the United States.

Patients with complete, chronic cervicothoracic SCI have also developed rhythmic flexor and extensor EMG activity in their leg muscles during manually assisted stepping with BWSTT (Fig. 8–3).[39a,44,46] The steplike

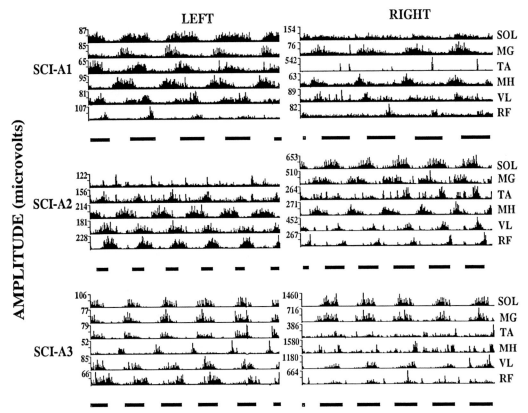

Figure 8–3. Electromyographic (EMG) recordings from each leg of three patients (A1, A2, A3) with a chronic, complete thoracic spinal cord injury (SCI). The solid bars show the timing of the stance phase during manually assisted stepping and body weight–supported treadmill training (BWSTT). Rhythmic bursts appear in most muscles, suggesting that the bursts are related to the response of the lumbosacral motor pools to the sensory inputs associated with the imposed locomotor activity. Muscles shown are the soleus (SOL), medial gastrocnemius (MG), tibialis anterior (TA), medial hamstrings (MH), vastus lateralis (VL), and rectus femoris (RF).[46]

EMG activity in the patients with complete SCI is similar to that seen in patients with incomplete lesions during passive, manually assisted stepping (Fig. 8–4). During attempted voluntary stepping, EMG bursts with similar waveforms increase in the patients with incomplete lesions. This finding suggests that supraspinal input amplifies the intrinsic spinal activity of motoneurons. Many of the patients with complete SCI have developed spontaneous hip flexion following hip extension at the end of stance. Greater sensory input such as increased loading of the joints enhances this EMG output and may evoke hip flexion at the end of stance. Although much of the muscle activity elicited is appropriate in its timing to the step cycle, it does not produce the torque needed for unassisted swing and stance. The exercise does increase muscle bulk in some muscle groups.[73] The inability of these patients with complete SCI to execute locomotor movements may be attributed to insufficient activation of motor pools to manage the muscular forces needed for bipedal stepping, to muscle atrophy, and to a greater dependence on supraspinal influences in humans than in lower animals that have undergone spinal transection. These studies of complete and incomplete SCI suggest, however, that therapeutic strategies can take advantage of the interneuron and motoneuron circuits that are still modulated by residual descending inputs and the segmental sensory feedbacks related to locomotor movements.

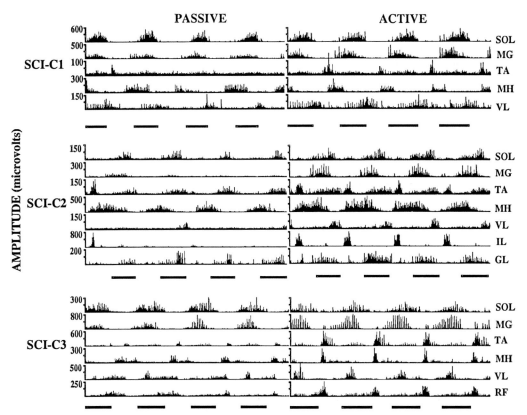

Figure 8–4. Electromyographic (EMG) recordings from the left legs of three patients with chronic, incomplete (ASIA C) thoracic spinal cord injury (SCI). The solid bars show the timing of the stance phase during passive, manually assisted stepping with body weight–supported treadmill training (BWSTT) and stepping at the same treadmill speed (0.8 mph) with the patients actively assisting. Because of marked paraparesis, the patients needed assistance to place each foot and to control the knee during the stance phase. Higher amplitude bursts appear in most muscles during active stepping, although they maintain a similar waveform, suggesting that they are derived from the same motor pools. Several muscles reveal additional bursts during active stepping, such as the tibialis anterior (TA) and medial gastrocnemius (MG) of C1 and the TA of C2 and C3.[46]

As an adjunct to traditional physical therapies, the combination of partial weight bearing on a treadmill belt and the use of a harness reduces the energy cost of locomotor training, serves as a safety measure to prevent falls, and allows therapists to step back to assess and correct gait deviations. For similar reasons, the technique may also aid in the training of stepping by FNS. Other theoretic benefits exist. In experiments with adult cats that have undergone low thoracic spinal transection, locomotion is enhanced by treadmill training and is adversely affected by a program of postural training for standing without stepping.[79] In neurologically impaired individuals, initial gait training, as a practical matter, is preceded by therapeutic exercise aimed at obtaining postural stability. This regimen may depress locomotor capability. Physical therapy proceeds beyond standing only if the patient has the strength required for weight support, weight shifting, and stepping. The BWSTT system facilitates a more rhythmic, reciprocal gait pattern without the requirements for good postural stability and full weight bearing. In addition, it is task-oriented therapy, which may provide an opportunity for problem solving as motor control is relearned. This therapy, in turn, may stimulate useful reorganization within residual descending pathways for locomotion. By providing a more typical locomotor pattern of cutaneous and proprioceptive input to the motor pathways during BWSTT locomotion, any residual cortical and subcortical representational maps within the distributed system for movement may come to more effective remodeling (see Fig. 1–6). The early initiation of even partially supported stepping that this training allows may also, as is sometimes claimed for FNS, help to prevent some of the medical complications of immobility such as joint contractures, muscle atrophy, deconditioning, dysautonomia, pressure sores, osteoporosis, heterotopic ossification, depression, and spasticity.

STRENGTHENING AND CONDITIONING

As already noted, the energy cost of locomotion is often too great for patients with paraparesis to be able to use walking in their ADLs. The rate of oxygen consumption between the ages of 20 to 59 years averages 12 mL/kg per minute at the casual walking velocity of 80 m per minute. The patient with paraplegia who wants to ambulate may use KAFOs and crutches with a swing-through gait to reach an average speed of 30 m per minute and an oxygen rate of 16 mL/kg per minute.[154] This rate is 160 percent higher than healthy persons use at that speed, and the oxygen cost per meter walked is six times normal. The energy cost for patients with paraparesis who have adequate motor control and strength to take steps may be reduced by interventions that decrease hypertonicity in the legs, including antispasticity medications and physical therapies such as stretching spastic hip adductor muscles.[109] In addition, some hormonal and drug interventions show promise in increasing the strength of paretic muscles (see Chapter 1).[133] The ability to meet the demands of walking with assistive devices and FNS is enhanced by a program of strengthening and cardiovascular conditioning.

For patients who cannot step, strengthening and fitness are potentially important goals to increase endurance for community tasks. For instance, routine wheelchair mobility uses 18 percent of the peak oxygen intake of athletes with paraplegia in their mid 20s, about 30 percent less than that used by sedentary patients with paraplegia of the same age, whereas sedentary patients with paraplegia who are in their 50s use over 50 percent of their peak oxygen intake for routine wheelchair mobility. Fitness training can increase reserves for midlife activities.

Risk factors for chronic disease can also probably be lowered with exercise. Several small-group comparisons have suggested that patients with quadriplegia and paraplegia have significantly lower high-density lipoprotein (HDL) levels than controls. A regimen of 8 weeks of wheelchair ergometer training in SCI subjects at the moderate intensity of about 60 percent of peak oxygen uptake for 20 minutes a day for 3 days a week increased HDL cholesterol levels by 20 percent and lowered low-density lipoprotein (LDL) levels by 15 percent. This training could lower the long-term risk of coronary artery disease by 20 percent.[80] Increased physical activity has also been shown in many studies of able-bodied persons to lower blood pressure and reduce the risks of heart disease and non–insulin-dependent diabetes.[105]

Exercise. Inactive patients with paraplegia have gained cardiorespiratory fitness by using arm crank training at 50 percent of peak oxygen intake on a schedule of three times a week for 40 minutes (although not for only 20 minutes) over both 8 and 24 weeks.[32] In able-bodied persons, workloads for the upper extremities should be about 50 percent of those used for leg training. The target heart rate should be 10 beats per minute lower than that prescribed for leg training. At a given submaximal workload, exercise of the arms is performed at a greater energy cost, but maximal physiologic responses including cardiac output and stroke volume are lower.[56] Using these guidelines, a central conditioning effect can be achieved by able-bodied and neurologically impaired people, especially in persons who are initially unfit. Freewheeling gamefield exercises including propelling a wheelchair over a rising power ramp and a ramp of uneven platforms and performing chin-ups from the chair produce heart rates and oxygen uptakes from arm exercise alone that are comparable to those necessary for a training effect in able-bodied persons.[19] Vigorous, enjoyable wheelchair sports and recreational activities may accomplish the same goal for the person with SCI.

Functional Electrical Stimulation (FES). Among all the neurologic disabilities, the most scientific attention to the limitations and benefits of fitness training and testing has been given to paraplegia and tetraplegia.[64] After SCI, cardiovascular conditioning can be limited by the use of only the upper body's small muscle mass, by pooling of blood in the leg muscles that reduces cardiac preloading, and by impaired cardiovascular reflexes. FES-induced leg cycle ergometry can improve both peripheral muscular and central cardiovascular fitness.[54] Resistive voluntary arm activity has been combined with electrical stimulation of leg muscles to further enhance aerobic conditioning.[55]

The responses to FES depend on many variables. With commercial devices such as the REGYS I and ERGYS I, computer-controlled stimulation of the quadriceps, gluteal, and hamstring muscle groups reaches 50 rpm, about 300 contractions per minute. Stimulation starts at 0 watts and aims to build by 6-watt increments for 30 minutes of exercise to a maximum, rarely achieved, of about 42 watts. On that schedule, the steady-state oxygen uptake reaches 2 L per minute, equivalent to about 50 percent of the maximum uptake of able-bodied joggers.[63] This schedule is too effortful for most patients with SCI, however. They tend to reach uptake levels of 1 L per minute, equivalent to walking in able-bodied persons.

Muscular contractions evoked solely by electrical stimulation or superimposed on contractions by paretic muscles can increase muscle bulk and strength.[91] For example, FES training of the quadriceps muscle, by stimulating full knee extension in sets of 5 to 15 repetitions against an increasing load resistance of 1 to 15 kg over 12 weeks, increases muscle bulk, improves strength, and reduces fatigability for the FES activity.[63] In a related study, FES appeared to reduce the rate of trabecular bone loss from the proximal tibia.[72] During FES, muscle fibers are activated synchronously at high, fatiguing frequencies with an undesirable recruitment order from large to small motor units. The optimal combination of stimulation fre-quency, pulse shape, duration of stimuli, and overall training regimen is uncertain. Much of the research in FES and in FNS gait systems aims to develop a method of stimulation that can reproduce the nervous system's smooth, low-fatiguing contractions.

Although psychologic and other physiologic benefits have been attributed to FES as a means to increase oxygen uptake, long-term home-based programs require at least as much motivation as needed by able-bodied people who bicycle for fitness. In a follow-up study of 28 patients with SCI who were trained on the ERGYS I for a median of 1 year before they purchased a home unit, one-third had stopped using the device a month later.[134] Moreover, some studies of participants in an FES program show that depression and hostility increase in patients who have had unrealistic expectations.[13] Ongoing studies will likely further develop methods of voluntary arm cranking and wheelchair ergometry.

Upper Extremity Function

In addition to the usual range of splints, orthotic devices, and strategies aimed at improving arm and hand function, patients with quadriplegia can benefit from some specific adaptations. For example, patients with a partial C-4 lesion with preserved elbow flexion or a C-5 injury with a functional deltoid or biceps can improve hand placement for feeding, writing, and typing activities by using a balanced forearm orthosis. If some wrist extension at the C-6 level is intact, finger flexion for a grasp will accompany extension, and finger opening will follow passive wrist flexion when the long finger flexors are allowed to become tight. A wrist-driven orthosis can assist in this action (Fig. 8–5). A well-designed elbow extension orthosis that corrects a torque imbalance between an active biceps and an inactive triceps can improve flexion and extension functions with or without the addition of FNS.[165] Overhead and counterbalance slings and mobile arm supports eliminate or use the force of gravity to assist in arm motion. Environmental controls, computers, and some simple robotic devices can enhance independence after

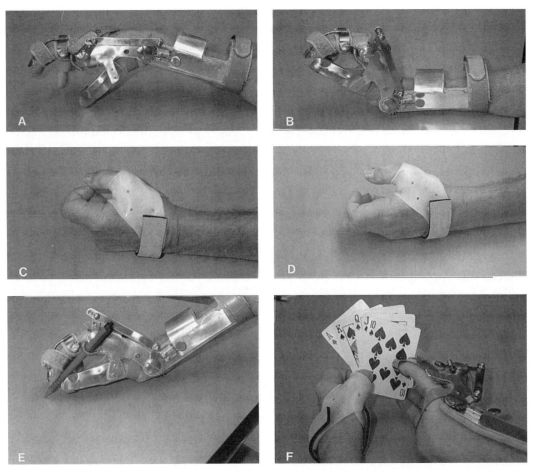

Figure 8–5. A man with an incomplete C-7 quadriparesis developed a syrinx and lost nearly all motor function of the hands. (*A*) The right hand was fitted with a wrist-driven orthosis that (*B*) opposes the thumb to the second and third digits for a pincer grasp when the wrist is extended. (*C*) A simpler plastic orthosis stabilized the proximal thumb of the left hand (*D*) to permit use of the patient's modest pincer motion. (*E*) Writing became possible with the right wrist-hand orthosis. (*F*) The combination of orthoses created a pair of winning hands.

more complete loss of upper extremity function.

EMG biofeedback for upper extremity muscles within or near the zone of partial preservation, perhaps combined with other physical therapies and electrical stimulation, may improve strength and function. In one study of patients with quadriparesis, biofeedback increased the peak EMG of several intrinsic hand muscles by two to five times.[139] The mechanism postulated from the investigators' single unit recordings and measures of twitch tensions was an increase in the firing rates of motor units that were already active. The increase seemed less likely to be due to recruitment of previously unavailable units, synchronization of additional units, a greater safety factor in neuromuscular transmission so that fibers might fire longer or at higher rates, sprouting of nerve terminals, or muscle fiber reinnervation. The patients had large numbers of motor units activated or deactivated after a prolonged latency of 10 seconds. A synergistic movement often elicited them. This finding suggests that a reticulospinal or other slower pathway substituted for a faster corticospinal pathway. Studies that make these physiologic distinctions could provide more selective and testable training methods. In a small clinical trial, however, the addition of at least one EMG biofeedback strategy to supervised physical therapies for patients with quadriparesis did not clearly improve arm and hand strength or use for self-care functions.[89]

RECONSTRUCTIVE SURGERY

Upper extremity function can sometimes improve by the following measures:

1. A surgical transfer of a tendon from its normal insertion to another tendon or to the insertion point of another muscle
2. Tenodesis, the division or attachment of a tendon to a bone or ligament to help stabilize or passively tether a joint during movement
3. Arthrodesis, to eliminate motion or realign, for example, a finger joint
4. Osteotomy, to reshape a bone

These techniques have been used alone and in combination, along with orthotics, physical training, and electrical stimulation.[6,145] Specific procedures for C-5 and lower functional levels are most commonly used to increase elbow extension, pronation and supination of the forearm, wrist extension, finger flexion, key grip pinch between the thumb and flexed fingers, and palmar prehension for the grasp of large objects, as well as for more subtle actions of the intrinsic hand muscles.[87] For example, active hand grasp may be achieved by a person with C-7 tetraplegia by means of surgical transfer of the brachioradialis to the flexor pollicis longus and transfer of the extensor carpi radialis longus to the flexor digitorum profundus. Surgeons prefer to wait at least 6 months after injury and use muscles with at least 4/5 strength across joints that are free of contractures. Postoperative immobilization of the limb can last for weeks. Activities such as wheelchair transfers and propulsion may be restricted for several months.

NEURAL PROSTHESES

Systems for FNS with visual and other sensory feedbacks are being developed especially to provide a hand grasp and release in patients with C-5 and C-6 quadriplegia. Some work also includes patients with C-4 and C-7 injuries. Electrodes are usually implanted in eight muscles. In an ongoing clinical trial, a hand neuroprosthesis allowed 40 percent more patients with C-5 and C-6 SCI to complete 10 ADLs with the upper limb.[66] FNS use may require one or more surgical reconstructions to optimize hand function. Computerized neuromuscular stimulation systems supplemented by splints have been triggered by voice and puff-and-suck commands to carry out hand and arm functions in a few patients with C-4 SCI.[117] Engineers are also trying to develop systems with sensory feedback controls to regulate the forces exerted by the grasp that is stimulated.[27] Simpler commercial systems are becoming available. In one design, electrodes for FNS are embedded in a wrist-hand orthosis that, by means of a control box, can stimulate a key grip or cylindrical grasp and release.

Spasticity

After the period of spinal shock from an acute SCI, a sequence of minimal reflex activity is often followed by flexor spasms, then flexor and extensor spasms, and then mostly extensor activity. Among 27 patients with a thoracic spinal cord transection verified by laminectomy, however, 5 patients with SCI at levels between T-3 and T-8 had a flaccid, areflexic paralysis with marked muscular atrophy 2 years after injury.[94] Most of the others had extensor spasms elicited by stretch of the iliopsoas muscle. Flexor responses typically followed plantar and genital stimuli.

Medication for spasticity is often given to patients whose flexor withdrawal and extensor spasms cause pain, interrupt sleep, and interfere with ADLs such as wheelchair transfers or driving. Of 466 patients entered into the Model Systems Program, 26 percent were discharged with an antispasticity agent an average of 105 days after injury, and 46 percent used medication by the 1-year follow-up.[111a] Further analysis of this cohort revealed that spasticity was related to the time from onset of injury and was most prominent in patients with cervical and upper thoracic SCI (90 percent in the University of Michigan subcohort and 57 percent in the national cohort at follow-up). Patients with Frankel grades A and D were less likely to have been treated than those with grades B and C. The data did not relate the use of antispasticity medication to any positive or negative effects on mobility. This clinical report and others,[99,128] however, add to the impression that spasticity is most prominent after incomplete, rather than complete, motor and sensory lesions. Partial preservation of supraspinal input on neurons below the lesion may be necessary for many of the clinical and physiologic manifestations of hypertonicity.[40]

Supported standing several times a day can reduce spasms in nonambulatory patients who have a myelopathy.[10] Variations in the excitability and patterns of muscle activation may be exaggerated by the stretch reflexes induced when ambulation loads a paretic limb at a dysfunctional angle, force, or point in the gait cycle. By controlling the magnitude of weight bearing with, for example, BWSTT, one may reduce the activation of spasticity and its functional sequelae. Although oral benzodiazepines, baclofen, and dantrolene can reduce extensor spasms, clonidine,[49] tizanidine,[116] and cyproheptadine[148] can be especially useful and may also improve the gait pattern of ambulatory patients. For refractory severe spasms and pain, intrathecal baclofen given by implanted, programmable pump infusion[101,123] has generally replaced intrathecal morphine, electrical spinal stimulation, selective dorsal rhizotomy, and myelotomy. For perineal care, hip flexor or adductor phenol blocks and neurectomies are occasionally necessary. The management of spasticity is discussed in Chapter 6.

LONG-TERM NEUROMEDICAL CARE

Health maintenance after inpatient rehabilitation becomes a lifelong challenge. Sensorimotor loss can mask awareness of infections, pressure sores, abdominal pain, and other medical and neurologic complications. Patients with SCI and their physicians have to pay attention to all organ systems. At the same time, physicians should be aware of the way in which their interventions may affect the lifestyle and real-world functioning of the patient. Table 8–8 lists the more common complications found in the second year and more than 30 years after SCI.[41] Although specific management is discussed in Chapter 6 and elsewhere,[33] some additional details about these problems put the health maintenance needs of the patient with SCI in perspective.

Pressure Sores

Model Systems Program data for patients admitted within 24 hours of traumatic SCI show that 4 percent subsequently developed

Table 8–8. **COMMON MEDICAL COMPLICATIONS LATE AFTER SPINAL CORD INJURY (PERCENTAGE OF PATIENTS PER YEAR)**

1 YEAR AFTER		30 YEARS AFTER	
Complication	**(%)**	**Complication**	**(%)**
Urinary tract infection	59	Pressure sore	17
Spasticity	38	Muscle and joint pain	16
Chills, fever	19	Gastrointestinal disorder	14
Pressure sore	16	Cardiovascular disorders	14
Dysautonomia	8	Urinary tract infection	14
Contractures	6	Infection, tumor	11
Heterotopic ossification	3	Genitourinary dysfunction	8
Azotemia	2	Renal stone, renal failure	6
Wound infection	2		

Source: Adapted from Ditunno J, Formal C.[41]

pressure sores, and 13 percent of these sores were graded as severe.[140] They occurred over the sacrum, heel, scapula, foot, and trochanter. Lower-grade skin lesions developed over nearly any bony prominence and over the genitals. A community study found 33 percent of patients with chronic SCI to have one or more lesions graded stage I to stage IV (see Table 6–8).[57] Indeed, 28 percent of these lesions were stages 3 and 4. Black patients had more severe ulcers than white patients. More severe lesions were incurred with injury in late life and in patients with the poorest mobility. Prevention after SCI requires daily examination of the skin, intermittent wheelchair push-ups, pressure-relieving cushions for the wheelchair, attention to bed coverings, and for the immobile patient, occasional repositioning during sleep.

Bowel and Bladder Complications

Fecal incontinence, constipation, and fecal impaction affect most patients with SCI until a practical bowel program is attained, usually during the inpatient stay. Digital stimulation of the anal sphincter and oral docusate sodium may be sufficient for evacuation timed to the patient's convenience. These are supplemented, as necessary, by glycerin or bisocodyl suppositories and other contact irritants, stool softeners, colonic stimulants, and bulk formers. Incontinence and dysreflexia can be helped by limiting the ingestion of gas-forming foods such as beans, large amounts of dairy products, fruit juices, and berries. Cisapride can improve bowel hypomotility.

The bladder is usually flaccid during the period of spinal shock. A detrusor reflex may not return for 6 weeks to 12 months. Bladder drainage requires some combination of intermittent catheterization, an external collection system, reflexive emptying, and, occasionally, a urethral or suprapubic catheter. The patient with paraplegia is trained to perform intermittent catheterization at least three times a day. If sensorimotor impairments persist, nearly all patients with SCI with a lesion that spares the S-2 to S-4 micturition center develop dyssynergia between the detrusor and the external sphincter.

These uncoordinated contractions lead to incontinence and outlet obstruction. Urodynamic studies and an intravenous pyelogram are indicated as a baseline and to assist in therapy. Urinary tract obstruction in a patient with quadriplegia is especially likely to lead to dysautonomia. If this condition is untreated, patients also develop recurrent infections, urosepsis, vesicoureteral reflux, urolithiasis, and hydronephrosis. Of course, one must optimize bladder emptying (see Chapter 6). Pharmacotherapy often helps in the management of dysfunction of the detrusor, bladder outlet, and striated urethral sphincter[169] (see Table 6–7). Electrical stimulation by implanted electrodes has been variably helpful for continence and voiding. Surgeons use a variety of electrodes, implant techniques, and placements that include the bladder and neck, the pudendal nerve, and sacral roots. Bowel and sexual function may be adversely affected.

Urinary tract infections are related to bladder overdistention, high-pressure voiding, large postvoid residuals, vesicoureteral reflux, and stones or outlet obstruction. Urine culture criteria for the diagnosis of bacteriuria include more than 10^2 colony-forming units per mL (cfu/mL) of urine from persons on intermittent catheterization, more than 10^4 cfu/mL from a clean void specimen in males using a condom collection device, and any bacteria from an indwelling catheter.[118] Prophylactic antimicrobial agents and attempts to change urine pH[141] are commonly used after repeated infections, but these drugs probably do not decrease bacterial colonization and symptomatic bacteriuria.

In a study of over 100 women and 400 men with SCI who were followed for at least 10 years, no significantly different rates for urologic complications and renal dysfunction were related to the system of drainage.[82] The majority of women were managed with an indwelling catheter, and the men, with a condom catheter. Only men with quadriplegia who used an ilioconduit had a significant decrease in one measure of renal perfusion. Model Systems Program data show that over 10 years, patients switched from intermittent catheterization to the use of condom and suprapubic catheters.[140] Condom catheters with leg drainage bags are used by many men with SCI to ensure continence, although these bags may loosen and may thereby allow accidents. For patients with a small, rectractile penis that lets a condom slip off, a semirigid penile hinge prosthesis can help to maintain continence and contribute to sexual function.

Drugs that diminish spasticity after SCI can have useful and negative effects on bladder activity. Diazepam, dantrolene, and baclofen can inhibit detrusor hyperreflexia to the point of areflexia and increased residual urine. Clonidine can reduce micturition reflex hyperactivity, presumably by alpha-2-receptor–mediated suppression of the polysynaptic vesicosomatic and pudendal reflexes released by the myelopathy.[77]

An individual's clinical course best determines the frequency of urologic evaluations. General recommendations include a urinalysis at 3-month intervals, urea nitrogen and creatinine determinations twice a year, a renal scan yearly, renal ultrasound every 3 years, and urodynamic studies if problems of urine storage and emptying arise.

Sexual Function

Although SCI is often accompanied by sexual dysfunction, most patients can be sexually active. About 40 percent of men with quadriplegia and 60 percent of those with paraplegia graded Frankel A to C reported having sexual intercourse in the previous 12 months.[162] Satisfaction with their sex lives ranked at the bottom of 12 life pursuits, although it was ranked the fifth most important to them. In a community-based sampling, women with SCI rated their sex lives tenth of 11 items in importance and satisfaction.[163] Counseling, education, and medical assistance are often necessary. In men and women, pain, spasms, dysautonomia, incontinence, feelings of unattractiveness, the effort of preparation, and concerns about satisfying a partner or oneself can interfere with foreplay and sexual intercourse.

Reflexogenic erections occur in over 90 percent of men with SCI with complete and incomplete lesions, but ejaculation may be functional in only 10 percent of patients with complete lesions and in one-third of those with incomplete lesions.[170] Severe headaches may accompany ejaculation. Reflexive paraspinal and cervical muscle spasm, dysautonomia with hypertension, and migraine may account for the paroxysmal pain. Prophylaxis depends on the mechanism. Erectile function and seminal ejaculation can be aided by many techniques. Intracavernous injections of papaverine and other substances work for some patients, but priapism is more likely in the patient with SCI. Vacuum techniques are often useful for maintaining an erection. Implanted, semirigid penile prostheses benefited 52 of 63 veterans with sexual dysfunction, some of whom had skin lacerations from external appliances, but they carried an initial 33 percent complication rate.[26] Infections occurred in 7 percent, and skin erosions evolved in 11 percent after 6 months. Penile vibration and subcutaneous administration of physostigmine with masturbation can elicit semen for insemination. Infertility can be related to the poor quality of semen. Some causes of infertility are treatable.[98] In addition to the technique of sacral anterior root stimulation, erectile function and ejaculation can be controlled by electrical stimulation of the hypogastric plexus or by a rectal probe.[122]

Women remain fertile after SCI. A vaginal lubricating jelly can aid sexual intercourse. Catheterization immediately after sexual intercourse helps to prevent bladder infections. Pregnancy can be complicated by hypertension and autonomic dysreflexia, pressure sores, urinary infections, central and dysesthetic pain, and failure to progress in labor. Term deliveries are common in patients who have close medical supervision, however.[28]

Dysautonomia

Autonomic reflexes may fail in persons with SCI at levels above T-6. Symptomatic postural hypotension is common in the first weeks after injury and may persist after quadriplegia. Plasma norepinephrine levels, which should at least double, do not rise appropriately with upright posture and hypotension in these patients, although renin, vasopressin, and aldosterone levels do reach normal levels.[71] Impaired norepinephrine release may cause denervation supersensitivity of alpha-1 and alpha-2 adrenoreceptors. Gradual reconditioning on a tilt table, sleeping in a reverse Trendelenburg position, full-leg hose, and an abdominal binder should be tried. In the inpatient setting, fluid loading with saline or albumin may aid the effort to compensate for venous pooling, decreased cardiac output, and impaired vasoconstriction and venoconstriction from interruption of sympathetic outflow. Fludrocortisone increases the intravascular volume and peripheral vascular resistance. The dosage can be pushed gradually to as high as 1 mg per day. Salt tablets should be added to the diet. Hypokalemia and edema with pressure sores can complicate the use of mineralocorticoids. While patients are upright, one can try ephedrine, 25 to 100 mg up to every 3 hours, or ergotamine, 2 mg up to several times daily. With denervation supersensitivity, clonidine, 0.1 mg twice a day, and midodrine, 10 mg every 8 hours, can increase venous return or have pressor effects.[131a]

Episodic autonomic hyperreflexia related to uninhibited sympathetic outflow may affect 30 to 90 percent of patients with high SCI, usually beginning several months after injury.[24] Paroxysmal hypertension is more common in ASIA A and B than in C or D patients with tetraplegia. This disorder is instigated by visceral and joint pain, oropharyngeal suctioning (which can also cause bradyarrhythmias), heterotopic ossification, pressure sores, bowel and bladder distention, fecal impaction, urinary infection and cystitis, epididymitis, any surgical procedure, ingrown toenails, pregnancy and labor, venous thrombosis, late development of a syrinx (Fig. 8–6), tight clothing, and a particular supine position, although it may have no evident cause. Hypertension, headache, diaphoresis, anxiety, reflexive bradycardia, nasal congestion, flushing above and pallor below the SCI level, extensor spasms, and piloerection can follow.

Treatment of sudden dysreflexia starts with removing the instigating cause. The patient is positioned upright, and the bladder is catheterized. Drug interventions include a calcium channel blocker such as nifedipine,

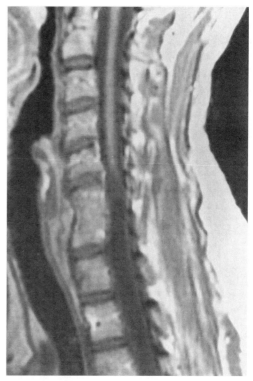

Figure 8–6. One-year after a diving injury that caused complete quadriplegia at C5, a young man developed increasing dysesthetic pain in the shoulders and arms. Bouts of autonomic dysreflexia also increased in frequency and severity. The T_1-weighted magnetic resonance imaging (MRI) scan revealed a syrinx surrounded by a thin perimeter of spinal cord that extended from the C5-C6 junction to the midthoracic region. Surgical venting collapsed the syrinx and greatly diminished his symptoms. (Courtesy of Ulrich Batzdorf, M.D., University of California Los Angeles.)

vasodilators such as hydralazine and nitroprusside, and occasionally phenoxybenzamine, prazosin, clonidine, nitroglycerin, oxybutynin, or diazoxide (Table 8–9). Some patients with quadriplegia have labile responses to antihypertensive drugs and suddenly become hypotensive. For frequent bouts of hypertension, maintenance therapy includes low doses of any of the foregoing oral agents. For paroxysmal bradycardia, propantheline or a pacemaker may be needed. Scopolamine can prevent bouts of sweating.

Table 8–9. REGIMEN FOR ACUTE AUTONOMIC DYSREFLEXIA

Sit patient up at 90 degrees.

Monitor blood pressure every 3 minutes.

Check urine collection system or catheterize the bladder using lidocaine gel.

Look for source of noxious stimulation.

If systolic blood pressure is higher than 170 mm Hg, apply nitropaste, 1 inch above spinal level.

Examine rectum with topical anesthetic and remove feces.

If no change, give 10 mg nifedipine; repeat in 10 minutes as needed.

Monitor for hypotension.

Start intravenous fluids if no change.

If hypertension and symptoms persist, give nitroglycerin 1/150 sublingually or hydralazine 10 mg intravenously.

If no change, give diazoxide, 300 mg intravenously.

Check blood pressure often.

For prophylaxis, give prazosin 5 mg orally up to three times daily.

Heterotopic Ossification

Ectopic bone may cause functional impairment in up to 20 percent of patients with SCI below the neurologic level of injury, usually in the first 4 months after injury. Patients with a complete lesion, pressure sores, and spasticity, and patients older than 30 years of age may be at greatest risk.[95] Ectopic bone develops when multipotential connective tissue cells transform to chondroblasts and osteoblasts, presumably under the influence of locally induced growth factors. The hips, knees, and shoulders are most often affected. Swelling, erythema, and decreasing range of motion are among the first clinical signs. A three-phase bone scan reveals focal uptake before radiographic visualization of bone. Early treatment with etidronate disodium suppresses mineralization of the osteoid. Range of motion exercises, aspirin, nonsteroidal anti-inflammatory drugs, and a wedge resection of mature heterotopic bone can decrease pain and immobility.[17]

Chronic Pain

Pain after SCI arises from contractures, osteoporotic fractures, extensor spasms, soft tissue injury, musculoligamentous strain, myofascial pain, and inflammation of tendons and bursae, especially from overuse of the upper extremities. In a survey of 450 patients with SCI, 72 percent reported chronic pain in the wrists or shoulders, especially during wheelchair propulsion and transfers.[142] Strain and cumulative trauma appeared to be the cause. Reflex sympathetic dystrophy after cervical SCI may be an underdiagnosed cause of pain.[1] Painful compression neuropathies such as carpal tunnel syndrome increase over time in patients with paraplegia who bear their weight through the upper extremities.

Pain at the level of injury may be radicular or central, with a sharp, burning, bandlike, or electric quality. Similar discomfort may develop in patches of skin anywhere below the lesion, particularly in the perineum. Visceral pain from the abdomen or pelvis is often difficult to localize, but it especially arises from a distended bladder or bowel. Late onset of pain, especially when associated with changes in the neurologic examination, suggests an expanding syringomyelia that may require venting (see Fig. 8–6). Neurogenic pain can be diminished by transcutaneous stimulation, tricyclic antidepressants, anticonvulsants, and analgesics (see Chapter 10). Spinal cord stimulation has not been effective for phantom pain below the sensory level.[25]

Disorders of Ventilation

Patients with high quadriplegia who require a tracheostomy and intermittent positive pressure ventilation have had an approximately 40 percent mortality over 5 years from pulmonary complications. Noninvasive methods have increasingly freed many patients from the problems of communication and swallowing and from the altered quality of life imposed by a tracheostomy.[4] These methods include intermittent positive pressure ventilation (IPPV) by mouth, nose, and acrylic strapless oronasal interface (SONI), glossopharyngeal breathing, and chest shell ventilation, supplemented by respiratory muscle training and consistent pulmonary toilet. Speaking tracheostomy tubes and devices such as the Venti-Voice or one of the models of an artificial larynx allow oral communication despite the presence of a tracheostomy. In patients with high tetraplegia at C-1 to C-3, phrenic nerve stimulation by radiosignal to an implanted electrode in the neck or second intercostal space can allow successful respiration for many years with good quality of life.[65,122] Intercostal and diaphragm muscle stimulation have also been used, but with less success. Persons with quadriparesis and high paraplegia who do not need assisted ventilatory support may be susceptible to feelings of breathlessness, airway hyperreactivity to aerosols, oxygen desaturation during sleep, and complications from atelectasis of lung tissue.

Endocrine Disorders

Immobilization can cause a 3 to 8 percent per month loss of bone calcium and rapid loss of trabecular bone by an average of 33 percent at 6 months after injury.[115] This accounts for the 2 to 6 percent incidence of long bone fractures in patients with paraplegia.[51] The disuse osteoporosis results from an initial increase in osteoclastic resorption and especially decreased osteoblastic formation. Although osteoclastic activity returns to normal, the osteoporosis may not recover. Increased calcium release from bones of paralyzed limbs also suppresses parathormone and downregulates calcitriol.[146] Drugs such as the antiosteoclastic bisphosphonates are being studied as a prophylactic measure to preserve bone mass.[21] FES, electrical fields, weight bearing, and trials of calcitonin and growth hormone have been tried with variable success.

Other endocrine abnormalities, particularly low triiodothyronine, high and low testosterone, hyperprolactinemia, and low growth hormone have been reported, although the relationship with paralysis is often uncertain.[149]

Cognitive Disorders

Up to half of patients with traumatic SCI have cognitive impairments from an associated traumatic brain injury (TBI) or substance abuse.[31] Formal neuropsychologic testing is usually needed to demonstrate the coincidence of SCI with deficits in attention, concentration, memory, mental flexibility, and problem solving. During inpatient rehabilitation and out-of-hospital living, these cognitive impairments can impede the patient's learning and execution of basic self-care skills, psychosocial adjustment, and vocational skills. This impairment may increase the likelihood of hospital readmission for recurrent medical complications. Routine screening and early intervention during inpatient rehabilitation can lessen complications and may improve outcomes in these doubly disabled people.

Aging

Our aging population will likely produce more patients with traumatic and nontraumatic SCI with the onset of injury beyond the age of 60 years. The elderly patient with acute SCI, like any older person, often has different values and rehabilitation goals than younger people who are beginning family life and careers. Slower progress and lower levels of independence may be associated with easy fatigability, overuse of muscles and joints, depression, more medical problems, and greater susceptibility to the side effects of medications. These factors complicate early therapeutic efforts and, as younger patients with SCI age, they will increasingly affect long-term management.

In one study, patients over the age of 61 years were compared with patients with acute SCI aged 16 to 30 years.[34] Older patients were over twice as likely to suffer pneumonia or a gastrointestinal hemorrhage, 5 times more likely to develop a pulmonary embolus, and 17 times more likely to have renal stones. During the second postinjury year, older patients were 4 times as likely to be rehospitalized, 72 times as likely to be living in a nursing home, and 7 times more likely to have hired an attendant. The 2-year survival rate of these patients was only 59 percent, compared with an expected 94 percent.

One-fourth of patients who sustained their injuries 20 to 40 years ago evolved a greater need for physical assistance over the years, especially for help with transfers.[62] These patients reported shoulder pain, fatigue, weakness, weight gain, and a decline in the quality of life more often than patients who did not require more assistance.

A study of military veterans with traumatic SCI found that those who survived at least 3 months had an additional 39-year survival, which is 85 percent of that of American men of similar ages.[131] Life expectancy for the first 20 years after injury was comparable to that of disabled veterans who did not have SCI, but then it declined. By 20 years, the causes of death were similar for both groups of veterans, with a falloff in SCI-related problems such as septicemia and renal failure. Complete quadriplegia was less predictive of poorer long-term survival than was older age at onset.

INTERVENTIONS AND OUTCOMES FOR PSYCHOSOCIAL PROBLEMS

Employment

Data from the Model Systems Program showed employment rates 5 years after SCI at 28 percent for patients with paraplegia and at 14 percent for patients with quadriplegia; patients with incomplete lesions have higher work rates in each category.[140] Although 64 percent of these patients were employed at the time of injury, 13 percent were working 2 years later, and 38 percent were working 12 years later. In the first year, previously employed patients often returned to their former jobs. After that time, these patients tended to find new employers or, having completed their education, joined the labor force. About 6 percent were Department of Vocational Rehabilitation clients before injury, 38 percent were clients at the time of rehabilitation discharge, and 8 percent were clients at 13 years after SCI.[35] In another sample of 286 patients with SCI who were interviewed an average of 18 years after injury, 48 percent were still working, and 75 percent had worked at some point.[92] Aside from level of injury, the most critical predictor of employment was education. Patients with at least 16 years of education had employment rates since injury of 95 percent, compared with 63 percent for those who had completed high school and 38 percent for those who had not. Creative problem solving by persons with SCI and the rehabilitation team often leads to inexpensive solutions for the adaptive equipment needs of patients and the architectural barriers that impede employment.

Marital Status

Five years after injury, 90 percent of unmarried patients with SCI followed in the Model Systems Program remained single, compared with 64 percent of noninjured persons of the same age. Of those already married, 78 percent remained so, compared with an expected rate of 89 percent. The risk of divorce was greater than in matched uninjured people, primarily in the second and third years after injury, but it was similar in the first, fourth, and fifth years.[35]

Adjustment and Quality of Life

Investigators have increasingly studied the gradual process by which patients with SCI psychologically assimilate changes in their bodies, their self-concepts, and their interactions with their environment.[100] Life satisfaction, on average, is lower for persons with SCI than for the general population of age-matched community dwellers. It is better in persons who have less handicap in social integration, occupation, and mobility, regardless of the degree of neurologic impairment and disability.[58] Subjective ratings of quality of life are strongly associated with perceived control, self-assessed health, and social support.

Depression is not an inevitable effect of SCI.[15] Suicide rates were about two to four times that of the general population within 5 years of SCI, however.[22] Measures of despondency both before and after SCI were higher in persons who later died of suicide than in a control group of persons who did not commit suicide. Feelings of shame and apathy were documented during the rehabilitation hospitalization. This situation poses an opportunity for intervention. Depressed or distressed patients with SCI reported spending more hours in bed and fewer days out of the house, and they received more personal care assistance compared with well-adjusted persons with SCI at 2 to 7 years after injury.[143] These patients also perceived having greater handicap with limitations, for example, in getting transportation. Again, by obtaining this information from the patient, clinicians can propose psychosocial interventions and possibly drug therapy for depression.

Anxiety and depression can also arise from a posttraumatic stress disorder associated with the event that led to the SCI. The symptoms and signs of this disorder should be sought in every patient in the first months after injury (see Chapter 3).[136]

Psychologic and social adjustments after SCI appear to be stronger predictors for long-term survival than antecedent medical complications. Using the Life Situation Questionnaire, one prospective study found that boredom, depression, loneliness, lack of transportation, conflicts with attendants, inability to control their lives, and alcohol and drug abuse characterized persons who died in the last 4 years of a 15-year follow-up.[93] Personality and mood disorders associated with self-destructive behaviors such as getting little exercise, letting bladder infections and skin sores go without attention, and abusing tobacco, alcohol, narcotics, and sedatives may contribute to this mortality. In one survey, 70 percent of patients with traumatic SCI reported substance abuse before or after injury. Although 16 percent believed they needed treatment, only 7 percent received specific help.[75]

Families, the rehabilitation team, and the physicians who provide long-term care must monitor the psychosocial adjustments, mood, and behavior of SCI-disabled persons and provide assistance as soon as a problem is identified. Over the long run, clues about potential problems may come from periodic administration of a standard quality-of-life questionnaire.

SUMMARY

The early and long-term rehabilitation assessment and management of patients with traumatic SCI or a myelopathy of any cause closely follow residual sensorimotor function, the potential for more independent function, and practical goals. The emphasis of training is on strengthening and conditioning and use of adaptive devices and strategies to regain control of personal care and of the home and work environment. Given near-normal upper extremity function, ambulation improves in relation to truncal and lower extremity strength and the energy cost of mobility. Assistive devices, from crutches and walkers with long leg braces to mechanical and electrical stimulation systems that foster reciprocal stepping, are useful for motivated patients. In the near future, biologic interventions and training that makes use of activity-dependent plasticity may enhance spinal cord function. Mechanical and computer-interfaced devices will increase functional independence across activities impeded by impairments and disabilities. These innovations will raise the quality of life for patients with SCI in concert with continuing modifications in approaches to spasticity, dysreflexia, skin and bladder care, and the psychosocial engineering engendered by the Americans with Disabilities Act.

REFERENCES

1. Aisen M, Aisen P. Shoulder-hand syndrome in patients with cervical spinal cord injury. Neurology 1992;42(Suppl 3):207.
2. Alstermark B, Lundberg A, Pinter M, et al. Subpopulations and functions of long C3–C5 propriospinal neurones. Brain Res 1987;404:395–400.
3. Apple D, Hudson L. Spinal cord injury: The model. Proceedings of the National Consensus Conference on Catastrophic Illness and Injury, December 1989. Atlanta: Shepherd Center for Treatment of Spinal Injuries, 1990:161.
4. Bach J. New approaches in the rehabilitation of

the traumatic high level quadriplegic. Am J Phys Med Rehabil 1991;70:13–19.

5. Barbeau H, Blunt R. A novel interactive locomotor approach using body weight support to retrain gait in spastic paretic subjects. In: Wernig A, ed: Plasticity of Motoneuronal Connections. Amsterdam: Elsevier, 1991:461–474.

6. Barbeau H, Fung J. New experimental approaches in the treatment of spastic gait disorders. Med Sport Sci 1992;36:234–246.

7. Blight A. Axonal physiology of chronic spinal cord injury in the cat: Intracellular recording in vitro. Neuroscience 1983;10:1471–1486.

8. Blight A. Cellular morphology of chronic spinal cord injury in the cat: Analysis of myelinated axons by line-sampling. Neuroscience 1983;10:521–543.

9. Blight A, Toombs J, Bauer M, et al. The effects of 4-aminopyridine on neurological deficits in chronic cases of traumatic spinal cord injury in dogs. J. Neurotrauma 1991;8:103–119.

10. Bohannon R. Tilt table standing for reducing spasticity after spinal cord injury. Arch Phys Med Rehabil 1993;74:1121–1122.

11. Bracken M. National Acute Spinal Cord Injury Study Group: Methylpredisone or naloxone treatment after acute spinal cord injury: 1-year follow-up data. J. Neurosurg 1992;76:23–31.

12. Bracken M, Shepard M. Collins W, et al. A randomized, controlled trial of methylprednisolone or naloxone in the treatment of acute spinal-cord injury. N Engl J Med 1990;322:1405–1411.

13. Bradley M. The effect of participating in a functional electrical stimulation exercise program on affect in people with spinal cord injuries. Arch Phys Med Rehabil 1994;75:676–679.

14. Brown P, Marino R, Herbison G, et al. The 72 hour examination as a predictor of recovery in motor complete quadriplegia. Arch Phys Med Rehabil 1991;72:546–548.

15. Buckelew S, Baumstark K, Frank R, et al. Adjustment after SCI. Rehabilitation Psychology 1990; 35:101–109.

16. Bunge R, Puckett W, Becerra J, et al. Observations on the pathology of human spinal cord injury. In: Seil F, ed: Spinal Cord Injury. New York: Raven Press, 1993:75–89.

17. Buschbacher R. Heterotopic ossification: A review. Crit Rev Phys Rehabil Med 1992;4:199–213.

18. Campbell J, Herbison G, Chen Y, et al. Spontaneous electromyographic potentials in chronic SCI patients. Arch Phys Med Rehabil 1991;72:23–27.

19. Cardius D, McTaggart W, Donovan W. Energy requirements of gamefield exercises designed for wheelchair-bound persons. Arch Phys Med Rehabil 1989;70:124–127.

20. Chaplin E, Winchester P, Habasevich R. FNS synthesized gait restoration following SCI (abstract). Journal of Neurologic Rehabilitation 1994;8:84.

21. Chappard D, Minaire P, Privat C, et al. Effects of tiludronate on bone loss in paraplegic patients. J Bone Miner Res 1995;10:112–117.

22. Charlifue S, Gerhart K. Behavioral and demographic predictors of suicide after traumatic SCI. Arch Phys Med Rehabil 1991;72:488–492.

23. Cohen L, Topka H, Cole R, et al. Paresthesias induced by magnetic brain stimulation in patients with thoracic spinal cord injury. Neurology 1991; 41:1283–1288.

24. Colachis S. Autonomic hyperreflexia wit spinal cord injury. J Am Paraplegia Soc 1992; 15:171–186.

25. Cole J, Illis L, Sedgwick E. Intractable central pain in spinal cord injury is not relieved by spinal cord stimulation. Paraplegia 1991;29:167–172.

26. Collins K, Hackler R. Complications of penile prostheses in the spinal cord injury population. J Urol 1988;140:984–985.

27. Crago P, Nakai R, Chizeck H. Feedback regulation of hand grasp opening and contact force during stimulation of paralyzed muscle. IEEE Trans Biomed Eng 1991;38:17–28.

28. Cross L, Meythaler J, Tuel S, et al. Pregnancy following SCI. West J Med 1991;154:607–611.

29. Crozier K, Graziani V, Ditunno Jr J, et al. Spinal cord injury: Prognosis for ambulation based on sensory examination in patients who are initially motor complete. Arch Phys Med Rehabil 1991; 72:119–121.

30. Daverat P, Sibrac M, Dartigues J, et al. Early prognostic factors for walking in spinal cord injuries. Paraplegia 1988;26:255–261.

31. Davidoff G, Roth E, Richards J. Cognitive deficits in SCI: Epidemiology and outcome. Arch Phys Med Rehabil 1992;73:275–284.

32. Davis G, Plyley M, Shephard R. Gains of cardiorespiratory fitness with arm-crank training in spinally disabled men. Can J Sport Sci 1991;16:64–72.

33. Department of Veterans Affairs. Care and Treatment of Spinal Cord Injury Patients. Washington, DC: Veterans Health Services, Spinal Cord Injury Service, 1991.

34. DeVivo M, Kartus P, Stover S, et al. The influence of age at time of spinal cord injury on rehabilitation outcome. Arch Neurol 1990;47:687–691.

35. DeVivo M, Richards J, Stover S, et al. Spinal cord injury: Rehabilitation adds life to years. West J Med 1991;154:602–606.

36. DeVivo M, Rutt R, Black K, et al. Trends in spinal cord injury demographics and treatment outcomes between 1973 and 1986. Arch Phys Med Rehabil 1992;73:424–430.

37. DeVivo M, Stover S, Black K. Prognostic factors for 12-year survival after SCI. Arch Phys Med Rehabil 1992;73:156–162.

38. DeVivo M, Whiteneck G, Stover S, et al. Indirect costs of spinal cord injury. J Am Paraplegia Soc 1993;16:92.

39. Dietz V, Colombo G, Jensen L. Locomotor activity in spinal man. Lancet 1994;344:1260–1263.

40. Dimitrijevic M. Residual motor functions in spinal cord injury. In: Waxman S, ed: Functional Recovery in Neurological Disease. New York: Raven Press, 1988:139–155.

41. Ditunno J, Formal C. Chronic spinal cord injury. N Engl J Med 1994;330:550–556.

42. Ditunno J, Stover S, Freed M, et al. Motor recovery of the upper extremities in traumatic quadriplegia. Arch Phys Med Rehabil 1992;73:431–436.

43. Dobkin B, Edgerton V, Fowler E. Sensory input during treadmill training alters rhythmic locomotor EMG output in subjects with complete spinal cord injury. In: Proceedings of the Annual Meet-

ing of the Society for Neuroscience. Anaheim, CA, Society for Neuroscience, 1992:1403.

44. Dobkin B, Edgerton V, Fowler E, et al. Training induces rhythmic locomotor EMG patterns in subjects with complete SCI. Neurology 1992;42(Suppl 3):207–208.

45. Dobkin B, Fowler E, Edgerton V, et al. Step-like electromyographic activity in the legs in subjects with complete and severe incomplete thoracic spinal cord injury. Ann Neurol 1994;36:298.

46. Dobkin B, Harkema S, Requejo P, et al. Modulation of locomotor-like EMG activity in subjects with complete and incomplete chronic spinal cord injury. Journal of Neurologic Rehabilitation 1995; 9:183–190.

47. Dobkin B, Taly A, Su G. Use of the audiospinal reflex to test for completeness of spinal cord injury. Journal of Neurologic Rehabilitation 1994; 8:187–191.

48. Donovan W. Operative and nonoperative management of spinal cord injury: A review. Paraplegia 1994;32:375–388.

49. Donovan W, Carter R, Rossi C, et al. Clonidine effect on spasticity: A clinical trial. Arch Phys Med Rehabil 1988;69:193–194.

50. Ducker T, Lucas J, Wallace C. Recovery from spinal cord injury. Clin Neurosurg 1983;30:495–513.

51. Elias A, Gwinup G. Immobilization osteoporosis in paraplegia. J Am Paraplegia Soc 1992;15:163–170.

52. Eschbach K, Herbison G, Ditunno J. Sensory root level recovery in patients with Frankel A quadriplegia. Arch Phys Med Rehabil 1992;73:618–622.

53. Evans R, Hendricks R, Connis R, et al. Quality of life after spinal cord injury: A literature critique and meta-analysis (1983–1992). J Am Paraplegia Soc 1994;17:60–66.

54. Faghri P, Glaser R, Figoni S. Functional electrical stimulation leg cycle ergometer exercise: Training effects on cardiorespiratory responses of SCI subjects at rest and during submaximal exercise. Arch Phys Med Rehabil 1992;73:1085–1093.

55. Figoni S. Perspectives on cardiovascular fitness and SCI. J Am Paraplegia Soc 1990;13:63–71.

56. Franklin B. Aerobic exercise training programs for the upper body. Med Sci Sports Exerc 1989; 21:S141–S148.

57. Fuhrer M, Garber S, Rintala D, et al. Pressure ulcers in community-resident persons with spinal cord injury: Prevalence and risk factors. Arch Phys Med Rehabil 1993;74:1172–1177.

58. Fuhrer M, Rintala D, Hart K, et al. Relationship of life satisfaction to impairment, disability, and handicap among persons with SCI living in the community. Arch Phys Med Rehabil 1992;73:552–557.

59. Fung J, Stewart J, Barbeau H. The combined effects of clonidine and cyproheptadine with interactive training on the modulation of locomotion in spinal cord injured subjects. J Neurol Sci 1990; 100:85–93.

60. Geisler F, Dorsey F, Coleman W. Recovery of motor function after SCI: A randomized, placebo-controlled trial with GM-1 ganglioside. N Engl J Med 1991;324:1829–1838.

61. Gellman H. Tendon transfer surgery after spinal cord injury. Crit Rev Phys Rehabil Med 1991; 3:147–153.

62. Gerhart K, Bergstrom E, Charlifue S, et al. Long-term spinal cord injury: Functional changes over time. Arch Phys Med Rehabil 1993;74:1030–1034.

63. Glaser R. Physiology of functional electrical stimulation-induced exercise: basic science perspective. Journal of Neurologic Rehabilitation 1991; 5:49–61.

64. Glaser R, Davis G. Wheelchair-dependent individuals. In: Franklin B, Gordon S, Timmis G, eds.: Exercise in Modern Medicine. Baltimore: Williams & Wilkins, 1989:237–267.

65. Glenn W, Brouilette R, Dentz B, et al. Fundamental considerations in pacing of the diaphragm for chronic ventilation insufficiency: A multicenter study. PACE 1988;11:2121–2170.

66. Gorman P, Peckham P. Upper extremity functional neuromuscular stimulation. Journal of Neurologic Rehabilitation 1991;5:3–11.

67. Granger C, Albrecht G, Hamilton B. Outcome of comprehensive rehabilitation: Measurement by PULSES and Barthel Index. Arch Phys Med Rehabil 1979;60:145–154.

68. Granger C, Hamilton B. The Uniform Data System for Medical Rehabilitation report of first admissions for 1992. Am J Phys Med Rehabil 1994;73:51–55.

69. Green D, Lee M, Ito V, et al. Fixed vs adjusted dose heparin in the prophylaxis of thromboembolism in SCI. JAMA 1988;260:1255–1258.

69a. Green D, Chen D, Chmiel J, et al. Prevention of thromboembolism in spinal cord injury: Role of low molecular weight heparin. Arch Phys Med Rehabil 1994;75:290–292.

70. Gresham G, Labi M, Dittmar S, et al. The Quadriplegia Index of Function: Sensitivity and reliability demonstrated in a study of thirty quadriplegic patients. Paraplegia 1986;24:38–44.

71. Groomes T, Huang C. Orthostatic hypotension after SCI: Treatment with fludrocortisone and ergotamine. Arch Phys Med Rehabil 1991;72:56–58.

72. Hangartner T, Rodgers M. Glaser R, et al. Tibial bone density loss in spinal cord injured patients: Effects of FES exercise. J Rehabil Res 1994;31:50–61.

73. Harkema S, Dobkin B. Requejo P, et al. Effect of assisted treadmill step training on EMG patterns and muscle volumes in spinal cord injured subjects. J Neurotrauma 1995;12:121.

74. Harvey C, Rothschild B, Asmann A, et al. New estimates of traumatic SCI prevalence: A survey based approach. Paraplegia 1990;28:537–544.

75. Heinemann A, Doll M, Armstrong M, et al. Substance use and receipt of treatment by persons with long-term SCI. Arch Phys Med Rehabil 1991; 72:482–487.

76. Heinemann A, Yarkony G, Roth E, et al. Functional outcome following spinal cord injury. Arch Neurol 1989;46:1098–1102.

77. Herman R, Wainberg M. Clonidine inhibits vesicosphincter reflexes in patients with chronic spinal lesions. Arch Phys Med Rehabil 1991;72:539–545.

78. Hirokawa S, Grimm M, Le T, et al. Energy consumption in paraplegic ambulation using the RGO

and electric stimulation of the thigh muscles. Arch Phys Med Rehabil 1990;71:687–694.

79. Hodgson J, Roy R, Dobkin B, et al. Can the mammalian spinal cord learn a motor task? Med Sci Sports Exerc 1994;26:1491–1497.

80. Hooker S, Wells C. Effects of low and moderate intensity training in spinal cord injured persons. Med Sci Sports Exerc 1989;21:18–22.

81. Isakov E, Douglas R, Berns P. Ambulation using the reciprocating gait orthosis and functional electrical stimulation. Paraplegia 1992;30:239–245.

82. Jackson A, DeVivo M. Urological long-term follow-up in women with spinal cord injury. Arch Phys Med Rehabil 1992;73:1029–1035.

83. Jackson A, Groomes T. Incidence of respiratory complications following spinal cord injury. Arch Phys Med Rehabil 1994;75:270–275.

83a. Jacobs SA, Yeaney N, Herbison E, et al. Future ambulation prognosis as predicted by somatosensory evoked potentials. Arch Phys Med Rehabil 1995; 76:635–641.

84. Jaeger R, Yarkony G, Roth E. Rehabilitation technology for standing and walking after spinal cord injury. Am J Phys Med Rehabil 1989;68:128–133.

85. Kakulas B, Taylor J. Pathology of injuries of the vertebral column and spinal cord. In: Frankel H, ed: Spinal Cord Trauma. Amsterdam: Elsevier, 1992:21–51.

86. Katz R, Toleikis R, Knuth A. Somatosensory evoked and dermatomal evoked potentials are not clinically useful in the prognostication of acute SCI. Spine 1991;16:730–735.

87. Keith M, Lacey S. Surgical rehabilitation of the tetraplegic upper extremity. Journal of Neurologic Rehabilitation 1991;5:75–87.

88. Kim S, Charallel J, Park K, et al. Prevalence of deep venous thrombosis in patients with chronic spinal cord injury. Arch Phys Med Rehabil 1994;75:965–968.

89. Klose E, Needham B, Schmidt D, et al. An assessment of the contribution of electromyographic biofeedback as an adjunct in the physical training of spinal cord injured persons. Arch Phys Med Rehabil 1993;74:453–456.

90. Klose K, Schmidt D, Needham B, et al. Rehabilitation therapy for patients with long-term spinal cord injuries. Arch Phys Med Rehabil 1990; 71:659–662.

91. Kramer J. Muscle strengthening via electrical stimulation. Crit Rev Phys Rehabil Med 1989;1:97–133.

92. Krause J. Employment after spinal cord injury. Arch Phys Med Rehabil 1992;73:163–169.

93. Krause J, Kjorsvig J. Mortality after SCI: A four-year prospective study. Arch Phys Med Rehabil 1992; 73:558–563.

94. Kuhn R. Functional capacity of the isolated human spinal cord. Brain 1950;73:1–51.

95. Lal S, Hamilton B, Heinemann A, et al. Risk factors for heterotopic ossification in spinal cord injury. Arch Phys Med Rehabil 1989;70:387–390.

96. Lazar R, Yarkony G, Ortolano D, et al. Prediction of functional outcome by motor capability after spinal cord injury. Arch Phys Med Rehabil 1989; 70:819–822.

97. Li C, Houlden D, Rowed D. Somatosensory evoked potentials and neurological grades as predictors of outcome in acute SCI. J Neurosurg 1990;72:600–604.

98. Linsenmeyer T, Perkash I. Infertility in men with SCI. Arch Phys Med Rehabil 1991;72:747–754.

99. Little J, Micklesen P, Umlauf R, et al. Lower extremity manifestations of spasticity in chronic spinal cord injury. Am J Phys Med Rehabil 1989; 68:32–36.

100. Livneh H, Antonak R. Psychosocial reactions to disability: A review and critique of the literature. Crit Rev Phys Rehabil Med 1994;6:1–100.

101. Loubser P, Narayan R, Sandin K, et al. Continuous infusion of intrathecal baclofen: Long-term effects on spasticity in spinal cord injury. Paraplegia 1991; 29:48–64.

102. Lyles M, Munday J. Report on the evaluation of the Vannini-Rizzoli stabilizing limb orthosis. J Rehabil Res 1992;29:77–104.

103. Macdonnell R, Donnan G. Magnetic cortical stimulation in acute spinal cord injury. Neurology 1995;45:303–306.

104. MacKenzie E, Shapiro S, Siegel J. The economic impact of traumatic injuries. JAMA 1988; 260:3290–3296.

105. Manson J, Nathan D, Krolewski A, et al. A prospective study of exercise and incidence of diabetes among US physicians. JAMA 1992; 268:63–67.

106. Marciello M, Flanders A, Herbison G, et al. Magnetic resonance imaging related to neurologic outcome in cervical spinal cord injury. Arch Phys Med Rehabil 1993;74:940–946.

107. Marsolais E, Kobetic R, Chizeck H, et al. Orthoses and electrical stimulation for walking in complete paraplegia. Journal of Neurologic Rehabilitation 1991;5:13–22.

108. Marsolais E, Kobetic R, Miller P. Status of paraplegic FNS-assisted walking. J Am Paraplegia Soc 1994;17:213.

109. Mattson E, Brostrom L, Karlsson J. Walking efficiency before and after long-term muscle stretch in patients with spastic paraparesis. Scand J Rehab Med 1990;22:55–59.

110. Maynard F. Immobilization hypercalcemia following SCI. Arch Phys Med Rehabil 1986;67:41–44.

111. Maynard F, Reynolds G, Fountain S. Neurological progress after traumatic quadriplegia. J Neurosurg 1979;50:611–616.

111a. Maynard FM, Karunas K, Waring W. Epidemiology of spasticity following traumatic spinal cord injury. Arch Phys Med Rehabil 1990;71:566–570.

112. Merli G, Crabbe S, Paluzzi R, et al. Etiology, incidence, and prevention of deep vein thrombosis in acute spinal cord injury. Arch Phys Med Rehabil 1993;74:1199–1205.

113. Meyers A, Branch L, Cupples L, et al. Predictors of medical care utilization by independently living adults with spinal cord injuries. Arch Phys Med Rehabil 1989;70:471–476.

114. Meythaler J, Steers W, Tuel S, et al. Intrathecal baclofen in hereditary spastic paraparesis. Arch Phys Med Rehabil 1992;73:794–797.

115. Minaire P. Immobilization osteoporosis. Clin Rheumatol 1989;852:95–103.

116. Nance P, Bugaresti J, Shellenberger K, et al. Efficacy and safety of tizanidine in the treatment of

spasticity in patients with spinal cord injury. Neurology 1994;44(Suppl 9):S44–S52.

117. Nathan R, Ohry A. Upper limb functions regained in quadriplegia: A hybrid computerized neuromuscular stimulation system. Arch Phys Med Rehabil 1990;71:415–421.

118. National Institute on Disability and Rehabilitation Research Consensus Statement. The prevention and management of urinary tract infections among people with spinal cord injuries. J Am Paraplegia Soc 1992;15:194–204.

119. Oakes D, Wilmot C, Hall K, et al. Benefits of early admission to a comprehensive trauma center for patients with SCI. Arch Phys Med Rehabil 1990; 71:637–643.

120. Ohshio I, Hatayama A, Kaneda K, et al. Correlation between histopathologic features and magnetic resonance images of spinal cord lesions. Spine 1993;18:1140–1149.

121. Patterson D, Miller-Perrin C, McCormick T, et al. When life support is questioned early in the care of patients with cervical-level quadriplegia. N Engl J Med 1994;328:506–509.

122. Peckham P, Creasey G. Neural prostheses: Clinical applications of functional electrical stimulation in SCI. Paraplegia 1992;30:96–101.

123. Penn R, Savoy S, Corcos D, et al. Intrathecal baclofen for severe spinal spasticity. N Engl J Med 1989; 320:1517–1521.

124. Penrod L, Hegde S, Ditunno J. Age effect on prognosis for functional recovery in acute, traumatic central cord syndrome. Arch Phys Med Rehabil 1990;71:963–968.

125. Petrofsky J, Smith J. Physiologic costs of computer controlled walking in persons with paraplegia using a reciprocating gait orthosis. Arch Phys Med Rehabil 1991;72:890–896.

126. Piepmeier J, Jenkins N. Late neurological changes following traumatic SCI. J Neurosurg 1988;69:399–402.

127. Reier P, Anderson D, Thompson F, et al. Neural tissue transplantation and CNS trauma: Anatomical and functional repair of the injured spinal cord. J Neurotrauma 1992;9(Suppl 1):S223–S248.

128. Riddoch G. The reflex functions of the completely divided spinal cord in man, compared with those associated with less severe lesions. Brain 1917; 40:264–402.

129. Roth E, Davidoff G, Haughton J, et al. Functional assessment in spinal cord injury: A comparison of the Modified Barthel Index and the "adapted" Functional Independence Measure. Clin Rehabil 1990;4:277–285.

130. Rubin R, Gold W, Kelley D, et al. The Cost of Disorders of the Brain. Washington, DC: National Foundation for Brain Research, 1992.

131. Samsa G, Patrick C, Feussner J. Long-term survival of veterans with traumatic spinal cord injury. Arch Neurol 1993;50:909–914.

131a. Senard JM, Arias A, Berlan M, et al. Pharmacological evidence of alpha-1 and alpha-2 adrenergic supersensitivity in orthostatic hypotension due to spinal cord injury. Eur J Clin Pharmacol 1991; 41:593–596.

132. Sherwood A, Dimitrijevic M, McKay W. Evidence of subclinical brain influence in clinically complete spinal cord injury: Discomplete SCI. J Neurol Sci 1992;110:90–98.

133. Signorile J, Banovac K, Gomez M, et al. Increased muscle strength in paralyzed patients after spinal cord injury: Effect of beta-2 adrenergic agonist. Arch Phys Med Rehabil 1995;76:55–58.

134. Sipski M, Alexander C, Harris M. Long-term use of computerized bicycle ergometry for SCI subjects. Arch Phys Med Rehabil 1993;74:238–241.

135. Sipski M, DeLisa J. Functional electrical stimulation in SCI rehabilitation: A review of the literature. NeuroRehabilitation 1991;1:46–57.

136. Solomon S, Gerrity E, Muff A. Efficacy of treatments for posttraumatic stress disorder. JAMA 1992;268:633–638.

137. Song Z, Cohen M, Vulpe M, et al. Two-point discrimination thresholds in spinal cord injured patients with dysesthetic pain. Paraplegia 1993; 31:485–493.

138. Stein R, Belanger M, Wheeler G, et al. Electrical systems for improving locomotion after incomplete spinal cord injury. Arch Phys Med Rehabil 1993;74:954–959.

139. Stein R, Brucker B, Ayyar D. Motor units in incomplete spinal cord injury: Electrical activity, contractile properties and the effects of biofeedback. J Neurol Neurosurg Psychiatry 1990;53:880–885.

140. Stover S. Spinal Cord Injury: The Facts and Figures. Birmingham: University of Alabama, 1986.

141. Stover S, Lloyd K, Waites K, et al. Urinary tract infection in SCI. Arch Phys Med Rehabil 1989; 70:47–54.

142. Subbarao J, Klopfstein J, Turpin R. Prevalence and impact of wrist and shoulder pain in patients with spinal cord injury. Journal of Spinal Cord Medicine 1995;18:9–13.

143. Tate D, Forchheimer M, Maynard F, et al. Predicting depression and psychological distress in persons with spinal cord injury based on indicators of handicap. Am J Phys Med Rehabil 1994;73:175–183.

144. Topka H, Cohen L, Cole R, et al. Reorganization of corticospinal pathways following spinal cord injury. Neurology 1991;41:1276–1283.

145. VandenBerghe A, VanLaere M, Hellings S, et al. Reconstruction of the upper extremity in tetraplegia: Functional assessment, surgical procedures and rehabiliation. Paraplegia 1991;29:103–112.

146. Vaziri N, Panadian M, Segal J, et al. Vitamin D, parathormone, and calcitonin profiles in persons with long-standing spinal cord injury. Arch Phys Med Rehabil 1994;75:766–769.

147. Visintin M, Barbeau H. The effect of body weight support on the locomotor pattern of spastic paretic patients. Can J Neurol Sci 1989;16:315–325.

148. Wainberg M, Barbeau H, Gauthier S. Quantitative assessment of the effect of cyproheptadine on spastic paretic gait: A preliminary study. J Neurol 1986; 233:311–314.

149. Wang Y-H, Huang T-S, Lien I-N. Hormone changes in men with spinal cord injuries. Am J Phys Med Rehabil 1992;71:328–332.

150. Waters R, Adkins R, Yakura J, et al. Motor and sensory recovery following complete tetraplegia. Arch Phys Med Rehabil 1993;74:242–247.

151. Waters R, Adkins R, Yakura J, et al. Motor and sen-

sory recovery following incomplete paraplegia. Arch Phys Med Rehabil 1994;75:67–72.

152. Waters R, Adkins R, Yakura J, et al. Motor and sensory recovery following incomplete tetraplegia. Arch Phys Med Rehabil 1994;75:306–311.

153. Waters R, Adkins R, Yakura J, et al. Prediction of ambulatory performance based on motor scores derived from standards of the American Spinal Injury Association. Arch Phys Med Rehabil 1994; 75:756–760.

153a. Waters RL, Sie I, Adkins R, et al. Injury pattern effect on motor recovery after traumatic spinal cord injury. Arch Phys Med Rehabil 1995;76:440–443.

154. Waters R, Yakura J. The energy expenditure of normal and pathological gait. Crit Rev Phys Rehabil Med 1989;1:183–209.

155. Waters R, Yakura J, Adkins R, et al. Determinants of gait performance following spinal cord injury. Arch Phys Med Rehabil 1989;70:811–818.

156. Waters R, Yakura J, Adkins R, et al. Recovery following paraplegia. Arch Phys Med Rehabil 1992; 73:784–789.

157. Weingarden S, Martin C. Independent dressing after spinal cord injury: A functional time evaluation. Arch Phys Med Rehabil 1989;70:518–519.

158. Wells J, Nicosia S. Scoring acute spinal cord injury. Journal of Spinal Cord Medicine 1995;18:33–41.

159. Wernig A, Muller S. Improvement of walking in spinal cord injured persons after treadmill training. In: Wernig A, ed: Plasticity of Motoneuronal Connections. Amsterdam: Elsevier, 1991:475–485.

160. Wernig A, Muller S. Laufband locomotion with body weight support improved walking in persons with severe spinal cord injuries. Paraplegia 1992; 30:229–238.

161. Wernig A, Muller S, Nanassy A, et al. Laufband therapy based on ''Rules of Spinal Locomotion'' is effective in spinal cord injured persons. Eur J Neurosci 1995;7:823–829.

162. White M, Rintala D, Hart K, et al. Sexual activities, concerns and interests of men with SCI. Am J Phys Med Rehabil 1992;71:225–231.

163. White M, Rintala D, Hart K, et al. Sexual activities, concerns and interests of women with SCI living in the community. Am J Phys Med Rehabil 1993; 72:372–378.

164. Whiteneck G. Outcome evaluation and spinal cord injury. NeuroRehabil 1992;2:31–41.

165. Wiegner A. Can basic science help improve arm function in C5 tetraplegia? J Am Paraplegia Soc 1993;16:75.

166. Wilmot C, Hall K. Evaluation of acute surgical intervention in traumatic paraplegia. Paraplegia 1986;24:71–76.

167. Wilmot C, Hall K. Evaluation of the acute management of tetraplegia: Conservative versus surgical treatment. Paraplegia 1986;24:148–153.

168. Woolsey R. Rehabilitation outcome following spinal cord injury. Arch Neurol 1985;42:116–119.

169. Wyndaele J. Pharmacotherapy for urinary bladder dysfunction in spinal cord injury patients. Paraplegia 1990;28:146–150.

170. Yarkony G. Enhancement of sexual function and fertility in spinal cord injured males. Am J Phys Med Rehabil 1990;69:81–87.

171. Yarkony G, Roth E, Heinemann A, et al. Functional skills after spinal cord injury rehabilitation: Three-year longitudinal follow-up. Arch Phys Med Rehabil 1988;69:111–114.

172. Yarkony G, Roth E, Heinemann A, et al. Benefits of rehabilitation for traumatic spinal cord injury. Arch Neurol 1987;44:93–96.

173. Yarkony G, Roth E, Meyer J, et al. Spinal cord injury care system: Fifteen-year experience at the Rehabilitation Institute of Chicago. Paraplegia 1990; 28:321–329.

174. Young W. Neurorehabilitation of spinal cord injury. Journal of Neurologic Rehabilitation 1994; 8:3–9.

CHAPTER 9

TRAUMATIC BRAIN INJURY

Patients with traumatic brain injury (TBI) test the rehabilitation mettle of clinicians, families, and community health, educational, social, and vocational providers. The impairments, disabilities, and residual abilities that follow a moderate to severe TBI vary across patients more than in any other acute neurologic disease. Within patients, these disabilities can differ widely over time. Early recovery can evolve from coma into confusion and agitation before more appropriate behavior begins. Even then, attention, recall, and insight may be poor. A patient's disabilities throughout the stages of restoration ebb and flow within the undertow of myriad dysfunctions in cognition and behavior. This flux especially challenges the therapeutic strategies of the rehabilitation team.

This chapter deals primarily with patients who suffer from a moderate to severe closed-head injury (CHI). Postinjury gains are related to the mechanisms of restitution, substitution, sparing, and compensation (Table 1–2). It touches upon issues related to mild TBI and penetrating head trauma as well. Many of the interventions described are also appropriate for managing the moderate to severe cognitive and behavioral sequelae found in 50 percent of 1-year survivors of cardiac arrest and in survivors of subarachnoid hemorrhage associated with diffuse vasospasm or subfrontal ischemia.[178,192]

EPIDEMIOLOGY

About a half-million persons in the United States receive hospital treatment for TBI yearly: 100,000 die and 75,000 have long-term impairments and disabilities. The peak incidences for TBI occur in males aged 16 to 25 years and in people over the age of 65 years.[193] Penetrating head injuries (PHI) from bullet wounds account for 10 percent and CHI for 90 percent of TBI. Significant associated factors include motor vehicle accidents, lower socioeconomic class, and alcohol or drug abuse (Table 9–1). In Great Britain, between 2000 and 3000 per million population are hospitalized each year with TBI.[140] On hospital admission, about 5 percent of these patients score less than 8 on the Glasgow Coma Scale (GCS; see Table 5–4), about 10 percent score between 9 and 12 in the moderate range of severity, and the rest have minor injuries, although 10 percent of these patients have skull fractures. Rates are about the same in United States studies.[101] Residual disability in newly hospitalized persons who survive a TBI is likely to require inpatient or outpatient rehabilitation in about 313 per million persons in a community each year (Table 9–2).[193] TBI also causes at least 5000 new cases of epilepsy and 2000 cases of persistent vegetative state (PVS) in the United States yearly.

Table 9–1. CAUSES OF TRAUMATIC BRAIN INJURY

Cause	Percentage (%)
Child abuse in infants	64
Motor vehicle accidents	52
Falls	21
Assaults and violence	14
Sports and recreation	10
Other	3

Table 9–2. ESTIMATED NEED FOR REHABILITATION SERVICES AFTER TRAUMATIC BRAIN INJURY

Severity	Incidence (Per Million Population)	Residual Disability (%)
Mild	1,360	10
Moderate	158	67
Severe	71	100

Source: Adapted from Sorenson S, Kraus J.[193]

Economic Impact

The economic impact of TBI is stunning. In 1983 dollars, a Maryland study found that the mean 1-year charge for a patient aged 16 to 45 years with severe head injury was $106,000, with 18 percent going to rehabilitation care.[123] Charges for serious to moderate TBI were about $57,000. TBI accounted for 19 percent of all hospital trauma discharges, but it contributed 26 percent to total charges. Based on a national study of estimated charges for all patients with head injury who were admitted to a hospital in 1 year,[131] the average direct and indirect lifetime cost in 1991 dollars for survivors was $111,600, whereas patients with fatal outcomes cost $454,700.[179] The total national cost was $48.25 billion; $31.7 billion supported the survivors. Inpatient rehabilitation accounted for $1.15 billion, nursing home care for $350 million, home modifications for $62 million, and vocational rehabilitation for $4 million.

Prevention

Rehabilitation specialists can appreciate the potential for preventing TBI. For example, the use of helmets has reduced deaths by motorcycle accidents by 18 percent, it has lowered acute care costs by 40 percent, and it has lessened disability.[143,150] National efforts could mandate the use of seat belts, air bags, and other highway safety measures, require sturdy helmets for bicyclists and skaters, regulate guns, promote programs to decrease alcohol and drug abuse, and continue to identify and manage predisposing causes of falls in the elderly. For some injuries, such as motorcycle-related TBI, 60 percent or more of the costs are borne by public funding.[175] Prevention, then, can have an impact on city, county, state, and federal shares of the economic burden of brain injury. A balance must be found between the personal freedom of individuals to choose whether to wear protective gear and their public responsibility.

PATHOPHYSIOLOGY

In patients with TBI, both immediate and delayed focal and diffuse injuries can unfold from a spectrum of interrelated pathophysiologic processes (Table 9–3). Expectations for neurorestoration are guided by the location and combination of these lesions, the severity of clinical consequences, and the clinicopathologic changes over time after the onset of TBI.

In CHI, acceleration and deceleration of the brain relative to the skull cause compressive, shearing, and tensile strains and displacements. The damage from PHI depends especially on the amount of energy imparted to the brain.[58] High-velocity bullets cause larger cavitations, more diffuse injury, and higher mortality than low-velocity bullets. Missile fragments, such as shrapnel, tend to produce focal injury. A cascade of cellular events can follow either CHI or PHI, including intracellular edema, calcium and other ionic fluxes, glutamate neurotoxicity, glial cell compromise, lipid peroxidation, cytokine production,[152] failure of protein synthesis, neurofilament degradation,[159] and other effects of early and delayed ischemia and mechanical injury.[84] The gross pathophysiologic sequelae are more readily imaged and monitored. Their identification can lead to early medical and neurosurgical interventions.[212] Compared with acute interventions for ischemic stroke, interventions that must be initiated within 6 or, better, within 3 hours of onset, the cascade of biologic events following TBI probably offers a longer window of opportunity. Some drug interventions that are being developed for acute TBI will likely prolong the therapeutic window. The period of compromise of functional plasticity may also have a longer duration after TBI, compared with stroke. Certain types of pathologic processes have particular consequences for rehabilitation.

Table 9–3. **PRIMARY AND SECONDARY PATHOPHYSIOLOGIC CONSEQUENCES OF TRAUMATIC BRAIN INJURY**

Focal Injury
　Contusion
　　Orbitofrontal, anterior temporal, basal
　　　ganglia
　Edema
　Hematoma
　　Intracerebral, subdural, epidural
　Hygroma

Diffuse Axonal Injury
　Petechial hemorrhages; edema; axotomy
　　Subcortical white matter, corpus callosum,
　　　brainstem
　Cytoskeletal damage
　Impaired axonal transport
　Delayed demyelination
　Retrograde neuronal death

Hypoxic-Ischemic Injury
　Systemic anoxia, hypotension
　　Laminar cortical necrosis
　　Arterial border zone
　　Vulnerable neurons, e.g., hippocampus,
　　　basal ganglia
　Microvascular injury
　　Loss of cerebrovascular autoregulation
　　Compression
　Arterial occlusion, e.g., posterior cerebral
　　artery
　Vasospasm

Increased Intracranial Pressure
　Focal and diffuse mass effect
　Hydrocephalus
　Herniation

Secondary Injury
　Excitotoxins
　Free radicals
　Lactic acidosis
　Arachidonic cascade
　Cytokines
　Inflammatory cells

Acceleration TBI, which often occurs in a motor vehicle accident, produces diffuse axonal injury (DAI). This disorder is characterized by swelling and retraction of the damaged ends of axons over days, followed by microglial infiltration and axonal degeneration over subsequent weeks. Trauma can cause initial axonal changes in larger areas than the mechanical disruption. These changes are related to axolemmal permeability, perturbations of the cytoskeleton with primary and secondary changes in the composition and alignment of neurofilaments, and other metabolic disturbances.[156] They lead to impaired axonal transport, to continued axonal swelling, and, over a course that can take more than 12 hours, to disconnection from the soma.[160] Thus, complex subsets of pathobiology follow traumatically induced axonal injury. Because this process evolves over the time of acute hospitalization, interventions to reverse axonal injury may be possible.

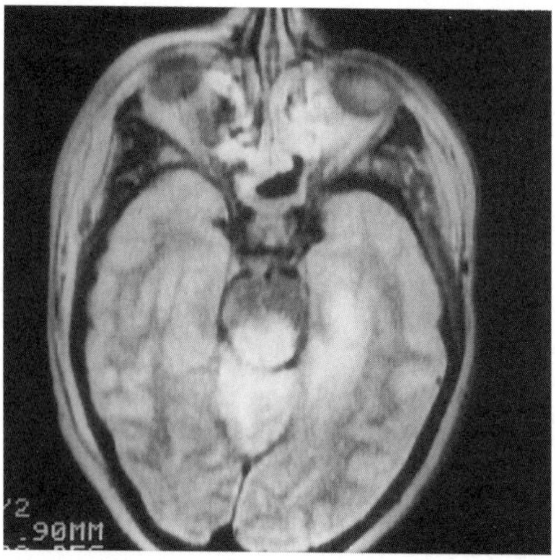

Figure 9–1. T$_2$-weighted scan at the level of the pons reveals hyperintensity of the dorsal pons, vermis of the cerebellum, and left medial temporal lobe (to the right of the brainstem) in a 40-year-old who survived a closed head injury (CHI) in a motor vehicle accident. The subcortical white matter had multiple petechial hemorrhages. The patient emerged from a Glasgow Coma Scale (GCS) score of 6, but 3 years later had permanent, debilitating cognitive and motor impairments.

Diffuse Axonal Injury

More severe trauma in a primate TBI model produces denser DAI in deeper and more diffuse regions of the cerebrum and dorsal brainstem, correlating with longer duration of coma and less clinical recovery.[51] The patient whose magnetic resonance imaging (MRI) scan is shown in Figure 9–1 had a similar distribution of lesions. DAI tends to be a midline process, with the rostral upper brainstem and corpus callosum involved in 90 percent of patients with serious TBI. The worst prognosis for functional recovery is found in patients with rostral brainstem lesions. The dorsal pons and midbrain are the repositories for serotonergic, cholinergic, and noradrenergic neurons. Damage to these projection systems can have widespread consequences for thalamocortical and frontal lobe function. For example, cholinergic neurons act upon the reticular nucleus of the thalamus, which gates the inputs and outputs from the dorsal thalamic nuclei and prefrontal cortex.[22] Dysfunction in this area may account for some of the attentional and other cognitive sequelae of TBI in patients with dorsal brainstem DAI.

Mortality, the duration of unconsciousness, the degree of posttraumatic amnesia (PTA), and the persistence of confusion appear to correlate best, although not linearly, with the severity of DAI. DAI is often accompanied by focal and diffuse edema and petechial hemorrhages with secondary loss of vascular autoregulation and increased intracranial pressure.

DAI is of special interest because it results in diffuse deafferentation of target sites. Positron emission tomography (PET) often reveals global cerebral hypometabolism soon after a severe TBI. Over time, partial deafferentation of target neurons can lead to denervation hypersensitivity and to the ingrowth of spared axonal inputs. Considerable focal DAI can lead to a more concentrated amount of target denervation, to less reinnervation by axons of the same pathway compared with a more diffuse process of DAI, and to more input from neighboring, but functionally different, axons. Adaptive or maladaptive plasticity may result in either situation. Potential rehabilitative biologic interventions include blocking the molecules that may inhibit the axonal growth cone and providing trophic factors that increase axonal extension to targets (see Chapter 2).

Hypoxic-Ischemic Injury

Other pathologic processes can also contribute to the effects of severe TBI. Systemic hypoxia and hypotension at the onset of TBI add to the insult up to the point of causing cortical laminar necrosis or damaging especially vulnerable neuronal populations, such as those of the hippocampus, cerebellum, and basal ganglia. Hypoxic-ischemic injury decreases cerebral blood flow and increases cortical hyperemia and intracranial pressure. These sequelae generally correlate with poorer cognitive and overall outcomes.[177,204] Both hypoxic-ischemic injury and high intracranial pressures that cannot be medically and surgically managed lead to the greater likelihood of morbidity, a vegetative state, and mortality. For example, the National Traumatic Data Bank found that intracranial pressure above 30 mm Hg was associated with a poor outcome regardless of the initial score on the GCS. Hypoxia on admission led to a 20 percent increase in mortality and vegetative state; blood pressure lower than 90 mm Hg was associated with a 30 percent increase.[107]

Focal Injury

Direct forces at the point of impact can produce focal coup and remote contracoup hematomas and contusions. Other focal contusions commonly occur within the anteroinferior temporal lobes and the orbitofrontal cortex, sites close to the bony skull, as shown in the computed tomographic (CT) scan in Figure 9–2. Damage and disruption of connections to and from these sites account for impairments in executive functions, drives, multimodal processing of information, mood, and memory. Hemorrhages develop in the distribution of sheared penetrating arteries, such as the lenticulostriates to the basal ganglia. Focal ischemia follows occlusion of small vessels by edema and of midsized posterior and anterior cerebral arteries if cerebral herniation ensues.

PHI also tends to cause focal tissue destruction, hematoma, and edema. Veterans followed in the Vietnam Head Injury Study of penetrating wounds were found to have lower global cognitive scores on the Wechsler Adult Intelligence Scale IQ test in relation to greater losses of brain volume.[59] Specific cognitive impairments developed more often with localized structural lesions. The study revealed the limitations of anatomic and functional correlations, however. Preinjury intelligence or education played a larger role than total volume loss or lesion location

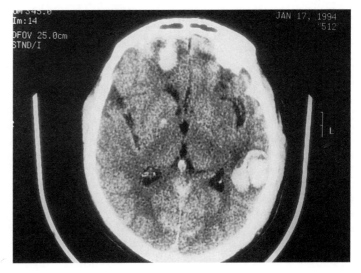

Figure 9–2. Computed tomography (CT) scan at the level of the internal capsule and thalamus of a 70-year-old woman who was knocked to the floor by a bookcase that fell upon her during the 1994 California Northridge earthquake. Her initial Glasgow Coma Scale (GCS) score was 8. Right frontal, right mesial globus pallidus, and left temporal lobe hematomas are shown. On higher cuts, a left subdural hematoma and cerebral edema were evident. She regained full motor function but was left with profound impairments in memory and behavior.

in predicting the persistence of cognitive deficits.

Neuroimaging

Neuroimaging with CT and MRI has been used to classify the disorders and outcomes of TBI. Focal injuries, DAI, and diffuse swelling can be identified by MRI with better confidence for nonhemorrhagic lesions.[199] Hemorrhages in the central white matter and at gray-white junctions, along with white matter edema, help to define DAI, although some patients have normal-appearing scans. These acute imaging categories have been related to outcomes.[203] For example, a PVS and mortality were most common in patients with DAI. On the Glasgow Outcome Scale (GOS; Table 5–13), good recovery occurred more often with focal injuries than after DAI. In a rehabilitation population after TBI, the GOS at 6 and 12 months post injury correlated significantly with the duration of PTA in patients with DAI, but not in those with primarily a focal brain injury.[93] Scores on neuropsychologic tests of memory, learning, and visuomotor speed were higher in patients with diffuse cerebral edema, although gains over the next 6 months were less than for patients with DAI. Deeper parenchymal lesions were associated with greater severity and duration of impaired consciousness; outcome at 6 months on the GOS was better in patients with more superficial lesions.[114]

In patients with a GCS of 13 to 15, the CT finding of an intracerebral contusion or hematoma alters the 6-month outcome from that found after mild CHI to a picture more like the consequences of moderate TBI.[213] Cortical lesions are especially likely to correlate with specific neuropsychologic impairments, but they are usually part of a heterogeneous group of injuries that may only modestly contribute to the clinical picture.[217] Aside from clinicopathologic relationships for focal injuries, anatomic imaging has not correlated well with neuropsychologic performance.[218] This lack of correlation may in part be reflected in the distributed representation of common TBI impairments, such as memory, executive functions, and attention.

Imaging during inpatient rehabilitation can uncover treatable structural causes of deterioration or of failure to improve in attention and cognition. For example, hydrocephalus and a cerebral hygroma or abscess can limit or reverse the patient's progress. Late imaging can yield prognostic indicators associated with an underlying pathologic process. For example, poor cognition at 1 year correlated with a wider third ventricle at 3 months after severe TBI; this finding suggests the impact of diencephalic atrophy associated with DAI and hypoxia.[173] Atrophy of the corpus callosum has been associated with DAI after severe TBI and with hemispheric disconnection syndromes.[116] Focal areas of encephalomalacia associated with persisting motor and cognitive impairments lead one to anticipate fewer functional gains related to those impairments.

Metabolic Imaging

Metabolic and blood flow imaging techniques show promise in revealing regional ischemia shortly after severe TBI.[128] This information could influence acute treatments. Metabolic imaging studies performed during rehabilitation offer other insights. PET has revealed focal and diffuse cortical hypometabolism in areas remote from, but transsynaptically connected to, subcortical regions affected by DAI. The degree of this metabolic diaschisis and overall metabolic depression for glucose metabolism has not clearly correlated with GCS at the time of the study.[11] Hypometabolism in the limbic and paralimbic areas, where MRI showed no lesion, has correlated with poorer outcome on the GOS.[46] Single-photon emission tomography (SPECT) studies have suggested several relationships. Low flow in the thalamus correlated with greater cognitive and neurologic impairment, and low frontal flow occurred in patients with disinhibited behavior.[149] PET studies performed more than 6 months after TBI suggest an association between persistent impairment of memory and executive functions with depression of glucose utilization in mesial temporal and orbitofrontal regions.[94a] The severity of neurologic impairment tends to correlate with the degree of metabolic depression. Additional studies are needed.

Identification of metabolically affected neural networks may provide insight into the causes of attentional, memory, and other cognitive and behavioral problems of patients. Metabolic studies correlated with particular outcomes may help to determine the likelihood of recovery at a particular point in time. In addition, activation paradigms and studies of markers for protein metabolism or of particular neurotransmitter pathways may reveal whether or not a patient is ready for cognitive information, able to learn novel information, or is likely to benefit from a particular rehabilitative intervention.

NEUROMEDICAL COMPLICATIONS

Many neurologic, general medical, and orthopedic derangements can complicate and interfere with the early and late rehabilitation of patients after a moderate or severe head injury.[81] TBI is often accompanied by injuries to bone, soft tissues, viscera, and the spinal cord and peripheral nerves. Deep vein thrombosis has been detected by serial testing in over 50 percent of patients after major TBI within 3 weeks of onset.[50] This incidence rose to over 75 percent in patients with associated femoral or tibial fractures. Many of the potential complications are outlined in Table 9–4. In a study of 180 patients with TBI who were admitted for rehabilitation, 56 percent had neurologic complications and 50 percent developed gastrointestinal complications, 45 percent had urinary complications, 34 percent had respiratory disorders, and 21 percent had dermatologic disorders.[90] We review the incidence and management of several of the more vexing problems.

Metabolic Sequelae

NUTRITION

Multiple interacting factors account for indices of malnutrition in about 60 percent of patients with TBI who are transferred to

a rehabilitation unit.[17,77] Acute trauma increases energy expenditure by an average of 40 percent. The highest metabolic energy expenditures and urinary nitrogen excretions affect patients with the lowest GCS, especially in the first several weeks after TBI.[222] Decerebration, spasms, seizures, agitation, and fever add to the hypermetabolic state. Mechanisms of hypercatabolism include acute-phase responses that also release cytokines, as well as autonomic hyperactivity and increases in blood catecholamines, glucagon, and cortisol. The likelihood of malnutrition increases when feedings are limited by gastric hypomotility, ileus, diarrhea, emesis, aspiration pneumonia, and a tracheal fistula. The use of corticosteroids and renal and liver failure contribute to this problem. Aphagia accompanies coma and poor attention, jaw and dental injuries, and central and peripheral causes of bulbar dysfunction, such as vocal cord paralysis. Later, during rehabilitation, cognitive and behavioral function and side effects of medications can affect the safety and quantity of oral intake and absorption. Better nutrition may improve functional outcomes.[222]

Several studies suggest that early parenteral hyperalimentation is better than nasogastric feeding for supplying needed calories, vitamins, and minerals including zinc. Regardless of the route of administration, the Quetelet Index of weight in kilograms, over height in square meters, should be brought into the range of 20 to 25. The serum albumin level should be kept well within the normal range, and attention should be given to providing a protein calorie contribution of 20 percent in the face of persistent hypercatabolism.

HYPOTHALAMIC-PITUITARY DYSFUNCTION

Severe, acute TBI can cause a rise in catecholamines, aldosterone, and cortisol, a fall in thyroid hormone release, diabetes insipidus or inappropriate secretion of antidiuretic hormone, and hypofunctioning of any component of the axis as a result of direct injury. The incidence varies from about 4 percent with symptoms appearing during rehabilitation to 60 percent in an autopsy se-

Table 9–4. SYSTEMIC COMPLICATIONS THAT CAN ACCOMPANY TRAUMATIC BRAIN INJURY

Skin

Decubitus ulcers
Acne; seborrhea; folliculitis
Sweat disorders
Drug reactions
Infections
Edema
Cosmetic deformity

Eye

Drying effect secondary to lid paralysis
Infection
Diplopia
Injuries: orbital fractures
Visual acuity; field cut; blindness; delayed optic neuropathy

Ear

Infection
Trauma
Drug toxicity
Hearing deficits, deafness

Nose

Trauma
Infection
Anosmia

Mouth and Throat

Dental-gingival disorders
  Jaw fractures
  Drug effects
  Bruxism
  Hygiene
  Dental injuries
Oral infections
Dysphagia

Larynx

Vocal cord trauma, paralysis
Infection

Trachea

With intubation: stenosis, erosion, fistula, excessive secretions
Tracheostomy dependence
Infection

Lungs

Emboli
Pneumonia
Atelectasis
Flail chest and lung trauma
Restrictive defects

Recurrent pneumothorax
Bronchopleural-cutaneous fistula
Adult respiratory distress syndrome
Pulmonary edema

Gastrointestinal Tract

Trauma; bowel ischemia
Gastroparesis
Reflux esophagitis
Peptic ulcer
Hepatitis; elevated liver function tests
Drug reactions
Diarrhea
Infection
Impaction
Incontinence
Complications of feeding tubes
Malnutrition
Bulimia and hyperphagia
Pancreatitis

Heart

Trauma; pericardial effusion
Heart failure
Arrhythmias

Peripheral Vascular System

Thrombophlebitis
Hypotension
Hypertension
Trauma with muscle or nerve ischemia

Genitourinary System

Infection
Catheter complication
Trauma of bladder or kidney
Incontinence
Sexual dysfunction

Female Reproductive System

Infection
Amenorrhea and oligomenorrhea
Organ trauma

Metabolic-Endocrine System

Hypothalamic-pituitary failure
Syndrome of inappropriate antidiuretic hormone
Salt-wasting syndrome
Hypothyroidism
Uremia
Electrolyte and fluid disorders
Malignant hyperthermia
Defective thermoregulation; central fever

Continued on following page

Table 9–4. *Continued*

Blood	Hydrocephalus
Anemia	Cerebrospinal otorrhea, rhinorrhea
Drug toxicity	Traumatic aneurysm, fistula
Clotting defects	Spasticity
Sepsis	Occult spinal cord injury
	Pain syndromes
Musculoskeletal System	Reflex sympathetic dystrophy
Osteoporosis	Headache
Weakness from drug reaction, disuse	Cervical musculoligamentous source
Contractures	Migraine
Heterotopic ossification	Radiculopathy
Osteomyelitis	Cutaneous neuroma
Fractures	Decerebration with autonomic "storm"
Soft tissue injuries	Movement disorders
	Cranial neuropathies
Central Nervous System	Vertigo, dysarthria, dysphagia, drooling,
Encephalopathy	diplopia
Drug reactions	
Metabolic disorders	*Peripheral Nervous System*
Infection	Neuropathies
Primary brain complications	Drug reaction
Recurrent or developing hematoma or	Metabolic disorders
hygroma	Local injury (peroneal, sciatic, ulnar nerves)
Infection; ventriculitis with a shunt	Compartment compression syndrome
Seizures	Brachial plexopathy

Source: Adapted from Horn L, Garland D,[81] pp 108–109.

ries.[90,100] Just how common occult and late endocrinopathies may be is uncertain.

PAIN

Head trauma is commonly associated with headache, perhaps most often after minor injuries. Cervical musculoligamentous and myofascial sources are common causes. Physical therapy with soft tissue techniques can lessen pain. During rehabilitation of patients who are less responsive and cognitively impaired or who have aphasia, pain due to undetected musculoskeletal injury and heterotopic ossification can add greatly to agitation and can limit participation. After TBI, heterotopic ossification especially tends to affect the proximal joints of patients in coma who have hypertonicity or fractures in those areas. Detection and management are covered in Chapter 8. In children, total body bone scans with technetium-99m MDP have

been recommended as a means of identifying some of these sources of pain.[187]

Nervous System Sequelae

SEIZURES

The incidence of seizures within the first week and later varies with the population reported. After a penetrating TBI, mostly resulting from shrapnel, 53 percent of veterans had a seizure, and half of them had ongoing epilepsy 15 years after the head injury.[181] In 18 percent, the first seizure happened more than 5 years after the PHI. Larger total brain volume loss detected by CT, hematoma, retained metal fragments, aphasia, hemiparesis, and organic mental disorder each increased the likelihood of a seizure. These risk factors did not necessarily lead to epilepsy, however. Phenytoin therapy in the first year had no prophylactic effect.

In a population study of over 2700 patients, mostly with CHI, 2 percent had a seizure in the first 2 weeks after injury. Patients with brain contusions, hematomas, or 24 hours of unconsciousness or amnesia had a 7 percent 1-year risk and an 11.5 percent 5-year risk of seizures.[2] Within the first 2 weeks in these patients with severe cases, children under the age of 15 years had a rate of seizures of 30 percent, compared with a 10 percent rate in adults. After a moderate injury defined as a skull fracture or 30 minutes to 24 hours of unconsciousness or amnesia, 0.7 percent at 1 year and 1.6 percent at 5 years had a seizure. The risk after a mild injury with briefer unconsciousness or amnesia was 0.1 and 0.6 percent, the same as in the general population.

Some of the best data on natural history come from a controlled trial of 400 patients admitted to a trauma center who were randomized to prophylactic phenytoin or placebo within 24 hours of injury.[200] Entry into the trial required a score of 10 or less on the GCS, a hematoma on CT scan, a penetrating skull wound, or a seizure within the first 24 hours. By day 7, 3.6 percent assigned to phenytoin had a seizure, compared with 14 percent on placebo. Between day 8 and 1 year, 21.5 percent of patients receiving phenytoin had a seizure, compared with 15.7 percent of patients receiving placebo. By year 2, 27.5 percent receiving phenytoin and 21 percent receiving placebo had seizures. Phenytoin levels were in a therapeutic range in 70 percent of patients. Thus, epilepsy is common after a serious TBI, and prophylaxis with phenytoin can reduce the incidence by about 70 percent in the first week, but not beyond that point. These findings are consistent with the results of a randomized trial that compared phenytoin, carbamazepine, and placebo for seizure prophylaxis after craniotomy for disorders other than malignant tumors.[47] Seizures were most frequent in the first month after surgery, but early and late seizures occurred at the same frequency, 37 percent, in all groups.

With a 25 percent rate of first seizures regardless of anticonvulsant prophylaxis, this approach does not seem productive beyond the first few weeks after a serious TBI. This conclusion has special impact for patients with TBI, because phenytoin, phenobarbital, and carbamazepine, perhaps more than valproate and newer drugs such as vigabatrin, can modestly impair motor and cognitive function.[39,185] In patients after TBI who were treated prophylactically with either phenytoin or carbamazepine and who were tested on and off the drugs, small effects were apparent on tests that required rapid motor and cognitive responses.[186] Some patients showed much greater slowing than others. Such individual variation may have an especially negative impact for some people during rehabilitation, academic work, and job training. Anticonvulsant management for at least 2 seizure-free years is a common practice when a primary or secondary generalized seizure occurs beyond the first week following an injury, however.

HYDROCEPHALUS

Acute obstructive hydrocephalus can be a complication of cerebral edema and of blood within the ventricles or the subarachnoid space. A ventricular shunt is indicated. After a subarachnoid hemorrhage, the development of symptomatic hydrocephalus is predicted by finding cisternal and ventricular blood or hydrocephalus on the initial CT scan.[207] Symptomatic nonobstructive or normal pressure hydrocephalus can develop insidiously over months, even years, after TBI. The incidence of hydrocephalus is probably no more than 5 percent.[69] Ventricular enlargement, however, develops in 30 to 70 percent of patients with severe TBI.[29,113] Most patients appear to have hydrocephalus ex vacuo, a passive enlargement from the loss of gray and white matter. No test predicts the response to a shunting procedure. Indium cisternography, features of the MRI scan, and a trial of lumbar drainage provide some insight.[205] Focal and diffuse brain disorders can account for all of a patient's impairments or may limit gains even after a shunt is placed for symptomatic hydrocephalus. As with other surgically accessible intracranial abnormalities that follow TBI, such as small residual subdural hematomas and hygromas, clinical acumen and the willingness of physicians, patient, and family to accept the risk of potential complications, such as an infection or shunt malfunction, guide decisions about intervention.

Enlarging ventricles with the triad of increasing gait apraxia, cognitive dysfunction, and incontinence are compelling indications for a ventricular shunt. Figure 9–3 shows the typical CT features in a patient with a positive response to a shunt. Excessively low ventricular pressures after placement of a ventriculoperitoneal shunt can also impair attention, alertness, and other cognitive processes, as well as produce headache.

In some patients, the ventricles may be only modestly enlarged in the presence of increased intracranial pressure (ICP) after a shunt malfunction. Brain elasticity is thought to be elevated, allowing the ICP to

be high or to rise precipitously with pressure waves and cause acute deterioration. Blood pressures in the low-normal range may diminish cerebral perfusion pressure in this circumstance and may cause more severe symptoms. In another variation, some patients have a low ventricular pressure after shunting, but the ventricular volume is not reduced, and symptoms persist or later worsen. To deal with this problem, external ventricular drainage at subzero pressures has been used to drain the ventricles over weeks.[153] In one patient, we drained 200 to 400 mL of fluid daily for 35 days at pressures of −10 to −25 cm H_2O. The ventricles diminished in size without inducing a subdural

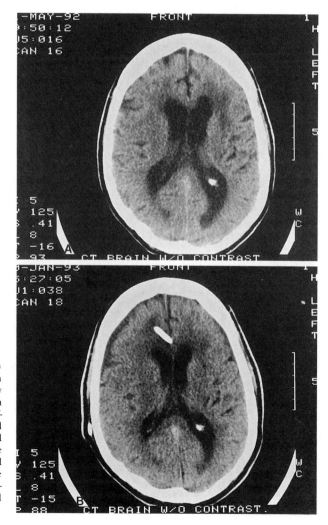

Figure 9–3. (*A*) Computed tomography (CT) scan of a patient who reached a plateau in cognition and gait during the first few months of rehabilitation for a traumatic brain injury (TBI) with multiple contusions and diffuse axonal injury (DAI). He then declined in his attention and spontaneous speech and developed a mild apraxia in his gait. (*B*) The shunt pictured in his left lateral ventricle led to only a modest decrease in the size of the ventricles but improved his mobility and cognition to a higher level than he had achieved prior to his decline.

hematoma or hygroma, and symptoms lessened. The procedure is followed by implanting a valveless shunt and by maintaining the patient slightly upright, even in bed. The proposed mechanism of this low-pressure hydrocephalic state is decreased viscoelasticity of the brain from expulsion of extracellular water and from distortion and ischemia of brain tissue from the radial compressive stresses of the large ventricles.[153] Slow drainage presumably allows rehydration and restores elasticity. Although no data are available to suggest the incidence of this phenomenon, rehabilitation specialists should consider the possibility that motor and cognitive deterioration, even after a low-pressure shunt produces smaller ventricles, may mean that the shunt is blocked or the intervention has not optimally shunted fluid. When a programmable shunt was used to test the effects of different intraventricular pressures in patients with hydrocephalus, great sensitivity to small pressure changes was found.[13] Thus, clinicians may have been too conservative in suggesting a shunt for patients who fail to improve during rehabilitation or whose condition deteriorates modestly. Moreover, shunts that are put into place may perform less than optimally.

MOVEMENT DISORDERS

Some posttraumatic movement disorders are common after serious TBI. These disorders include tremors, myoclonic jerks, and parkinsonism, particularly the punch-drunk syndrome of boxers. Less often, patients develop akinetic-rigid syndromes, chorea and ballismus, focal and more general dystonia, tics, psychogenic jerks, and other movements.[99] These disorders can develop within weeks, months, or as long as 10 years after injury. Late evolution of movement disorders raises the possibility of ongoing changes within the basal ganglia and their connections, such as denervation hypersensitivity and axonal sprouting onto partially denervated target cells.

Both peripheral and central injuries are associated with the dystonias. An initial focal finger or foot dystonia or a hemidystonia can progress to a multifocal hemidystonia or a generalized dystonia.[104] Lesions in the contralateral basal ganglia and the thalamus have been imaged by CT and MRI in most patients with acquired hemidystonia. In several reported cases, scans were normal, but PET revealed metabolic abnormalities.[99] Metabolic imaging has also pointed to reorganization of motor activity. Contralateral to a hemidystonia of the arm, frontal overactivity with movement was found. The investigators suggested that the acquired hemidystonia resulted from thalamofrontal disinhibition due to structural disruption of inhibitory control by the basal ganglia.[24a]

Therapy for movement disorders associated with TBI does not differ from drug interventions for the same disorders from other causes.[91] Patients with head injury may be especially susceptible to the cognitive side effects of high-dose anticholinergic, dopaminergic, or dopamine receptor–blocking agents, however. Stereotactic thalamotomy has been used in rare instances to improve function.

PERSISTENT VEGETATIVE STATE

A PVS follows TBI with coma in 1 to 14 percent of 1-month survivors, and it follows nontraumatic coma in about 12 percent.[142] Nontraumatic causes of PVS in adults are mostly from hypoxic-ischemic injury, but they include cerebral hemorrhages, infections, and degenerative diseases. In children, metabolic disorders and developmental anomalies contribute to the problem. These patients tend to have an even worse prognosis than patients with anoxia from drowning and cardiac arrest. Diffuse or multifocal laminar cortical necrosis and thalamic necrosis due to anoxia, along with extensive subcortical DAI, produce a PVS. The electroencephalogram usually reveals diffuse slowing, and PET reveals a marked reduction in global glucose utilization. In patients who are most likely to die or to remain vegetative, sensory-evoked potentials are absent.

Rehabilitation specialists are often called upon to help in prognostication, to provide maintenance care, and to try interventions that may improve the patient's awareness. The natural history of PVS is dismal, however. Tables 9–5 and 9–6 summarize outcomes from several studies.[142] Families and coma-stimulation therapists often find hope

Table 9–5. **GLASGOW OUTCOME SCALE (GOS) CLASSIFICATION FOR RECOVERY OF CONSCIOUSNESS AND FUNCTION IN ADULTS IN A PERSISTENT VEGETATIVE STATE (PVS) BEYOND 1 MONTH**

Outcomes (GOS)	3 Months (%)	6 Months (%)	12 Months (%)
Traumatic Brain Injury			
Death	15	24	33
PVS	52	30	15
Consciousness	33	46	52
Severe disability			28
Moderate disability			17
Good recovery			7
Nontraumatic Brain Injury			
Death	24	40	53
PVS	65	45	32
Consciousness	11	15	15
Severe disability			11
Moderate disability			3
Good recovery			1

Source: Adapted from Multi-Society Task Force on PVS,[142] p 1574.

Table 9–6. **GLASGOW OUTCOME SCALE (GOS) CLASSIFICATION FOR RECOVERY OF CONSCIOUSNESS AND FUNCTION IN CHILDREN IN A PERSISTENT VEGETATIVE STATE (PVS) BEYOND 1 MONTH**

Outcomes (GOS)	3 Months (%)	6 Months (%)	12 Months (%)
Traumatic Brain Injury			
Death	4	9	9
PVS	72	40	29
Consciousness	24	51	62
Severe disability			35
Moderate disability			16
Good recovery			11
Nontraumatic Brain Injury			
Death	20	22	22
PVS	69	67	65
Consciousness	11	11	13
Severe disability			7
Moderate disability			0
Good recovery			6

Source: Adapted from Multi-Society Task Force on PVS,[142] p 1574.

for recovery in the inconsistent, nonpurposeful movements derived from reflex responses to modest stimulation and the patterned, innate responses related to internally driven, subcortical activity. With their intact brainstem functions, some patients have inconsistent auditory or visual orienting reflexes, but no clear-cut visual pursuit or fixation. Some patients grunt, cry, moan, and grimace to internal and, on occasion, to external stimuli; however, PVS means that patients are unaware of self or environment and cannot interact in any purposeful way. They do retain irregular sleep-wake cycles and hypothalamic and brainstem-controlled vital functions.

In case reports, rare patients have recovered spontaneously several years after the onset of PVS. Interventions to reverse coma or a PVS either early or late after onset have generally not been successful, although a few reports have claimed recovery of consciousness by using bromocriptine and amphetamine, by using electrical stimulation of the reticular formation and its connections, and by implementing sensory stimulation programs (see the discussion on coma stimulation later in this chapter). Families and clinicians tend to try sensory stimulation in previously competent adults and in children who have no underlying disease. By 1 year after onset, the real dilemma is how much medical and nutritional support to continue. Mortality rates for patients in PVS are 70 percent at 3 years and 84 percent at 5 years.[142]

ASSESSMENTS AND OUTCOME MEASURES

For purposes of early and ongoing assessment, prognostication, and outcome, certain measurement tools and descriptors have been recommended.[75] The range of physical, behavioral, and cognitive disabilities is so great in the patient with moderate to severe TBI that we elaborate upon some of the tools described in Chapter 5. Some scales are used almost exclusively in studies of TBI or hypoxic-ischemic injury to describe the stage of recovery and the level of disability and to categorize behavior.

Stages of Recovery

The GCS is used most often to define the depth and duration of coma.[86] The GCS has been used in most outcome studies of TBI, is in routine clinical use, and allows distinctions about severity that have some prognostic meaning when the test is given 6 hours after the onset of TBI. The test should be performed daily if the score is less than 15, until the patient is discharged from the hospital. On the GCS, the sum score of 13 to 15 is considered evidence of a mild injury, 9 to 12 is evidence of a moderate injury, and 8 or less indicates severe injury.

The Galveston Orientation and Amnesia Test (GOAT) is a simple, reliable assessment of PTA that separates patients into normal, borderline, and impaired groups. The test is given as soon as the patient is alert, at hospital discharge, and at 6 months (see Table 5–5). A score of 75 or higher on 2 consecutive days suggests normal functioning,[110] although the GOAT may not measure the consolidation of memory in that time.

Stages of recovery beyond coma are often described by the subjectively defined Rancho Los Amigos Levels of Cognitive Functioning (Table 9–7).[71] These levels take into account early, middle, and late stages in the evolution of recovery from DAI.[92,197]

The initial stages go from coma to an unresponsive vigilant or vegetative state with sleep-wake cycles. Purposeful wakefulness with limited nonverbal or brief, hypophonic responses to commands often evolves in patients who do not remain in a vegetative state. Simple yes-no answers may be possible to elicit. A confusional stage follows with PTA, limited attention, and easy distractibility. Agitation, hostility, perseveration, and confabulation are often found. Behavioral interventions are more likely to be of value at this stage, compared with interventions that deal with specific cognitive processes. The middle period, which can last from 3 to 12 months, takes the patient from the end of PTA to a gradually increasing awareness of deficits, independence in ADLs with self-initiation, work on specific cognitive dysfunctions, goal setting, and resocialization. Neuropsychologic and language testing batteries for monitoring and planning

Table 9–7. **RANCHO LOS AMIGOS SCALE OF COGNITIVE FUNCTIONING**

I. No response
Complete lack of response to any stimuli.

II. Generalized Response
Reaction to stimuli inconsistent and nonpurposeful. Responses often same regardless of stimuli. Responses possibly including physiologic changes, gross body movements, or vocalization. Delayed responses likely.

III. Localized Response
Reaction to stimuli specific, but inconstant, and directionally related to stimulus, e.g., turning head toward sound. Possible following of simple commands such as closing eyes, squeezing or extending extremity in inconsistant, delayed manner. Possible vague awareness of self and body by responding to discomfort. Possible response to some persons but not to others.

IV. Confused, agitated response
Heightened state of activity with severely decreased ability to process information. Behavior frequently bizarre and nonpurposeful. Verbalization frequently incoherent or inappropriate. Possible confabulation. Possible hostility or euphoria. Short gross attention to environment. Selective attention often nonexistent. Inability to perform self-care without maximum assistance.

V. Confused, inappropriate, nonagitated response
Appearance of alertness and response to simple commands. Responses nonpurposeful to more complex commands. Possible agitated behavior. Gross attention to environment, but high level of distractibility. Inability to focus on specific tasks. Inappropriate verbalization. Severe memory impairment with confusion of past and present. Lack of initiation of functional tasks and, often, inappropriate use of objects without external direction. Possible performance of previously learned tasks when structured, but inability to learn new information. Best response to self, body, comfort, and sometimes family members. Usual ability to perform self-care activities with assistance. Possible wandering.

VI. Confused, appropriate response
Goal-directed behavior, but dependence on external input for direction. Appropriate response to discomfort. Consistent following of simple directions and remembering of relearned tasks such as self-care. Responses appropriate to situation.

VII. Automatic, appropriate response
More goal-directed and self-initiated everyday behavior.

VIII. Purposeful, appropriate response
Self-directed behavior that accomplishes basic and more skilled tasks. Supervision still possibly necessary.

interventions become more valuable at this stage than previously. The last stage can subsume many behavioral, cognitive, and mood problems, both serious and subtle, that may last for years. Structured assessments can produce different results than are found in real-life situations. For example, disturbances in personality and in the ability to attend to multiple environmental stimuli and to shift logically from one concept to another may not be brought out by routine testing.

Disability

The GOS is a global physical, economic, and social measure (see Table 5–13).[85] As a rehabilitation tool, it has shortcomings. The GOS is too global to be sensitive to gradual functional progress. It does not attempt to indicate changes in specific functional, cognitive, and behavioral abilities or in neurologic impairments.

The Disability Rating Scale (DRS)[171] is easy to use and is reliable. It has concurrent and predictive validity in assessing patients with moderate to severe TBI from onset through up to 10 years of follow-up.[171] The domains of this scale include the opening of the eye, verbalization, and motor responsiveness of the GCS, the cognitive skills needed for feeding, toileting, and grooming, and the overall level of dependence and employability. The summated disability score falls within 1 to 10 categories that range from no disability (0) to death (30). The DRS ap-

Table 9–8. **FUNCTIONAL ASSESSMENT MEASURE ITEMS ADDED TO THE FUNCTIONAL INDEPENDENCE MEASURE**

Swallowing
Car transfer
Community mobility
Reading
Writing
Speech intelligibility
Emotional status
Adjustment to limitations
Orientation
Attention
Safety judgment

pears fairly sensitive to change in patients with a hospital admission GCS score of 4 to 12 who are transferred to rehabilitation. It is least sensitive to functional levels for patients with mild TBI and for those with severe impairment, whose DRS exceeds 22. The DRS is more sensitive to change than the GOS.[73] In follow-up, four additional 5-point scores can assess the impact of physical and mental impairment on work and on living.[171] DRS scores higher than 15 on admission to rehabilitation, higher than 7 on discharge, and higher than 4 at follow-up 3 months after discharge predict the likely inability of the patient to return to work.[74] Thus, scores give an indication of employability. The DRS is so quick to use that it may also serve as a way to stratify rehabilitation inpatients for clinical trials and to help track changes in outpatients.

The Functional Assessment Measure (FAM) is a 12-item addendum to the Functional Independence Measure (FIM) that reflects more community-based activities, so it may increase sensitivity to outpatient levels of functional recovery (Table 9–8). The DRS, FIM, and FAM correlate highly with each other and with duration of coma, length of PTA, and the Rancho Los Amigos scale. Lesser correlations were found with the GCS and with presence or absence of CT abnormalities in one analysis of patients with TBI.[74] The Mayo-Portland Adaptability In-

ventory, which was developed for patients with TBI, has also been correlated with the DRS and Rancho Los Amigos scales and adds useful ratings of emotional behavior to those of functional abilities and physical disabilities.[125]

Behavior

The Katz Adjustment Scale–Relatives Form has been used often in TBI studies to assess the way in which the family perceives the patient in the home, but its reliability and validity are uncertain.

The Neurobehavioral Rating Scale is a structured interview with a formal mental status examination. It includes 27 variables that can be grouped as loading on four factors (Table 9–9). Interrater reliability and

Table 9–9. **NEUROBEHAVIORAL RATING SCALE**

Cognition/Energy
Disorientation
Emotional withdrawal
Conceptual disorganization
Memory
Fatigue
Motor retardation
Blunted affect

Metacognition
Disinhibition
Agitation
Self-appraisal
Thought content
Excitement
Poor planning

Somatic/Anxiety
Somatic concern
Anxiety
Depression
Hostility
Suspiciousness
Tension

Language
Expressive deficit
Comprehension deficit

sensitivity to the severity and chronicity of CHI have been shown.[111]

The Agitated Behavior Scale is a 14-item instrument for documenting agitated behaviors.[31] It has good interrater reliability and at least face validity. It includes, for example, short attention span, easy distractibility, and inability to concentrate as one item and impulsivity, impatience, and low tolerance for pain or frustration as another.

Cognition

No specific battery of neuropsychologic tests has been put into general use for patients with TBI. Specialized tests or normative data for the tools listed in Chapter 5 are needed in assessing pediatric and geriatric patients. In addition to the revised Wechsler Adult Intelligence Scale, the Halstead-Reitan test[121] and the Luria-Nebraska test often serve as core batteries. Timed tasks in real-world settings such as the Rivermead Behavioral Memory Test[126] and the Multiple Errands and the Six Elements Tests[184] are especially useful for assessing memory, initiation, and planning in this population of patients.

PREDICTORS OF FUNCTIONAL OUTCOME

Predictors and measures of functional outcome continue to undergo methodologic refinements. The GCS has become the most widely used acute predictor. Of course, alcohol, drugs, and acute neurosurgical and medical care affect scoring and interpretation. Global and specific measures of functional disability, neurobehaviors, and physical and cognitive impairments are likely to vary in reliability, validity, and sensitivity to change across the spectrum of initial severity of TBI and across subsequent curves of recovery. Other factors that contribute especially to the behavioral effects of TBI include premorbid education and psychiatric and behavioral disorders, age, socioeconomic factors, and the variety of disorders characterized by neuroimaging.

Level of Consciousness

The Traumatic Coma Data Bank related the GCS taken following nonsurgical resuscitation to the GOS at hospital discharge.[129] For mortality, lower scores combined with pupillary abnormalities and age over 40 years accounted for most of the variance. With an initial GCS of 3, 78 percent died, compared with a mortality of 18 percent in patients with a score of 6 to 8. Higher scores increase the likelihood of a viable rehabilitation effort. With a GCS lower than 6, 16 percent of patients reached a level of good recovery or moderate disability by the GOS. With scores between 6 and 8, 64 percent did so; however, only 4 percent of patients over the age of 45 years with scores below 9 had a good recovery by 6 months, compared with 29 percent of younger patients. The lowest early GCS and absent pupil reactivity were much more predictive of a poor outcome than a high intracranial pressure or, by CT scan, the presence of diffuse cerebral swelling or a mass lesion.[107] Consistent with the Traumatic Coma Data Bank study, the International Coma Data Bank of patients with acute neurosurgical disorders found that only 11 percent of patients with a best GCS of 5 by 3 days after injury reached levels of good recovery or moderate disability.[87]

One TBI inpatient rehabilitation facility reported that patients who had a GCS of 3 to 7, compared with patients with higher scores when admitted to the acute care hospital, had significantly longer acute hospital stays and lower admission and discharge motor and cognitive FIM scores for the rehabilitation stay.[33a] Total hospital days were greater for patients with a skull fracture and intracranial bleed compared with the group with normal CT scans. The rehabilitation admission FIM motor score helped predict the duration of inpatient rehabilitation and its cost, which could prove useful in anticipating resource utilization, if confirmed by larger studies.

Duration of Coma and Amnesia

Duration of coma and time to recovery have a rather linear relationship, especially when neuroimaging suggests DAI as the primary pathologic process.[118] As coma extends from 1 month to beyond 2 months, the likelihood of recovery to moderate disability or better falls to about 40 percent.[16] After an anoxic injury, coma that lasts beyond 1 week leaves almost no chance of recovery to better than severe disability.[117] Duration of PTA also has a telling effect, although measures of the inability to acquire and retrieve information vary among studies. In the International Coma Data Bank, duration of less than 2 weeks was associated with good recovery in over 80 percent of patients, and no patient was left with severe disability, whereas PTA for longer than 4 weeks was associated with a good recovery in 25 percent and with severe disability in 30 percent.[87]

These relationships were similar for patients referred to one rehabilitation unit. In a group of 243 consecutive admissions, a significant inverse relationship was found between GCS and length of coma (LOC), and a strong positive relationship was observed between LOC and PTA.[93] For DAI, a regression analysis showed that duration of PTA (in weeks) was equal to [0.4 × LOC (in days)] + 3.6. PTA was especially prolonged for the LOC in patients over the age of 40 years. Of 119 patients with likely DAI, no one in a coma for more than 2 weeks or with PTA for over 12 weeks had a good recovery by the GOS at 1 year post injury. Two-thirds of the small subgroup with LOC longer than 2 weeks improved to moderate disability when LOC was 2 to 4 weeks. Only one-third achieved this level if coma persisted for more than 4 weeks. Half of the rehabilitation patients with PTA lasting 2 to 8 weeks reached the level of moderate disability, and 80 percent of those with PTA for less than 2 weeks had a good recovery. PTA was longer with advancing age. Outcomes were worse in patients over the age of 60 years.[94]

Several studies have provided other useful information using the length of PTA.[105] As PTA diminishes, orientation tends to recover in the sequence of person, place, and then time. Retrograde amnesia tends to recede from more remote to more recent chronologic information after moderate and severe CHI. During PTA, memory rapidly decays. Procedural memory, however, is better. During rehabilitation, patients with severe CHI were able to acquire motor and pattern analyzing skills, even when they recalled little about the way they came to learn the skills. In children, the duration of PTA correlated with verbal learning and memory at the time of resolution and at 12 months post injury.

LEVELS OF REHABILITATIVE CARE

Rehabilitation programs for TBI rely on a continuum of treatment options built on medical, neurobehavioral, social, educational, and vocational models.[136] Medically stable patients who remain in a coma are usually placed in a nursing facility where techniques such as coma stimulation may be tried. Patients emerging from coma and those who are still disabled by problems in mobility, ADLs, confusion, agitation, and cognitive dysfunction are appropriate candidates for an interdisciplinary inpatient effort. Patients who become mobile but who are unable to control their wandering require a locked unit. Patients often graduate to one of several therapy options other than routine outpatient rehabilitation services.

A *day treatment program* helps to relieve the family of full-time care. Along with therapies for physical disabilities, patients are trained in skills for independent living, socialization, vocation, and school re-entry. If behavioral and cognitive dysfunctions dominate, a *residential program* designed especially for behavioral modification can lead to better socialization and more independence. A supervised, homelike *transitional living* setting helps to train patients in skills for independent living, community activity, and employment. Any type of milieu or therapeutic community can provide the structure to resolve psychosocial and behavioral problems. Programs emphasize social competence and dealing with the limitations imposed by brain injury. Group interactions, counseling, psychotherapy, and behavioral modification are provided within the context of ADLs and leisure activities. Vocational rehabilitation centers and academic programs, which are often governmental efforts, provide useful resources, but they may not be able to cater to the needs of young patients with brain injury. In a *protected work trial*, the patient works under the supervision of a therapist and a job supervisor or coach. The setting tolerates the cognitive and behavioral impairments that are ordinarily not permitted at a workplace. Task-oriented skills are reinforced. Supportive counseling and behavior modification techniques help to ease the patient into volunteer, protected, or competitive work.

After a moderate to severe TBI, most patients who meet criteria for rehabilitation improve in their skills and become less disabled as they move through non–hospital-based programs.[28] No studies have been undertaken that allow clinicians to know which settings and services are most efficacious and which are of little value. Type, intensity, and duration of services at any of these levels of care depend on judgments about needs and about whether a plateau in gains has been reached. The provision of services also depends on the perceived obligations of insurers or the financial resources of families. Moreover, any study of postacute rehabilitation faces problems in sampling, in defining outcomes, in showing the way in which a treatment can be generalized, and in calculating cost-effectiveness.[20]

REHABILITATION INTERVENTIONS

Survivors of a serious TBI tend to make their greatest gains in mobility, functional skills, and language over the first 3 to 6 months, much like patients after stroke. Performance measures, such as the ability to accomplish a timed or novel task, recover more slowly. Some patients continue to improve for several years in distinct cognitive and behavioral measures. Indeed, young patients with fixed impairments probably learn new skills and make adaptations with supervised help and on their own indefinitely, as the need arises.

Organized inpatient rehabilitation services provided within the first months post injury are likely to benefit patients and families who actively participate. Overall, patients clearly make functional gains during inpatient care. Table 9–10 shows Uniform Data System (UDS) data for changes between admission and discharge in FIM scores across several hundred inpatient rehabilitation programs. No randomized trials of a well-defined program with a control group have been undertaken, however.

A few studies have been invoked as presumptive evidence that programs do benefit patients. One small study suggested that patients admitted to rehabilitation within 35 days of TBI spent half the number of days in therapy as patients admitted later.[30] The late-admission group had more patients with a tracheostomy, so the patients may have been more severely impaired. Outcomes on a scale of social function did not differ at the 2-year follow-up. Another report found that a formal program of rehabilitation assessment and intervention begun within a few days of hospitalization was associated with one-third the duration of coma and length of rehabilitation stay, compared with patients who were not provided an early program.[122] The level of cognition and the number of discharges home were also significantly higher in the early-therapy group.

Table 9–10. **NATIONAL UNIFORM DATA SERVICE FIRST ADMISSIONS FOR TRAUMATIC BRAIN INJURY (3360 PATIENTS)**

	Admission	Discharge
Mean onset (days)	34	
Mean subscore		
Self-care	3.7	5.6
Sphincter control	4.0	5.8
Mobility	3.4	5.4
Locomotion	2.7	5.0
Communication	3.8	5.2
Social cognition	3.0	4.5
Mean FIM total	62 (S.D. 29)	95 (S.D. 28)
Median FIM total	63	105
Length of stay		40 (S.D. 44)
Discharge (%)		
Community		83
Long-term care		8
Acute care		5
Mean age (yr)	40 (S.D. 21)	

FIM = Functional Independence Measures.

Aside from physical, occupational, and speech therapies, the formalized program provided family support and sensory stimulation for patients in coma. Coma stimulation is not of proven value, however, as discussed later. This study is likely flawed by differences in the initial severity of TBI in the groups of patients studied. The length of coma was 20 days for the early-intervention group versus 54 days for the late-intervention group. Like many studies, it also suffers from using retrospective data, in this instance from 10 facilities. Indeed, methodologic flaws hamper the interpretation of all reported studies of programs of inpatient and outpatient rehabilitation.[72]

Most clinical studies report on a particular type of program or on a specific type of problem, such as cognitive or behavioral dysfunction. Most often, these studies are carried out beyond the usual duration of inpatient care. We examine the approaches that differ from interventions already described for the impairments and disabilities of other neurologic diseases. Much of the emphasis in rehabilitation of patients with TBI is, of course, on cognitive, behavioral, and vocational function.

Physical Disability

Although physical impairments that cause disability are common after a moderate to severe TBI at the time of transfer into a rehabilitation program (Table 9–11), these impairments most often improve within 6 months. Cognitive and behavioral sequelae linger. The Vietnam Head Injury Study examined 420 veterans who suffered PHI, mostly from low-velocity shrapnel that caused a focal injury. At 1 week after injury, 21 percent had a hemiparesis and 11 percent had a hemisensory impairment.[181] Fifteen years later, 10 percent were hemiparetic and 21 percent (a greater number because the examination was presumably more reliable) had a residual sensory loss.

Contractures and spasticity associated with flexor and extensor posturing and traumatic injuries to the limbs require special attention during acute medical and rehabilitation inpatient stays. Early interventions include proper positioning, exercises for range of

Table 9–11. IMPAIRMENTS IN 1-MONTH SURVIVORS OF SEVERE TRAUMATIC BRAIN INJURY

Impairment	Percentage (%)
Cognition	60–90
Hemiparesis, diparesis	60
Dysarthria	50
Cranial neuropathy	30
Dysphagia	30
Ataxia	10
Aphasia	10
Hemianopia	5
Optic neuropathy	1
No physical signs	25

Source: Adapted from Levin H, Hamilton W, Grossman R.[109]

motion for joints, orthoses, serial casting, and even temporary motor point blocks. These interventions may prevent later complications and the need for surgical management when the patient has regained enough cognitive and motor function to participate in movement therapies. In addition to the spectrum of physical therapeutic approaches, many patients with TBI need ongoing encouragement and a structured program to maintain general fitness. An individualized aerobic training program can improve motor skills, decrease fatigability, and improve mood.[219]

Activities of Daily Living and Independent Living

Most patients admitted for inpatient rehabilitation after TBI improve in their self-care and community reintegration skills over time. Studies have generally not been designed to distinguish a treatment effect from the natural history of recovery. In general, after moderate to severe TBI, self-care and mobility improve from admission to discharge, and gains are maintained or continue to increase for about 6 months.[78] About 50 percent of patients return to work at 6 months. Socialization and leisure activities generally do not return to premorbid levels. Most reports from facilities include small numbers of cases. They also describe wide ranges in time from the onset of TBI to admission for rehabilitation, in level of initial function, and in length of inpatient stay. These studies vary in their measures of functional outcome. The UDS data in Table 9–10 provide a bird's-eye view of first admission and discharge function for a large population using the FIM.[61]

Brain injury often interferes with the ability to generalize a functional skill from one situation to another. Functional training in the face of cognitive dysfunction requires an approach that is skill-specific and often context-specific. Adaptations are often required by the family, by the workplace, and by other aspects of the patient's social system.

Psychosocial Recovery

Problems in social, leisure, work, and family role performances are related more to the cognitive, behavioral, and emotional sequelae of TBI than to physical impairments. The nature and severity of postinjury psychosocial difficulties vary with measures of severity of TBI and time from injury to observation. These problems tend to improve over the first year.[135] The Sickness Index Profile has been a useful tool, along with measures of social networks and checklists of physical and psychologic symptoms. Negative attitudes and poor socialization increase the level of stress of patients and their caregivers.[64] Counseling, education, and psychotherapy can assist families.

Residential and work or school placements are important goals for therapy and as outcome measures. Successful vocational outcomes must be considered in terms of premorbid work abilities and postinjury hours of supervision and level of productivity. After PHI, 56 percent of the military veterans in one study were employed at 15-year follow-up, compared with 82 percent of controls.[183] The researchers found a linear association between work status and the number of residual impairments. These impairments included epilepsy, paresis, visual field loss, losses in verbal memory and learning and in visual memory, psychologic problems, and self-reported violent behavior.

Table 9–12. **PREDICTORS OF SUCCESSFUL EMPLOYMENT**

Duration of coma and posttraumatic amnesia

Cognition: verbal memory, speed of information processing, language

Behavior: mood, self-control

Family and employer support: coachability

Preinjury intellectual and work status

General predictors of employability after CHI are shown in Table 9–12. Impaired verbal memory and slow information processing strongly relate to unemployment 7 years after a severe CHI.[21] The DRS, Patient Evaluation and Conference System (PECS), and other scales have been of value in predicting return to work when other factors such as social need, drug abuse, and social supports are also taken into account.[169] Employment status can be independent of other measures of social performance, so it can be a separate outcome. Welfare benefits, economic conditions, and intangible factors often play a role in who returns to work, however. After a severe TBI, most follow-ups beyond 2 years reveal that about 10 percent of patients return to former jobs, and fewer than 30 percent are employed.[210] With supported employment services in the workplace, provided for under the Rehabilitation Act Amendments of 1992,[56] more patients are able to gain permanent work in warehouse, clerical, and service-related occupations, although the cost can be considerable. In one well-organized interventional study, a mean of 250 hours of supportive staff time was necessary to return 67 percent of patients to work at a mean of 6 years after severe TBI.[210]

Cognitive Impairments

The amount and rate of recovery of neuropsychologic functions vary with the measure and type of function, with the type and severity of lesions, and with the patient's age. Other more subtle factors, such as the interactions of pathologic processes, impairments, and premorbid intellect and education, also confound the prediction of outcomes. For example, severe CHI can compromise the patient's ability to make cohesive discourse. A left prefrontal injury can produce disorganized sentences and an impoverished narrative, whereas a right prefrontal lesion may cause tangential, socially inappropriate expression.[1] Consequences for eventual employment are hard to predict, especially after adding in other cognitive abnormalities that may affect expression and comprehension of language and the patient's range of premorbid communicative abilities.

As noted earlier, impairments tend to plateau faster in patients with focal lesions than in those with DAI. In one study, verbal IQ scores on the Wechsler Adult Intelligence Scale plateaued 5 months after TBI, whereas performance scores that reflect more global cognitive function did so at 13 months.[127] Other patterns have been found, however.[33] In general, measured functions improve over the first year. Gains in the second year are limited to fewer functions, mostly in patients with the most severe injuries.[35]

Table 9–13 describes some of the varied cognitive dysfunctions found after TBI.[206] The individual patient's profile often reveals a preponderance of frontal lobe impairments in attention and executive functions.

More than 700 programs for neuropsychologic rehabilitation are in place in the United States.[146] Although these clinical services are in high demand, especially for patients with TBI, they are delivered without much empiric support. Uncertainty about their efficacy arises in part from methodologic problems and from evolving theories about cognitive processing. Services are provided by physical, occupational, speech, and vocational therapists within the context of mobility and spatial orientation, self-care and community activities, communication, and work or schooling. These therapists often work on specific cognitive domains along with a neuropsychologist. Trained aides can assist in computer work.

A few general approaches have been taken to ameliorate the cognitive difficulties of patients with head injury. These approaches include functional adaptation and compensatory techniques, general cognitive stimulation, training of specific cognitive processes, and behavioral conditioning. In practice, various approaches are taken. Counseling about strengths and weaknesses, providing emotional and social support, and compensatory problem solving are standard team interventions. Multimodal programs have stressed the learning of task-specific skills by remedial techniques while they teach self-awareness of impairments and build toward independent living and work.[8] The contribution of a program that includes

Table 9–13. COMMON AREAS OF COGNITIVE IMPAIRMENT AFTER TRAUMATIC BRAIN INJURY

Attention
Alertness
Mental processing (slow)
Selective attention during distraction
Divided attention
Sustained attention
Awareness of disability and impairment

Perception
Visual
Auditory
Visuospatial

Memory
Retrograde, anterograde
Immediate, delayed, cued, and recognition recall
Visual and verbal learning

Executive Functions
Planning
Initiation
Maintaining goal or intention
Conceptual reasoning
Hypothesis testing and shifting response
Self-appraisal
Self-regulation

Intelligence
Verbal expression
Performance
Problem solving
Abstract reasoning

Language
Speech (aphasia; vague, tangential, confabulatory speech; verbose or impoverished speech)
Affective expression

remediation of particular cognitive domains is especially difficult to determine because many interventions are simultaneous and outcome measures often reflect broad functional categories, rather than those specific domains. At the same time, spontaneous recovery and practice effects can make it seem that an approach is working when it is not.

COMPENSATORY APPROACH

With the adaptive approach, therapy takes place in a real setting or in a simulated functional setting, such as the home, place of work, or school. These programs try to lessen or circumvent the effects of cognitive impairments on daily activities. The underlying notion is that addressing specific cognitive impairments is unlikely to improve functional outcomes more than specifically training patients in the desired functions. Instead of treating impairments, therapists manage the more important disabilities and handicaps that impairments impose. Adaptive techniques tend to rely on repetition, cues, overlearning, and cognitive assistive devices, much like the routine compensatory interventions for ADL training. In addition, the environment should be structured so that it is predictable and cues the patient.

Functional remediation, as well as specific cognitive process remediation, should try to use learning principles (see Chapter 3). Ideally, the therapist should provide an optimal schedule of feedback during performance and related to results. Overlap of the elements and the organization of a task, as well as practice in a variable context, can increase the likelihood that the patient will learn a skill. The diverse cognitive sequelae of TBI may counteract this reinforcement, however. Learning one strategy to perform a task may not generalize to novel circumstances or even transfer to another related task or setting. Careful attention to the components of a task and to the setting can improve function.[155]

BEHAVIORAL TRAINING

Behavioral training targets discrete behaviors or tasks and reinforces them with rewards. Behavioral modification protocols must be structured and used by the entire team, especially when the goal is to eliminate disruptive behavior. For example, a token economy in which the patient is given chits or tokens that can be spent like money or given direct or monetary incentives can be used to reward patients during inpatient rehabilitation or in a transitional living setting for completing a self-care task or for reducing aggressive actions.[154]

COGNITIVE REMEDIATION

General cognitive stimulation training assumes that any stimulation may improve function. Therapists may draw upon workbooks, art, computer programs, and other stimuli to encourage cognitive processing. Mental jumping jacks, however, are not likely to recondition the patient's brain for the acquisition and retention of skills and strategies that reduce disability.

Cognitive remediation has many nuances, but it usually includes a cognitive process–specific approach that articulates subroutines of a mental process. Therapists aim to ameliorate impairments in problem solving, they often use feedback, and they consider that the therapeutic methods used may reorganize the function of the patient's cognitive neural networks.[120,164,191] The approach targets distinct, if theoretic, components of separable cognitive processes. Repetition of a task at one level of difficulty or related to one subcomponent of the cognitive process continues until the goal is reached. Then the task is enlarged within its presumed hierarchic organization. For example, once two-dimensional constructions are copied, three-dimensional drawings may be undertaken. Once auditory attention is learned, auditory encoding is practiced. Gains are expected to generalize to related tasks and to transfer into real-world functioning.

In practice, when cognitive impairments are mapped by neuropsychologic testing, early interventions are often designed to boost the efficiency of a domain for which the patient has demonstrated some capacity, rather than to tackle domains for which the patient's ability is poor. When possible, a relatively intact cognitive skill may be used to compensate for a severely impaired skill. For example, impaired auditory encoding may be compensated for by writing what was said and by using a visual memory strategy.

Cognitive remediation techniques have been used to treat many of the common sequelae of TBI. These techniques are less successful as the severity of impairments increases. Specific approaches, based on inexact theories of cognitive processing, have been outlined for generic disorders of orientation, attention, memory, visuoperception, language, executive functions, and problem solving.[8,54,191] For example, selective attention, which is the ability to focus on a particular stimulus or response, can be reinforced behaviorally, compensated for by placing the patient in a nondistracting environment, possibly improved by withdrawing medications that reduce arousal, attention, and the speed of mental processing, and possibly remediated by dealing individually with the poorly understood processes that reflect goal-directed controls by the frontal lobes. To illustrate these possibilities and problems, we examine some of the approaches to amnestic disorders.

Approaches to Amnestic Disorders

Natural History of Recovery. Residual memory disturbances are apparent in about 25 percent of patients after moderate CHI and in about 50 percent of patients after severe CHI.[108] After mild TBI, memory usually recovers by 3 months.[36,112] This recovery varies with the test used to measure the severity of CHI, with the amount of time from injury to testing, with the indicator tests used, and with the comparison group.[37] One year after severe CHI, patients followed in the Traumatic Coma Data Bank had greater impairments in verbal and visual memory and in other neurobehaviors, such as naming to confrontation and block construction, compared with normative data.[107] Selective, rather than global, cognitive impairments were likely at 1 year. Memory was disproportionately impaired compared with overall intellectual functioning in 15 percent of patients with moderate CHI and 30 percent of patients with severe CHI. In another group, 25 percent of 1-year to 3-year survivors of moderate and severe CHI who were able to be tested showed defective memory on visual and auditory measures, despite normal verbal and performance IQs.[108] Of course,

other cognitive impairments, especially in attention and language, can amplify the disability of any memory loss. Moreover, a visual or auditory sensory loss may limit initial registration.

One prospective study found that memory impairments were related to the time from injury to assessment, to the nature of the memory task, and to the severity of the injury. A group of 102 patients with TBI aged 10 to 60 years, who were hospitalized after any period of unconsciousness, PTA of more than 1 hour, or evidence of cerebral trauma, were examined at 1 and 12 months post injury.[38] At 1 month, the patients with TBI performed significantly worse on the Wechsler Memory Scale (WMS) and the Selective Reminding Test than did a control group. Patients who could not follow a command for the longest times beyond 24 hours post injury had more subtests of the WMS below the control scores. Tests of orientation and short-term memory were inferior in their ability to reveal memory deficits compared with tests that required storage of new information for later use. At 1 year, patients performed better than they had 1 month after onset. The group most severely impaired at 1 year initially had been unable to follow a command for more than a day, had PTA for over 14 days, and had a GCS score of 8 or less.

A long-term follow-up study of 26 patients who had a TBI and who had undergone rehabilitation 5 to 10 years earlier found that 58 percent were unchanged, 31 percent performed better, and 11 percent performed worse on the Rivermead Behavioral Memory Test and the WMS.[214] Their mean length of coma had been 5 weeks, with a range of 1 hour to 24 weeks. Many patients relied on memory aids.

Memory Mechanisms. Experimental neuropsychology,[3,157,194,202] as well as neurophysiology,[139] and anatomic and neuroimaging studies[79,137,161,191] point to certain systems and subsystems with a variety of operating characteristics that contribute to memory. This work has begun to specify the way in which these serial and parallel, distributed systems may function under normal circumstances. For example, Table 9–14 shows the activation pattern for a series of PET subtraction studies for low-capacity, short-dura-

Table 9–14. PROCESSES OF SHORT-TERM MEMORY (STM) STUDIED BY FUNCTIONAL IMAGING

Cognitive Process	Cortical Regions Activated
Verbal STM	
Phonologic buffer storage	Left inferior parietal
Rehearsal/inner speech scratchpad	Left inferoposterolateral frontal
Visuospatial STM	
Visuospatial buffer	Right inferior parietal
Visuospatial sketchpad	Right prefrontal, parietal, dorsolateral occipital

tion tasks that reflect short-term memory (STM).[48] Recall of fewer than seven letters or line drawings, which is the approximate encoding capacity of STM, was compared with control tasks. Rehabilitation specialists may be able to apply this information to see the ways in which, in vivo, processing of STM is altered by a brain injury and the way in which its network may reorganize. If, for instance, a patient undergoing rehabilitation after TBI cannot activate part of the network by the same verbal or visuospatial task used in healthy persons, then interventions that rely on the impaired network may have to be altered by methods that activate the impaired component or an uninjured component.

With an eye on the increasingly fine details produced by investigations about memory, rehabilitation specialists have drawn upon some of the tentative organizational schemes of memory to create theory-based practices.

After TBI, tests can reveal impairments of short-term memory, which is about capacity rather than time-related recall; working memory, which is on-line, rehearsing recall; and anterograde and retrograde long-term memory for verbal, visuospatial, and declarative information.[4] Particular stages in memory processing may be impaired. Some of the more easily described stages include attention, organizational strategy, registration, encoding, storage, and retrieval. The maintenance of stored memories and the ability to return them for use depend, among other processes, on widespread interactions among primary sensorimotor cortex, association cortex, and frontal executive func-

tions. Frontal executive functions organize storage and an efficient, selective search at the time of retrieval. *Prospective memory*, which is the ability to remember to carry out a task in the future, often falters after TBI. Patients may recall what they were supposed to do when cued or asked, but they do not do it otherwise because the executive functions that maintain a goal state over time fail them.[184]

Recent studies also suggest that some memory functions may be divided by their qualities, much as separable neurons and pathways in the visual system subserve qualities such as motion, shape, recognition of an object, and awareness of placement in space. Primate prefrontal cortex is segregated into object and spatial domains. By function and by region of the cortex, different neurons code information related to stimulus identity and the visual location of the stimulus.[216] In this model, then, the memory for the "what" and "where" of an object is dissociable. Given these separable modules, and perhaps others, memories must form in parallel fashion. One implication for memory and cognitive rehabilitation is that therapists must more finely diagnose whether particular modules are functioning and develop strategies to make use of surviving or alternate modules.

Taxonomies of memory distinguish between declarative and nondeclarative memory. *Declarative* or *explicit memory* depends on limbic and diencephalic structures. These networks receive new sensory information about facts and events and sketch a memory trace until it is bound onto the remote cortical modules that consolidate the memory.[225] The circuit allows for the conscious recollection of facts and events. It is lost in patients with amnesia with hippocampal and midline diencephalic injuries. *Implicit* or *nonconscious memory* supports the learning of skills and habits, simple conditioning, and the phenomenon of priming. This memory process is a more diverse aggregation of systems. The striatum is important for skills and habits, the neocortex for priming, the amygdala for emotional conditioning, the cerebellum for skeletal muscle conditioning, and reflex pathways for nonassociative learning.[196] Knowledge about the qualities of items that place them in the same category can be acquired implicitly, so that even a patient with amnesia can learn the pattern that classifies items.[98]

Often, procedural memory and implicit learning are relatively well preserved after TBI. Patients can use this rule-based recall and their ability to learn automatic behavioral sequences for a motor, perceptual, or cognitive skill, even though they may have only nonspecific knowledge about having learned or having carried out the task. During the period of PTA, patients with CHI have learned motor and pattern analysis skills while they have impaired memory for word lists and recent events. They carry over some of this procedural memory into the period of recovery from PTA.[42] During PTA, many patients show an increased rate of forgetting over the course of 30 hours on a visual recognition test compared with patients with CHI who are past PTA.[110] This finding suggests that therapy during PTA should emphasize skills learning and should spend less effort on repetitive mental exercises that seek to improve the episodic and semantic components of declarative memory.

Semantic memory, the knowledge of word meanings and factual knowledge or ideas and information, is usually superior to episodic memory after TBI. *Episodic memory* is personally experienced, time-specific, and place-specific recollection. Semantic processing of information, however, often declines. For example, patients tend not to use strategies such as clustering related words in a list to organize the information for retention. They recall better with cues. Indeed, previous exposure to verbal and, especially,

to nonverbal information can, with cues and prompts, allow many patients with amnesia after TBI to recall that information, a phenomenon called *priming*. Tests of recognition memory are especially sensitive methods for detecting residual memory in patients with severe amnesia. This implicit memory neocortical mechanism can even support the rapid acquisition of novel verbal and nonverbal material. It is independent of the hippocampal and diencephalic structures that cause amnesia.[144] Priming seems especially useful during rehabilitation to enhance procedural memory.

Priming systems are thought to handle information about physical form and structure, rather than about the meanings and associative properties of objects and words.[182] These systems are insensitive to semantic processing for encoding. Priming is specific to the particular properties of the input and relies on perceptual representations stored by modality-specific memory subsystems, such as those that process word forms and visual objects. Each hemisphere may store different representations. For example, changing the font of typed letters does not affect word-stem priming when the fragments are presented to the left hemisphere, but it does impair recognition when the partial word fragments are presented to only the right hemisphere.[130] PET activation studies have begun to reveal the cortical localization of some forms of priming.[195]

Interventions for Amnestic Disorders. Cognitive rehabilitation specialists have begun to teach skills through procedural memory processes, to improve recall with priming techniques, and to develop more specific semantic strategies to enhance episodic memory. These more sophisticated attempts at memory remediation cannot be isolated endeavors. For example, even when recovery is generally good, the memory performance of many patients declines during a distracting task.[198] After severe CHI, patients tend to underestimate their memory and emotional impairments, even as they acknowledge physical and other cognitive problems. Without this insight or concern about their sense of knowing what they know, these patients may deny any impairment and may withdraw or become angry during attempts at rehabilitation. Lack of insight and loss of the sense of familiarity may result in confabulation that interferes with therapy.

After moderate to severe TBI, repetitive drills can have little impact on general recall or on enhancing memory outside the training session.[166] The styles of practice and methods of reinforcement of learning need further exploration in patients with various memory impairments. For example, severely amnestic patients learned more in one study when errors during training were minimized and performed worse when allowed to generate guesses that produced incorrect responses.[215a] These patients relied on their implicit memory, which may respond best to errorless learning.

External aids such as a calendar and appointment diary and internal strategies such as the mnemonic devices of rehearsal, visual imagery, and peg words help some patients. The most frequently deployed memory devices still used by patients with TBI 5 or more years after being trained in their use are listed in Table 9–15.[124] Touch-screen pocket computers with memory prompts and ''help'' software, pagers that receive typed messages, alarm wristwatches, calendars, and a place for phone numbers and notes can be adapted for some patients. Although internal aids may be of value within a structured task, their postinjury use often cannot become generalized to real-world settings.[174] The person with TBI has to remember to invoke these aids and must hurdle past other impairments such as concrete thinking, which impedes the strategy.

One randomized, controlled trial of patients with CHI found that a group given memory strategy training and another given drill and repetitive practice training on memory tasks subjectively rated their everyday memory as improved, compared with a group that received no treatment.[9] Only the strategy-training group showed objective gains in memory performance, more clearly apparent at a 4-month follow-up than at the end of two 3-week sessions of training. These patients were a mean of 5 years post injury, half were employed, and they had experienced a mean of 30 days of PTA. Thus, therapists can attempt to teach memory strategies to patients with residual cognitive dysfunction and to determine whether the techniques will become generalized to other

Table 9–15. **AIDS AND STRATEGIES FOR COPING WITH MEMORY IMPAIRMENT**

External
  Reminders by others
  Tape recorder
  Notes written on hand
  Time reminders
    Alarm clock/phone call
    Personal organizer/diary; calendar/wall
      planner
    Orientation board
  Place reminders
    Labels; codes: colors, symbols
  Person reminders
    Name tags
    Clothes that offer a cue
  Organizers
    Lists; items grouped for use
    Electronic or written calendar organizer
    Posted numbered series of reminders
  Radiopagers

Internal
  Mental retracing of events; rehearsal
  Visual imagery
  Alphabet searching; first-letter mnemonics
  Associations with items already recalled
  Chunking or grouping of items

material or to a novel context. If trained skills cannot be generalized, then therapy may concentrate on strategies that lead to a transfer of learning. In a successful transfer, the patient uses the same organizational approach to a task that is nearly the same as the trained-for task.

Another method builds upon these approaches, although more on the basis of intuition than on the grounds of adequate testing. First, it deals with attentional impairments that can interfere with memory training. This approach addresses focused, sustained, selective, alternating, and divided attention with a program called Attention Process Training.[188,190] It then addresses impairments in encoding and recall of information with another standardized treatment program called Prospective Memory Process Training.[189] This program uses associative and external cues meant to prompt an action after increasingly longer intervals. It also makes use of a memory notebook. Attempts at generalized use of the notebook depend most heavily on sparing of procedural memory.[191] Although single-case studies suggest modest gains with these techniques, whether success can be maintained over time and become generalized to related tasks in the aftermath of moderate to severe TBI is unclear. These standardized protocols provide a testable approach that will no doubt molt many times as theories and practices evolve, however.

A more modest goal for the patient with amnesia focuses on the acquisition of knowledge about a particular task or subject, so-called domain-specific knowledge. It draws upon the ability of patients with amnesia to learn and to show relatively good priming effects that can allow them to make new associations. This technique also draws upon the relative sparing of procedural memory. The technique includes the method of vanishing cues. For example, patients are taught new computer terms by gradually reducing the number of letters in the new words and by training them to complete the word fragment.[54] Eventually, some patients are able to provide the word without any letter cues when given its definition. With this technique, some patients have learned to enter data into a computer by acquiring specific rules and procedures that do not readily transfer to novel documents.

In summary, the approach to the cognitive remediation of amnestic disorders draws upon the various modules of memory networks being defined by neuroscientific studies. Techniques aim to train patients in the use of the subcomponent processes that underlie declarative and nondeclarative memory. Therapists can then take a substitutive or compensatory approach to improving particular memory skills for functionally important activities. The same approach can be developed for other cognitive impairments. In most programs, cognitive remediation itself is only one of the components of the rehabilitation of patients with brain injury.

MULTIMODAL SKILLS TRAINING

Most acute and postacute rehabilitation programs combine cognitive remediation with other organized services.[76] The content of training includes the skills that the patient needs for ADLs, socialization, or work. These lengthy programs have had an impact on some important outcomes, although the optimal type of patient, the content and duration of therapy, and the setting of realizable goals are debatable issues.

In one interdisciplinary program, 18 highly selected patients received cognitive and psychologic therapies that emphasized awareness of deficits, along with social, work, and family training.[166] These patients had good family support, no premorbid psychiatric history, and moderate to severe cognitive dysfunction. Mostly one-on-one therapies were given 6 hours a day for 4 days a week and lasted at least 6 months. In a comparison with 17 matched patients who received a traditional approach, 50 percent of the intensively treated group and 36 percent of the control group were employed at a 6-month to 26-month follow-up. The group receiving intensive therapy also tended to do better in some cognitive tests, including the WMS. The self-selection of these patients for participation in the experimental group may have been an uncontrolled factor that accounted for the modest findings. A similar scheme of therapy was used in a larger group of patients who had completed traditional therapy and had failed to regain employment.[7] These patients received about 400 hours of cognitive remediation, instruction on interpersonal communication and social skills, and counseling to understand and accept their disability. The patients continued with 3 to 9 months of supervision in a work setting. Six months later, 84 percent were employed, about half in a competitive setting. At a 3-year follow-up, 76 percent of a smaller available group still was employed, half in a competitive job. Other single-institution reports of late rehabilitation have also found positive effects on posttreatment work status, attendant care, and independent living that the authors believed were cost-effective.[28,88]

Much has been written about the confusing and poor methods of studies of multimodal programs of rehabilitation.[10,80] For example, the proponents of a lengthy outpatient program that has emphasized cognitive, social, and vocational interventions describe statistically significant improvements without a control group, using a scale of functional performance of uncertain reliability and validity related to work status.[145] Although the data show a change from pretreatment to posttreatment, the differences seem to have no practical meaning for employability. Publications from single institutions about their results in uncontrolled trials must be viewed with caution; however, the effects of programs that use multiple, simultaneous interventions can be evaluated systematically.

In one approach, three matched groups were assigned to three different mixes of remedial interventions.[172] All subjects received the same number of hours of therapy, counseling, and interaction with peers in group activities. One group received cognitive remediation using a hierarchy of training procedures for constructional and visual analysis tasks and verbal reasoning. Another group received this therapy, plus training in interpersonal skills that emphasized acceptance of disability and awareness of deficits. The third group received interpersonal skills training without cognitive remediation. Measures specific to each type of training improved in those who received one or both. Thus, gains could be attributed to more than the overall milieu of rehabilitation. Other comparisons of different packages of therapies would have ethical, scientific, and practical benefits while taking advantage of the supportive milieu.

COMPUTER APPLICATIONS

Enthusiasm for computer-assisted cognitive rehabilitation (CACR) was initially great. CACR methods and goals have been undergoing a reassessment, however.[95] Most therapy programs include CACR. Computer software allows clinicians to make serial measurements of the patient's progress in what are usually repetitive tasks. The computer is rigid in its demands and so offers the consistency needed by many patients with TBI. Partial and complete visual and auditory cues can be built in to aid declarative and nondeclarative learning. Reinforcement schedules for knowledge of performance and knowledge of results can be set. Pleasurable visual and auditory reinforcers are

easy to create. In general, patients can work with intermittent supervision, and this feature should lessen the expense of therapy.

Although computer technology provides environmental control systems and external aids, perhaps enough to be considered a mental prosthesis, the value of this technology in cognitive remediation and skills training is less certain. Some patients have been trained in tasks such as data entry, database management, and word processing by taking advantage of preserved cognitive abilities, including the ability to respond to partial cues and to acquire procedural information.[53] As noted earlier, this knowledge is specific to the patient's training and does not readily generalize to even modest changes in requirements. Using a similar technique, verbal and visual mnemonic strategies have been used to teach a computer graphics program.[162] Other patients have been trained to do cooking and vocational tasks with an interactive guidance system that cues each subtask and builds up to the required task.[96] Computer-based cognitive remediation software programs have also shown promise for special education classes in a school setting.[201]

These limited, but interesting successes suggest that the computer can assist in skills training as a kind of learning or reminding prosthesis. The computer may eventually find use as a means to help remedy specific cognitive processes by allowing systematic practice on their subcomponents. Although some modest successes have been published in small-group or single-case studies, clear gains by CACR in, for example, patients with attentional deficits have often failed.[63,158] Even the most powerful computer has to await our knowledge of these cognitive processes and their modulation. With greater computing power, the CD-ROM, easier interfaces, voice recognition, and the growing ability of software to simulate real-world settings, the possibilities for computers in cognitive rehabilitation will require continuous reassessment.

PHARMACOLOGIC FACILITATION

Rehabilitation physicians have probably tried more neuropharmacologic agents in individual patients with TBI in an attempt to modify cognition and behavior than for any other disease. On occasion, a positive experience or a single-case study design has led to a randomized clinical trial. Drugs for postinjury behavioral and psychiatric disorders have been more clearly efficacious. They are discussed later in this chapter.

The disruption of the cholinergic pathway in Alzheimer's disease, the negative effect on recall by the cholinergic antagonist scopolamine, and the mediation of declarative, but not procedural, memory by the cholinergic system have made cholinergic agonists a favorite drug to try in patients with memory disorders.[147] Positive results, however, have been less reproducible and of more limited consequence than the modest effects of tacrine on the dementia of Alzheimer's disease. After a dorsal pontine and midbrain DAI, which can damage any of at least three neurotransmitter pools, replacement with agonists of serotonin, norepinephrine, and acetylcholine has some rationale.

Catecholamine agonists and vasopressin have had occasional benefit in increasing arousal, attention, and initiation. A vasopressin analog studied in a double-blind, placebo-controlled, matched-pairs trial, however, had no effect on cognitive recovery in the 3 months following mild TBI.[15] Bromocriptine at 2.5 to 10 mg three times a day, carbidopa-levodopa at 25/100 to 25/250 mg four times a day, or amantadine at 100 mg up to three times a day has occasionally improved mutism, akinesia, a flat affect, goal-directed behavior, and aspects of memory in some patients with frontal lobe injuries.

The effects of a drug intervention are not readily predictable. Clinicians might anticipate that positive effects on one aspect of cognition could have an adverse effect on another. For example, amphetamines may increase attention, but they may also produce hypervigilance to extraneous stimuli, stereotyped behavior, and paranoia. Drug trials must take into consideration that short-term crossover designs may mask an effect that lasts longer than the time allowed for withdrawal from the medication. Moreover, the optimal dose, the amount of time on a drug, and the type of practice in cognitive tasks while receiving a drug all factor into assessing a measurable change.

Table 9–16. POSSIBLY USEFUL DRUG CLASSES FOR COGNITIVE DISORDERS IN TRAUMATIC BRAIN INJURY

Cholinergic Agonists
  Physostigmine
  Tacrine
  Cytidine diphosphate (CDP) choline[115]
  Choline/lecithin precursors

Catecholamine Agonists
  d-amphetamine
  Methylphenidate[66]
  L-dopa[102]
  Amantadine[67]
  Bromocriptine[40]
  Desipramine

Nootropic Agents
  Pramiracetam[134]

Neuropeptides
  Vasopressin

Table 9–16 lists some of the more commonly used classes of drugs tried in patients with TBI in North America and Europe.[24,151,220] Individual drug trials should include gradual dose escalations, specific tests of efficacy for specified goals, and monitoring for side effects. These medications may have a differential effect across the stages of recovery. If a benefit seems to be present, a drug holiday after several weeks can help to determine ongoing need for the agent. At present, patients are probably more likely to show a decline in cognition as an adverse reaction to centrally acting medications than they are apt to benefit from a drug.

EFFICACY OF COGNITIVE THERAPIES

Does cognitive rehabilitation work for patients with moderate and severe TBI? Although clinicians have argued about this question from the point of view of theory, methodology, interventions, and measures of outcome,[8,12,23,52,57,208,215] the studies that may provide an answer have not been attempted. Treatment aimed at the subcomponents of cognitive processes requires many hours of therapy. So far, at least for patients with serious TBI, treatments considered to be cognitive remediation techniques produce equivocal or very modest measurable changes. These changes, with a few exceptions, do not translate into functional gains. For a large effort, multimodal skills acquisition training seems to offer some gains, such as the ability of the patient to be employed in a structured environment.

The methods and benefits of rehabilitation that aims to lessen cognitive disability after TBI have not been questioned any more rigorously than have the methods and benefits of rehabilitation for other neurologic diseases and associated disabilities. Therapy programs seem worthwhile, because efforts protect patients from medical and emotional complications that can limit spontaneous gains. Programs can also promote adaptive functional gains, create compensatory strategies, train practical and social skills, improve behavior, reduce psychosocial and neuropsychiatric problems, and help patients to reintegrate into home, school, or work. The most effective approaches to these goals for most patients are still uncertain. The most controversial issue for rehabilitation of patients with TBI is whether specific cognitive approaches can be identified and applied so that they change what they aim to treat, as well as related functional outcomes.

At present, a thorough neuropsychologic evaluation helps to describe the loci of cognitive impairments within the neurocognitive architecture. This information clearly influences the way in which therapists understand the impairments and disabilities of their patients. It also influences the interventional choices made by the rehabilitation team. Rehabilitation interventions are determined by the details of analysis, by available treatments, and by overriding goals. The present contribution of cognitive remediation may be in defining what is right and what is wrong with a patient in a systematic way, so that existing tools and techniques can be applied as appropriately as the state of knowledge allows. Progress in cognitive remediation, as in any aspect of rehabilitation, follows what is learned from the ongoing interactions among initial assessment, generation of hypotheses, and monitoring of consequences of interventions. Informed clinicians who take a heuristic approach that leads to clinical trials may produce an array of cognitive remediation innovations.

Cognitive remediation is one of the newest neurorehabilitation endeavors. It was once bounded by approaches from education and behavioral psychology. It now extends toward experimental work related to neurocognitive networks and neuroplasticity. In this expanding universe of data, clinicians can hope to develop theory-driven practices that demonstrate efficacy upon rigorous testing.

Neurobehavioral Disorders

If cognitive dysfunction is the powerful undertow that threatens to pull down efforts at rehabilitation of TBI, then behavioral and personality changes are the waves that crash against patients and their supporters. Some of these puzzling, demanding behaviors are listed in Table 9–17. Changes in personality have been reported in up to 75 percent of patients from 1 to 15 years after TBI, and they tend not to improve beyond 2 years after onset.[205]

Frontolimbic injuries can be associated with agitated, aggressive, out-of-control behavior that stresses the family, rocks relationships, and prevents acceptance into work and society. Agitated motor and verbal behaviors were found in 11 percent of patients during acute inpatient rehabilitation.[19] Another 35 percent of these patients were restless. Many patients quickly evolve away from the confused, agitated behavior of level IV on the Rancho Los Amigos scale in the first weeks after they emerge from coma. As cognition improves, agitation declines.[32] Other patients exhibit directed and nondirected aggressive, impulsive behavior. Interventions include a medical assessment for exacerbating problems such as pain and drug-induced confusion, behavioral modification, structuring of the environment, individual and group psychotherapy, and medication trials.

Table 9–17. **COMMON CHANGES IN BEHAVIOR AND PERSONALITY AFTER TRAUMATIC BRAIN INJURY**

Disinhibition
Impulsiveness
Aggressiveness
Irritability
Lability
Euphoria
Paranoia
Lack of self-criticism and insight
Irresponsibility, childishness
Egocentricity, selfishness
Sexual deviation, inappropriateness
Substance abuse
Self-abuse
Poor personal habits
Indecision
Lack of initiation
Blunted emotional responses
Poor self-worth
Apathy, inertia
Indifference
Passive dependency

BEHAVIORAL MODIFICATION

Behavioral modification of maladaptive conduct requires consistent and attentive care. Important target behaviors and their antecedent events or conditions are identified and are counted. The team designs positive reinforcers and rewards and applies them on a consistent schedule of reinforcement. Rewards can be as simple as special foods, breaks from therapy, phone calls, passes, praise, and some time alone. A token economy, in which credits are earned for appropriate behaviors and are exchanged for treats and privileges, can provide powerful incentives. The rehabilitation milieu for these patients should be supportive, peaceful, and nonthreatening. Negative reinforcement paradigms are rarely used.

PHARMACOLOGIC INTERVENTIONS

Some centrally acting medications can alter neurotransmitter activity and, in turn, can affect disorders of behavior and personality (Table 9–18). Hypoarousal sometimes improves with stimulants such as methylphenidate and amphetamine, as well as with dopamine agonists. Blocking dopaminergic and noradrenergic receptors and increasing serotonin levels can sometimes reduce aggressive behavior. Most of the agents with antimanic effects are worth trying in the patient who is difficult to control. Hypomanic behavior may respond best to lithium, which is an especially effective agent for the mood-related symptoms of bipolar, manic-depressive disorder.[163] The drug requires considerable monitoring for side effects and for optimizing the dose. Anticonvulsants such as carbamazepine sometimes prevent outbursts related to episodic dyscontrol. Lithium and the anticonvulsants should be titrated into their usual therapeutic serum levels. Beta-blockers can decrease feelings of irritability. A randomized trial of propranolol with a dose escalation to 420 mg a day showed a reduction in the intensity of agitation, but not in the frequency of episodes, compared with a placebo.[18] In both treatment groups, the episodes dropped sharply by week 6 after admission for rehabilitation. Indeed, the frequency of symptoms and the bouts of loss of control tend to decline over time. Thus, medication that reduces symptoms should be tapered off on a trial basis after 2 months of use. Premorbid personality and mood disorders may contribute to the persistence of symptoms and need for drug therapy.

Table 9–18. **DRUG INTERVENTIONS FOR AGGRESSIVE BEHAVIOR, RESTLESSNESS, AND EPISODIC DYSCONTROL**

Anticonvulsants (carbamazepine, valproate)
Beta-blockers
Lithium carbonate
Antidepressants (amitriptyline, fluoxetine)
Stimulants (*d*-amphetamine, methylphenidate, pemoline)
Neuroleptics
Benzodiazepines
Clonidine
Verapamil

Neuropsychiatric Disorders

Premorbid psychopathologic features may be common in patients who suffer a TBI. In one study of patients who suffered trauma without head injuries, 56 percent had this history, especially when alcohol and a violent act were associated with their injuries.[211] The prevalence of psychosis has been estimated at up to 5 percent after moderate TBI and at 10 percent after severe TBI.[68] Mania with delusions, often associated with frontal lesions, has been managed with carbamaze-

DEPRESSION

The prevalence of depression after TBI ranges from 25 to 60 percent.[68] Depression has been related to lesion location in some correlative studies. Left anterior injuries, as in unilateral stroke, are associated with an early, transient depression.[89] Other focal and diffuse injuries make it difficult to relate mood disorders to specific sites, however. In the Vietnam Head Injury Study, anxiety and depression were associated with a right orbitofrontal lesion, and anger and hostility were related to a left dorsofrontal penetrating injury.[60] Late-onset depression in patients with CHI is more closely associated with a premorbid psychiatric history and lower psychosocial function than with lesion location.[89] Long-term depression and anxiety seem more closely related to problems in social adjustment.

A randomized trial comparing cognitive remediation with supportive day treatment for 8 weeks found that depression improved with both approaches.[180] Cognitive remediation, which tends to confront patients with their impairments, did not worsen their emotional state or their psychosocial adjustment. The effectiveness of psychotherapy is uncertain in patients with memory or language dysfunction and limited awareness of deficits. Antidepressant medication may improve symptoms.

PSYCHOSEXUAL DISORDERS

Psychosexual dysfunction evolves in up to 50 percent of patients after TBI. Infrequent sexual intercourse is the most common problem.[148] Neuroendocrine dysfunction, pain, neurologic impairments, cognitive and behavioral dysfunction, alterations in libido, bowel and bladder incontinence, and psychosocial issues can often be managed.[223] Hypersexuality and disinhibition of sexual activity sometimes follow a medial basalfrontal or diencephalic injury. Klüver-Bucy syndrome is associated with bitemporal injuries. Change in sexual preference has been related to limbic lesions.[138]

SLEEP DISORDERS

Sleep disturbances are common in the first few months and late after injury.[27] Up to half of patients after TBI have difficulty in initiating and maintaining sleep. About one-third complain of somnolence. Management of sleep dysfunction is an important part of any rehabilitation effort, especially for patients who have disorders of memory, attention, and mood. As noted in earlier chapters, an abnormal sleep cycle can prevent consolidation of newly learned information.

POSTTRAUMATIC STRESS DISORDER

Although the incidence of posttraumatic stress disorder after TBI has not been reported, clinicians may expect that patients who suffer violent injuries and who witness the injury or death of a companion are at risk. Anterograde and retrograde amnesia probably protects most patients with moderate to severe TBI from this disorder.

Role of Psychotherapy

Psychotherapy has been recommended for nonpsychotic symptoms and for general support as a part of rehabilitation of TBI.[26,165] Practices of psychotherapeutic techniques differ widely, and measures of efficacy are less than striking. These techniques can be used to help patients understand what has happened to them and to improve self-awareness and insight. Problems in awareness and acceptance of disability can affect the patient's motivation for rehabilitation and can impede progress on cognitive, social, and emotional fronts. At some stage of recovery, patients often underestimate their difficulties in memory and emotional control. Lack of insight, however, as accurately as it may be measured, does not necessarily correlate with failure to make gains in rehabilitation.[124] Psychotherapy can also help patients to control anger and other affective responses, to achieve self-acceptance and find hope, to make realistic commitments, and to assess their role in the family. Spousal and family therapy can contribute to domestic tranquility, understanding, and the patient's reintegration. Although some patients after TBI may be too impaired cognitively to participate, patients who seem to need the intervention usually can work with a therapist.

SPECIAL POPULATIONS

Pediatric Patients

The severity of brain injury and neurobehavioral impairment have a dose-response relationship in children and adolescents, as in adults.[106] Duration of PTA, as measured by the Children's Orientation and Amnesia Test (COAT), time to a 75 percent score on the COAT, time to reach a GCS of 15, initial GCS, and duration of loss of consciousness are all directly proportional to neurobehavioral outcomes.[133]

Eight months after children aged 4 months to 5 years suffered a severe head injury, cognitive functions tended to recover more completely than motor skills.[43] Compared with a group of matched peers, however, children who were 6 to 15 years old at the time of moderate to severe TBI (based on the GCS) showed significant neurocognitive, academic, and functional deficits at 1 and 3 years post injury.[45] The children with head injury scored lower in 40 of 53 variables tested, including measures of intelligence, adaptive reasoning, memory, and psychomotor, motor, and academic performance. Their rate of improvement was strong in the first year after TBI, but it slowed markedly over the next 2 years, especially in the most severely injured youngsters.[83] The group also scored inferiorly on parent ratings of behavior and social competence. The ability to engage in abstract concept learning was seriously reduced, and this impairment could, when combined with other impairments, disrupt the acquisition of cognitive skills. These findings, along with the plateau reached by the more severely affected children, pose a major challenge for cognitive rehabilitation and schooling.

Rehabilitation for the pediatric age group must take into account age-specific neurologic, cognitive, and psychosocial development. Hyperactivity, poor attention, impulsivity, and apathy are common behavioral problems generally treated with behavioral strategies. Preinjury family and child functioning can explain many behavioral and academic outcomes.[176] Family adjustment and return to school require planning, support services, and long-term monitoring.[103,221] Attempts at early management of physical, intellectual, and emotional sequelae seem especially important in children. For example, after mild TBI, symptoms present 5 years post injury tended to persist 18 years later. These symptoms correlated with diminished psychosocial adaptation.[97] Early intervention may mitigate this situation.

Geriatric Patients

The incidence of TBI rises beyond the age of 70 years, especially because of falls. Subdural hematomas, which are associated with the rapid acceleration of the brain during falls and with cerebral atrophy that allows greater stretch of bridging veins, accompany 25 percent of CHI in the elderly.[119] Few long-term studies of late middle-aged and elderly people have been conducted. A well-designed, prospective study of outcomes related to mild and moderate TBI in patients over the age of 50 years is in progress and should provide useful insights.[55] Studies suggest that greater disability and less likelihood of returning home follow equivalent severity of TBI in the elderly compared with younger patients.[34] Cognition may be at special risk. At a mean follow-up of 10 months post injury, half of 70 consecutive hospitalized patients over the age of 50 years had cognitive dysfunction not closely related to the initial severity of CHI.[132] Remarkably, 21 percent had what appeared to be dementia secondary to the trauma. After severe TBI, the risk of developing dementia later in life was four times that of the general population in one study.[68] Case-control and epidemiologic studies are inconsistent in pointing to a single episode of TBI with loss of consciousness as a risk factor for subsequent Alzheimer's disease, however.[25,62]

Postdischarge support is especially necessary for many elderly patients who return home. Help is often needed for bathing, housework, shopping, and pain and medication management. With cognitive dysfunction, the elderly often require full-time supervision.

Patients with Mild Injury

Mild TBI generally refers to injury severity with a GCS of 13 to 15, loss of consciousness for less than 20 minutes, and PTA for less than 24 hours. The category includes patients who have any alteration of consciousness or mentation at the time of injury or who persist with any memory, cognitive, or brain-related physical symptoms.[14] The designation is often synonymous with the terms *concussion* and *postconcussional* or *posttraumatic* syndrome.

The posttraumatic syndrome can include headache, vertigo and dysequilibrium, irritability, malaise, and impaired concentration and memory. Many clinicians believe that emotional factors and compensation through litigation play a role in aggravating or prolonging these symptoms. Neuropsychologic testing of memory, attention, and speed of information processing at 1 week post injury, however, shows significant impairments compared with matched controls, although most patients improve 1 month later.[112] About 20 percent of patients have some disability after mild TBI.[109] Although symptoms can interfere with vocational activity for an average of 3 months, some patients take 18 months or more to recover. In a matched-peer control study, mild head injury in children and adolescents did not cause measurable differences in neuropsychologic and academic or social performance at 1 or 3 years post injury.[44]

Cognitive dysfunction can also accompany a whiplash injury in patients without a direct head injury.[41] Headache and neck pain are common associated symptoms. Results of neuropsychologic testing can be abnormal, especially for complex attentional tasks. Cognitive symptoms tend to fade by 6 months after injury, but when they persist, centrally acting medications and pain may be contributing factors.[167]

Slowness in mental processing is less after mild, compared with more severe, TBI, but divided attention often suffers. For example, 1 week after relatively mild TBI with a mean duration of PTA of 5 days, 89 percent of patients were impaired on the Paced Auditory Serial Addition Task, compared with controls.[65] At 6 months, 56 percent were impaired. In this test, the patient is instructed to listen to a random string of digits from 1 to 9 and to add the last digit spoken to the preceding one. For example:

$$\begin{array}{lcccccc} \text{stimulus} & 2 & 7 & 4 & 3 & \dots \\ \text{response} & - & 9 & 11 & 7 & \dots \end{array}$$

Management of mild TBI and the postconcussional syndrome includes protecting the patient from the emotional repercussions of memory impairment, inefficient information processing, and difficulty in dealing with simultaneous and distracting stimuli. Education, reassurance, and stress management can reduce the time needed to be able to return to work.[109] For patients with memory dysfunction, compensatory strategies and aids can limit adverse consequences on daily activities. For problems in divided attention, students may find it easier to tape record lectures than to try to listen in class and write notes. At home and at work, the patient should try to structure tasks so that only one is tackled until completed. Physical therapies for headache related to cervical soft tissue injury, antimigraine medications for posttraumatic vascular headache, and antidepressants are among the more frequently prescribed interventions.

Coma Sensory Stimulation

Patients in a coma or a vegetative state are often given structured sensory stimulation as therapy that augments neuromedical care and family counseling. Input to the reticular activating system and notions about enriching the environment for the sensory-deprived patient have served as theoretic rationales.

Electrical stimulation of the nonspecific thalamic nuclei and of the high cervical spinal cord with implanted electrodes was used in six patients for 12 hours a day at 30 percent of the threshold that elicited eye opening and pupil dilation.[82] Although the details are unclear, two patients who had a GCS of less than 6 for about 10 months became able to handle oral feedings and made simple responses to verbal commands over 10 months of stimulation. Less invasively, therapists have tried vestibular, tactile, auditory, olfactory, visual, and gustatory stimuli.[49] Sensory stimulation for periods up to 3 months has had no apparent effect on arousal or recovery.[168] Even in those extraordinary instances in which coma stimulation seemed to shorten the time to arousal relatively early after onset of coma,[141] the effect on subsequent disability is unclear. Although some investigators have begun to define the level of dysfunction of patients by more reliable scales[170] and to monitor for specific physiologic or behavioral responses, reports of sensory stimulation do not yet offer evidence that promotes its efficacy.[224] On the other hand, family and friends should be encouraged by the rehabilitation team to talk to patients while touching their faces or briefly opening the eyelids if necessary to make contact. These personal actions have general therapeutic effects for everyone.

ETHICAL ISSUES

Ethical issues arise often during rehabilitation of patients with TBI. The medicolegal demands related to a personal injury, the assessment of competence of the patient to make small and large decisions,[70] the use of behavioral modification techniques, the application of interventions of borderline acceptance (such as coma stimulation), and the provision of appropriate postacute rehabilitation services are among the issues that must be considered. Perhaps more so than in the rehabilitation of patients with other neurologic diseases, TBI brings out the issue of what constitutes a good or an acceptable outcome.[6] Survivors of TBI who have persisting disabilities are central to the social, economic, and political activities of the movement for independent living.

Studies of the efficacy of rehabilitation of TBI are often hampered by a pseudoethical dilemma. European and North American studies of cognitive rehabilitation techniques too often state, "Given the constraint that in a rehabilitation setting it is, for ethical reasons, not acceptable to assign patients randomly to treatment groups or to control groups, . . . [we used] quasi-experimental group studies . . . alternative design."[209] This constraint is iatrogenic nonsense. The process of obtaining informed consent from cognitively impaired patients poses ethical problems, but progress in developing cost-effective programs and specific interventions, whether cognitive or neurobiologic, eventually depends on controlled, randomized comparison trials.

SUMMARY

Rehabilitation of the patient with TBI takes a broad, holistic approach. The range of disabilities, many of them tied to cognitive and neurobehavioral impairments, and the age spread of subjects demand alternatives for therapy settings, styles, and goals. As described in this chapter, the rehabilitation team has many strategies. Some attempt to build recovery from our present understanding of the architecture of neurocognitive networks. Most have not been tested for their efficacy. New approaches may benefit from insights provided by activation studies during functional neuroimaging. Additional pharmacologic and training strategies that pass the test of clinical trials can be expected to return more patients with TBI to their home, community, school, and work.

REFERENCES

1. Alexander M, Benson D, Stuss D. Frontal lobes and language. Brain Lang 1989;37:656–691.
2. Annegers J, Grabow J, Groover R, et al. Seizures

after head trauma: A population study. Neurology 1980;30:683–689.

3. Baddeley A. Working memory. Science 1992; 255:556–559.

4. Baddeley A, Harris J, Sunderland A, et al. Closed head injury and memory. In: Levin H, Grafman J, Eisenberg H, eds: Neurobehavioral Recovery from Head Injury. New York: Oxford University Press, 1987:295–317.

5. Bakchine S, Lacomblez L, Benoit N, et al. Manic-like state after bilateral orbitofrontal and right temporoparietal injury. Neurology 1989;39:777–781.

6. Banja J, Johnston M. Ethical perspectives and social policy. Arch Phys Med Rehabil 1994;75:SC19–SC26.

7. Ben-Yishay J, Silver S, Plasetsky E, et al. Relationship between employability and vocational outcome after intensive holistic cognitive rehabilitation. Journal of Head Trauma Rehabilitation 1987;2:35–48.

8. Ben-Yishay Y, Diller L. Cognitive remediation in traumatic brain injury: Update and issues. Arch Phys Med Rehabil 1993;74:204–213.

9. Berg I, Koning-Haanstra M, Deelman B. Long-term effects of memory rehabilitation. Neuropsychological Rehabilitation 1991;1:97–111.

10. Bergquist T, Boll T, Harley J, et al. Neuropsychological rehabilitation: Proceedings of a consensus conference. Journal of Head Trauma Rehabilitation 1994;9:50–61.

11. Bergsneider M, Kelly D, Shalmon E, et al. Remote metabolic depression following human traumatic brain injury: A PET study. J Neurotrauma 1995; 12:110.

12. Berrol S. Issues in cognitive rehabilitation. Arch Neurol 1990;47:219–224.

13. Black P, Hakim R, Bailey N. The use of the Codman-Medos programmable Hakim valve in the management of patients with hydrocephalus. Neurosurgery 1994;34:1110–1113.

14. Boake C, Bobetic K, Bonke C. Rehabilitation of the patient with mild traumatic brain injury. NeuroRehabilitation 1991;1:70–78.

15. Bohnen N, Twijnstra A, Jolles J. A controlled trial with vasopressin analogue (DGAVP) on cognitive recovery immediately after head trauma. Neurology 1994;43:103–106.

16. Bricolo A, Turazzi S, Feriotti G. Prolonged post-traumatic unconsciousness. J Neurosurg 1980; 52:625–634.

17. Brooke M, Barbour P, Cording L, et al. Nutritional status during rehabilitation after head injury. Journal of Neurologic Rehabilitation 1989; 3:27–33.

18. Brooke M, Patterson D, Questad K, et al. Treatment of agitation during initial hospitalization after traumatic brain injury. Arch Phys Med Rehabil 1992;73:917–921.

19. Brooke M, Questad K, Patterson D, et al. Agitation and restlessness after closed head injury: A prospective study of 100 consecutive admissions. Arch Phys Med Rehabil 1992;73:320–323.

20. Brooks N. The effectiveness of post-acute rehabilitation. Brain Inj 1991;5:103–109.

21. Brooks N, McKinlay W, Simington C, et al. Return to work within the first 7 years of severe brain injury. Brain Inj 1987;1:5–19.

22. Brooks V. The Neural Basis of Motor Control. New York: Oxford University Press, 1986:330.

23. Butler R, Namerow N. Cognitive retraining in brain-injury rehabilitation: A critical review. Journal of Neurologic Rehabilitation 1988;2:97–101.

24. Cardenas D. Cognition-enhancing drugs. J Head Trauma Rehabil 1993;8:112–114.

24a. Ceballos Baumann AO, Passingham R, Marsden CD, Brooks D. Motor reorganization in acquired hemidystonia. Ann Neurol 1995;37:746–757.

25. Chandra V, Kokmen E, Schoenberg B, et al. Head trauma with loss of consciousness as a risk factor for Alzheimer's disease. Neurology 1989; 39:1576–1578.

26. Christensen A-L, Rosenberg N. A critique of the role of psychotherapy in brain injury rehabilitation. Journal of Head Trauma Rehabilitation 1991;6:56–61.

27. Cohen M, Oksenberg A, Snir D, et al. Temporally related changes of sleep complaints in traumatic brain injured patients. J Neurol Neurosurg Psychiatry 1992;55:313–315.

28. Cope D, Cole J, Hall K, et al. Brain injury: Analysis of outcome in a post-acute rehabilitation system. Brain Inj 1991;5:111–139.

29. Cope D, Date E, Mar E. Serial computed tomographic evaluations in TBI. Arch Phys Med Rehabil 1988;69:483–486.

30. Cope D, Hall K. Head injury rehabilitation. Arch Phys Med Rehabil 1982;63:433–437.

31. Corrigan J. Development of a scale for assessment of agitation following traumatic brain injury. J Clin Exp Neuropsychol 1989;11:261–277.

32. Corrigan J, Mysiw J. Agitation following traumatic head injury: Equivocal evidence for a discrete stage of cognitive recovery. Arch Phys Med Rehabil 1988;69:487–492.

33. Crosson B, Greene R, Roth D, et al. WAIS-R pattern clusters after blunt head injury. Clinical Neuropsychology 1990;4:255–262.

33a. Cowen TD, Meythaler J, DeVivo M, et al. Influence of early variables in TBI on Functional Independence Measure scores and rehabilitation length of stay and charges. Arch Phys Med Rehabil 1995;76:797–803.

34. DeMaria E, Kenney P, Merriam M, et al. Aggressive trauma care benefits the elderly. J Trauma 1987;27:1200–1206.

35. Dikmen S, Machamer J, Temkin N, et al. Neuropsychological recovery in patients with moderate to severe head injury: Two years' follow-up. J Clin Exp Neuropsychol 1990;12:507–517.

36. Dikmen S, McLean A, Temkin N. Neuropsychological and psychosocial consequences of minor head injury. J Neurol Neurosurg Psychiatry 1986; 49:1227–1232.

37. Dikmen S, McLean A, Temkin N, et al. Neuropsychologic outcome at one-month postinjury. Arch Phys Med Rehabil 1986;67:507–513.

38. Dikmen S, Temkin N, McLean A, et al. Memory and head injury severity. J Neurol Neurosurg Psychiatry 1987;50:1613–1618.

39. Dikmen S, Temkin N, Miller B, et al. Neurobe-

havioral effects of phenytoin prophylaxis of post-traumatic seizures. JAMA 1991;265:1271–1277.

40. Dobkin B, Hanlon R. Dopamine agonist treatment of antegrade amnesia from a mediobasal forebrain injury. Ann Neurol 1992;33:313–316.

41. Ettlin T, Kischka U, Reichmann S, et al. Cerebral symptoms after whiplash injury of the neck: A prospective clinical neuropsychological study. J Neurol Neurosurg Psychiatry 1993;55:943–948.

42. Ewert J, Levin H, Watson M, et al. Procedural memory during posttraumatic amnesia in survivors of severe closed head injury. Arch Neurol 1989;46:911–916.

43. Ewing-Cobbs L, Miner M, Fletcher J, et al. Intellectual, motor and language sequelae following head injury in infants and preschoolers. J Pediatr Psychol 1989;14:531–547.

44. Fay G, Jaffe K, Polissar N, et al. Mild pediatric trauma brain injury: A cohort study. Arch Phys Med Rehabil 1993;74:895–901.

45. Fay G, Jaffe K, Polissar N, et al. Outcome of pediatric traumatic brain injury at three years: A cohort study. Arch Phys Med Rehabil 1994;75:733–741.

46. Fontaine A, Bazin B, Mangin J-F, et al. Metabolic correlates of poor outcome in severe closed head injury: A high resolution FDG-PET study. Neurology 1994;44(Suppl 2):A175.

47. Foy P. Do prophylactic anticonvulsant drugs alter the pattern of seizures after craniotomy? J Neurol Neurosurg Psychiatry 1992;55:753–757.

48. Frackowiak R. Functional mapping of verbal memory and language. Trends Neurosci 1994; 17:109–115.

49. Freeman E. Coma arousal therapy. Clinical Rehabilitation 1991;5:241–249.

50. Geerts W, Code K, Jay R, et al. A prospective study of venous thromboembolism after major trauma. N Engl J Med 1994;331:1601–1606.

51. Gennarelli T, Thibault L, Adams J. Diffuse axonal injury and traumatic coma in the primate. Ann Neurol 1982;12:564–574.

52. Gianutsos R. Cognitive rehabilitation: A neuropsychological specialty comes of age. Brain Inj 1991;5:353–368.

53. Glisky E. Computer-assisted instruction for patients with traumatic brain injury: Teaching of domain-specific knowledge. Journal of Head Trauma Rehabilitation 1992;7:1–12.

54. Glisky E, Schacter D. Extending the limits of complex learning in organic amnesia: Computer training in a vocational domain. Neuropsychologia 1989;27:107–120.

55. Goldstein F, Levin H. Neurobehavioral outcome of traumatic brain injury in older adults: Initial findings. Journal of Head Trauma Rehabilitation 1995;10:57–73.

56. Goodall P, Lawyer H, Wehman P. Vocational rehabilitation and traumatic brain injury: A legislative and public policy perspective. Journal of Head Trauma Rehabilitation 1994;9:61–81.

57. Gordon W, Hibbard M, Kreutzer J. Cognitive remediation: Issues in research and practice. Journal of Head Trauma Rehabilitation 1989;4:76–84.

58. Grafman J, Salazar A. Methodological considerations relevant to the comparison of recovery

from penetrating and closed head injuries. In: Levin H, Grafman J, Eisenberg H, eds: Neurobehavioral Recovery from Head Injury. New York: Oxford University Press, 1987:43–54.

59. Grafman J, Salazar A, Weingartner H, et al. The relationship of brain-tissue loss volume and lesion location to cognitive deficit. J Neurosci 1986; 6:301–307.

60. Grafman J, Vance S, Weingartner H, et al. The effects of lateralized frontal lesions on mood regulation. Brain 1986;109:1127–1148.

61. Granger C, Hamilton B. The Uniform Data System for Medical Rehabilitation report of first admissions for 1992. Am J Phys Med Rehabil 1994; 73:51–55.

62. Graves A, White E, Koepsell T, et al. The association between head trauma and Alzheimer's disease. Am J Epidemiol 1990;131:491–501.

63. Gray J, Robertson I, Pentland B, et al. Microcomputer-based attentional retraining after brain damage: A randomised group controlled trial. Neuropsychol Rehabil 1992;2:97–115.

64. Gray J, Shepherd M, McKinlay W, et al. Negative symptoms in the traumatically brain-injured during the first year postdischarge. Clinical Rehabilitation 1994;8:188–197.

65. Gronwall D. Paced auditory serial-addition task: A measure of recovery from concussion. Percept Mot Skills 1977;44:367–373.

66. Gualtieri C, Evans R. Stimulant treatment for the neurobehavioral sequelae of traumatic brain injury. Brain Inj 1988;2:273–290.

67. Gualtieri T, Chandler M, Coons T, et al. Amantadine: A new clinical profile for traumatic brain injury. Neuropharmacology 1989;12:258–270.

68. Gualtieri T, Cox D. The delayed neurobehavioral sequelae of traumatic brain injury. Brain Inj 1991; 5:219–232.

69. Gudeman S, Kishore P, Becker D, et al. Computed tomography in the evaluation of incidence and significance of post-trauma hydrocephalus. Radiology 1981;141:397–402.

70. Haffey W. The assessment of clinical competency to consent to medical rehabilitative interventions. Journal of Head Trauma Rehabilitation 1989; 4:43–56.

71. Hagen C, Malkmus D, Durham P. Levels of Cognitive Functioning. Downey, CA: Rancho Los Amigos Hospital, 1972.

72. Hall K, Cope D. The benefit of rehabilitation in traumatic brain injury: A literature review. Journal of Head Trauma Rehabilitation 1995;10:1–13.

73. Hall K, Cope D, Rappaport M. Glascow Outcome Scale and Disability Rating Scale: Comparative usefulness in following recovery in traumatic brain injury. Arch Phys Med Rehabil 1985;66:35–37.

74. Hall K, Hamilton B, Gordon W, et al. Characteristics and comparisons of functional assessment indices: Disability Rating Scale, Functional Independence Measure, and Functional Assessment Measure. Journal of Head Trauma Rehabilitation 1993;8:60–74.

75. Hall K, Johnston M. Measurement tools for a nationwide data system. Arch Phys Med Rehabil 1994;75(Suppl 12):SC10–SC18.

76. Hayden M, Hart T. Rehabilitation of cognitive and behavioral dysfunction in head injury. Adv Psychosom Med 1986;16:194–229.

77. Haynes M. Nutrition in the severely head-injured patient. Clinical Rehabilitation 1992;6:153–158.

78. Heinemann A, Sahgal V, Cichowski K, et al. Functional outcome following traumatic brain injury rehabilitation. Journal of Neurologic Rehabilitation 1990;4:27–37.

79. Heiss W-D, Pawlik G, Holthoff V, et al. PET correlates of normal and impaired memory functions. Cerebrovasc Brain Metab Rev 1992;4:1–27.

80. High W, Boake C, Lehmkuhl L. Critical analysis of studies evaluating the effectiveness of rehabilitation after traumatic brain injury. Journal of Head Trauma Rehabilitation 1995;10:14–26.

81. Horn L, Garland D. Medical and orthopedic complications associated with traumatic brain injury. In: Rosenthal M, Griffith E, Bond M, et al, eds: Rehabilitation of the Adult and Child with Traumatic Brain Injury. Philadelphia: FA Davis, 1990:107–126.

82. Hosobuchi Y, Yingling C. The treatment of prolonged coma with neurostimulation. In: Devinsky O, Beric A, Dogali M, eds: Electrical and Magnetic Stimulation of the Brain and Spinal Cord. New York: Raven Press, 1993.

83. Jaffe K, Polissar N, Fay G, et al. Recovery trends over three years following pediatric traumatic brain injury. Arch Phys Med Rehabil 1995;76:17–26.

84. Jane J, Torner J, Young W. NIH CNS Trauma Status Report 1991. J Neurotrauma 1992;9(Suppl 1):S1–S416.

85. Jennett B, Bond M. Assessment of outcome after severe head injury: A practical scale. Lancet 1975;1:480–484.

86. Jennett B, Teasdale G. Aspects of coma after severe head injury. Lancet 1977;1:876–881.

87. Jennett B, Teasdale G, Braakman R, et al. Prognosis in a series of patients with severe head injury. Neurosurgery 1979;4:283–289.

88. Johnston M. Outcomes of community reentry programmes for brain injury survivors. Brain Inj 1991;5:141–168.

89. Jorje R, Robinson R, Arndt S, et al. Comparison between acute and delayed onset depression following traumatic brain injury. J Neuropsychiatry Clin Neurosci 1993;5:43–49.

90. Kalisky A. Medical problems encountered during rehabilitation of patients with head injury. Arch Phys Med Rehabil 1985;66:25–29.

91. Katz D. Movement disorders following traumatic head injury. Journal of Head Trauma Rehabilitation 1990;5:86–90.

92. Katz D. Neuropathology and neurobehavioral recovery from closed head injury. Journal of Head Trauma Rehabilitation 1992;7:1–15.

93. Katz D, Alexander M. Traumatic brain injury: Predicting course of recovery and outcome for patients admitted to rehabilitation. Arch Neurol 1994;51:661–670.

94. Katz D, Kehs G, Alexander M. Prognosis and recovery from traumatic head injury: The influence of advancing age. Neurology 1990;40(Suppl 1):276.

94a. Kelly D, Bergsneider M, Shalmon E, et al. Following TBI, long-term neuropsychologic deficits are associated with regionally specific local depression of cerebral glucose utilization. J Neurotrauma 1995;12:370.

95. Kirsch N, Levine S. Technology and head injury rehabilitation. Journal of Head Trauma Rehabilitation 1992;7:1–80.

96. Kirsch N, Levine S, Lajiness-O'Neill R, et al. Computer-assisted interactive task guidance: Facilitating the performance of a simulated vocational task. Journal of Head Trauma Rehabilitation 1992;7:13–25.

97. Klonoff H, Clark C, Klonoff P. Long-term outcome of head injuries: A 23 year follow up study of children with head injuries. J Neurol Neurosurg Psychiatry 1993;56:410–415.

98. Knowlton B, Squire L. The learning of categories: Parallel brain systems for item memory and category knowledge. Science 1993;262:1747–1749.

99. Koller W, Wong G, Lang A. Posttraumatic movement disorders: A review. Mov Disord 1989;4:20–36.

100. Kornblum R, Fisher R. Pituitary lesions in craniocerebral injuries. Arch Pathol 1969;88:242–248.

101. Kraus J, Black M, Hessol N, et al. The incidence of acute brain injury and serious impairment in a defined population. Am J Epidemiol 1984;119:186–201.

102. Lal S, Merbitz C, Grip J. Modification of function in head-injured patients with Sinemet. Brain Inj 1988;2:225–233.

103. Lash M, Scarpino C. School reintegration for children with traumatic brain injuries. NeuroRehabilitation 1993;3:13–25.

104. Lee M, Rinne J, Marsden C, et al. Dystonia after head trauma. Neurology 1994;44:1374–1378.

105. Levin H. Neurobehavioral recovery. J Neurotrauma 1992;9(Suppl 1):S359–S373.

106. Levin H, Eisenberg H, Wigg N, et al. Memory and intellectual ability after head injury in children and adolescents. Neurosurgery 1982;11:668–673.

107. Levin H, Gary H, Eisenberg H, et al. Neurobehavioral outcome one year after severe head injury: Experience of the Traumatic Coma Data Bank. J Neurosurg 1990;73:699–709.

108. Levin H, Goldstein F, High W, et al. Disproportionately severe memory deficit in relation to normal intellectual functioning after closed head injury. J Neurol Neurosurg Psychiatry 1988;51:1294–1301.

109. Levin H, Hamilton W, Grossman R. Outcome after head injury. In: Braakman R, ed: Handbook of Clinical Neurology. Amsterdam: Elsevier, 1990:367–395.

110. Levin H, High W, Eisenberg H. Learning and forgetting during post-traumatic amnesia in head injured patients. J Neurol Neurosurg Psychiatry 1988;51:14–20.

111. Levin H, High W, Goethe K, et al. The neurobehavioral rating scale: Assessment of the behavioural sequelae of head injury by the clinician. J Neurol Neurosurg Psychiatry 1987;50:183–193.

112. Levin H, Mattis S, Ruff R, et al. Neurobehavioral outcome following minor head injury: A three center study. J Neurosurg 1987;66:234–243.

113. Levin H, Meyers C, Grossman R, et al. Ventricular enlargement after closed head injury. Arch Neurol 1981;38:623–629.

114. Levin H, Williams D, Crofford M, et al. Relationship of depth of brain lesions to consciousness and outcome after closed head injury. J Neurosurg 1988;69:861–866.

115. Levin H, Williams D, Eisenberg H. Treatment of postconcussional symptoms with CDP-choline. Neurology 1990;40(Suppl 1):326.

116. Levin H, Williams D, Valastro M, et al. Corpus callosum atrophy following closed head injury: Detection with magnetic resonance imaging. J Neurosurg 1990;73:77–81.

117. Levy D, Carona J, Singer B, et al. Predicting outcome from hypoxic-ischemic coma. JAMA 1985; 253:1420–1426.

118. Lobato R, Cordobes F, Rivas J, et al. Outcome from severe head injury related to the type of intracranial lesion: A computed tomography study. J Neurosurg 1983;59:762–774.

119. Luerssen T, Klauber M, Marshall L. Outcome from head injury related to patient's age: A longitudinal prospective study. J Neurosurg 1988; 68:409–416.

120. Luria A, Naydin V, Tsvetkova L, et al. Restoration of higher cortical function following local brain damage. In: Vinken P, Bruyn G, eds: Handbook of Clinical Neurology: Disorders of Higher Nervous Activity. Amsterdam: North-Holland Publishers, 1969:368–433.

121. Macciocchi S. Neuropsychological assessment following head trauma using the Halstead-Reitan Neuropsychological Battery. Journal of Head Trauma Rehabilitation 1988;3:1–11.

122. Mackay L, Bernstein B, Chapman P, et al. Early intervention in severe head injury: Long-term benefits of a formalized program. Arch Phys Med Rehabil 1992;73:635–641.

123. MacKenzie E, Shapiro S, Siegel J. The economic impact of traumatic injuries. JAMA 1988; 260:3290–3296.

124. Maila K, Torode S, Powell G. Insight and progress in rehabilitation after brain injury. Clinical Rehabilitation 1993;7:23–29.

125. Malec J, Thompson J. Relationship of the Mayo-Portland Adaptability Inventory to functional outcome and cognitive performance measures. J Head Trauma Rehabil 1994;9:1–15.

126. Malec J, Zweber B, Depompolo R. The Rivermead Behavioral Memory Test, laboratory neurocognitive measures, and everyday functioning. J Head Trauma Rehabil 1990;5:60–68.

127. Mandelberg I. Cognitive recovery after severe head injury. J Neurol Neurosurg Psychiatry 1976; 39:1001–1007.

128. Marion D, Darby J, Yonas H. Acute regional cerebral blood flow changes caused by severe head injuries. J Neurosurg 1991;74:407–414.

129. Marshall L, Gautille T, Klauber M, et al. The outcome of severe closed head injury. J Neurosurg 1991;75:S28–S36.

130. Marsolek C, Kosslyn S, Squire L. Form-specific visual priming in the right hemisphere. J Exp Psychol 1992;18:492–508.

131. Max W, MacKenzie E, Rice D. Head injuries: Costs and consequences. J Head Trauma Rehabil 1991;6:76–91.

132. Mazzucchi A, Cattelani R, Misale G, et al. Head-injured subjects over age 50 years: Correlations between variables of trauma and neuropsychological follow-up. J Neurol 1992;239:256–260.

133. McDonald C, Jaffe K, Fay G, et al. Comparison of indices of traumatic brain injury severity as predictors of neurobehavioral outcome in children. Arch Phys Med Rehabil 1994;75:328–337.

134. McLean A, Cardenas D, Burgess D, et al. Placebo-controlled study of pramiracetam in young males with memory and cognitive problems resulting from head injury and anoxia. Brain Inj 1991; 5:375–380.

135. McLean A, Dikmen S, Temkin N. Psychosocial recovery after head injury. Arch Phys Med Rehabil 1993;74:1041–1046.

136. McMillan T, Greenwood R. Models of rehabilitation programmes for the brain-injured adult. Clin Rehabil 1993;7:346–355.

137. Mesulam M-M. Large-scale neurocognitive networks and distributed processing for attention, language, and memory. Ann Neurol 1990; 28:597–613.

138. Miller B, Cummings J, McIntyre H, et al. Hypersexuality or altered sexual preference following brain injury. J Neurol Neurosurg Psychiatry 1986; 49:867–873.

139. Miller E, Li L, Desimone R. A neural mechanism for working and recognition memory in inferior temporal cortex. Science 1991;254:1377–1379.

140. Miller J. Head injury. J Neurol Neurosurg Psychiatry 1993;56:440–447.

141. Mitchell S, Bradley V, Welch J, et al. Coma arousal procedure: A therapeutic intervention in the treatment of head injury. Brain Inj 1990;4:273–279.

142. Multi-Society Task Force on PVS. Medical aspects of the persistent vegetative state (second of two parts). N Engl J Med 1994;330:1572–1579.

143. Murdock M, Waxman K. Helmet use improves outcomes after motorcycle accidents. West J Med 1991;155:370–372.

144. Musen G, Squire L. Nonverbal priming in amnesia. Memory Cognition 1992;20:441–448.

145. Namerow N. Cognitive and behavioral aspects of brain-injury rehabilitation. Neurol Clin 1987; 5:569–583.

146. National Head Injury Foundation. National Directory of Head Injury Services. Southborough, MA: National Head Injury Foundation, 1992.

147. Nissen M, Knopman D, Schacter D. Neurochemical dissociation of memory systems. Neurology 1987;37:789–794.

148. O'Carroll R, Woodrow J, Maroun F. Psychosexual and psychosocial sequelae of closed head injury. Brain Inj 1991;5:303–313.

149. Oder W, Goldenberg G, Spatt J, et al. Behavioural and psychological sequelae of severe closed head injury and regional cerebral blood flow: A SPECT study. J Neurol Neurosurg Psychiatry 1992; 55:475–480.

150. Offner P. The impact of motorcycle helmet use. J Trauma 1992;32:636–642.

151. O'Shanick G. Cognitive function after brain in-

jury: Pharmacologic interference and facilitation. NeuroRehabilitation 1991;1:44–49.

152. Ott L, McClain C, Gillespie M, et al. Cytokines and metabolic dysfunction after severe head injury. J Neurotrauma 1994;11:447–472.

153. Pang D, Altschuler E. Low-pressure hydrocephalic state and viscoelastic alterations in the brain. Neurosurgery 1994;35:643–656.

154. Parente R. Effect of monetary incentives on performance after traumatic brain injury. Neuro-Rehabilitation 1994;4:198–203.

155. Parente R, Twum M, Zoltan B. Transfer and generalization of cognitive skill after traumatic brain injury. NeuroRehabilitation 1994;4:25–35.

156. Pettus E, Christman C, Giebel M, et al. Traumatically induced altered membrane permeability: Its relationship to traumatically induced reactive axonal change. J Neurotrauma 1994;11:507–522.

157. Polster M, Nadel L, Schacter D. Cognitive neuroscience analyses of memory: An historical perspective. Journal of Cognitive Neuroscience 1991; 3:95–116.

158. Ponsford J, Kinsella G. Evaluation of a remedial programme for attentional deficits following closed head injury. J Clin Exp Neuropsychol 1988;10:693–708.

159. Posmantur R, Hayes R, Dixon C, et al. Neurofilament 68 and neurofilament 200 protein levels decrease after traumatic brain injury. J Neurotrauma 1994;11:533–545.

160. Povlishock J. Traumatically induced axonal injury: Pathogenesis and pathobiological implications. Brain Pathol 1992;2:1–12.

161. Press G, Amaral D, Square L. Hippocampal abnormalities in amnesic patients revealed by high-resolution magnetic resonance imaging. Nature 1989;341:54–57.

162. Prevey M, Delaney R, De I'Aune W, et al. A method of assessing the efficacy of memory rehabilitation techniques using a "real-world" task. J Rehabil Res 1991;28:53–60.

163. Price L, Heninger G. Lithium in the treatment of mood disorders. N Engl J Med 1994;331:591–598.

164. Prigatano G. Neuropsychological Rehabilitation after Brain Injury. Baltimore: Johns Hopkins University Press, 1986.

165. Prigatano G. Disordered mind, wounded soul: The emerging role of psychotherapy in rehabilitation after brain injury. J Head Trauma Rehabil 1991;6:1–10.

166. Prigatano G, Fordyce D, Zeiner H, et al. Neuropsychological rehabilitation after closed head injury in young adults. J Neurol Neurosurg Psychiatry 1984;47:505–513.

167. Radanov B, Stefano G, Schnidrig A, et al. Cognitive functioning after common whiplash. Arch Neurol 1993;50:87–91.

168. Radar M, Alston J. Sensory stimulation of severely brain-injured patients. Brain Inj 1989;3:141–148.

169. Rao N, Kilgore K. Predicting return to work in traumatic brain injury using assessment scales. Arch Phys Med Rehabil 1992;73:911–916.

170. Rappaport M, Dougherty A, Kelting D. Evaluation of coma and vegetative states. Arch Phys Med Rehabil 1992;73:628–634.

171. Rappaport M, Herrero-Backe C, Rappaport M, et

172. Rattok J, Ben-Yishay Y, Ezrachi O, et al. Outcomes of different treatment mixes in a multidimensional neuropsychological rehabilitation program. Neuropsychology 1992;6:395–415.

173. Reider-Groswasser I, Cohen M, Costeff H, et al. Late CT findings in brain trauma: Relationship to cognitive and behavioral sequelae and to vocational outcome. AJR Am J Roentgenol 1993; 160:147–152.

174. Richardson J. Imagery mnemonics and memory remediation. Neurology 1992;42:283–286.

175. Rivara F, Dicker B, Bregman A, et al. The public cost of motorcycle trauma. JAMA 1988;260:221–223.

176. Rivara J, Jaffe K, Polissar N, et al. Family functioning and children's academic performance and behavior problems in the year following traumatic brain injury. Arch Phys Med Rehabil 1994; 75:369–379.

177. Robertson C, Contant C, Narayan R, et al. Cerebral blood flow, AVDO$_2$, and neurologic outcome in head-injured patients. J Neurotrauma 1992; 9(Suppl 1):S349–S358.

178. Roine R, Kajaste S, Kaste M. Neuropsychological sequelae of cardiac arrest. JAMA 1993;269:237–242.

179. Rubin R, Gold W, Kelley D, et al. The Cost of Disorders of the Brain. Washington, DC: National Foundation for Brain Research, 1992.

180. Ruff R, Niemann H. Cognitive rehabilitation versus day treatment in head-injured adults: Is there an impact on emotional and psychosocial adjustment? Brain Inj 1990;4:339–347.

181. Salazar A, Jabbari B, Vance S, et al. Epilepsy after penetrating head injury: Clinical correlates. Neurology 1985;35:1406–1414.

182. Schacter D, Cooper L, Tharan M, et al. Preserved priming of novel objects in patients with memory disorders. Journal of Cognitive Neuroscience 1991;3:117–130.

183. Schwab K, Grafman J, Salazar A, et al. Residual impairments and work status after penetrating head injury. Neurology 1993;43:95–105.

184. Shallice T, Burgess P. Deficits in strategy application following frontal lobe damage in man. Brain 1991;114:727–741.

185. Smith D, Mattson R, Cramer J, et al. Results of a nationwide Veterans Administration Cooperative Study comparing the efficacy and toxicity of carbamazepine, phenobabital, phenytoin and primidone. Epilepsia 1987;28(Suppl):S50–S58.

186. Smith K, Goulding P, Wilderman D, et al. Neurobehavioral effects of phenytoin and carbamazepine in patients recovering from brain trauma. Arch Neurol 1994;51:653–660.

187. Sobus K, Alexander M, Harcke H. Undetected musculoskeletal trauma in children with TBI or spinal cord injury. Arch Phys Med Rehabil 1993; 74:902–904.

188. Sohlberg M, Mateer C. Attention Process Training. Puyallup, WA: Association for Neuropsychological Research and Development, 1986.

189. Sohlberg M, Mateer C. Prospective Memory Process Training. Puyallup, WA: Association for Neu-

ropsychological Research and Development, 1986.

190. Sohlberg M, Mateer C. Effectiveness of an attention training program. Journal of Clinical Experimental Psychology 1987;9:117–130.

191. Sohlberg M, Mateer C. Introduction to Cognitive Rehabilitation. New York: Guilford Press, 1989: 414.

192. Sonesson B, Ljunggren B, Saveland H, et al. Cognition and adjustment after late and early operation for ruptured aneurysm. Neurosurgery 1987; 21:279–287.

193. Sorenson S, Kraus J. Occurrence, severity, and outcomes of brain injury. Journal of Head Trauma Rehabilitation 1991;6:1–10.

194. Squire L. Mechanisms of memory. Science 1986; 232:1612–1619.

195. Squire L, Ojemann J, Mezin F, et al. Activation of the hippocampus in normal humans: A functional anatomical study of memory. Proc Natl Acad Sci USA 1992;89:1837–1841.

196. Squire L, Zola-Morgan S. Memory: Brain systems and behavior. Trends Neurosci 1988; 11:170–175.

197. Stuss D, Buckle L. Traumatic brain injury: Neuropsychological deficits and evaluation at different stages of recovery and in different pathologic subtypes. Journal of Head Trauma Rehabilitation 1992;7:40–49.

198. Stuss D, Ely P, Hugenholtz H. Subtle neuropsychological deficits in patients with good recovery after closed head injury. Neurosurgery 1985; 17:41–47.

199. Teasdale G, Teasdale E, Hadley D. Computed tomographic and magnetic resonance imaging classification of head injury. J Neurotrauma 1992; 9(Suppl 1):249–257.

200. Temkin N, Dikmen S, Wilensky A, et al. A randomized, double-blind study of phenytoin for the prevention of post-traumatic seizures. N Engl J Med 1990;323:497–502.

201. Thomas-Stonell N, Johnson P, Schuller R, et al. Evaluation of a computer-based program for remediation of cognitive-communication skills. Journal of Head Trauma Rehabilitation 1994; 9:25–37.

202. Tulving E, Schacter D. Priming and human memory systems. Science 1990;247:301–306.

203. Uzzell B, Dolinskas C, Wiser R, et al. Influence of lesions detected by computed tomography on outcome and neuropsychological recovery after severe head injury. Neurosurgery 1987;20:396–402.

204. Uzzell B, Obrist W, Dolinskas C, et al. Relationship of acute CBF and ICP findings to neuropsychological outcome in severe head injury. J Neurosurg 1986;65:630–635.

205. Vanneste J. Three decades of normal pressure hydrocephalus: Are we wiser now? J Neurol Neurosurg Psychiatry 1994;57:1021–1025.

206. Van Zomeran A, Saan R. Psychological and social consequences of severe head injury. In: Braakman R, ed: Handbook of Clinical Neurology: Head Injury. Amsterdam: Elsevier, 1990.

207. Vermeij F, Hasan D, Vermeulen M, et al. Predictive factors for deterioration from hydrocephalus after subarachnoid hemorrhage. Neurology 1994;44:1851–1855.

208. Volpe B, McDowell F. The efficacy of cognitive rehabilitation in patients with traumatic brain injury. Arch Neurol 1990;47:220–222.

209. Von Cramon D, von Cramon G, Mai N. Problem-solving deficits in brain-injured patients: A therapeutic approach. Neuropsychological Rehabilitation 1991;1:45–64.

210. Wehman P, Sherron P, Kregel J, et al. Return to work for persons following severe traumatic brain injury. Am J Phys Med Rehabil 1993;72:355–363.

211. Whetsell K, Patterson C, Young D, et al. Preinjury psychopathology in trauma patients. J Trauma 1989;29:422–428.

212. White R, Likavec M. The diagnosis and initial management of head injury. N Engl J Med 1992; 327:1507–1511.

213. Williams D, Levin H, Eisenberg H. Mild head injury classification. Neurosurgery 1990;27:422–428.

214. Wilson B. Recovery and compensatory strategies in head injured memory impaired people several years after insult. J Neurol Neurosurg Psychiatry 1992;55:177–180.

215. Wilson B, Patterson K. Rehabilitation and cognitive neuropsychology. Applied Cognitive Psychology 1990;4:247–260.

215a. Wilson BA, Baddeley A, Evans J, et al. Errorless learning in the rehabilitation of memory impaired people. Neuropsychological Rehabilitation 1994;4:307–326.

216. Wilson F, Schalaidhe S, Goldman-Rakic P. Dissociation of object and spatial processing domains in primate prefrontal cortex. Science 1994; 260:1955–1958.

217. Wilson J, Wiedmann K, Hadley D, et al. Early and late magnetic resonance imaging and neuropsychological outcome after head injury. J Neurol Neurosurg Psychiatry 1988;51:391–396.

218. Wilson J, Wyper D. Neuroimaging and neuropsychological functioning following closed head injury: CT, MRI, and SPECT. Journal of Head Trauma Rehabilitation 1992;7:29–39.

219. Wolman R, Cornall C, Fulcher K, et al. Aerobic training in brain-injured patients. Clinical Rehabilitation 1994;8:253–257.

220. Wroblewski B, Glenn M. Pharmacological treatment of arousal and cognitive deficits. Journal of Head Trauma Rehabilitation 1994;9:19–42.

221. Ylvisaker M, Hartwick P, Stevens M. School reentry following head injury: Managing the transition from hospital to school. Journal of Head Trauma Rehabilitation 1991;6:10–22.

222. Young B, Ott L, Yingling B, et al. Nutrition and brain injury. Journal of Neurotrauma 1992; 9(Suppl 1):S375–S383.

223. Zasler N, Horn L. Rehabilitative management of sexual dysfunction. Journal of Head Trauma Rehabilitation 1990;5:14–24.

224. Zasler N, Kreutzer J, Taylor D. Coma stimulation and coma recovery. NeuroRehabilitation 1991; 1:33–40.

225. Zola-Morgan S, Squire L. Neuroanatomy of memory. Annual Review of Neuroscience 1993; 16:547–563.

CHAPTER 10

OTHER NEUROLOGIC DISORDERS

The rehabilitation team has opportunities to enhance the function of patients stricken with other monophasic illnesses, such as acute inflammatory polyradiculoneuropathy, as well as progressive, fluctuating, or chronic diseases, such as Duchenne muscular dystrophy (DMD) and multiple sclerosis (MS). Ideally, a rehabilitation life-management plan can be developed for patients whose course is not static. As impairments and disabilities increase, patients and families need disease-related and disability-related information, assistive devices, counseling, and advice for caregivers. Home and workplace needs can be anticipated within the goals for long-term management of chronic diseases. A brief outpatient effort can provide guidance and interventions to maintain an optimal level of mobility, personal and community activities, nutrition, speech, and respiratory function. A physician and rehabilitation team may manage outpatients individually, in a disease-oriented group, or in a disability-oriented program, such as a comprehensive outpatient rehabilitation facility (CORF) with day care. The approach must offer flexible, coordinated care. Education and problem solving are especially important undertakings. Patients, families, physicians, and therapists all help to identify realistic short-term goals that are important to patients and caregivers, decide on a treatment plan, and monitor functional outcomes. Inpatient therapy can help return home the patient with MS who suffers an exacerbation or the patient with Parkinson's disease whose mobility deteriorates during an intercurrent illness. Disease-specific, philanthropic, and government-affiliated regional and national organizations

299

provide educational materials, Internet mailboxes, and newsletters with updates on medical advances. Some organizations, such as the Muscular Dystrophy Association, offer clinics, supportive services for equipment, and therapies. Members of the rehabilitation team often join or initiate support groups that offer activities to improve fitness, psychosocial interactions, and quality of life.

This chapter supplements earlier chapters as it touches on rehabilitative practices for disabilities not yet discussed that are common to certain neurologic disorders. Very few controlled trials of a rehabilitative intervention have been undertaken. Despite this shortcoming, neurorehabilitation specialists should participate in the design of clinical trials of drug and implant interventions to ensure that optimal functional outcome measures and general disability management are provided to the study.

NEUROPATHIC PAIN

Pain has been defined by the International Association for the Study of Pain as the subjective "unpleasant sensory and emotional experience associated with actual or potential tissue damage or described in terms of such damage."[112] Neurorehabilitation specialists often participate in the diagnosis and management of painful conditions, as well as in related basic and clinical research. Mechanisms of acute and chronic pain are becoming better understood, particularly regarding modulation of neural plasticity. Culture, motivation, cognition, mood, and other factors unrelated to injury affect experience and communication about nociception. Pain also has direct and indirect effects on physical and psychosocial functioning. Thus, success in pain intervention often requires personnel from multiple disciplines working as a rehabilitation team. A brief chapter section cannot extend far past the "Imaginot Line" that bounds the intellectual property of neurologic rehabilitation related to pain. We can review some of the biologic mechanisms that reveal the neurophysiologic plasticity associated with chronic neurogenic pain and the assess-ments and therapeutic approaches used by the rehabilitation team.

Mechanisms of Central and Peripheral Pain

The ascending and descending components of the pain transmission and the modulation systems are complex in their connectivity, parallel pathways, use of neurotransmitters and peptides, and functional and structural plasticity.[181] Within these systems, rehabilitation specialists can find some solid and many indirect rationales for physical, pharmacologic, and surgical interventions for neuropathic pain.

Acute nociceptive pain most often begins with the release of algesiogenic and inflammatory substances by injured tissue. Prostaglandins, substance P, bradykinin, catecholamines, leukotrienes, and other purines and indoleamines activate nociceptors and sensitize them to synthesized and released substances. Therapies are aimed at the injured tissue and at dorsal horn, opiate receptor, and other spinal and more central sites. Physical modalities such as cold and massage can reduce some sources of tissue pain. The nonsteroidal anti-inflammatory drugs (NSAIDs) attenuate pain by inhibiting cyclooxygenase, which decreases production of the prostanoids that facilitate pain activity in C-fiber afferents. The NSAIDs also appear to have a central effect in inhibiting nociceptive processing in the spinal cord and brain.[100] Thus, inflammation itself need not exist for these drugs to have an effect on nociception. Opioids also have a peripheral effect, perhaps by blocking the release of substance P in tissue, as they do within the spinal cord.[162] The sites of action of most drugs for pain are likely to be at multiple levels.

Neuropathic pain commands more attention for neurorehabilitation. Chronic neuropathic pain is a maladaptive modification. In many instances, it develops from the activation of low-threshold mechanoreceptive fibers whose ordinarily innocuous sensations come to be processed abnormally in a spinal somatosensory system that has developed increased excitability, decreased inhibition, and structural reorganization.[189]

Pain can arise from primary afferents in peripheral nerves and in dorsal and ventral roots with, for example, diabetic neuropathy or root compression by vertebral disk protrusion. These afferent fibers release excitatory amino acids, particularly aspartate and glutamate, and a variety of neuropeptides, endogenous opioids, and substance P. Within the layers of the dorsal horn, inhibitory amino acids such as glycine and γ-aminobutyric acid (GABA), monoamine neurotransmitters including histamine, serotonin, norepinephrine, and dopamine, and other peptides, especially opioids, become involved in the first spinal stage of pain transmission. Descending pathways contribute the nociceptive inhibitory monoamines that modulate pain signals in direct and indirect ways. These pathways arise from the cortex, hypothalamus, and thalamus, projecting to the periaqueductal gray (PAG) of the midbrain, and descend from the PAG and reticular formation. Within the dorsal horn, nociceptive-specific neurons encode information about the location and nature of the pain stimulus.[42] Neurons with wide dynamic range encode intensity, but they are also inhibited by surrounding receptive fields for inputs that are not noxious. This differentiation contributes to a separation in the ascending circuits for discriminative pain and for the affective-motivational aspects of pain.[42]

Potentially long-standing changes in the spinal cord are brought about by the activation of N-methyl-D-aspartate (NMDA) receptors, second-messenger protein kinases, and oncogenes that direct protein metabolism. Moreover, pain inputs at one dermatome can spread to other dorsal spinal segments and can thereby produce widespread painful sensations. This plasticity leads to changes in the spinothalamic and spinoreticular inputs and representational maps for pain within the somatotopically organized thalamus. For example, repeated pain signals sensitize spinal neurons to future signals, in part by their effects on the NMDA receptor. The pain response is enhanced. Pain signals then may fail to trigger the GABA-producing neurons in the thalamus that ordinarily mute incoming pain sensation.[13] Changes in responsiveness of pronociceptive projecting neurons that lead to the thalamus can subsequently

Table 10–1. PREVALENCE OF CENTRAL PAIN

Disorder	Percentage (%)
Stroke	5
Parkinson's disease	10
Multiple sclerosis	20
Spinal cord injury	30

Source: Data from Casey K.[33]

cause pain independent of afferent input or of inputs previously unassociated with pain.[109]

With such changes in just this one modulation system, intrinsically generated and other sensory inputs such as touch are allowed to reach the cortex, interpreted as nociceptive signals. The results are as follows: allodynia, a low pain threshold; hyperalgesia, an increased response to a painful stimulus; and hyperpathia, a greater reaction especially to a repetitive stimulus. Dysesthetic thalamic pain can also arise from damage to the pain and temperature representations in the ventral part of the ventral medial nucleus of the thalamus.[41] Cell loss in this area appears to disinhibit specific spinothalamic signals that reach the anterior cingulate by a neighboring thalamic nucleus. Thus, within the spinal cord, the thalamus, and the thalamocortical projections to the somatosensory and anterior cingulate cortex,[141] pronociceptive and antinociceptive plasticity is found. These changes presumably account for peripheral neurogenic pain and the common syndrome of central pain that develops within a variety of neurologic diseases (Table 10–1).

Management of Neurogenic Pain

Pain can be managed with medications, physical therapies and modalities, behavioral interventions and counseling, and by anesthesia and surgical approaches. The aims are to eliminate pain or at least to make discomfort tolerable and to restore physical and social functioning. People with chronic, debilitating pain are sometimes best managed as inpatients, especially if they need to be withdrawn from high doses of narcotic analgesics and have poor exercise tolerance. Outpatient management programs for chronic pain include a rehabilitation team that can carry out behavioral modification, relaxation, and cognitive, physical, and occupational therapies to increase activity and to reduce pain behaviors, such as anxiety, social withdrawal, sedentary lifestyle, and demands for pain medication. In addition, the team may adjust medications, deal with mood disorders, and provide education. Claims about the efficacy of pain treatments and team management programs that have not been subjected to a clinical trial must be considered in relation to the nonspecific placebo effects provided by the team's interest, attention, and overall approach to the patient.[176] For example, although many drug, biofeedback, and neurostimulation techniques for phantom limb pain seem to work, clinical trials have not revealed a response greater than a placebo effect.[154]

The dimensions of pain that are unique to each individual include quality, intensity, duration, course, personal meaning, and impact on function and roles. The measurement of these dimensions poses challenges. Although some potential physiologic measures are available,[35] subjective personal assessments of pain are used most often. These assessments are supported by scales of motor performance, ADLs, work history, mood, and quality of life. Clinicians most often record the frequency of pain-related behaviors and employ visual analog scales for pain, verbal pain rating scales, the McGill Pain Questionnaire,[111] the Minnesota Multiphasic Personality Inventory, and the Sickness Index Profile (see Chapter 5).

NONANALGESIC MEDICATIONS

Details about the use of medications for pain are readily available.[127] We emphasize the nonanalgesic drugs that act within the inhibitory neurotransmitter mechanisms for pain control just discussed (Table 10–2). These medications can cause central nervous system and systemic side effects that increase if combinations of drugs become necessary. They should be initiated at low doses and gradually increased.

Antidepressants. Norepinephrine has a marked tonic inhibitory effect on nociceptive neurons in the dorsal horn. Indeed, because all of the monoamines released by descending pain pathways inhibit pain, the tricyclic antidepressants that affect norepinephrine and serotonin uptake have been valuable for the treatment of chronic neuropathic pain. These drugs also have local anesthetic effects and potentiate opioid-induced analgesia. Doses are usually much lower than needed for antidepressant therapy. All these agents are worth trying for peripheral and central causes of neuropathic pain. Amitriptyline has been studied the most thoroughly. When this drug is taken about an hour before bedtime, its sedating action becomes useful for patients who sleep poorly. Trazodone can also be sedating. Desipramine tends to have the fewest anticholinergic side effects, so it is better for patients with prostatic hypertrophy that causes outlet obstruction and for patients who dislike a dry mouth. The more selective serotonergic nontricyclic antidepressants tend to have a similar profile for pain relief, are generally less sedating, and can be included among first-line drugs. Placebo-controlled trials have shown the efficacy of these agents in the treatment of tension and migraine headache, diabetic neuropathy,[104] postherpetic neuralgia,[182] and myofascial pain.

Anticonvulsants. Phenytoin and carbamazepine probably act on pain mechanisms by suppressing paroxysmal discharges, by blocking ion channels, by preventing the spread of discharges, and by other commonly invoked anticonvulsant effects. These drugs seem especially effective in reducing the lancinating and dysesthetic pain of trigeminal and glossopharyngeal neuralgia, postherpetic neuralgia, traumatic neuropathies, MS, and spinal cord injury (SCI). Some patients respond to clonazepam or valproate. Several of the newer anticonvulsants that tend to increase GABA availability, such as gabapentin and vigabatrin, may be used following a trial of carbamazepine and valproate or may be used with one of these two agents. Side effects of the anticonvulsants can be limited by building up doses slowly and by keeping blood levels in the usual therapeutic range.

Anesthetics. Local injection of short-act-

Table 10–2. **CLASSES OF MEDICATION FOR NEUROGENIC PAIN**

Class	Possible Mechanisms	Range of Daily Dosage (mg)
Anticonvulsants		
Carbamazepine	Blockade of voltage-dependent sodium channel	400–1600
Phenytoin	Blockade of voltage-dependent sodium channel	200–500
Valproate	Enhancement of GABA; blockade of voltage-dependent sodium channel	500–1500
Vigabatrin	Inhibition of GABA transaminase	500–2000
Antidepressants		
Amitriptyline	Blockade of uptake of norepinephrine, serotonin; anticholinergic effects	10–200
Desipramine	Blockade of uptake of norepinephrine, serotonin	25–200
Fluoxetine	Blockade of uptake of serotonin	10–60
Venlafaxine	Blockade uptake of norepinephrine, serotonin	50–150
Adrenergics		
Clonidine	Alpha-receptor agonist	0.1–0.4
Anesthetics		
Mexiletine	Sodium channel blockade	75–750
Benzodiazepines		
Clonazepam	GABA receptor binding	0.5–10
Calcium channel blockers		
Nifedipine	Inhibition of calcium entry	30–120
GABAergics		
Baclofen	GABA receptor binding	30–120
Nonsteroidal anti-inflammatory drugs	Prostaglandin inhibition; potentiation of opioids	
Opiates	Binding of receptors	

GABA = γ-aminobutyric acid.

ing anesthetic agents such as procaine, with or without a corticosteroid, often helps to relieve painful trigger points, tender areas, and taut bands associated with myofascial pain.[83] As little as 1 mL of 1 percent procaine is injected, enough to eliminate each palpably tender or referred pain area. This drug presumably alters C-fiber activity. Physical therapy should follow. Intravenous administration of local anesthetics and antiarrhythmics can limit chronic peripheral neuropathic pain.[7] These agents are less likely to affect pain caused by a central injury.[69] The analgesic mechanism may be the suppression of ectopic impulse generators in the damaged peripheral nerve. In postherpetic neuralgia, both injection and topical application of lidocaine into the sensitive, painful skin has reduced the pain in some patients, an effect that suggests that the cutaneous terminals play a role.[143] Mexiletine, given orally at up to 750 mg per day, has also shown a benefit in, for example, diabetic neuropathy.[34]

Sympatholytics. Sympathetically maintained pain has been associated with stroke, MS, SCI, radiculopathies, and peripheral neuropathies. Trauma and immobilization are other predisposing causes. Reflex sympathetic dystrophy (RSD) is characterized by poorly localized burning, boring pain, hyperesthesia, and autonomic dysfunction. After a peripheral nerve injury, the syndrome is often called causalgia. Table 10–3 describes the common clinical stages of this disorder. Diagnostic tests include skin plethysmography, skin conductance, thermography, and x-ray studies. The three-phase technetium bone scan has a sensitivity of 45 to 95 percent and a specificity of 85 to 92 percent for RSD.[45] It may also have predictive value about subsequent symptoms in asymptomatic patients with upper extremity sensorimotor loss after stroke.[185]

Successful treatment of RSD by intravenous regional sympathetic blockade with drugs such as reserpine and guanethidine, or with stellate ganglion blockade and surgical sympathectomy, reflects the sense that the pain of RSD is maintained by the sympathetic nervous system. One possible mechanism is that a peripheral nerve injury results in the sprouting of normal postganglionic sympathetic fibers around large, axotomized dorsal root ganglion neurons, which are myelinated, low-threshold mechanoreceptors.[108] Innocuous inputs become noxious. An injury also releases nerve growth factor, which allows the growth of these sympathetic connections in animal models. Nerve growth factor (NGF)–neutralizing compounds are being studied to try to reduce the proliferation and, in turn, to diminish pain.

A sympathetic mechanism for RSD is not necessarily the only mechanism, however. For example, a controlled trial of infusions of a placebo, an agonist (phenylephrine), and an antagonist (phentolamine) to the alpha-1–adrenergic receptor revealed no influence on pain, including neuropathic pain due to polyneuropathy.[179] Other explanations for RSD have been offered. On the painful side of patients with allodynia and hyperhidrosis, norepinephrine levels are lower, suggesting possible supersensitivity to sympathetic neurotransmitters.[52]

Initial therapies for RSD include joint range of motion, reduction of edema with massage and skin compression, graduated exercises, and NSAIDs or corticosteroids such as 20 to 40 mg of prednisone for up to 3 weeks. Beta-blockers, calcium channel blockers, tricyclic antidepressants, anticonvulsants, local anesthetic blockade, and transcutaneous electrical nerve stimulation (TENS) are potential adjunctive treatments. When these treatments fail, a pain-management team may initiate invasive pharmacologic interventions such as intravenous or regional reserpine, hydralazine, bretylium, labetalol, phentolamine, or guanethidine[186] or surgical sympathectomy.

Other Agents. Neuroleptic agents are often tried in patients with otherwise unresponsive central and peripheral pain. The efficacy of these agents is unclear, and side effects inhibit their wide use. Their monoamine blocking effects can alter cortical ap-

Table 10–3. **STAGES OF REFLEX SYMPATHETIC DYSTROPHY**

Stage	Onset and Duration	Clinical Features
Stage I	Develops in first month; lasts 3 to 6 months	Edema, burning, warm and dry or cold and sweaty skin
Stage II	Follows stage 1; lasts 3 to 6 months	Atrophic skin, osteoporosis, spreading pain, joint fibrosis, muscle wasting
Stage III	Duration varies	Resolving pain, contractures, cool skin, atrophy

preciation of pain. The use of clonidine is in part based on its modulation of dorsal horn sensory inputs by an adrenergic effect. Baclofen has GABAergic effects that have been especially useful for neuralgic pain. Intrathecal baclofen (50 to 150 μg) has been reported to rapidly relieve central pain after subcortical and thalamic strokes.[166] Capsaicin cream lessens the pain of postherpetic neuralgia and peripheral neuropathies by depleting substance P. This cream must be applied at least three times a day, and, for best results, the area must be covered by a nonabsorbing material such as plastic wrap.

Oral and epidural corticosteroids can reduce root pain from compressive radiculopathy. Corticosteroids injected into one cervical zygapophyseal joint, however, have not significantly reduced pain compared with bupivacaine in patients with chronic localized cervical pain associated with a whiplash injury.[14] Corticosteroid injections into the lumbar facets have not reduced pain or improved function compared with saline solution in patients with chronic low back pain.[32]

In general, the pharmacotherapy of chronic neuropathic pain is most often initiated with anticonvulsant or antidepressant medications, depending on the anticipated tolerance of side effects, followed by baclofen or by a sympatholytic agent when RSD is diagnosed. The clinician may try two different classes of drugs that act by similar putative mechanisms to amplify their effect or may try bringing several different mechanisms into play (see Table 10–2). Capsaicin for postzoster or diabetic neuropathic pain is a first-line intervention, and mexiletine is for a second-line trial. NSAIDs, aspirin, propoxyphene, and acetaminophen can be tried in concert with any drug trial. When combined with physical therapies, these analgesics will lessen peripheral musculoligamentous and joint sources of pain, which may reduce noxious inputs that help drive central pain mechanisms. Muscle relaxants, benzodiazepines, antihistamines, L-tryptophan to raise serotonin levels, levodopa, calcium channel blockers, alpha-blockers, and beta-blockers can be used as second-line interventions. Doses tend to be equal to or lower than those recommended by the manufacturer. Narcotic analgesia, when practi-

cal, should be limited to nighttime use to aid sleep.

NEUROSTIMULATION

TENS stimulates large nonnociceptive sensory afferents that inhibit nociceptive activity in the dorsal horn. The combination of TENS and vibratory stimulation at 100 Hz, thought to recruit a larger number of large-diameter afferents or to increase their discharge frequency, alleviated pain better than either technique alone or when compared with sham stimulation in one trial.[77] In a study of chronic low back pain, however, TENS was no more effective than a placebo and added no benefit to exercise.[49] TENS has been most useful in treating pain due to musculoskeletal disorders and peripheral nerve damage.[124] Individual patients come to prefer continuous or burst-pulse patterns at a variety of intensities and frequencies.

Dorsal column stimulation has a similar, if more direct, effect on afferents. Stimulation of the PAG also inhibits dorsal horn neurons that have been activated by C fibers. Much of this inhibition involves the release of monoamines and endogenous opiates. Acupuncture with or without electrical stimulation may also release opioids.[46] Invasive, central stimulation techniques carry the risk of infection and displacement of electrodes, seldom work over the long run, and should be considered as a last resort before a central ablation procedure.

PHYSICAL THERAPIES

Common modalities for soft tissue and joint pain include ultrasound, electrical stimulation, heat and cold application, and hydrotherapy. These therapeutic techniques can increase range of motion and tissue mobility.[80] Used alone, they are unlikely to benefit the patient with chronic neuropathic pain. Orthotics and braces can reduce pain associated with, for example, a carpal tunnel syndrome or a lumbar disorder. Cervical and lumbar traction is often tried in patients with cervical and lumbar pain with or without signs of a radiculopathy. Although some systems can greatly reduce intradiskal pressure,[136] whether such treatment results in less dysfunction at a nerve root, relaxes soft tissues and muscle spasm, or, more important, lessens pain is not clear. A randomized trial of traction without any other intervention did not show significant pain reduction or increased cervical range of motion in patients with chronic neck pain.[115] As in other attempts at studying physical interventions, however, the specific details of the treatment and the certainty of the diagnosis can vary within a study and may not be generally applicable. For example, the source of pain, the technique for traction, the amount of weighted traction applied, and the associated therapies administered by the therapist and by the patient at home can play a confounding role in trying to understand what place, if any, the intervention may have.

Hands-on therapies can be of great value in patients with tension headache, myofascial pain, and many of the musculoligamentous causes of neck and back pain. Traditional physical therapies such as muscle stretching and flexibility exercises, traction, deep pressure and massage, strengthening exercises, fitness programs, postural education, and physical modalities are a mainstay of treatment of these conditions. Passive movement techniques that aim for cervical and lumbar joint mobilization to localize and treat pain have been advocated by many schools of physical therapy. These techniques can have a great impact in reducing pain when they are applied with skill.[61,98,99]

Swedish manual therapy and corticosteroid injections were found to improve outcomes, compared with traditional treatment for low back pain.[23] The McKenzie method[51] was superior to back care education in another randomized trial.[161] Chiropractic styles of high-velocity and low- or high-amplitude manipulations also benefit some patients.[94] The effects may be on joint and mechanoreceptors and Golgi tendon and Ia afferents that inhibit pain inputs, but the mechanisms are unclear. Manipulative therapy for chronic neck and back pain appeared better than placebo and routine outpatient management, although not clearly better than physical therapy, in two randomized trials.[88,110]

Myofascial pain is characterized by chronically, palpably painful areas within muscle, fascia, and ligaments. Common sites in patients undergoing neurorehabilitation are the suboccipital musculoligamentous tissues; the upper trapezius, levator scapulae, supraspinatus, paraspinal, and rhomboid muscles; the upper outer buttocks; the area around the sacroiliac joints; and the transverse and interspinous ligaments from C-4 to C-7 and L-3 to S-1. Treatments include injection into tender areas, tissue stretching and manipulation, postural education, exercise conditioning and strengthening, the administration of amitriptyline or other modulators of monoamines and serotonin, the use of muscle relaxants such as cyclobenzaprine, and regimens of medication and psychotherapy for depression.[169,188]

The causes of and therapy for episodic and chronic tension-type headache remain controversial.[102,156] Myofascial and cervical joint and nerve sources have been considered[56] and, perhaps, underappreciated. The loads and electromyographic (EMG) levels induced in cervical and shoulder girdle muscles increase markedly with head-forward postures.[151] These tense postures are common in stressed people. Thus, these muscles and their related structures may be expected to fatigue from overuse and to become a source of pain. Skillful physical therapies similar to those mentioned for neck pain can help many patients. Simple exercises[165] that reduce an exaggerated cervical lordosis and increase cervical flexion and rotation, postural education about positions that increase cervical dysfunction, and passive joint mobilization techniques are often used with success. Improved head and neck positioning was associated with reduced neck pain in one controlled trial.[137] Too often, physical therapy is limited to ultrasound, hot packs, and a little massage, which are unlikely to help the patient with chronic neck and headache pain.

Rehabilitation approaches have also played an important role in managing patients with the multiple causes of acute and chronic low back pain.[48,68] Although diagnostic ambiguity permeates attempts at studying specific interventions, the evidence points to improved outcomes for pain and function with physical therapies. Programs emphasize mobilization; back extension over flexion exercises; stretching of back, hip, and leg soft tissues; strengthening of abdominal, back, and other weak muscles; conditioning; psychologic support; and training in work-related activities with work modifications.[105,114,177,180] Exercise to improve back and abdominal strength and overall conditioning also reduces the risk of developing low back pain.[92]

SURGICAL PROCEDURES

For patients with chronic peripheral nerve and spinal pain, interventions have included anterolateral cordotomy, cordectomy, lesioning of the dorsal root entry zone, various tractotomies, and creation of thalamic and hypothalamic lesions.[149] The value of these interventions is unclear, and the risks of pain, complications of anesthesia, and surgical morbidity are significant. Controlled trials have not been undertaken, even of popular techniques such as microvascular decompression for trigeminal neuralgia.

DISORDERS OF THE MOTOR UNIT

The rehabilitation of patients with diseases of the anterior horn cell, peripheral nerve, neuromuscular junction, and muscle depends especially on the temporal course of the specific illness, the distribution of weakness, and its natural history. Neuromuscular rehabilitation has far more similarities than differences, however, whether the disease primarily affects muscle or nerve.[18,139] Gene therapies, trophic factors, immune therapies, and transplants of, for example, myoblasts have raised the hopes of physicians and patients for cures. In the interim, care aims to prevent complications of immobilization, improve selective muscle strength and limb function, optimize ventilation and oral nutrition, provide orthoses and assistive and communicative devices to make ADLs more independent, manage pain, restore sensation in the case of neuropathies, educate and counsel, and solve problems that limit the patient's independence or add to the burdens of caregivers.

Exercise

Small-group and case studies have shown that selective muscle strengthening and general conditioning can be achieved by modest levels of exercise, almost regardless of the pathophysiology of the neurologic disease.[50] The type, intensity, and duration of a muscle contraction and the frequency and duration of exercise sessions determine whether strength will increase. In healthy persons, strength improves significantly by the combination of isometric resistance against 60 percent of the person's maximum load, 10 repetitions each performed for 5 seconds, and training three times a week for 6 weeks.[24] Strengthening of atrophic muscle has occurred by training with forces of only 20 to 30 percent of the patient's maximum resistance, however. The goal is to recruit a large percentage of the musculature at an intensity that stimulates morphologic, biochemical, and histochemical adaptations. For patients with neurologic diseases, the potential confounding problem is that impaired function along the motor unit can cause rapid fatigue or can interfere with the muscle cell's metabolic and contractile functions.[95]

A program of moderate-resistance exercise starting at 10 to 30 percent of each person's maximum resistance enabled a group of patients with myotonic dystrophy, hereditary sensorimotor neuropathies, spinal muscular atrophy, and limb-girdle syndromes to increase strength for handgrip, knee extension, and elbow flexion.[1] Over 12 weeks, these patients gradually increased the amount of resistance and the number of repetitions during isotonic exercise of one side. At follow-up, both the exercised and unexercised homologous muscles had improved, up to 20 percent for the knee extensors. Gains have been the same in healthy control subjects. A neural adaptation probably accounts for the improvement in the unexercised muscles.[193] The same patients were given a high-resistance exercise program 3 days a week for 12 weeks.[86] These patients worked out with the maximum weight each could lift 12 times and gradually increased the number of sets of 10 repetitions and the weight used. Patients had mixed responses. A measure of exercise work increased more than with the moderate-resistance protocol, but the elbow flexors developed what may have been overwork weakness.

Across diseases of muscle and nerve, stronger muscles tend to improve more dramatically than weaker ones with resistance training, and patients with less severe paresis have a greater improvement in cardiovascular conditioning.[28] Even in patients with the postpolio syndrome (PPS), in which fatigue from overuse of muscles is a common complaint, leg ergometry with interval training improved maximal oxygen uptake by 15 percent and increased knee extensor strength by 30 percent.[84] In another study of PPS, resistance exercise led to muscle strengthening by a combination of neural and muscular adaptations.[57] Strength training also has improved maximal muscle force and endurance in patients with myasthenia gravis.[96] When strength improves, functional performance related to that gain may or may not change. Strength training should be combined with functional training.[95a] In any of the neuromuscular diseases, patients with very weak muscles will have to initiate selective muscle strengthening against manual resistance. Some patients with weak muscles may generate their maximum force in daily activities, however, so that additional resistance training adds little and can overwork a muscle.[113]

In the absence of neurologic disease, muscle and nerve change with aging. The number of motor and sensory axons drops by up to 50 percent by age 80; large, fast motor units especially decrease; cross-sectional area of muscle progressively declines; and a delay in recovery follows fatiguing exercises.[112a] As a consequence, strength reductions of up to 40 percent have been found in leg muscles by age 70. Despite these effects of aging, even frail elderly people can improve strength in, for example, their quadriceps muscles with resistance exercises. Although some of this gain is due to improved neural control (see Chapter 1), it is associated with greater walking speed.[64,112a]

Modestly disabled patients tend to prefer exercise that is more practical or pleasurable than resistance training. Walking, swimming, stationary bicycling, rowing, and resisting the tension of a stretchable rubber material such as a Theraband as part of a flexibility and conditioning program may be more motivating and may lead to greater compliance.

Ventilation

Respiratory dysfunction is a prominent feature of many disorders of the motor unit.[5] Acute respiratory failure due to a neuromuscular disease occurs most often in myasthenia gravis and the Guillain-Barré syndrome. Symptoms may not develop until the vital capacity falls to 25 percent of predicted. Mechanical ventilation is usually begun when the vital capacity falls to 15 mL/kg body weight.

In DMD, the vital capacity starts to fall by about the age of 15 years, when the child is wheelchair dependent. At that point, nighttime nasal intermittent positive-pressure ventilation (IPPV) can prevent the symptoms of hypercarbia.[43,81] During the day, customized adaptive seating can improve the patient's vital capacity. A variety of respiratory aids can prolong independence before intubation and mechanical support become necessary.[8] In patients with amyotrophic lateral sclerosis (ALS), initial nocturnal hypoventilation can also be managed with mouth or nasal IPPV or by continuous positive airway pressure (CPAP) with a mask, as well as intermittent abdominal pressure ventilation or a negative pressure ventilator. In the latter, air is removed from under a thoracic shell, which expands the chest and sucks air into the lungs. Exercises for the diaphragm or chest wall muscles are of equivocal benefit. In one study of patients with ALS, tracheostomy was not necessary until the peak cough expiratory flow fell below 3 L/sec and the maximum insufflation capacity fell below the vital capacity.[9a] These measures reflect bulbar muscle function.

Many reports show that severely disabled ventilator-assisted individuals with a neuromuscular disease are satisfied with their lives.[9] Much of the satisfaction relates to social relations and the ability to communicate with computer-assistive devices. In one community study, however, only 10 percent of patients with ALS chose intubation and home ventilation, but 90 percent said they would choose it again.[116] Family caregivers reported significant burdens. The yearly cost was $150,000.

Motoneuron Diseases

In addition to range of motion and mild resistive and walking exercises, patients with ALS may need rehabilitative interventions for spasticity, footdrop, hand paresis, and dysphagia. The inertia of a spastic paretic gait and spasms sometimes respond to drugs such as baclofen, dantrolene, clonidine, and the benzodiazepines. These medications can worsen bulbar function. Standing can reduce leg tone temporarily. Anticholinesterase medications such as pyridostigmine, 30 to 120 mg, can modestly increase strength and decrease muscle fatigue. This effect may be partly owing to structural and functional abnormalities of the neuromuscular junction.[101] Quinine gluconate or sulfate, 250 to 325 mg before bed or a few times a day, can relieve cramping.

An ankle-foot orthosis (AFO) for footdrop, a frequent early impairment, improves the safety of gait. Many patients use a scooter before they require full-time use of a wheelchair. Wrist and finger orthotics can prolong a useful grasp and pincer movement. Any residual movement can be used to run a computerized augmentive communication device and a voice synthesizer (see Chapter 3).

Symptoms and signs of dysphagia may respond to oromotor exercises and compensatory strategies. A modified barium swallow can suggest therapeutic approaches. Head control and the safety of oral intake can improve by using a cervical collar, a steel spring head support, or a high-back wheelchair with head rest. A suctioning machine in the home may be necessary. Glycopyrrolate, 1 mg, or 2.5 mg of methscopolamine taken up to three times daily, and amitriptyline, 10 to 25 mg at night, can reduce salivation. Caregivers should learn the Heimlich maneuver and should assist the patient with oral hygiene. Before they have to make a decision about using a ventilator, most patients must decide whether they will agree to a gastrostomy feeding tube.

The maximal voluntary isometric contraction of each affected muscle appears to be the most reliable technique for monitoring the progress of the disease.[119] The Tufts Quantitative Neuromuscular Examination (see Chapter 5) is a useful tool to measure overall impairment over time.[4]

Postpolio Syndrome

The 300,000 survivors of the poliomyelitis epidemic of the 1950s and older victims are at risk for PPS. Based on a community study, 40 or more years after the poliovirus attack, new symptoms evolve in about 65 percent, and these symptoms change the lifestyle of 20 percent.[187] Symptoms include fatigue, weakness, joint pain, muscle cramps, and a decline in mobility.[74] New symptoms of weakness arise in muscles that were acutely affected. For example, previously involved bulbar muscles can again cause oropharyngeal dysfunction and dysphagia.[159] Fractures are also more frequent in a weak limb.[72] PPS does not result in the degree of decline that produces the level of disability suffered in the initial illness, however. Indeed, the functional consequences are usually modest and may be improved with rehabilitation efforts.

The cause of new dysfunction is uncertain, but it includes several possible biologic mechanisms.[118,163] New and ongoing denervation has been found in initially weak muscles and in uninvolved or asymptomatic muscles. Ongoing reorganization and age-related dropout of normal or previously injured motor neurons and of reinnervated muscles may contribute to the problem. Evidence of immunologic abnormalities and perhaps of a new viral offensive has been found. Longitudinal studies of patients with PPS are needed to understand the magnitude of the biologic and functional changes.

One site of muscle fatigability in PPS appears to be at the level of excitation-contraction coupling. Weakening as a result of exertion seems less likely to be due to energy depletion, an accumulation of metabolites such as hydrogen ion, central fatigue, fatigue at the nerve or neuromuscular junction, or impaired excitability of the muscle membrane.[153] Muscle may also be affected by endocrine changes associated with disease and immobility. The nocturnal secretion of growth hormone was low in a group of survivors of poliomyelitis, compared with healthy young men, but replacement therapy for 3 months, without any exercise, did not improve strength.[78]

Late decline in function can also be related to imbalances in muscle strength and musculotendon length across joints, overuse of compensatory muscle actions, faulty biomechanics, overstretch of ligaments, abnormal stresses on joints, pain, and increased energy expenditure caused, in part, by these impairments. For example, years of ambulation with gait deviations such as a hip hike to clear the foot or a genu recurvatum would be expected to result in mechanical dysfunction with back, hip, or knee joint pain and overuse weakness.

Physical therapies aim to improve postural alignment during gait and sitting to place muscles in an optimal position for contractions. Gait deviations are improved with orthotic and assistive devices that decrease the energy cost of ambulation. Therapists can also treat soft tissue and joint sources of pain with modalities such as ultrasound and with hands-on techniques. Assistive devices and splints can reduce pain and lessen overuse of the weak upper extremities. Pain from a carpal tunnel syndrome associated with use of a cane or wheelchair can often be treated with a cock-up wrist splint. Surgery is considered when weakness and sensory loss are increasing in an already weak hand, however. Work and home modifications and support groups are especially valued by many patients with PPS.

Neuropathies

Despite the enormous range of causes of the neuropathies,[50] a few types of rehabilitative interventions apply to most of these disorders. Some generalizations can be made using the acute polyneuropathy of the Guillain-Barré syndrome (GBS) and focal nerve injuries[17] as models.

Rehabilitation efforts are supportive during the early stage of an acute inflammatory polyradiculoneuropathy.[142] Hand and ankle dorsiflexion splinting and proper positioning help to avoid skin sores, contractures, and pain. Range of motion exercises should be performed unless they worsen uncomfortable paresthesias or induce pain after completion. Once the patient's condition is stable, particularly following completion of plasmapheresis or use of immunoglobulin, work on bed mobility and movement against gravity can begin. A week to several months after plasma exchange, some patients suffer an exacerbation, often while in rehabilitation. During inpatient rehabilitation, fatigue and dysautonomia can slow progress in mobility and ADLs. Selective strengthening exercises must avoid overworking muscles and causing discomfort. In the presence of orthostatic hypotension, tilt-table exercise can help to re-establish postural cardiovascular reflexes and to increase vascular volume. Failure to improve may be an indication to give intravenous immunoglobulin for 5 days (2.4 g/kg/day) to severely affected patients during their stay. Residual motor impairments affect 15 to 60 percent of patients and tend to be the primary limitation on ADLs and leisure and work activities.[93] The anticholinesterase inhibitors sometimes decrease muscle fatigability. The conduction block of the Guillain-Barré syndrome was not reversed, nor was a clinical benefit seen, when a group of patients was treated with 3,4-diaminopyridine (3,4-DAP) (see the discussion in this chapter on MS).[19]

Chronic motor and sensory impairments may lessen by one of several mechanisms after a mononeuropathy or peripheral polyneuropathy. Reinnervation of muscle and of sensory receptors can follow denervation. Centrally, the motor and sensory representational maps for movements and sensation can change at levels from the spinal cord to the thalamus and the sensorimotor cortices (see Chapter 1). To improve functional movement, the patient may relearn to accomplish the act without the complete use of the affected muscle group. Successful substitution results from practice and may be enhanced by an orthotic device that puts active muscles at an advantage. These approaches may be effective in patients with, for example, a median, ulnar, or radial nerve injury or a partial brachial plexopathy.

For sensory re-education, several methods have been suggested. In one method for the hand,[190] the patient manipulates blocks with and without visual input and builds up a tactile-visual image of the edges and sizes. Next, the patient works with various textures. All along, the therapist trains the patient in touch localization. Then, the patient slowly explores everyday objects with feedback about size, weight, and shape. The approach depends heavily on the kinesthetic input of motor manipulation. Another therapeutic technique stresses retraining of specific sensory inputs by rapid and slow adapting mechanoreceptors.[97] The sequence of inputs goes from pinprick to vibration at 30 Hz, followed by moving touch, constant touch, and then vibration at 256 Hz. Visual inputs are also used to help in recognition. These tasks should be combined with the application of learning principles. Both techniques aim to train the somatosensory areas to recognize what may be a new pattern of sensory coding. Case reports of improvement with these techniques are intriguing, especially in the way in which they support experimental notions of experience-induced neuroplasticity.[123]

Management of the thoracic outlet syndrome includes physical therapy. Paresthesia and pain often respond to postural education and exercises that stretch the scalene muscles and increase cervical and shoulder range of motion. Magnetic resonance imaging of the outlet and brachial plexus[39,126] may provide insight into the best physical therapeutic approach based on anatomic detail, as well as the potential for relief by surgery.

The most frequent cause of chronic polyneuropathy is diabetes mellitus. Rehabilitative interventions include medications and TENS for painful dysesthesias, bracing that does not chafe the skin, and conditioning and tilt-table exercises for dysautonomia that produces fatigue and postural hypotension.

Myopathies

The most common hereditary myopathy is DMD, with its dystrophin deficiency. In DMD, weakness evolves in the hip flexors and gluteal muscles and leads to a lordotic stance. The plantarflexors are stronger than the tibialis anterior, so children walk on their toes. Tendon shortening gradually increases across all joints. Gait becomes unsafe. Some patients choose to use a wheelchair, whereas others choose to use a polypropylene knee-ankle-foot orthosis (KAFO) to prolong ambulation for 1 or 2 years. Contractures may require tendon lengthening or casting before fitting the braces, however. A spinal fusion for scoliosis is less likely to be used in patients with DMD than in patients with spinal muscular atrophy, congenital myopathy, or poliomyelitis, because of the inexorable course of DMD. A few other procedures have a place in the treatment of long-lasting myopathies. For example, patients with facioscapulohumeral dystrophy benefit from a thoracoscapular fusion that allows the deltoid muscle to assist in abduction, elevation, and flexion of the arm.

In treating the inflammatory myopathies or when using corticosteroids to manage other immune-mediated diseases, a steroid myopathy can confound the determination of whether the drug or the disease is producing proximal weakness. Disuse also augments paresis from a neuromuscular disease. Modest resistive exercise[44] and a reduction to low-dose or alternate-day corticosteroids can allow strength to recover. Disability from the disuse myopathy and polyneuropathy of a critical illness,[25] such as sepsis, also tends to respond quickly to functionally oriented exercise.

PARKINSON'S DISEASE

Although dopaminergic and anticholinergic drug therapy dominates the approach to Parkinson's disease,[129] modest rehabilitative interventions can lessen impairments and disabilities. In contrast, patients with other movement disorders are much more likely to respond to drug and surgical interventions than to traditional rehabilitative efforts. Physical therapy was the only treatment for Parkinson's disease before the discovery of L-dopa, although one of the first controlled trials revealed no benefit on global outcome measures.[71] The interventions were based on neurodevelopmental therapies, however. When training strategies take into account some of the pathophysiologic impairments of these patients, outcomes can improve, at least during the intervention.

Bradykinesia, or slow ongoing movements, and akinesia, or inability to make willed movements, compromise the activities of many patients with Parkinson's disease. The problem arises in part from within the subcortical processes that precede and support motor cortex activation, the pattern of muscle firing, and the production of simultaneous and sequential movements.[16] Patients can, however, be trained to increase the speed of a skilled movement such as buttoning, although with more practice than healthy controls require.[158] Moreover, practice twice a week for 3 months in whole body movements such as sitting, kneeling, standing up, and throwing, along with problem solving for these activities, has improved the speed of movements needed for mobility in moderately disabled patients with Parkinson's disease.[192]

Although large-amplitude limb and truncal movements and general fitness and flexibility exercises may be expected to improve function, few studies have offered proof or insight into how best to accomplish this goal.[82] A randomized, crossover study compared regular activity to 1 hour of repetitive stretching, endurance, balance, gait, and fine motor exercises. These exercises were performed three times a week, with a progressive number of repetitions for 4 weeks.[40] The patients with Parkinson's disease had moderate disability ratings on the United Parkinson's Disease Rating Scale (UPDRS). The total UPDRS score and the ADLs and motor subscores, particularly the bradykinesia and rigidity components, significantly improved with exercise. Depression scores and medications did not change. Without an ongoing formal exercise program, these gains were lost 6 months later.

Another study found that the combination of drug treatment and physical therapy improved some measures of motor performance, although overall gains did not differ.[65] Associated with passive, active, and walking exercises, the walking speed of the treated patients improved. Range of motion activities can be an important component of exercise, because up to 12 percent of patients have a frozen shoulder,[138] and many have limited hip flexion and reduced leg strength that can slow gait speed.[26]

Other approaches need testing. For example, the mechanical and multisensory effects of practice in walking on a moving treadmill belt may enhance the rhythmicity of locomotion or, at least, may allow step training for balance, strengthening, and fitness. For patients at risk for falls, an overhead support device can be attached to a harness worn by the patient. Visual, auditory, and somatosensory stimuli of an appropriate intensity, frequency, and timing during gait can be used to trigger muscle activation to improve locomotion. In one study, visual cues such as stepping to reach targets did improve several measures of gait.[10] Rhythmic music has this benefit for some patients. A solidly balanced rolling walker can improve step automaticity, but it can also encourage unsafe festination in some.

Fatigue, orthostatic hypotension, cognitive dysfunction related to the disease or to anticholinergic medication, depression, bladder dysfunction, dysphagia,[30] pain, and sleep disturbances are among the more common problems that can be managed by a rehabilitation team. Speech therapy can improve prosody.[152] Tremor during reaching may lessen with weighting the upper extremity, but drug therapies that include beta-blockers are more likely to help. Assistive devices and removal of environmental hazards to walking enhance safety.

MULTIPLE SCLEROSIS

MS is one or more immune-mediated diseases of white matter with still uncertain endogenous and exogenous predisposing causes.[155] For the patient, it carries a lifetime of prognostic uncertainty with regard to subsequent impairments, disabilities, and handicaps. For rehabilitation specialists, long-term monitoring and flexibility in considering therapies are necessary. Opportunities for therapeutic intervention depend on the frequency and severity of attacks, the duration of remissions, the rate of progression, the secondary medical complications, and the side effects of pharmacologic treatments.

Epidemiology

Although prevalence rates vary considerably among populations and studies, the sex-adjusted and age-adjusted prevalence of probable and definite MS was 167 per 100,000 in Olmsted County, Minnesota.[140] The direct and indirect yearly costs in the United States related to the disease are $7.5 billion.[145] About 50 percent of patients with MS have a progressive disease 10 to 15 years after onset, and 50 percent of all patients have reached a Disability Status Scale score (see Chapter 5) of 6, which includes the need to use a cane to walk half a block.[183] By 15 years, about 20 percent are confined to a wheelchair. More favorable prognostic characteristics include onset at age less than 40 years in females, optic neuritis or sensory symptoms at onset, a relapsing-remitting course, and a low frequency of attacks over the first 5 years.

In the Olmstead County population, one-third of patients with MS had a marked paraparesis or quadriparesis, 25 percent required intermittent or continuous bladder catheterization, 4 percent required supervision for cognitive dysfunction, 53 percent worked full time, and 28 percent needed outside financial support. Fatigue was a significant problem for 43 percent. Table 10–4 shows the level of disability based upon the Incapacity Status Scale of the Minimal Record of Disability for Multiple Sclerosis.

Table 10–4. **PERCENTAGE OF POPULATION WITH MULTIPLE SCLEROSIS NEEDING ASSISTANCE FOR ACTIVITIES OF DAILY LIVING**

Activity	Assistive Device	Human Assistance
Stair climbing	31	26
Ambulation	13	28
Transfers	14	18
Bathing	18	23
Dressing	10	20
Feeding	12	9

Source: Data from Rodriguez M, Siva A, Ward J, et al.[140]

Table 10–5. **SYMPTOMS IN 656 PATIENTS WITH MULTIPLE SCLEROSIS**

Symptom	No Difficulty in Activities of Daily Living (%)	Interferes With Activities of Daily Living (%)
Fatigue	21	56
Imbalance	24	50
Paresis	18	45
Sensory	39	24
Bladder	25	34
Spasticity	23	26
Bowel	19	20
Memory	21	16
Depression	18	18
Pain	15	21
Lability	24	8
Visual	14	16
Tremor	14	13
Speech	12	11

Source: Adapted from Kraft G, Freal J, Coryll J.[89]

Symptoms reported by clinic patients with MS often interfere with ADLs (Table 10–5) Quality of life has been correlated negatively with signs of pyramidal tract, brainstem, and visual impairment.[146] The Functional Independence Measure (FIM) will likely find increasing use as a reliable and valid measure of the physical care needs of patients with MS.[29,73]

Rehabilitative Interventions

Problems such as spasticity, paresis, sensory loss, dysphagia, the commonplace neurogenic bladder that is most often hyperreflexic with sphincter dyssynergia, sexual dysfunction, and functional disabilities are managed much as they would be for patients with stroke or SCI. Tizanidine, clonidine, and oral and intrathecal baclofen have been especially useful in lessening lower extremity spasms (see Chapter 6). TENS sometimes decreases painful spasms when it is placed over the affected muscles.[103] As in SCI, the advent of intermittent bladder catheterization by a clean technique has probably reduced morbidity and mortality more than any other recent intervention. Although cognitive dysfunction accompanies white matter plaques in up to 50 percent of people with MS, global intellectual impairment is unusual.[47] Compensatory memory strategies (see Table 9-15) can aid patients who develop mild subcortical dementia-like impairments.

Some problems are more nearly unique to patients with MS. Heat sensitivity is especially prominent, although muscle fatigue and lassitude can follow heat exposure in any patient with a neurologic disease, especially patients with stroke or myasthenia gravis. Visual impairment from optic neuritis can require magnifying lenses or braille materials. Diplopia sometimes responds to a prism, but patients more often prefer to cover one of their eyes, unless the resulting loss of depth perception is disabling. Pendular nystagmus causing oscillopsia is more likely to interfere with ADLs. It has been successfully reduced with isoniazid in some patients.[174] An action tremor may also respond to up to 1200 mg of isoniazid[54] or to propranolol, acetazolamide, glutethimide, benzodiazepines, or primidone, although functional gains are generally modest. Limb ataxia can be dampened by slightly weighting the distal limb or the utensils used by the patient. Paroxysmal pain can be treated with carbamazepine and other interventions for central pain and dysesthesia.

Fatigability is especially common. Its possible origins include impaired central conduction that increases paresis with activity, slowed neural processing before the activation of primary motor pathways,[148] increases in body temperature, exhaustive efforts related to impairments, and malaise associated with a mood disorder. Cooling, energy-conservation techniques during activities, and assistive devices can reduce fatigue in some patients. During resistive and aerobic exercises, persons with MS should drink cold fluids, work out under a fan or in an air-conditioned environment, and, if very sensitive to overheating, try wearing a cooling jacket device.

Medications may reduce fatigability and lassitude, and they may improve impairments due to a conduction block. Amantadine,[31] 100 mg per day, and pemoline,[184] 75 mg per day, have lessened fatigue in short-term controlled trials.[90] Long-term oral treatment with 4-aminopyridine (4-AP) at 0.5 mg/kg has also reduced fatigue.[133] Both 4-AP and 3,4-DAP, 40 to 100 mg per day, block potassium channels in demyelinated axons to improve conduction (see Chapter 1). Digitalis also restores high-frequency impulse transmission in demyelinated central and peripheral fibers and may reverse a conduction block in patients with MS.[85] The aminopyridines have improved some neurologic impairments, particularly those sensitive to heat.[20] In controlled trials using different methods, 4-AP has improved ADLs and neurophysiologic parameters in some patients,[178] but it has not clearly decreased disability in others.[21] It has not benefited neuropsychologic performance either, at least not in small-group crossover trials.[157] Potential adverse reactions include paresthesias, imbalance, and dizziness. Seizures have occurred at a high serum concentration. Gastrointestinal pain is more frequent with 3,4-DAP administration.[132]

Aerobic training by arm-leg bicycle ergometry significantly decreased fatigue, depression, and anxiety and improved fitness in a controlled trial of ambulatory patients with MS.[131] These patients exercised for 30 minutes at 60 percent of their maximal aerobic capacity four times a week for 15 weeks. A fan helped to cool them during exertion. Some neurologic symptoms worsened during and shortly after exercise, but no exacerbations of MS were related to the program. Disease severity and disability complicate training to improve muscle strength and cardiopulmonary fitness,[135] but an individual exercise prescription can often overcome these limitations. Muscle weakness tends to be greater with concentric than with eccentric muscle contractions, with alternating flexion-extension compared with isolated flexion movements, and with high-speed compared with low-speed contractions. This pattern is typical of upper motoneuron dysfunction. Many patients prefer pool exercise at cool temperatures, which takes advantage of the patient's buoyancy for support while allowing work against the resistance of the water.

Immune suppression and immunomodulating therapies, such as the oral administration of basic myelin protein antigen[36] and treatment with beta interferon, copolymer-1, and other agents, offer hope for amelioration of MS. In the future, remyelination by transplantation of oligodendrocytes or Schwann cells, perhaps with protein growth factors,[75] may stimulate repair of plaques. These approaches should be combined with measures of impairment and disability and ongoing rehabilitation-related problem solving to optimize recovery of function.

PEDIATRIC DISEASES

The rehabilitation of infants and children requires clinicians to establish goals based partly on needs at a particular chronologic and developmental stage. Realistic motor, psychosocial, educational, lifestyle, and vocational objectives must be considered throughout the disabled person's life.

Ethical issues about disabled children are especially vexing. Children depend on the values and beliefs of parents, clergy, physicians, and other rehabilitation specialists. From the moment of diagnosis of cerebral palsy or meningomyelocele, decisions must be made in the best interest of the infant or child amid clinical and moral uncertainty about treatments and their alternatives.[12] Psychologic and financial burdens and familial stress also affect decision making. Family counseling and support groups can help the child's caregivers to work through their obligations, beliefs, and course of action. One of the dilemmas is that families, patients, and therapists often demand more physical therapy when, in the absence of good clinical trials and outcome measures, the potential benefit is unclear.

Cerebral Palsy

Over 100,000 persons in the United States under the age of 18 years have the symptom complex of cerebral palsy, which can include motor and cognitive impairments and epilepsy in about one-third of patients.[91] The direct and indirect costs for the 275,000 persons in the United States with serious disability from cerebral palsy is about $5 billion per year.

For rehabilitation, the most practical classification is based on which limbs are affected, the presence of hypotonia or spasticity, and the presence of a movement disorder such as athetosis. These differences among individuals increase the difficulty of studying a particular intervention. For example, in patients with hemiplegic cerebral palsy, studies suggest abnormal spinal branching of corticospinal axons from the undamaged motor cortex to ipsilateral motoneurons.[60] This novel path may account for mirror movements. More important, this developmental neuroplasticity may offer therapeutic approaches that are not relevant to the patient with a spastic diplegia from bicerebral periventricular leukomalacia.

Although many styles of intervention have had allure for parents and therapists, their benefits have generally not been evaluated. Most formal studies of rehabilitative interventions have been undertaken in infants and children with spastic diplegia. One controlled trial compared a program of motor, sensory, language, and cognitive stimulation with physical therapy with a neurodevelopmental approach.[125] The infants were 12 to 19 months old and received either 12 months of physical therapy (PT) or 6 months of PT followed by the stimulation. Over this short run, patients in the stimulation program were more likely to walk and had a higher mental quotient. The small sample size, the uncertain longer-term implications, and the possibility that physical therapy may delay walking when it is aimed at altering tone and pushing the child toward more normal patterns of movement leave rehabilitation specialists with intriguing questions about the best therapeutic approach. In another small study, infants who received weekly neurodevelopmental therapy had higher scores on tests of motor development than did infants who received monthly therapy for 6 months.[106] This modest intervention with uncertain between-treatment care cannot be considered a clear-cut efficacy study. In older children and in adults, EMG biofeedback,[37] fitness training,[61] and a short pulse of therapy for specific limb and trunk impairments and singular disabilities can benefit persons with well-defined problems. No trials that apply motor learning principles have been reported.

Much of the rehabilitation work in cerebral palsy concerns the management of spasticity and ambulation.[22] One study showed that contractures of the soleus muscle could be prevented if dorsiflexion of the ankles is maintained with a slight force for at least 6 hours within every 24 hours.[167] Splinting can be done during sleep. Inhibitive casting and AFOs and KAFOs are often used to limit tone or to compensate for paresis. Hypertonicity in children can be lessened with antispasticity medications, but their side effects and the potential to excessively reduce the extensor tone needed for stance limits their use. Intrathecal baclofen has reduced tone and has improved ADLs for both the upper and lower extremities and can be titrated to allow enough tone to stand and walk.[2] Nerve and motor point blocks, especially at the hip adductors, hamstrings, and triceps surae, allow a more localized approach. So would intramuscular botulinumtoxin. Tendon releases must not overcorrect the shortening. EMG studies should precede these approaches, so that the optimal muscle can be chosen to try to correct the deviations that affect ambulation. Rhizotomy of selected dorsal lumbar roots in carefully chosen children with spastic diplegia, followed by extensive physical therapy, can decrease tone and improve functional mobility,[53,128] although the ultimate role and efficacy of the procedure are still equivocal.[38] These approaches are discussed in Chapter 6.

Other efforts by the rehabilitation team include improving oromotor function, speech, and swallowing disorders associated with a pseudobulbar palsy, managing cognitive and behavioral problems, and monitoring for potential orthopedic issues such as scoliosis and hip dislocation.

Myelomeningocele

This neural tube defect occurs in about 1 per 1000 births. About 75 percent of these infants also have progressive hydrocephalus, and all have an Arnold-Chiari type II malformation with caudal displacement of the cerebellar vermis and aqueductal stenosis.

A defect within the thoracic spine or at the L-1 to L-2 level generally prevents assisted ambulation in older children. At the L-3 level, about 50 percent of patients can walk, at L-4, about 67 percent can walk, and at the L-5 and sacral levels, 80 percent walk sometimes.[15] A syrinx or syringomyelia, symptomatic Chiari malformation, scoliosis, advancing age, and hip flexion contractures interfere with ambulation, especially in children with lesions below L-2. Overall, only about 30 percent of children become functionally independent. Early bracing can allow a child with a high lesion to walk, perhaps through adolescence. Walking can result in fewer bone fractures and pressure sores and more independent ADLs, but it can also increase the need for orthopedic interventions and physical therapy.[107] Some devices can extend the age for walking despite high lesions by reducing the energy requirement.[160] Scoliosis, clubfoot, hip dislocation, shunt failure, tethered spinal cord, and bladder dysfunction are among the complications that may require surgical intervention.[3]

BALANCE DISORDERS

Falls in the Elderly

Much clinical research has gone into the issues of geriatric rehabilitation, particularly related to the prevention of falls and the management of the disabilities that can accompany aging. The yearly incidence of falls increases from 25 percent among 70-year-old persons living in the community to 35 percent after the age of 75 years; half of these elderly patients fall repeatedly.[172] About 5 percent of falls cause a fracture, and another 10 percent result in serious injury. Many of the predisposing causes that may respond to rehabilitation efforts involve disease or age-related declines in neurologic and musculoskeletal function (Table 10–6). For many geriatric patients, the cause of falls is multifactorial. Although tests of postural instability and gait have become a growth industry for those trying to predict who is at risk, the simplest physical tests are the manual examination of leg muscle strength, balance on standing, and observation of a short walk and turning. A prospective study of persons over the age of 70 years found that timed tests of standing in semitandem and

Table 10–6. **RISKS IDENTIFIED BY STUDIES OF NONSYNCOPAL FALLS IN THE ELDERLY**

Environmental hazards

Use of sedatives and antidepressants

Cognitive impairment

Postural hypotension, often related to medication

Impaired vision

Decreased hip or knee strength

Difficulty in standing up or tandem walking

Foot, knee, and hip pain or limited range of motion

Neurologic disease
  Parkinsonism
  Cervical myelopathy
  Vitamin B_{12} deficiency
  Polyneuropathy
  Vestibular disorder
  Stroke with hemiparesis
  Multiple subcortical infarcts
  Normal pressure hydrocephalus
  Toxic-metabolic encephalopathy
  Seizures
  Syncope

Source: Data from references 76, 120, 144, 164, 172, and 173.

tandem stance, walking 8 feet, and rising from a chair and sitting down five times could be used to predict subsequent disability in mobility and ADLs by 4 years later.[79]

Most rehabilitation interventions are straightforward. Environmental hazards such as steps, loose rugs, slick floors, loose slippers, pets, poor lighting, low beds and toilets, and raised floor thresholds can be corrected. The use of drugs that sedate, confuse, or cause postural hypotension should be reconsidered. As noted earlier, resistance exercises can improve leg strength and mobility even in frail, elderly patients.[63,64] A special effort should be made to assess the hip, knee, and ankle muscle groups and to strengthen those muscles that are weak. Patients who are predisposed to fall should develop the strength and balance needed to arise from the floor.[171] Supplements of human growth hormone may also increase muscle mass, but side effects, so far, outweigh physical benefits and costs.[147] Older

patients may experience a carpal tunnel syndrome, fluid retention, and arthralgias.[191] Growth hormone–releasing drugs are in clinical trials. Stretching for hip and ankle flexibility and practicing balance exercises can help to defray some of the risks of falling. Pain management for arthritis and other sources of discomfort with exercise and assistive devices, such as canes and walkers, can also reduce this risk. No particular gait characteristics during formal gait analysis separate patients who fall from those who do not,[70] but a visual inspection of ambulation may reveal an individual's problem.

The intensity of an intervention depends on the patient's setting. During the acute hospital stays of elderly patients, a geriatric rehabilitation unit was shown to improve function, decrease nursing home placements, and potentially reduce mortality.[6] On the other hand, a 4-month trial of physical therapy for frail nursing home residents, including range of motion and strengthening and endurance exercises, balance and coordination training, and work on mobility, revealed modest improvements, but not fewer falls.[117]

A physical therapy evaluation should be part of a falls assessment for the elderly person who lives at home. A controlled community trial of 301 people who had risk factors for falling and were over the age of 70 years showed a significant reduction for falls during a 1-year intervention.[170] The risk dropped from 47 percent in the controls to 35 percent in the group managed for targeted risk factors by a nurse and physical therapist. Targeted findings included postural hypotension, use of sedatives, use of more than four medications, inability to perform a safe toilet or tub transfer, home environmental hazards, and impaired gait, balance, and strength.

Thus, exercise, particularly a selective program of strengthening, conditioning, stretching, and balance for physical impairments, along with practice in ADLs and community activity tasks, may reduce falls. In turn, confidence in physical skills can ease the fear of falling that puts self-limitations on the lives of frail, elderly patients. By designing interventions for specific physical disabilities, as well as for depressive symptoms, the rehabilitation team can help to prevent a downward spiral in the quality of life of elderly patients.

Vestibular Dysfunction

Dizziness is a common and disabling symptom. Dizziness and episodic vertigo have many causes that can be managed by medications and, for a few pathologic conditions, by surgical procedures of the inner ear.[11] Vertigo from acute vestibular dysfunction generally improves over time, but some patients have residual unsteadiness, symptoms that can be related to mismatches in vestibulo-ocular gain, and episodic vertigo that does not respond to niacin, diuretics, meclizine, or benzodiazepines. Debilitating psychiatric symptoms that include anxiety are often associated with vestibular dysfunction.[55] These symptoms require management if the vertigo persists. Rehabilitative movement therapies can reduce or eliminate symptoms related to unilateral vestibular hypofunction and benign positional vertigo (BPV).[121]

Patients with ongoing vestibular dysfunction or episodic BPV tend to limit their movements. The rehabilitative approach encourages activity and specific exercises for balance, proprioceptive feedback, and head movements. Vestibular habituation training offers a detailed method of evaluation and exercise aimed at encouraging adaptation within the connections of the vestibular pathways.[122] Three specific positioning exercises have been recommended for treating BPV.[27]

The incidence of BPV is 141 per 100,000 at the age of 50 years and about 190 per 100,000 by the age of 85 years.[67] The attacks are triggered by debris within an otolith that gravitates through the endolymph during head positional changes.[175] When the floating material reaches the most dependent part of the canal, it settles on the cupula and produces forces that initiate short-duration vertigo. A single maneuver or a series of rapid head-tilting and trunk-tilting maneuvers can loosen the debris and can disperse it into the cavity of the utricle.[27] For example, patients begin in a seated position and then rapidly lean to the side until their head touches the bed. They remain there until the vertigo ceases and return to the upright position until all symptoms stop. The maneuver is repeated toward the opposite side, and 10 to 20 repetitions are done 3 times a day. In the single Semont liberatory maneuver for BPV arising from the posterior canal, patients start seated with the head turned 45 degrees toward the unaffected ear. They are taken from the sitting to the side-lying position with the head tilted back about 105 degrees toward the affected ear, a position that induces vertigo. They hold this position for 3 to 20 minutes. Then they are swung quickly to the opposite side with the nose down. If this maneuver induces the typical nystagmus of BPV, they hold this position for at least 5 minutes and then sit up slowly. Some clinicians recommend that the head be held upright for 48 hours.

MISCELLANEOUS DISORDERS

Motor Conversion Disorders

Hemiparesis, paraparesis, or monoparesis with no neuropathologic basis can arise from a conversion disorder and from malingering. The suspicion of hysterical paralysis evolves from a history of injury that is not expected to produce profound impairments. Sometimes, the astute clinician can discern the special psychologic meaning that the symptoms and signs hold for the patient. The examination may reveal odd patterns of sensory loss and paresis, changing examination findings, giveway weakness, unilateral loss of sensation to pinprick or vibration that splits the midline of the sternum or forehead, remarkably better use of the limb in a functional setting than on specific testing, and an indifferent affect. Although malingerers may behave in a similar fashion, they try to convince the clinician of how disabled they are and how much they depend on a financial settlement or other secondary gain. For nonmalingerers, psychotherapy and behavioral approaches can lead to motor recovery.[168] The physician and therapist should set definite goals with the patient, provide positive feedback and support for each small accomplishment, and not reinforce symptoms and signs of disability.

Alzheimer's Disease

Modest functional benefits result from intake of the centrally acting acetylcholinesterase inhibitor tacrine.[59] Quality of life can improve for patients who can tolerate the drug.[87] Physical therapy can improve mobility despite the dementia.[134] The approach to ADLs and social activities can take advantage of the ability of many patients with Alzheimer's disease to learn skills by procedural memory.[58] This motor learning depends on corticocerebellar and striatal structures, rather than on the mesial temporal networks that bear the brunt of the degeneration.

Epilepsy

After surgery for epilepsy, psychosocial rehabilitation can help patients to reintegrate into the community and to find employment.[66] Cognitive and behavioral rehabilitation is needed for a minority of patients. A quality-of-life inventory has been developed for use in daily practice.[130]

Chronic Fatigue Syndrome

General conditioning exercises and energy conservation techniques may improve daily functioning for patients given this diagnosis, which probably includes a variety of causes. The syndrome may be associated with neurally mediated hypotension, which can respond to sodium loading.[25a]

Organ Transplantation

Organ transplantation accompanied by serious pretransplant and posttransplant complications can leave patients quite debilitated. Deconditioning is common, along with disuse paresis, steroid myopathy, and chronic illness or drug-induced polyneuropathy. Patients who undergo lung, heart, or liver transplantation tend to have developed the greatest disability for mobility tasks. Patients respond within a few weeks, once they are medically stable, to a program of light resistance exercises and walking for balance and conditioning.

AIDS

The myriad neurologic complications of infection by the human immunodeficiency virus (HIV) require ongoing assessment and management. Rehabilitative efforts can optimize strength, mobility, fitness, ADLs, and cognition for the neurobehavioral problems, dementia, myelopathy, mononeuritis or polyneuropathy, and myopathy that can compromise patients with this infection.

SUMMARY

Rehabilitation specialists can find opportunities to diminish disabilities associated with every neurologic disease and any neurologic complication of a medical illness. The rehabilitation physician can serve patients well by acting as the general practitioner or quarterback for the person's long-term care as it relates to the disease. In patients with a chronic or progressive central or peripheral neurologic disease, proactive interventions can sometimes delay or prevent deterioration in the quality of a patient's life.

REFERENCES

1. Aitkens S, McCrory M, Kilmer D, et al. Moderate resistance exercise program: Its effect in slowly progressive neuromuscular disease. Arch Phys Med Rehabil 1993;74:711–715.
2. Albright A, Barron W, Fasick M, et al. Continuous intrathecal baclofen infusion for spasticity of cerebral origin. JAMA 1993;270:2475–2477.
3. Alexander M, Steg N. Myelomeningocele: Comprehensive management. Arch Phys Med Rehabil 1989;70:637–641.
4. Andres P, Finison L, Conlon T, et al. Use of composite scores (megascores) to measure deficit in ALS. Neurology 1988;38:405–408.
5. Annoni J-M, Chevrolet J, Kesselring J. Respiratory problems in chronic neurological disorders. Crit Rev Phys Rehabil Med 1993;5:155–192.
6. Applegate W, Miller S, Graney M, et al. A randomized, controlled trial of a geriatric assessment unit in a community rehabilitation hospital. N Engl J Med 1990;322:1572–1578.

7. Bach F, Jensen T, Kastrup J, et al. The effect of intravenous lidocaine on nociceptive processing in diabetic neuropathy. Pain 1990;40:29–34.

8. Bach J. Pulmonary rehabilitation considerations for Duchenne muscular dystrophy. Crit Rev Phys Rehabil Med 1992;3:239–269.

9. Bach J, Barnett V. Ethical considerations in the management of individuals with severe neuromuscular disorders. Am J Phys Med Rehabil 1994; 73:134–140.

9a. Bach J. Amyotrophic lateral sclerosis: Predictors for prolongation of life by noninvasive respiratory aids. Arch Phys Med Rehabil 1995;76:828–832.

10. Bagley S, Kelly B, Tunnicliffe N, et al. The effect of visual cues on the gait of independently mobile Parkinson's disease patients. Physiotherapy 1991; 77:415–420.

11. Baloh R, Honrubia V. Clinical Neurophysiology of the Vestibular System. Philadelphia: FA Davis, 1991.

12. Banja J, Jann B. Ethical issues in treating pediatric rehabilitation patients. NeuroRehabilitation 1993;3:44–52.

13. Barinaga M. Playing "telephone" with the body's message of pain. Science 1992;258:1085.

14. Barnsley L, Lord S, Wallis B, et al. Lack of effect of intra-articular corticosteroids for chronic pain in the cervical zygapophyseal joints. N Engl J Med 1994;330:1047–1050.

15. Beaty J, Canele S. Orthopedic aspects of myelomeningocele. J Bone Joint Surg Am 1990;72:626–630.

16. Benecke R, Rothwell J, Dick J, et al. Disturbance of sequential movements in patients with Parkinson's disease. Brain 1987;110:361–379.

17. Berger A, Schaumburg H. Rehabilitation of focal nerve injuries. Journal of Neurologic Rehabilitation 1988;2:65–91.

18. Berger A, Schaumburg H. Rehabilitation of the peripheral neuropathies. Journal of Neurologic Rehabilitation 1988;2:25–36.

19. Bergin P, Miller D, Hirsch N, et al. Failure of 3,4-diaminopyridine to reverse conduction block in inflammatory demyelinating neuropathies. Ann Neurol 1993;34:406–409.

20. Bever C. The current status of studies of aminopyridines in patients with multiple sclerosis. Ann Neurol 1994;36:S118–S121.

21. Bever C, Young D, Anderson P, et al. The effects of 4-aminopyridine in multiple sclerosis patients. Neurology 1994;44:1054–1059.

22. Binder H, Eng G. Rehabilitation management of children with spastic diplegic cerebral palsy. Arch Phys Med Rehabil 1989;70:481–489.

23. Blomberg S, Tibblin G. A controlled, multicentre trial of manual therapy with steroid injections in low-back pain. Clinical Rehabilitation 1993;7:49–62.

24. Bohannon R. Exercise training variables influencing the enhancement of voluntary muscle strength. Clinical Rehabilitation 1990;4:325–331.

25. Bolton C, Young G, Zochodne D. The neurological complications of sepsis. Ann Neurol 1993; 33:94–100.

25a. Bou-Holaigah I, Rowe P, Kann J, et al. The relationship between neurally mediated hypotension and the chronic fatigue syndrome. JAMA 1995; 274:961–967.

26. Bowes S, Charlett A, Dobbs R, et al. Gait in relation to ageing and idiopathic parkinsonism. Scand J Rehabil Med 1992;24:157–160.

27. Brandt T, Steddin S, Daroff R. Therapy for benign paroxysmal positioning vertigo, revisited. Neurology 1994;44:796–800.

28. Brinkmann J, Ringel S. Effectiveness of exercise in progressive neuromuscular disease. J Neuro Rehab 1991;5:195–199.

29. Brosseau L, Wolfson C. The inter-rater reliability and construct validity of the Functional Independence Measure for multiple sclerosis subjects. Clinical Rehabilitation 1994;8:107–115.

30. Bushmann M, Dobmeyer S, Leeker L, et al. Swallowing abnormalities and their response to treatment in Parkinson's disease. Neurology 1989; 39:1309–1314.

31. Canadian MS Research Group. A randomized controlled trial of amantadine in fatigue associated with multiple sclerosis. Can J Neurol Sci 1987;14:273–278.

32. Carette S, Marcoux S, Truchon R, et al. A controlled trial of corticosteroid injections into facet joints for chronic low back pain. N Engl J Med 1991;325:1002–1007.

33. Casey K. Central pain syndromes: Current view on pathophysiology, diagnosis, and treatment. Reg Anesth 1992;17:59–68.

34. Chabal C, Jacobson J, Mariano A, et al. The use of oral mexiletine for the treatment of pain after peripheral nerve injury. Anesthesiology 1992; 76:513–517.

35. Chapman C, Casey K, Dubner R, et al. Pain measurement: An overview. Pain 1985;22:1–31.

36. Chen Y, Kuchroo V, Inobe J, et al. Regulatory T cell clones induced by oral tolerance: Suppression of autoimmune encephalomyelitis. Science 1994;265:1237–1240.

37. Colborne G, Wright V, Naumann S. Feedback of triceps surae EMG in gait of children with cerebral palsy: A controlled study. Arch Phys Med Rehabil 1994;75:40–45.

38. Cole H. Dorsal rhizotomy: Diagnostic and therapeutic technology assessment. JAMA 1990; 264:2569–2574.

39. Collins J, Shaver M, Disher A, et al. Compromising abnormalities of the brachial plexus as displayed by magnetic resonance imaging. Clinical Anatomy 1995;8:1–16.

40. Comella C, Stebbins G, Brown-Toms N, et al. Physical therapy and Parkinson's disease: A controlled clinical trial. Neurology 1994;44:376–378.

41. Craig A, Bushnell M, Zhang E-T, et al. A thalamic nucleus specific for pain and temperature sensation. Nature 1994;372:770–773.

42. Cross S. Pathophysiology of pain. Mayo Clin Proc 1994;69:375–383.

43. Curran F, Colbert A. Ventilator management in DMD and postpoliomyelitis syndrome: Twelve years' experience. Arch Phys Med Rehabil 1989; 70:180–185.

44. Czerwinski S, Kurowski T, O'Neill T, et al. Initiating regular exercise protects against muscle at-

rophy from glucocorticoids. J Appl Physiol 1987; 63:1504–1510.

45. Davidoff G, Werner R, Cremer S, et al. Predictive value of the three-phase technetium bone scan in diagnosis of reflex sympathetic dystrophy syndrome. Arch Phys Med Rehabil 1989;70:135–137.

46. Debreceni L. Chemical releases associated with acupuncture and electric stimulation. Crit Rev Phys Rehabil Med 1993;5:247–275.

47. DeLuca J, Johnson S. Cognitive impairments in multiple sclerosis. NeuroRehabilitation 1993;3:9–16.

48. Deyo R, Rainville J, Kent D. What can the history and physical examination tell us about low back pain? JAMA 1992;268:760–765.

49. Deyo R, Walsh N, Martin D, et al. A controlled trial of transcutaneous electrical nerve stimulation and exercise for chronic low back pain. N Engl J Med 1990;322:1627–1634.

50. Dobkin B. Exercise fitness and sports for individuals with neurologic disability. In: Gordon S, Gonzalez-Mestre X, Garrett W, eds: Sports and Exercise in Midlife. Rosemont, IL: American Academy of Orthopedic Surgeons, 1993;235–252.

51. Donelson R. The McKenzie approach to evaluating and treating low back pain. Orthop Rev 1990; 19:681–686.

52. Drummond P, Finch P, Smythe G. Reflex sympathetic dystrophy: The significance of differing plasma catecholamine concentrations in affected and unaffected limbs. Brain 1991;114:2025–2036.

53. Dudgeon B, Libby A, McLaughlin J, et al. Prospective measurement of functional changes after selective dorsal rhizotomy. Arch Phys Med Rehabil 1994;75:46–53.

54. Duquette P, Pleines J, duDouich P. Isoniazid for tremor in multiple sclerosis: A controlled trial. Neurology 1985;35:1772–1775.

55. Eagger S, Luxon L, Davies R, et al. Psychiatric morbidity in patients with peripheral vestibular disorder. J Neurol Neurosurg Psychiatry 1992; 55:383–387.

56. Edmeads J. The cervical spine and headache. Neurology 1988;38:1874–1878.

57. Einarsson G. Muscle conditioning in late poliomyelitis. Arch Phys Med Rehabil 1991;72:11–14.

58. Eslinger P, Damasio A. Preserved motor learning in Alzheimer's disease: Implications for anatomy and behavior. J Neurosci 1986;6:3006–3009.

59. Farlow M, Gracon S, Hershey L, et al. A controlled trial of tacrine in Alzheimer's disease. JAMA 1992;268:2523–2529.

60. Farmer S, Harrison L, Ingram D, et al. Plasticity of central motor pathways in children with hemiplegic cerebral palsy. Neurology 1991;41:1505–1510.

61. Farrell J. Cervical passive techniques. Physical Medicine Rehabilitation: State of the Art Reviews 1990;4:309–334.

62. Fernandez J, Pitetti K. Training of ambulatory individuals with cerebral palsy. Arch Phys Med Rehabil 1993;74:468–472.

63. Fiatarone M, Marks E, Ryan N, et al. High-intensity strength training in nonagenarians. JAMA 1990;263:3029–3034.

64. Fiatarone M, O'Neill E, Ryan N, et al. Exercise training and nutritional supplementation for physical frailty in very elderly people. N Engl J Med 1994;330:1769–1775.

65. Formisano R, Pratesi I, Modarelli F, et al. Rehabilitation and Parkinson's disease. Scand J Rehabil Med 1992;24:157–160.

66. Fraser R, Gumnit R, Thorbecke R, et al. Psychosocial rehabilitation: A pre- and post-operative perspective. In: Engel J, ed: Surgical Treatment of the Epilepsies. New York: Raven Press, 1993.

67. Froehling D, Silverstein M, Mohr D, et al. Benign positional vertigo: Incidence and prognosis in Olmsted County, Minnesota. Mayo Clin Proc 1991;66:596–601.

68. Frymoyer J. Back pain and sciatica. N Engl J Med 1988;318:291–300.

69. Galer B, Miller K, Rowbotham M. Response to intravenous lidocaine infusion differs based on clinical diagnosis and site of nervous system injury. Neurology 1993;43:1233–1235.

70. Gehlsen G, Whaley M. Falls in the elderly. Part 1: Gait. Arch Phys Med Rehabil 1990;71:735–738.

71. Gibberd F, Page N, Spencer K, et al. Controlled trial of physiotherapy and occupational therapy for Parkinson's disease. BMJ 1981;282:1196.

72. Goerss J, Atkinson E, Winderbank A, et al. Fractures in an aging population of poliomyelitis survivors: A community based study in Olmstead County. Mayo Clin Proc 1994;69:333–339.

73. Granger C, Cotter A, Hamilton B, et al. Functional assessment scales: A study of persons with multiple sclerosis. Arch Phys Med Rehabil 1990; 71:870–875.

74. Grimby G, Einarsson G. Post-polio management. Crit Rev Phys Rehabil Med 1991;2:189–200.

75. Grinspan J, Stern J, Franceschini B, et al. Protein growth factors as potential therapies for central nervous system demyelinative disorders. Ann Neurol 1994;36:S140–S142.

76. Grisso J, Kelsey J, Strom B, et al. Risk factors for falls as a cause of hip fracture in women. N Engl J Med 1991;324:1326–1331.

77. Guieu R. Analgesic effects of vibration and TENS applied separately and simultaneously to patients with chronic pain. Can J Neurol Sci 1991;18:113–119.

78. Gupta K, Shetty K, Agre J, et al. Human growth hormone effect on serum IGF-I and muscle function in poliomyelitis survivors. Arch Phys Med Rehabil 1994;75:889–894.

79. Guralnik J, Ferrucci L, Simonsick E, et al. Lower-extremity function in persons over the age of 70 years as a predictor of subsequent disability. N Engl J Med 1995;332:556–561.

80. Hayes K. The use of ultrasound to decrease pain and improve mobility. Crit Rev Phys Rehabil Med 1992;3:271–287.

81. Heckmatt J, Dubowitz V. Night-time nasal ventilation in neuromuscular disease. Lancet 1990; 1:579–581.

82. Homberg V. Motor training in the therapy of Parkinson's disease. Neurology 1993;43(Suppl 6):S45–S46.

83. Hong C-Z. Myofascial trigger point injection. Crit Rev Phys Rehabil Med 1993;5:203–217.

84. Jones D, Speier J, Canine K, et al. Cardiorespira-

tory responses to aerobic training by patients with postpoliomyelitis sequelae. JAMA 1989;261:3255–3258.

85. Kaji R, Happel L, Sumner A. Effect of digitalis on clinical symptoms and conduction variables in patients with multiple sclerosis. Ann Neurol 1990; 28:582–584.

86. Kilmer D, McCrory M, Wright N, et al. The effect of a high resistance exercise program in slowly progressive neuromuscular disease. Arch Phys Med Rehabil 1994;75:560–563.

87. Knapp M, Knopman D, Solomon P, et al. A 30-week randomized controlled trial of high-dose tacrine in patients with Alzheimer's disease. JAMA 1994;271:985–991.

88. Koes B, Bouter L, Essers A, et al. Randomized clinical trial of manipulative therapy and physiotherapy for persistent back and neck complaints: Results of one year follow-up. BMJ 1992;304:601–604.

89. Kraft G, Freal J, Coryll J. Disability, disease duration and rehabilitation service needs in multiple sclerosis: Patient perspectives. Arch Phys Med Rehabil 1986;67:164–178.

90. Krupp L, Coyle P, Doscher C, et al. A comparison of amantidine, pemoline and placebo on the treatment of MS fatigue. Neurology 1993; 43(Suppl):281.

91. Kuban K, Leviton A. Cerebral palsy. N Engl J Med 1994;330:188–195.

92. Lahad A, Malter A, Berg A, et al. The effectiveness of four interventions for the prevention of low back pain. JAMA 1994;272:1286–1291.

93. Lennon S, Koblar S, Hughes R, et al. Reasons for persistent disability in Guillain-Barré syndrome. Clinical Rehabilitation 1993;7:1–8.

94. Lewett K. Manipulative Therapy in Rehabilitation of the Motor System. London: Butterworth, 1985.

95. Lewis S, Haller R. Skeletal muscle disorders and associated factors that limit exercise performance. In: Holloszy J, ed: Exercise and Sports Science Reviews. Baltimore: Williams & Wilkins, 1991;67–113.

95a. Lindeman E, Leffers P, Spaans F, et al. Strength training in patients with myotonic dystrophy and hereditary motor and sensory neuropathy: A randomized clinical trial. Arch Phys Med Rehabil 1995;76:612–620.

96. Lohi E-L, Lindberg C, Andersen O. Physical training effects in myasthenia gravis. Arch Phys Med Rehabil 1993;74:1178–1180.

97. Mackinnon S, Dellon A. Surgery of the Peripheral Nerve. New York: Thieme, 1988:521–533.

98. Maigne R. Diagnostic et traitment des douleurs communes d'origine rachidienne. Paris: Expansion Scientifique Francaise, 1989:515.

99. Maitland G. Vertebral Manipulation. London: Butterworth, 1986.

100. Malmberg A, Yaksh T. Hyperalgesia mediated by spinal glutamate or substance P receptor blocked by spinal cyclooxygenase inhibition. Science 1992;257:1276–1278.

101. Maselli R, Wollman R, Leung C, et al. Neuromuscular transmission in amyotrophic lateral sclerosis. Muscle Nerve 1993;16:1193–1203.

102. Mathew N. Chronic refractory headache. Neurology 1993;43(Suppl 3):S26–S33.

103. Mattison P. Transcutaneous electrical nerve stimulation in the management of painful muscle spasm in multiple sclerosis. Clin Rehabil 1993; 7:45–48.

104. Max M, Lynch S, Muir J, et al. Effects of desipramine, amitriptyline, and fluoxetine on pain in diabetic neuropathy. N Engl J Med 1992;326:1250–1256.

105. Mayer T, Gatchel R, Mayer H, et al. A prospective two-year study of functional restoration in industrial low back injury. JAMA 1987;258:1763–1767.

106. Mayo N. The effect of physical therapy for children with motor delay and cerebral palsy. Am J Phys Med Rehabil 1991;70:258–267.

107. Mazur J, Shurtleff D, Menelaus M, et al. Orthopedic management of high-level spinal bifida. J Bone Joint Surg Am 1989;71:56–61.

108. McLachlan E, Janig W, Devor M, et al. Peripheral nerve injury triggers noradrenergic sprouting within dorsal root ganglia. Nature 1993;363:543–545.

109. McMahan S, Koltzenburg M. Novel classes of nociceptors: Beyond Sherrington. Trends Neurosci 1990;13:199–201.

110. Meade T, Dyer S, Browne W, et al. Low back pain of mechanical origin: Randomised comparison of chiropractic and hospital outpatient treatment. BMJ 1990;300:1431–1437.

111. Melzack R. The McGill pain questionnaire: Major properties and scoring methods. Pain 1975; 1:275–299.

112. Merskey H. Classification of chronic pain. Pain 1986;3(Suppl):1–225.

112a. Miller RG. The effects of aging upon nerve and muscle function and their importance for neurorehabilitation. Journal of Neurologic Rehabilitation 1995;9:175–181.

113. Milner-Brown H, Miller R. Muscle strengthening through high-resistance weight training in patients with neuromuscular disorders. Arch Phys Med Rehabil 1988;69:14–19.

114. Mitchell R, Carmen G. Results of a multicenter trial using an intensive active exercise program for the treatment of acute soft tissue and back injuries. Spine 1990;15:514–521.

115. Moffett J, Hughes G, Griffiths P. An investigation of the effects of cervical traction. Clin Rehabil 1990;4:205–211, 287–290.

116. Moss A, Casey P, Stocking C, et al. Home ventilation for ALS patients. Neurology 1993;43:438–443.

117. Mulrow C, Gerety M, Kanten D, et al. A randomized trial of physical rehabilitation for very frail nursing home residents. JAMA 1994;271:513–524.

118. Munsat T. Poliomyelitis: New problems with an old disease. N Engl J Med 1991;324:1206–1207.

119. Munsat T, Andres P, Finison L, et al. The natural history of motoneuron loss in amyotrophic lateral sclerosis. Neurology 1988;38:409–413.

120. Nevitt M, Cummings S, Kidd S, et al. Risk factors for recurrent nonsyncopal falls. JAMA 1989; 261:2663–2668.

121. Norre M. Rehabilitation treatments for vertigo and related syndromes. Crit Rev Phys Rehabil Med 1990;2:101–120.

122. Norre M, De Weerdt W. Treatment of vertigo based on habituation. II. Technique and results of habituation training. J Laryngol Otol 1980; 94:971–980.

123. O'Leary D, Ruff N, Dyck R. Development, critical period plasticity, and adult reorganization of mammalian somatosensory systems. Curr Opin Neurobiol 1994;4:535–544.

124. Oosterwijk R, Meyler W, Henley E, et al. Pain control with TENS and TEAM nerve stimulators: A review. Crit Rev Phys Med Rehabil 1994;6:219–258.

125. Palmer F, Shapiro B, Wachtel R, et al. The effects of physical therapy on cerebral palsy. N Engl J Med 1991;318:803–808.

126. Panegyres P, Moore N, Gibson R, et al. Thoracic outlet syndromes and magnetic resonance imaging. Brain 1993;116:823–841.

127. Payne R, Pasternak G. Pain. In: Johnston M, MacDonald R, Young A, eds: Principles of Drug Therapy in Neurology. Philadelphia: FA Davis, 1993:268–293.

128. Peacock W, Staudt L. Spasticity in cerebral palsy and the selective posterior rhizotomy procedure. J Child Neurol 1990;5:179–185.

129. Penney J, Young A. Movement disorders. In: Johnston M, MacDonald R, Young A, eds: Principles of Drug Therapy in Neurology. Philadelphia: FA Davis, 1992:50–80.

130. Perrine K. A new quality-of-life inventory for epilepsy patients. Epilepsia 1993;34:S28–S33.

131. Petajan J, Gappmaier E, Spencer M, et al. Aerobic exercise for persons with multiple sclerosis. Ann Neurol 1994;36:298.

132. Polman C, Bertelsmann F, de Wall R, et al. 4-Aminopyridine is superior to 3,4-diaminopyridine in the treatment of patients with multiple sclerosis. Arch Neurol 1994;51:1136–1139.

133. Polman C, Bertelsmann F, van Loenen A, et al. 4-Aminopyridine in the treatment of patients with MS. Arch Neurol 1994;51:292–296.

134. Pomeroy V. The effect of physiotherapy input on mobility skills of elderly people with severe dementing illness. Clin Rehabil 1993;7:163–170.

135. Ponichtera-Mulcare J, Glaser R. Evaluation of muscle performance and cardiopulmonary fitness in patients with multiple sclerosis. Neuro-Rehabilitation 1993;3:17–29.

136. Ramos G, Martin W. Effects of vertebral axial decompression on intradiscal pressure. J Neurosurg 1994;81:350–353.

137. Revel M, Minguet M, Gergoy P. Changes in cervicocephalic kinesthesia after a proprioceptive rehabilitation program in patients with neck pain. Arch Phys Med Rehabil 1994;75:895–899.

138. Riley D, Lang A, Blair R, et al. Frozen shoulder and other shoulder disturbances in Parkinson's disease. J Neurol Neurosurg Psychiatry 1989; 52:63–66.

139. Ringel S, Neville H. The rehabilitation of muscular disorders. Journal of Neurologic Rehabilitation 1990;4:203–215.

140. Rodriguez M, Siva A, Ward J, et al. Impairment, disability, and handicap in multiple sclerosis: A population-based study in Olmsted County, Minnesota. Neurology 1994;44:28–33.

141. Roland P. Cortical representation of pain. Trends Neurosci 1992;15:3–5.

142. Ropper A. The Guillain-Barré syndrome. N Engl J Med 1992;326:1130–1136.

143. Rowbotham M. Managing post-herptic neuralgia with opioids and local anesthetics. Ann Neurol 1994;35(Suppl):S46–S49.

144. Rubenstein L, Robbins A, Schulman B, et al. Falls and instability in the elderly. J Am Geriatr Soc 1988;36:266–278.

145. Rubin R, Gold W, Kelley D, et al. The Cost of Disorders of the Brain. Washington, DC: National Foundation for Brain Research, 1992.

146. Rudick R, Miller D, Clough J, et al. Quality of life in multiple sclerosis. Arch Neurol 1992;49:1237–1242.

147. Rudman D, Feller A, Nagraj H, et al. Effects of human growth hormone in men over 60 years old. N Engl J Med 1990;323:1–6.

148. Sandroni P, Walker C, Starr A. Fatigue in patients with multiple sclerosis: Motor pathway conduction and event-related potentials. Arch Neurol 1992;49:517–524.

149. Sano K. Neurosurgical treatments of pain. Acta Neurochir Suppl 1987; 38:86–96.

150. Schaumburg H, Berger A, Thomas P. Disorders of Peripheral Nerves. Philadelphia: FA Davis, 1992.

151. Schuldt K. On neck muscle activity and load reduction in sitting postures. Scand J Rehabil Med Suppl 1988;19:1–49.

152. Scott S. Speech therapy for Parkinson's disease. J Neurol Neurosurg Psychiatry 1983;46:140–144.

153. Sharma K, Kent-Braun J, Miller R, et al. Excessive muscular fatigue in the postpoliomyelitis syndrome. Neurology 1994;44:642–646.

154. Sherman R. Phantom limb pain: mechanisms, incidence, and treatment. Crit Rev Phys Rehabil Med 1992;4:1–26.

155. Silberberg D. Multiple sclerosis: Approaches to management. Ann Neurol 1994;36(Suppl):S1–S162.

156. Silberstein S. Tension-type and chronic daily headache. Neurology 1993;43:1644–1649.

157. Smits R, Emmen H, Bertelsmann F, et al. The effects of 4-aminopyridine on cognitive function in patients with multiple sclerosis. Neurology 1994;44:1701–1705.

158. Soliveri P, Brown R, Jahanshahi M, et al. Effect of performance of a skilled motor task in patients with Parkinson's disease. J Neurol Neurosurg Psychiatry 1992;55:454–460.

159. Sonies B, Dalakas M. Dysphagia in patients with the post-polio syndrome. N Engl J Med 1991; 324:1162–1167.

160. Stallard J, Major R, Butler P. The orthotic ambulation performance of paraplegic myelomeningocele children using the ORLAU ParaWalker treatment system. Clin Rehabil 1991;5:111–114.

161. Stankovic R, Johnell O. Conservative treatment of low-back pain. Spine 1990;15:120–123.

162. Stein C, Comisel K, Haimerl E, et al. Analgesic effect of intraarticular morphine after arthroscopic knee surgery. N Engl J Med 1991; 325:1123–1126.

163. Stone R. Post-polio syndrome. Science 1994; 264:909.

164. Sudarsky L. Geriatrics: Gait disorders in the elderly. N Engl J Med 1990;322:1441–1446.

165. Sweeney T, Prentice C, Saal J, et al. Cervicothoracic muscular stabilization techniques. Physical Medicine Rehabilitation: State of the Art Review 1990;4:335–359.

166. Taira T, Tanikawa T, Kawamura H, et al. Spinal intrathecal baclofen suppresses central pain after a stroke. J Neurol Neurosurg Psychiatry 1994; 57:381–382.

167. Tardeu C, Lespargot A, Tabary C, et al. For how long must the soleus muscle be stretched each day to prevent contracture? Dev Med Child Neurol 1988;30:3–10.

168. Teasell R, Shapiro A. Rehabilitation of chronic motor conversion disorders. Crit Rev Phys Rehabil Med 1993;5:1–13.

169. Thompson J. Tension myalgia as a diagnosis at the Mayo clinic and its relationship to fibrositis, fibromyalgia, and myofascial pain syndrome. Mayo Clin Proc 1990;65:1237–1248.

170. Tinetti M, Baker D, McAvay G, et al. A multifactorial intervention to reduce the risk of falling among elderly people living in the community. N Engl J Med 1994;331:821–827.

171. Tinetti M, Liu W-L, Claus E. Predictors and prognosis of inability to get up after falls among elderly persons. JAMA 1993;269:65–70.

172. Tinetti M, Speechley M. Prevention of falls among the elderly. N Engl J Med 1989;320:1055–1059.

173. Tinetti M, Speechley M, Ginter S. Risk factors for falls among the elderly living in the community. N Engl J Med 1988;319:1701–1707.

174. Traccis S, Rosati C, Monaco M. Successful treatment of acquired pendular elliptical nystagmus in multiple sclerosis with isoniazid and base-out prisms. Neurology 1990;40:492–494.

175. Troost B, Patton J. Exercise therapy for positional vertigo. Neurology 1992;42:1441–1444.

176. Turner J, Deyo R, Loesser J, et al. The importance of placebo effects in pain treatment and research. JAMA 1994;271:1609–1614.

177. Twomey L, Taylor J. Age-related changes of the lumbar spine and spinal rehabilitation. Crit Rev Phys Rehabil Med 1991;2:153–169.

178. Van Dieman H, Polman C, van Dongen T, et al. The effect of 4-aminopyridine on clinical signs in multiple sclerosis. Ann Neurol 1992;32:123–130.

179. Verdugo R, Ochoa J. Sympathetically maintained pain. Neurology 1994;44:1003–1014.

180. Walker W, Chiappini R, Buschbacher R. Rational prescription of exercise in managing low back pain. Crit Rev Phys Rehabil Med 1993;5:219–226.

181. Wall P, Melzack R. Textbook of Pain. Edinburgh: Churchill Livingstone, 1989:1664.

182. Watson C, Chipman M, Reed K, et al. Amitriptyline versus maprotiline in postherpetic neuralgia. Pain 1992;48:29–36.

183. Weinshenker B, Bass B, Rice G, et al. The natural history of multiple sclerosis: A geographically based study. Brain 1989;112:133–146.

184. Weinshenker B, Penman M, Bass R, et al. A double-blind, randomized crossover trial of pemoline in fatigue associated with multiple sclerosis. Neurology 1992;42:1468–1471.

185. Weiss L, Alfano A, Bardfeld P, et al. Prognostic value of triple phase bone scanning for reflex sympathetic dystrophy in hemiplegia. Arch Phys Med Rehabil 1993;74:716–719.

186. Werner R, Priebe M, Davidoff G. Reflex sympathetic dystrophy syndrome associated with hemiplegia. NeuroRehabilitation 1992;2:16–22.

187. Windebank A, Litchy W, Daube J, et al. Late effects of paralytic poliomyelitis in Olmsted County, Minnesota. Neurology 1991;41:501–507.

188. Wolfe F. Fibrositis, fibromyalgia, and musculoskeletal disease. Arch Phys Med Rehabil 1988; 69:527–531.

189. Woolf C, Doubell T. The pathophysiology of chronic pain. Curr Opin Neurobiol 1994;4:525–534.

190. WynnParry C. Rehabilitation of the Hand. London: Butterworth, 1981.

191. Yarasheski K, Zachwieja J. Growth hormone therapy for the elderly. JAMA 1993;270:1694.

192. Yekutiel M, Pinhasov A, Shahar G, et al. A clinical trial of the re-education of movement in patients with Parkinson's disease. Clinical Rehabilitation 1991;5:207–214.

193. Yue G, Cole K. Strength increases from the motor program: Comparison of training with maximal voluntary and imagined muscle contractions. J Neurophysiol 1992;67:1114–1123.

INDEX

An "f" following a page number indicates a figure; a "t" indicates a table.

ISBN 0-8036-0169-7